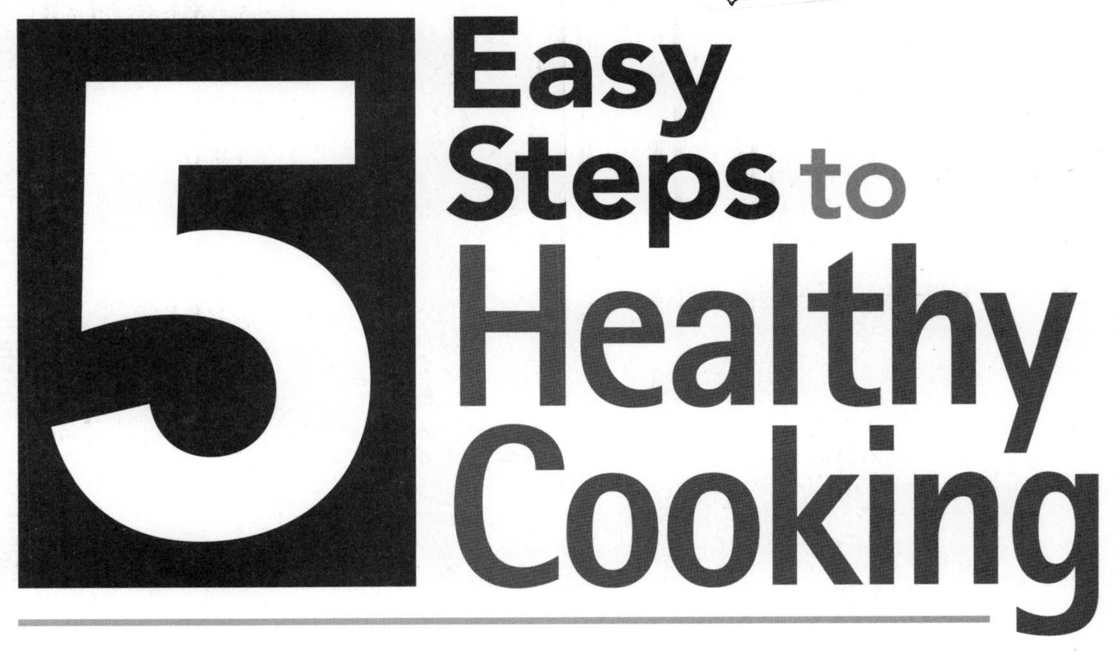

500
Recipes for Lifelong Wellness

Camilla V. Saulsbury

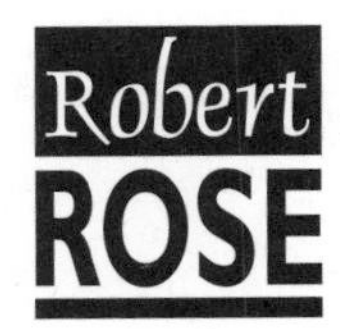

For complete cataloguing information, see page 544.

Disclaimer

The recipes in this book have been carefully tested by our kitchen and our tasters. To the best of our knowledge, they are safe and nutritious for ordinary use and users. For those people with food or other allergies, or who have special food requirements or health issues, please read the suggested contents of each recipe carefully and determine whether or not they may create a problem for you. All recipes are used at the risk of the consumer.

We cannot be responsible for any hazards, loss or damage that may occur as a result of any recipe use.

For those with special needs, allergies, requirements or health problems, in the event of any doubt, please contact your medical adviser prior to the use of any recipe.

Design and production: Kevin Cockburn/PageWave Graphics Inc.
Editor: Sue Sumeraj
Recipe editor: Jennifer MacKenzie
Proofreader: Kelly Jones
Indexer: Gillian Watts
Photographer: Colin Erricson
Associate photographer: Matt Johannsson
Food stylist: Kathryn Robertson
Prop stylist: Charlene Erricson

Additional photography:
© iStockphoto.com/largeformat4x5 (Assorted Nuts)
© iStockphoto.com/Jasmina (Colorful Vegetables in Basket)
© iStockphoto.com/FotografiaBasica (Green Vegetables and Legumes)
© iStockphoto.com/terradesign (Citrus Fruits)

Cover image: Stir-Fried Pork and Peppers with Buckwheat Noodles (page 329)

We acknowledge the financial support of the Government of Canada through the Book Publishing Industry Development Program (BPIDP) for our publishing activities.

Published by Robert Rose Inc.
120 Eglinton Avenue East, Suite 800, Toronto, Ontario, Canada M4P 1E2
Tel: (416) 322-6552 Fax: (416) 322-6936
www.robertrose.ca

Printed and bound in Canada

1 2 3 4 5 6 7 8 9 TGILBF 20 19 18 17 16 15 14 13 12

For my sister, Rebecca Saulsbury,
and my brother, Sean Saulsbury

Contents

Introduction 6
The Five Steps 8
Common Nutrition Terms 15
About the Nutrient Analyses 18
Ingredients for Healthy Cooking 19

Breakfasts 42
Power Snacks, Spreads and Nibbles 78
Salads 112
Soups, Stews and Chilis 164
Sandwiches, Wraps, Burgers and Pizzas 214
Meatless Main Dishes 248
Poultry and Lean Meat Main Dishes 296
Fish and Seafood Main Dishes 340
Multigrain Pasta and Noodles 380
Side Dishes 432
Breads 460
Natural Sugar Sweets 492

Index 533

Introduction

A good diet helps our bodies run smoothly throughout the day — it improves our brain function, increases our energy levels and helps us relax and sleep well.

Auguste Escoffier, the great French chef, urged cooks to keep it simple. The adage is particularly apt for healthy cooking and eating in the modern era.

With our daily exposure to a constant stream of conflicting information about nutrition and health, it can be a challenge to discern which foods really do form the components of a healthy diet, let alone how to turn them into delicious dishes that can be prepared without too much time, fuss and expense. And when a new diet is touted every other week, each with its unique set of strict tangents (many of which are diametrically opposed), the notion of finding a simplified, healthy way to eat may seem out of reach.

But a solution is here: *5 Easy Steps to Healthy Cooking: 500 Recipes for Lifelong Wellness.* Vastly different from a diet book, this simplified, five-step approach to healthy eating is holistic and flexible. This book approaches healthy cooking from a very different perspective: because it is first and foremost a cookbook, not a diet book, it focuses on enticing, easy-to-prepare recipes that make following the five steps simple and doable, with good health and great eating as the delicious compensation.

The choices we make at the market, in our kitchens and around the dining table can affect our health — for better or for worse. Knowing that is one of the most powerful steps we can take toward well-being. Today, most of us understand the importance of providing good, healthy meals for ourselves and our families. Healthy eating helps our children grow and thrive, developing strong bodies. Healthy foods can boost the immune system and offer protection from cancers, diabetes and cardiovascular disease. Most noticeably, a good diet helps our bodies run smoothly throughout the day — it improves our brain function, increases our energy levels and helps us relax and sleep well.

Nutrition Claims and Standards

The nutrition claims and standards in this book are based on U.S. recommendations and guidelines from the following sources:

- The USDA MyPlate Guidelines, 2011.
- The USDA Nutrient Database for Standard Reference, Release 18. U.S. Department of Agriculture, 2011.
- The Healthy Eating Plate Guidelines, created by the Department of Nutrition at Harvard School of Public Health, 2011.
- The USDA Dietary Guidelines for Americans, 2010.
- Dietary Reference Intakes (DRI Report) for Energy, Carbohydrate, Fiber, Fat, Fatty Acids, Cholesterol, Protein, and Amino Acids (Macronutrients), created by the National Academy of Sciences, U.S. Institute of Medicine and the U.S. Food and Nutrition Board, 2005.
- The USDA Food and Nutrition Information Center (FNIC).

What Is a Healthy Recipe, Anyway?

This book offers simple, delicious recipes that use ingredients with a proven track record in enhancing health or offering protection from diseases. The positive health benefits of the foods used in the recipes have been well established and confirmed in trials across the world over a period of years.

That being said, even a book with 500 recipes cannot be definitive, and there are many foods not featured in this collection that are healthy and nutritious in their own right. If your favorite vegetable, fruit, grain or other healthy food is not found in these pages, that doesn't mean it won't add positive nutrition to your overall diet.

Remember, no one food can make you healthy on its own — aim instead for a varied and balanced diet. The diversity of recipes in this collection offers ways to enjoy a wide variety of nutritious foods throughout the day — from breakfast to dessert, and everywhere in between. This book will help you build your own perfect diet while you learn more about the wonderful world of healthy, natural foods.

Enjoy choosing which recipe to try first. Whichever one it is, I wish you a happy, healthy, and very delicious experience!

No one food can make you healthy on its own — aim instead for a varied and balanced diet.

The Meatless Monday Movement

Born almost 100 years ago, the Meatless Monday Movement began in the United States during the First World War as a voluntary effort to reduce consumption of key staples such as meat. The campaign was a huge success, and was repeated during the Second World War. The program was relaunched in 2003 by Johns Hopkins Bloomberg School of Public Health as a non-profit initiative to help Americans cut down on saturated fat, and has since become a full-blown social movement to improve individual health as well as the health of the planet.

The premise is simple: one day a week, cut out the meat. Are you ready to join the phenomenon? For more information, visit www.meatlessmonday.com.

The Five Steps

Step 1: Choose Fresh, Whole Foods

Choose foods that are fresh and natural over refined, highly processed foods. Whenever possible, opt for local, seasonal, organic products.

Whole foods are just what they sound like: foods that are unprocessed (or processed and refined as little as possible) and as close to their natural state as possible. Fruits and vegetables are perfect examples. You can eat them fresh from the garden, skin and all. By contrast, processed foods have been significantly altered from their natural state; they typically have fewer vitamins and minerals and less fiber, not to mention a laundry list of unpronounceable additives that serve as fillers, enhancers or preservatives.

Eating a diet rich in whole foods supports optimum health and the loss of extra pounds.

Eating a diet rich in whole foods — notably fruits, vegetables, whole grains and lean protein — supports optimum health and the loss of extra pounds and will fuel your body for all of your daily activities. Additionally, an increasing body of research indicates that the vitamins, minerals and phytonutrients derived from whole foods can protect the body against a variety of chronic diseases, including cancer and heart disease.

The simplest first step is to avoid processed foods — including fast foods — as much as possible. But that does not mean all packaged foods are off-limits: whole-grain cereals and breads, dried beans and legumes, whole-grain pasta, brown rice and canned tomatoes are all examples of healthy, minimally processed foods. The key when choosing packaged foods at the grocery store is to look for short ingredient lists; the more "stuff" in the list, the more processed it is. Watch out for words like "enriched" and ingredients that sound like they were created by a mad scientist. And avoid packaged foods containing high-fructose corn syrup and products with any kind of sweeteners near the top of the ingredient list; these are good signs that the item is highly processed.

Once your grocery cart is stocked with minimally processed dry goods, the second step is to concentrate your shopping in the fresh foods sections of the grocery store: the produce section, filled with delicious fruits and vegetables, the meat section (look for lean cuts of meat), the fish counter, and the dairy and eggs section. And don't forget the frozen foods section: fresh fruits and vegetables are flash-frozen at their peak and are a convenient and affordable way to add produce to your meals.

Third, shop at farmers' markets, particularly from late spring to late fall. Not only do farmers' markets offer a broad range of fresh, local whole-food options, these foods are also typically available at a great price. When your favorite food is in season, you can buy extra to freeze for the winter months. Check your local newspaper, as well as city or county websites, for listings of markets, including their locations and opening dates.

Incorporating more whole foods into your diet and weaning yourself off processed foods will greatly improve your overall health. Start small, with changes that are easy to handle: add fresh fruit and vegetables to your daily meals and enjoy an apple and cheese as your snack instead of chips and a soda. Take your time, and soon enough you will have a pantry full of fresh and whole foods that will nourish your body and mind.

Step 2: Eat Mostly Vegetable- and Fruit-Based Foods

Make plant foods — vegetables, fruits, legumes and whole grains — the largest part of your diet each day. Eat a colorful variety of such foods to ensure that you're getting the best nutrients.

Eating an abundance of fruits and vegetables is essential to a healthy diet and lifelong wellness. Many organizations — including the U.S. Department of Agriculture, the National Institutes of Health, the American Heart Association and the Harvard School of Public Health — recommend eating a minimum of 5 cups (1.25 L) of fruits and vegetables (raw volume) each day.

The health benefits of a diet rich in plant foods are extensive and well documented. For starters, fresh fruits and vegetables are low in calories and packed with nutrients. In addition, they have many important phytochemicals — typically related to the colors of the produce — that promote wellness and protect the body from illness and disease. Further, the high levels of fiber found in plant foods slow the absorption rate of sugars and carbohydrates, which helps normalize blood sugar levels and prevent diabetes.

Fresh fruits and vegetables are low in calories and packed with nutrients.

Fruits and vegetables also tend to be naturally low in sodium and high in potassium, a combination that helps reduce high blood pressure. Large population studies show that the higher the intake of fruits and vegetables, the lower the risk for heart disease and stroke, and when large studies (such as the INTERHEART study, which included 52 nations) have looked at heart disease, the results showed that those individuals who ate the most vegetables and fruits had 30% fewer heart attacks.

Finally, hundreds of research studies indicate that people who consume an abundance of fruits and vegetables have the lowest rates of cancers. The World Health Organization (WHO) estimates that as many as 30% of all cancers are caused by poor eating habits. They recommend that everyone eat an abundance of fruits and vegetables. The first recommendation by the World Cancer Research Fund and the American Institute for Cancer Research regarding cancer prevention is "Choose a predominantly plant-based diet rich in fruits, vegetables, and legumes."

Here are some easy ways to add more fruits and vegetables to your diet:

- Keep ready-to-eat raw vegetables handy in a clear container in the front of your refrigerator (easily within view).
- Keep a supply of fresh fruit — oranges, apples, grapes, kiwis, bananas, etc. — on the table or counter.
- Stock up on dried, frozen and canned fruits and vegetables.
- Encourage children to help select fruits and vegetables on grocery shopping trips.
- Eat more vegetable salads, including a variety of raw vegetables: broccoli, peppers, green onions, carrots, cucumbers, tomatoes, cauliflower, celery, beets and greens such as kale, spinach and Swiss chard.
- Add a variety of vegetables to soups (both homemade and store-bought).
- Eat fruit salads often. Finish a meal with fresh or dried fruit, such as berries, melons, dates, grapes, pineapple or papaya.
- Add vegetables to dishes you already love, such as sandwiches, pizza, pasta, ethnic foods and egg dishes like omelets and scrambles.
- Drink ready-made vegetable juices (preferably reduced-sodium) and vegetable-fruit juices. Or create your own by blending carrot juice with fruit juice. Or drink a smoothie made with frozen unsweetened fruit and lower-fat dairy or non-dairy milk.
- Add strawberries, blueberries, bananas and other brightly colored fruits to your waffles, pancakes, cereal, oatmeal, yogurt or toast.

Add vegetables to dishes you already love.

Step 3: Opt for Healthy Fats and Proteins

Enjoy healthy fats from plant sources and minimize extracted oils and processed fats. Choose lean and lower-fat meats, seafood and dairy products, and also incorporate plant-based proteins, such as whole grains and legumes.

Fats

We have become a culture obsessed with low-fat foods. From low-fat diets to low-fat chips, ice cream, salad dressings, cookies and cakes, "low-fat" is part of the modern mantra when it comes to what we put in our mouths and how we evaluate food. Yet despite the prodding from doctors, nutritionists and food manufacturers that eating foods low in fat is the answer, obesity rates in North America have soared.

The latest — and ever-mounting — research on the subject indicates the flaw in the groupthink: it turns out that quality is far more important than quantity when it comes to dietary fats. Simply cutting out fat is not the solution. Saturated and trans fats increase blood cholesterol and the risk of certain diseases, while good fats have the opposite effect, protecting the heart, lowering cholesterol and supporting overall health. In fact, good fats — such as omega-3 fats — are absolutely essential not only to overall physical health but to mental and emotional well-being.

The bottom line on fats is simple: don't go no-fat; go good fat. Instead of avoiding fat, replace saturated fats and trans fats with good fats. For example, serve vegetables with a drizzle of olive oil instead of butter, or eat fatty fish such as salmon or mackerel in place of red meat. In addition:

- Try to eliminate trans fats from your diet. Check food labels for trans fats. Avoiding commercially baked goods and fast foods is one of the most important first steps.
- Limit your intake of saturated fats by cutting back on red meat and full-fat dairy foods.
- Eat omega-3 fats often. Good sources include fish, walnuts, ground flax seeds, flaxseed oil, canola oil and soybean oil.
- Keep total fat intake in the range of 20% to 35% of total calories per day.

Don't go no-fat; go good fat.

Good Fats

Monounsaturated fats and polyunsaturated fats are known as the "good fats" because they are good for your heart, your cholesterol level and your overall health. The following foods are good sources of these beneficial fats:

- Plant-based oils (e.g., olive oil, canola oil, sunflower oil, peanut oil, sesame oil, walnut oil, flaxseed oil)
- Avocados
- Olives
- Peanuts and nuts (e.g., almonds, walnuts, pecans, macadamia nuts, hazelnuts, pecans, cashews)
- Seeds (e.g., pumpkin, sunflower, sesame, flax, hemp)
- Natural nut and seed butters (e.g., peanut butter, cashew butter, sunflower seed butter)
- Fatty fish (e.g., salmon, tuna, mackerel, herring, trout, sardines)
- Non-dairy milks (e.g., soy, almond, hemp, rice)
- Tofu

Protein

Proteins are part of every cell, tissue and organ in our bodies, but these proteins are constantly being broken down and replaced. Because protein cannot be stored in the body (fat and carbohydrates can), it must be derived from what we eat. Once consumed, it can be digested into amino acids that are later used to replace the proteins in our bodies.

What makes some proteins preferable to others is the saturated fat content. Proteins that are high in saturated fats can raise cholesterol levels, which in turn can lead to a higher risk for heart disease. Fifteen percent of the calories adults consume should come from protein. And though most North Americans already eat more protein than they need, they do not necessarily eat enough good-quality protein. Experts recommend lean, high-quality protein choices such as fish, skinless poultry, lean cuts of meat, egg whites, low-fat dairy foods, legumes, nuts, whole grains and seeds. Studies show that the consumption of high-quality protein does everything from staving off hunger (often for hours) to regulating blood sugar and insulin levels to enhancing fat-burning.

It turns out that even a little bit of change in protein consumption can make a big difference. Researchers at Johns Hopkins Medical Center have shown that eating a slightly increased amount of high-quality protein foods, when coupled with a small decrease in starchy carbohydrates (think potatoes and white rice), can dramatically impact heart health. And researchers at the Optimal Macronutrient Intake Trial to Prevent Heart Disease (OmniHeart) project found that people who replace just 10% of their carbohydrate calories with high-quality protein can significantly lower blood pressure, cholesterol and triglyceride levels.

Focus on adding a wide variety of high-quality protein sources to your diet throughout the day.

In practical terms, focus on adding a wide variety of high-quality protein sources to your diet throughout the day. For example, at breakfast, top a bowl of cereal or yogurt with chopped walnuts, or scramble some eggs (part whole eggs, part egg whites) with vegetables; at lunch, layer a sandwich with lean turkey breast or baked tofu, or create a quick bean and vegetable burrito; for a mid-afternoon snack, nibble a mix of seeds, nuts and dried fruit; at dinner, opt for variety, from salmon to lean cuts of meat to vegetarian entrées focusing on legumes and whole grains.

Step 4: Select Superfoods (Nutrient-Dense Foods)

Choose foods that are rich in nutrients when compared to their total caloric content (also known as "superfoods" or foods with a high nutrient density). The healthiest foods have a wide spectrum of vitamins, minerals, phytonutrients and antioxidants.

It's usually fairly obvious if a food item is a healthy option. A spinach salad or bowl of berries: healthy. A banana split or chili cheese dog: not so much. Far less obvious is whether a given food is exceptionally healthful. Such foods have become known as "superfoods" — nutrient-dense, multi-tasking foods brimming with various nutrients that increasing numbers of nutritionists, doctors and researchers contend can dramatically improve our general health and simultaneously ward off disease. Another catchphrase applied to such foods is "nutrient density," an assessment of the amount of nutrients a food contains in comparison to the number of calories. In short, the greater the level of nutrients in comparison to the level of calories, the greater the nutrient density.

When you increase your consumption of superfoods, the inevitable result is a more nutrient-dense, lower-calorie, health-promoting diet.

The best thing is that an endless variety of nutritious and delicious recipes can be made from superfoods. The list of superfoods is vast: in fact, just about every brightly colored fruit and vegetable fits the category, as do nuts, beans, seeds, aromatic and brightly colored herbs and spices, and oily fish (such as salmon). The health benefits of many of these superfoods are highlighted in "Superfood Spotlight" boxes throughout the book.

A mountain of scientific evidence supports a varied, nutrient-dense approach to eating, and the end result — a "superdiet" — is an indisputable path to lifelong wellness.

Step 5: Eat More Whole Grains

Eat whole grains — as opposed to refined grains — the majority of the time. Compared to refined grains, whole grains are superior sources of fiber and other important nutrients, such as selenium, potassium, magnesium and even protein.

Whole grains help form the foundation of a healthy diet: they are great sources of carbohydrates and provide fiber, vitamins, minerals and antioxidants to prevent disease and help keep blood sugar and energy levels strong and steady. Whole grains have as much as four times the amount of dietary fiber as their refined counterparts (baked goods made with white flours, white rice, white pasta, etc). High-fiber foods, including whole grains, take longer to digest, stabilizing blood sugar levels and hunger, and keeping you full on fewer calories. Fiber helps regulate digestion and reduces the risk of digestive diseases, cancer, high blood pressure, heart disease, diabetes and obesity. Yet most North Americans eat less than one serving of whole grains per day.

All grains begin as whole grains; they are the seeds or kernels of a plant in its complete form. Grains have three parts: the endosperm, which contains starch and protein; the bran, rich in fiber, minerals and phytonutrients; and the germ, full of B vitamins, vitamin E and other antioxidants and minerals. Refined grains, such as white flours and white rice, are stripped of the most nutritious elements, notably the bran and the germ.

Aim for at least three servings of whole grains per day.

If you're ready to go for the grain, take heart: it's easier than ever before, even if you don't cook. It's all about choice, and there are so many new, deliciously healthy whole-grain products out there. Aim for at least three servings of whole grains per day. Here are a few simple ways to add whole grains to your diet:

- **Begin the day with a high-fiber cereal.** When choosing a cereal, look for the word "whole" in the first ingredient and at least 3 grams of fiber per serving. Next, look at the sugar content: aim for sugar grams per serving in the low single digits. Such cereals will keep you feeling full throughout the morning due to the high fiber content. Serve your cereal with fresh fruit (bananas, berries, apples) and, for a protein boost, with dairy or non-dairy milk, or sprinkled atop yogurt.

If a product is truly whole-grain, whole grains will be first in the ingredient list.

- **Choose bread products with whole grains at the top of the ingredient list.** Don't be fooled by the statement "made with whole grains" on the front of a package; unless "whole grains" is preceded by "100%," the whole grains may be second to last on the ingredient list, with refined white flour at the top. It's the fine print on the package (specifically the ingredient list) that matters. If a product is truly whole-grain, whole grains (e.g., wheat, whole oats or some other whole grain) will be first in the ingredient list.
- **Switch pastas.** Try whole-wheat pasta, especially the new high-fiber, high-protein varieties; they're even friendlier to your blood sugar. Some are made from grains such as oats, spelt and barley in addition to durum wheat, which means they're higher in soluble fiber. And yet their taste and texture is surprisingly close to regular pasta choices.
- **Bake with whole-grain flours.** Give a boost to homemade baked goods by replacing one-third to one-half of the white flour with whole wheat flour or other whole-grain flours (e.g., spelt, quinoa, millet or amaranth flour).
- **Make cooked whole grains your new sides.** In place of white rice, white pasta or potatoes on the side, try whole grains. Many varieties can be prepared in the same amount of time as white rice or pasta, and the flavors are fantastic (see page 438 for a whole grains cooking chart).

Consider Becoming a Flexitarian

A growing segment of the population is inclined toward eating less meat and more vegetables, fruits and whole grains. They want the health benefits of eating vegetarian without having to give up meat altogether. They are part of the growing flexitarian health movement. Declared the most useful and innovative word of 2003 by the American Dialect Society, "flexitarian" comes from a combination of the words "flexible" and "vegetarian." Following a flexitarian diet simply means eating more plant-based meals and less meat, most notably for reasons of good health and well-being. Ample scientific evidence supports the healthfulness of a diet made up mostly of plant foods. As a bonus, eating less meat and more plant-based foods is both environmentally and economically smart.

Given the confusion consumers face when it comes to eating more healthfully, going flexitarian, with its healthful emphasis on grains, lean proteins, vegetables and legumes, is an extremely appealing option.

Common Nutrition Terms

Amino acids: Amino acids are the chemical compounds that comprise plant and animal proteins. They are classified into two categories: essential and non-essential. The eight essential amino acids are those that must be obtained from food sources because the body cannot synthesize them on its own. Non-essential amino acids are those that the body can manufacture on its own.

Antioxidants: Antioxidants protect the body from damage caused by harmful molecules called free radicals. Many experts believe this damage is a factor in the development of blood vessel disease (atherosclerosis), cancer and other conditions. Exposure to free radicals most often comes about through by-products of normal processes that take place in the body, such as the breakdown of nutrients, but it can also be through pollutants in the environment. Antioxidants include some vitamins (such as vitamins C and E), some minerals (such as selenium) and flavonoids, which are found in plants. The best sources of antioxidants are fruits and vegetables.

Calories: A calorie is a measurement of the amount of energy released when the body breaks down food; calories are provided by carbohydrates, proteins and fats. The more calories a food has, the more energy it can provide the body. When more calories are eaten than are needed for energy, the body stores the extra calories as fat.

Carbohydrates: Carbohydrates provide fuel for the body in the form of glucose. Glucose is a sugar that is the primary source of energy for all of the body's cells. Adults should get about 45% to 65% of their calories from carbohydrates. Carbohydrate sources include many foods that are nutrient-rich, such as whole grains, fruits, vegetables and legumes, as well as foods such as candy, pastries, cookies and flavored beverages (soft drinks and fruit drinks), which provide insignificant amounts of vitamins, minerals and other essential nutrients.

Adults should get about 45% to 65% of their calories from carbohydrates.

Carotenoids: Carotenoids, a type of phytonutrient (see page 17), are the red, orange and yellow pigments in fruits and vegetables. Some of the most familiar carotenoids are alpha carotene, beta carotene, lycopene and lutein. Fruits and vegetables that are high in carotenoids appear to protect against certain cancers, heart disease and age-related macular degeneration.

Cholesterol: Cholesterol is a waxy, fat-like substance made in the liver and other cells and is found in certain foods, such as dairy products, eggs and meat. The body needs some cholesterol to function properly. Its cell walls, or membranes, need cholesterol to produce hormones, vitamin D and the bile acids that help digest fat. But the body needs only a limited amount of cholesterol to meet its needs. When too much is present, health problems such as heart disease may develop.

Cholesterol moves through the bloodstream by attaching to a protein; in combination, these are called lipoproteins. Low-density lipoproteins (LDL), also known as "bad" cholesterol, can cause buildup of plaque on artery walls, which can lead to heart disease and other ailments. High-density lipoproteins (HDL), also known as "good" cholesterol, help the body rid itself of LDL. Hence, the higher the body's HDL cholesterol, the better; the lower the HDL, the greater the chance of heart disease.

Fat: Fat is made up of compounds called fatty acids, or lipids. Depending on their chemical structure, these fatty acids can be monounsaturated, polyunsaturated, saturated or trans fats. Trans fats and saturated fats are the unhealthiest fats.

Trans fats are formed when manufacturers turn liquid oils into solid fats (hydrogenation), such as with shortening and hard margarine. Trans fats can also be found in many processed foods, including crackers (even healthy-sounding ones), cereals, baked goods, snack foods, salad dressings and fried foods.

Saturated fats are found in meats and whole dairy products such as milk, cheese, cream and ice cream. They are also present in some plant foods, such as tropical oils (for example, coconut or palm kernel oil). When margarine or vegetable shortening is made from soybean oil, corn oil or other vegetable oils, hydrogen atoms are added, making some of the fat molecules "saturated." This also makes the fat solid at room temperature.

Eating unsaturated fat instead of saturated fat may improve your cholesterol levels.

Unsaturated fat is liquid at room temperature. It is found mostly in plant oils. Eating unsaturated fat instead of saturated fat may improve your cholesterol levels. Try to eat mostly unsaturated fats. Monounsaturated fat and polyunsaturated fat are both types of unsaturated fat. Monounsaturated fat is found in vegetable oils such as canola, olive and peanut oil. Eating foods high in monounsaturated fat may help lower your "bad" LDL cholesterol. Monounsaturated fat may also keep "good" HDL cholesterol levels high. Polyunsaturated fat is found mainly in vegetable oils such as safflower, sunflower, sesame, soybean and corn oil. Polyunsaturated fat is also the main fat in seafood. Eating polyunsaturated fat in place of saturated fat may lower LDL cholesterol. Omega-3 fatty acids are a type of polyunsaturated fat that may reduce the risk of heart disease. To get the health benefits of omega-3s, eat a 3-ounce (90 g) serving of fatty fish, such as salmon or mackerel, twice a week. Ground flax seeds, flaxseed oil, nuts and seeds also provide omega-3 fatty acids.

Fiber: Dietary fiber is found naturally in edible plants. It does not break down in the gastrointestinal system and instead passes through the body undigested. Dietary fiber is either soluble or insoluble, and both forms are needed for optimal health.

Soluble fiber attracts water and forms a gel, which slows down digestion. Soluble fiber delays the emptying of your stomach and makes you feel full, which helps control weight. Slower stomach emptying may also affect blood sugar levels and have a beneficial effect on insulin sensitivity, which may help control diabetes. In addition, soluble fiber can help lower LDL ("bad") blood cholesterol by interfering with the absorption of dietary cholesterol. Sources of soluble fiber include oats, oat bran, psyllium, nuts, flax seeds, lentils, beans, dried peas, apples, oranges, pears, strawberries, blueberries, cucumbers, celery and carrots.

Insoluble fiber has a laxative effect and adds bulk to the diet, helping prevent constipation. It does not dissolve in water, so it passes through the gastrointestinal tract relatively intact. Insoluble fiber is found mainly in whole grains and vegetables. Sources of insoluble fiber include whole wheat, wheat bran, corn bran, bulgur, barley, couscous, brown rice, seeds, nuts, raisins, grapes, zucchini, celery, broccoli, cabbage, onions, tomatoes, carrots, cucumbers, green beans, dark leafy vegetables and root vegetable skins.

Flavonoids: Flavonoids are polyphenols, natural components in thousands of plants that give them their beautiful colors. Most flavonoids function in the human body as antioxidants, helping to neutralize and prevent overly reactive oxygen-containing molecules from damaging cells. Foods rich in flavonoids include onions, apples, red grapes, strawberries, raspberries, blueberries, cranberries, grape juice, tea, red wine and certain nuts.

Micronutrients: Vitamins and minerals are called micronutrients because the body needs them in small amounts. Micronutrients are vital to the body's ability to process macronutrients — fats, proteins and carbohydrates.

Minerals: Minerals, like vitamins, must come from diet; the body does not make them. Many minerals, such as calcium, potassium and iron, are vital to the body's proper function and must be consumed in relatively large amounts. Others, including the trace minerals zinc, selenium and copper, are needed only in small amounts to maintain good health.

Minerals, like vitamins, must come from diet; the body does not make them.

Phytonutrients: The prefix "phyto-" comes from a Greek word meaning "plant." Phytonutrients are organic components of plants — such as beta carotene, lycopene and resveratrol — that are thought to promote human health. Fruits, vegetables, grains, legumes, nuts and teas are rich sources of phytonutrients. Unlike the traditional nutrients (protein, fat, carbohydrates, vitamins and minerals), phytonutrients are not "essential" for life, so some people prefer the term "phytochemicals."

Protein: Proteins are nutrients that are essential to the building, maintenance and repair of body tissue, such as the skin, internal organs and muscles. They are also the major components of the immune system and hormones. Proteins are made up of substances called amino acids, 22 of which are considered vital for health. Of these, the adult body can make 14; the other eight (the essential amino acids) can only be obtained from diet. Proteins are found in all types of food, but (with the exception of quinoa) only fish, meat, poultry, eggs, cheese and other foods from animal sources contain "complete" proteins, meaning they provide the eight essential amino acids.

The RDA is the amount of nutrients most people need daily to prevent the development of disease.

Recommended Dietary Allowance (RDA): A subset of assessment values for the Dietary Reference Intakes (DRI), a new means of assessing dietary needs for healthy individuals, the RDA is the amount of nutrients most people need daily to prevent the development of disease, as outlined by the USDA. As an example, the RDA for vitamin C is 70 milligrams; if you consume less than that each day, you run the risk of developing scurvy.

Vitamins: Vitamins help with chemical reactions in the body. In general, vitamins must come from the diet; the body doesn't make them. Thirteen vitamins are essential to the body. They are divided into two categories: water-soluble (vitamin C and all the B vitamins) and fat-soluble (vitamins A, D, E and K). The fat-soluble vitamins are more easily stored by the body. Because the water-soluble vitamins aren't stored for long in the body, they must be consumed daily.

About the Nutrient Analyses

Computer-assisted nutrient analysis of the recipes was prepared by Kimberly Zammit, HBSc (the project supervisor was Len Piché, PhD, RD, Division of Food & Nutritional Sciences, Brescia University College, London, ON), using Food Processor® SQL, version 10.9, ESHA Research Inc., Salem OR (this software contains over 35,000 food items based largely on the latest USDA data and the entire Canadian Nutrient File, 2007b). The database was supplemented when necessary with documented data from reliable sources.

The analysis was based on:

- imperial weights and measures (except for foods typically packaged and used in metric quantities);
- the smaller ingredient quantity when there was a range;
- the first ingredient listed when there was a choice of ingredients.

Calculations involving meat and poultry use lean portions without skin and with visible fat trimmed. A pinch of salt was calculated as ⅛ tsp (0.5 mL). All recipes were analyzed prior to cooking. Optional ingredients and garnishes, and ingredients that are not quantified, were not included in the calculations.

Ingredients for Healthy Cooking

Consider this your go-to list of quality ingredients that will help you pull together healthful, nourishing meals and snacks at any time. Don't feel like you need to purchase everything listed here at once. Building up kitchen staples is a process that happens over time, with weekly shopping trips. Enjoy the journey and the delicious results it yields.

Stock your pantry with nutritious, delicious grains and wholesome whole-grain flours.

Flours and Grains

Eating more whole grains (Step 5) begins right here when you stock your pantry with nutritious, delicious grains and wholesome whole-grain flours.

Flours

Whole wheat flour is the most obvious choice when it comes to whole-grain flour, but other delicious options are available and are every bit as easy to use in a broad range of recipes. Here are my top picks for flours to keep at the ready.

Whole Wheat Pastry Flour

A fine-textured, soft wheat flour, whole wheat pastry flour can be used interchangeably with all-purpose flour in most recipes. Most, but not all, whole wheat pastry flours include the wheat germ; for optimum nutrition, select a variety that includes 100% of the wheat berry.

In many recipes in this book, I've used whole wheat pastry flour in combination with all-purpose flour, but feel free to increase the proportion of whole wheat pastry flour to replace more or all of the all-purpose flour.

It is extremely important not to substitute regular whole wheat flour for the whole wheat pastry flour; the results will be coarse, leaden and possibly inedible.

You can find whole wheat pastry flour at well-stocked supermarkets and at natural food stores. Store it in a sealable plastic bag in the refrigerator.

Whole Wheat Flour

Whole wheat flour is milled from hard red wheat; it has a fuller flavor and is far more nutritious than all-purpose flour because it contains the wheat bran and sometimes the germ. Because of its higher fat content, it should be stored in the refrigerator to prevent rancidity.

Brown Rice Flour

Brown rice flour contains no gluten, so it is a boon for those who are gluten-intolerant, as well as for anyone looking to cut back on wheat. It is milled from unpolished brown rice and has a higher nutrient value than white rice flour. Since it contains bran, it has a short shelf life and should be stored in the refrigerator.

Buckwheat Flour

Despite its name, buckwheat is related to rhubarb, not wheat; it is naturally gluten-free. The small seeds of the plant are ground to make a strongly nutty-flavored flour that works well in a wide variety of baked goods. You can easily replace anywhere from a quarter to half of the amount of wheat flour in a recipe with buckwheat flour (with the exception of yeast breads).

Whole-Grain Spelt Flour

Whole-grain spelt flour is a nutritious, delicious flour that can be used interchangeably with wheat flour in most recipes. Although it is not wheat, spelt is a cereal grain in the wheat family and does contain gluten. Spelt flour has a nutty and slightly sweet flavor similar to that of whole wheat flour. It has slightly fewer calories than wheat flour and is somewhat higher in protein. The flour is easy to digest but is lower in fiber than whole wheat flour. Be sure to choose a whole-grain variety, as opposed to refined white spelt flour, in which the germ and the endosperm have been removed to create flour with a smoother texture.

Cornmeal

Cornmeal is simply ground dried corn kernels. There are two methods of grinding. The first is the modern method, in which milling is done by huge steel rollers, which remove the husk and germ almost entirely; this creates the most common variety of cornmeal found in supermarkets. The second is the stone-ground method, in which some of the hull and germ of the corn is retained; this type of cornmeal is available at health food stores and in the health food sections of most supermarkets. The two varieties can be used interchangeably in most of the recipes in this collection, but I recommend sticking with the stone-ground variety where specified, as it has a much deeper corn flavor and is far more nutritious.

Keeping a variety of whole grains on hand is a convenient, economical and, most importantly, delicious way to make healthy dishes for every meal of the day.

Whole Grains

Keeping a variety of whole grains on hand is a convenient, economical and, most importantly, delicious way to make healthy dishes for every meal of the day. As a general rule, buy only what you anticipate being able to use within a 6-month period, to maximize freshness. Whole grains should be stored in airtight containers in a cool, dark place.

Amaranth

Amaranth is quite sticky when cooked; hence, it can be used to thicken soups and stews while simultaneously adding whole-grain goodness.

It can also be toasted in a skillet until it pops, like popcorn, and then sprinkled over salads and entrées for a nutty flavor and delicate crunch.

Brown Rice (Short- or Medium-Grain)

Brown rice is an excellent source of manganese and a good source of selenium, magnesium and fiber. When cooked, short-grain brown rice tends to stick together, making it an ideal component to vegetarian burgers, risotto or rice balls.

Brown Jasmine Rice

Brown jasmine rice is an aromatic long-grain rice originally grown in Thailand. It is particularly delicious when paired with Asian flavors.

Brown Basmati Rice

Brown basmati rice is an extra-long-grain aromatic rice cultivated primarily in India. It can be used interchangeably with brown jasmine rice or any other long-grain brown rice.

Buckwheat Groats

Technically, buckwheat isn't a grain; rather, it is a distant relative of rhubarb. The groats are the hulled, crushed kernels. They are often sold toasted (in which case they are called kasha). Buckwheat can be used in the same variety of recipes that grains can, whether left whole or ground into a flour. It is a gluten-free grain, making it a perfect choice for those who have celiac disease or any kind of gluten sensitivity.

Buckwheat can be used in the same variety of recipes that grains can, whether left whole or ground into a flour.

Bulgur Wheat

Bulgur is partially cooked cracked wheat. It is quick and easy to prepare for main dishes, porridges and salads.

Farro

Farro, a member of the wheat family, has a luscious, chewy texture. It can be used to make farrotto (a farro version of risotto), soups, stews and breakfast porridge. It is particularly rich in fiber, magnesium and vitamins A, B, C and E.

Kamut

Considered by some to be the great-great-grandfather of grains, Kamut is a variety of high-protein wheat that has never been hybridized. The kernels are two to three times the size of most wheat kernels. Kamut has both a deliciously nutty flavor and an impressive nutritional profile.

Millet

Millet is a tiny, mild-flavored grain that can be prepared in multiple ways with completely different outcomes. Toast it and it makes a crunchy, delicious alternative to nuts in baked goods. Cook it with a small amount of liquid and it has a pilaf-like texture that's a cross between couscous and bulgur. Or cook it with a large amount of liquid to create a soft porridge akin to polenta (for suppertime) or creamy oatmeal (for breakfast).

Pearl Barley

Pearl barley is a deliciously chewy grain that is lightly milled to retain all of the germ and at least two-thirds of the bran, making it a healthy choice for both sweet and savory recipes.

Quinoa

Classified as a whole grain but technically a seed, quinoa was a staple of the ancient Incas and is still an important food in South American cuisine. It contains more protein than any other grain and is considered a "complete protein" because it contains all eight essential amino acids. The tiny kernels cook like rice and expand to four times their original volume. Quinoa's flavor is delicate and is often compared to couscous.

Rolled Oats

Two types of rolled oats are called for in these recipes: large-flake (old-fashioned) rolled oats are oat groats (hulled and cleaned whole oats) that have been steamed and flattened with huge rollers; quick-cooking rolled oats are groats that have been cut into several pieces before being steamed and rolled into thinner flakes. For the best results, it is important to use the type of rolled oats specified in the recipe.

Spelt

Spelt is similar to wheat in texture and flavor, but it's worth adding to your cooking repertoire because it has 30% more protein than wheat. It's particularly well tolerated by wheat-sensitive folks, too.

Swapping regular pasta for whole-grain pasta is one of the easiest ways to add whole grains to your diet.

Wheat Berries

Wheat flour may be common, but most people are far less familiar with whole wheat berries, which are the whole kernels, or grains, of wheat. They have an addictive, chewy texture and a nutty flavor, and are filling and delicious in a wide variety of soups, salads and entrées.

Whole-Grain Pasta

Swapping regular pasta for whole-grain pasta is one of the easiest ways to add whole grains to your diet. An added plus? These pastas typically have a subtle, toasted flavor that adds to the overall flavor of the dish.

Whole Wheat and Multigrain Pasta

Both whole wheat pasta and multigrain pasta (made from a whole-grain blend) are readily available in supermarkets these days, in many different shapes and sizes. Check the label to make sure the pasta is made with 100% whole grains. Keep large, medium and small sizes on hand, as well as whole wheat couscous.

Quinoa Pasta

Quinoa pasta is made from a nutritious blend of quinoa flour and corn and is available in several shapes and sizes. Given that quinoa is so high in protein (and a complete protein, at that), swapping quinoa pasta for regular pasta is a convenient way to make meatless pastas — as well as meatless soups that contain pasta — extra-filling and nutritious. Quinoa pasta is 100% gluten-free, and its flavor, texture and appearance are very close to those of regular pasta.

Soba Noodles

These traditional Japanese buckwheat noodles are long, thin and flat. They are high in protein and other nutrients. If you are gluten-sensitive, be sure to read the package label; some varieties of soba noodles are made with a combination of buckwheat and wheat flours.

Fruits and Vegetables

Study after study indicates that diets heavy in fruits and vegetables are healthier for our hearts, help prevent cancer, keep weight in check, keep us looking and feeling younger and help us live longer. Best of all, fruits and vegetables are delicious and are far easier to add to your diet than you might think. Here are some of the terrific options to consider when you're building your fruit and vegetable reserves.

Diets heavy in fruits and vegetables are healthier for our hearts, help prevent cancer, keep weight in check, keep us looking and feeling younger and help us live longer.

Fresh Fruits and Vegetables

Fresh fruits and vegetables are packed with essential vitamins and nutrients, so it's a good idea to always have some on hand. Place a bowl of fresh fruit on the counter, and keep washed and cut vegetables in the refrigerator for ready-to-eat snacks. Store hardy vegetables, such as onions, potatoes, carrots and celery, in the pantry and crisper — they're a great foundation for countless recipes.

For the freshest fruits and vegetables at the best prices, buy what is in season. In most cases, you can buy fruits a few days before their peak ripeness and let them ripen at home before use. If you choose to buy them at or past peak, use them right away — within a day or two.

Which Fruits Ripen, Which Do Not

- *Ripen only after picking:* avocados
- *Never ripen after picking:* soft berries, cherries, citrus, grapes, pineapple, watermelon
- *Ripen in color, texture and juiciness but not in sweetness after picking:* apricots, blueberries, figs, melons (except watermelon), nectarines, passion fruit, peaches, persimmons
- *Get sweeter after picking:* apples, kiwi, mangos, papayas, pears
- *Ripen in every way after picking:* bananas

Delicate fruits and vegetables, such as berries, cherries, plums, asparagus, bell peppers, corn, cucumbers, mushrooms, yellow summer squash and zucchini, should be used close to the day of purchase. The following, by contrast, keep well:

- Apples
- Bananas
- Citrus fruits (such as oranges, lemons and grapefruits)
- Cabbage
- Carrots
- Celery
- Garlic
- Onions
- Potatoes (yellow and russet)
- Sweet potatoes

Ask your grocery store's produce manager what the delivery days are, so you can purchase your favorite fruits and vegetables before their quality declines. Alternatively, buy your produce at a local farmers' market. Many communities sponsor weekly farmers' markets to provide a central, in-town site for small farms to sell their produce directly to consumers.

Frozen Fruits and Vegetables

In addition to its convenience, frozen produce can sometimes be more nutritious than fresh.

Keeping a selection of frozen fruits and vegetables in the freezer is a wise move for healthy cooking and eating, whether for quick soups or for morning smoothies.

In addition to its convenience, frozen produce can sometimes be more nutritious than fresh. When fresh fruits and vegetables are shipped long distances, they rapidly lose vitamins and minerals thanks to exposure to heat and light; by contrast, frozen fruits and vegetables are frozen immediately after being picked, ensuring that all of the vitamins and minerals are preserved.

Whenever possible, choose organic frozen fruits and vegetables. Some varieties to keep on hand include:

- Winter squash purée (typically a blend of acorn and butternut squash)
- Petite peas
- Chopped greens (e.g., spinach, Swiss chard, mustard greens)
- Chopped onions
- Vegetable stir-fry blends
- Broccoli florets
- Shelled edamame
- Corn
- Lima beans
- Berries (blueberries, blackberries, raspberries, strawberries)
- Diced mangos
- Diced pineapples
- Sliced peaches

The Dirty Dozen and the Clean 15

The Environmental Working Group (EWG), a non-profit organization, created the *Shoppers Guide to Pesticides in Produce*. The 2011 edition of the guide is based on the results of 51,000 tests for pesticides on produce, conducted from 2000 to 2009 by the U.S. Department of Agriculture and the federal Food and Drug Administration. It's important to note that the EWG states that almost all of the tests were performed on produce that had been rinsed or peeled. For more information, visit www.ewg.org.

The Dirty Dozen

Here are the top 12 most pesticide-contaminated fruits and vegetables in America. When shopping for these items, buy organic whenever possible.

1. Apples
2. Celery
3. Strawberries
4. Peaches
5. Spinach
6. Nectarines (imported)
7. Grapes (imported)
8. Bell peppers
9. Potatoes
10. Blueberries
11. Lettuce
12. Kale/collard greens

The Clean 15

These fruits and vegetables are the least contaminated by pesticides, so it's not as crucial to buy organic.

1. Onions
2. Sweet corn
3. Pineapples
4. Avocados
5. Asparagus
6. Sweet peas
7. Mangos
8. Eggplants
9. Cantaloupe (domestic)
10. Kiwifruit
11. Cabbage
12. Watermelon
13. Sweet potatoes
14. Grapefruit
15. Mushrooms

Interpreting Organic Labels

Understanding the various organic labels can be a challenge. Here's what the four most common labels and claims mean:

"100% Organic" USDA ORGANIC	For a food product to be 100% organic and be able to bear the USDA organic seal, it must be made with 100% organic ingredients. The food product also must have an ingredient list and list the name of the certifying agency.
"Organic" USDA ORGANIC	For a food product to be labeled as "organic" and be able to bear the USDA organic seal, it must be made with 95% organic ingredients. The food product also must list the name of the certifying agency and have an ingredient statement on the label where organic ingredients are identified as organic.
"Made with Organic Ingredients"	To make this claim, a food product must be made with at least 70% organic ingredients. The food product also must list the name of the certifying agency and have an ingredient statement on the label where organic ingredients are identified as organic.
"Some Organic Ingredients"	Food products with less than 70% organic ingredients cannot bear the USDA seal nor have information about a certifying agency, or any reference to organic content.

Canned tomatoes retain almost all of their nutrients and actually contain more lycopene than raw tomatoes.

Shelf-Stable Tomato Products

Canned tomatoes may sound nutritionally benign (if not bereft), but nothing could be further from the truth. Unlike many canned vegetables, canned tomatoes retain almost all of their nutrients (including substantial amounts of vitamins A and C) and actually contain more lycopene than raw tomatoes. Choose organic whenever possible, as they tend to be lower in sodium and residual chemicals.

Diced Tomatoes

Canned diced tomatoes can replace diced fresh tomatoes in most recipes, especially soups and stews. Stock up on diced fire-roasted tomatoes, too, as they add a subtle smoky flavor to dishes.

Crushed Tomatoes

Canned crushed tomatoes (sometimes called ground tomatoes) are a convenient way to add fresh tomato flavor to soups, stews and pastas without the separate step of puréeing.

Tomato Sauce

Tomato sauce can be used to make delicious sauces, stews and soups when you want to give them a distinct tomato flavor. For true tomato flavor with minimal processing, be sure to select a variety of tomato sauce that is low in sodium and has no added seasonings.

Tomato Paste

Tomato paste is made from tomatoes that have been cooked for several hours, then strained and reduced to a deep red, richly flavored concentrate. It is available in both cans and convenient squeeze tubes. Just a tablespoon or two (15 or 30 mL) can greatly enrich a wide variety of dishes, adding acidity, depth and a hint of sweetness. Select a brand that is low in sodium and has no added seasonings.

Sun-Dried Tomatoes

Sun-dried tomatoes are a flavorful and nutritious way to add an extra bit of zest to your recipes. Look for organic sun-dried tomatoes, which are often processed at a lower temperature than most commercial varieties, preserving some of the nutrients.

Marinara Sauce

Jarred marinara sauce — a highly seasoned Italian tomato sauce made with onions, garlic, basil and oregano — is typically used on pasta and meat, but it is also a great pantry staple for creating meals in minutes. For the best tomato flavor and the most versatility, choose a variety with minimal ingredients and low sodium.

Chunky Tomato Salsa

Like marinara sauce, ready-made chunky salsa — rich with tomatoes, peppers, onions and spices but low in calories — packs tremendous flavor into recipes in an instant. For the best flavor and nutrition, select a brand that is low in sodium and has a short list of easily identifiable ingredients.

Dried Fruit

Dried fruit is essential to a well-stocked pantry. Keep a variety of dried fruits at the ready for cooking, baking or eating out of hand (especially when a craving for sweets strikes). Whenever possible, opt for organic dried fruit. The following are top picks:

Keep a variety of dried fruits at the ready for cooking, baking or eating out of hand.

- Raisins (both dark and golden)
- Dried currants (sometimes labeled Zante currants)
- Dried cranberries (preferably sweetened with fruit juice)
- Dried cherries
- Dried apricots
- Dried apples
- Dried figs
- Prunes (dried plums)

Legumes

Legumes are nutritional powerhouses. One cup (250 mL) of cooked legumes has an average of 200 to 300 calories, next to no fat (with the exception of soybeans), about one-third of the protein you need in a day and lots of fiber. In addition, legumes are very low in cost and easy to prepare in a wide variety of recipes.

With their high protein content, wide availability, low cost and convenience, canned beans are ideal for a wide range of quick, healthy meals and snacks.

Canned Beans

With their high protein content, wide availability, low cost and convenience, canned beans are ideal for a wide range of quick, healthy meals and snacks. For the best flavor and versatility, select varieties that are low in sodium and have no added seasonings. The following varieties are great choices to keep on hand for everything from dips to entrées:

- Black beans
- White beans (e.g., cannellini and white navy beans)
- Pinto beans
- Red kidney beans
- Chickpeas

Dried Beans

The recipes in this collection call for canned beans because they are a convenient option that saves time and effort in the kitchen. However, I encourage you to prepare dried beans when you can. I have provided a cooking chart for a broad range of dried legumes on page 436. Once prepared, they can be substituted in any recipe calling for canned beans. In general, substitute 1⅔ cups (400 mL) cooked beans for each can of beans.

Dried Split Peas (Green and Yellow)

A variety of yellow and green peas are grown specifically for drying. These peas are dried and split along a natural seam (hence, "split peas"). Split peas are very inexpensive and are loaded with good nutrition, including a significant amount of protein. They are available packaged in supermarkets and in bulk in health food stores. Unlike dried beans, they do not require presoaking.

Dried Lentils

Lentils are inexpensive, require no presoaking, cook in about 30 to 45 minutes and are very high in nutrients (soybeans are the only legume with more protein). Lentils come in a variety of sizes and colors: common brown lentils and French green lentils can be found in supermarkets, and increasingly, so can red and black lentils.

Soybean Products

Just a short while back, soybean products — tofu, soy milk, tempeh, soy cheese and soy yogurt — were considered health food oddities. Now, most of these items have gone mainstream and are usually available in well-stocked grocery stores.

Tofu

All of the recipes in this collection were tested with refrigerated tofu. Although shelf-stable tofu is convenient, the flavor and texture are markedly inferior.

Tofu, or bean curd, is made from soy beans that have been cooked, made into milk and then coagulated. The soy milk curdles when heated, and the curds are skimmed off and pressed into blocks. Tofu can be found in extra-firm, firm and soft varieties in the refrigerated section of the supermarket. Be sure to use the variety specified in the recipe for optimal results.

Tempeh

Tempeh (pronounced *TEM-pay*) is a traditional Indonesian food. It is made from fully cooked soybeans that have been fermented with a mold called rhizopus and formed into cakes. Some varieties have whole grains added to the mix, creating a particularly meaty, satisfying texture. Tempeh, like tofu, takes on the flavor of whatever it is marinated with, and also needs to be stored in the refrigerator.

Nuts, Seeds and Nut/Seed Butters

Nuts and seeds — including natural nut and seed butters — are very nutritious. In addition to being excellent sources of protein, nuts and seeds contain vitamins, minerals, fiber and essential fatty acids (such as omega-3 and omega-6). Although many people are hesitant to eat nuts and seeds because of their high fat content, nuts and seeds can provide a sense of fullness and satisfaction that actually causes you to eat less of other high-calorie, high-fat foods.

Although many people are hesitant to eat nuts and seeds because of their high fat content, nuts and seeds can provide a sense of fullness and satisfaction that actually causes you to eat less of other high-calorie, high-fat foods.

Nuts

A wide variety of nuts is used in this collection, including walnuts, cashews, pecans, almonds, peanuts, hazelnuts and pistachios. Many of the recipes call for the nuts to be toasted before they are used. Toasting nuts deepens their flavor and makes them crisp. To toast whole nuts, spread the amount needed for the recipe on a rimmed baking sheet. Bake in a preheated 350°F (180°C) oven for 8 to 10 minutes or until golden and fragrant. Alternatively, toast the nuts in a dry skillet over low heat, stirring constantly for 2 to 4 minutes or until golden and fragrant. Transfer the toasted nuts to a plate and let them cool before chopping.

Ground Flax Seeds (Flaxseed Meal)

Flax seeds are highly nutritious, tiny seeds from the flax plant. They have gained tremendous popularity in recent years thanks to their high levels of omega-3 fatty acids. But to reap the most benefits from the seeds, they must be ground into meal. Look for packages of ready-ground flax seeds, which may be labeled "flaxseed meal," or use a spice or coffee grinder to grind whole flax seeds to a very fine meal. The meal adds a nutty flavor to a wide range of recipes. Store ground flax seeds in an airtight container in the refrigerator for up to 5 months or in the freezer for up to 8 months.

Green Pumpkin Seeds (Pepitas)

Pepitas are pumpkin seeds with the white hull removed, leaving the flat, dark green inner seed. They are subtly sweet and nutty, with a slightly chewy texture when raw and a crisp, crunchy texture when toasted or roasted. They can be used much as nuts are used — sprinkled atop salads, soups and entrées for a pleasant, contrasting crunch, or added to muffins, cookies or breads.

Shelled Sunflower Seeds

Sunflower seeds are highly nutritious and have a mild, nutty flavor and texture. The recipes in this collection call for seeds that have been removed from their shells. They can be used in place of nuts in both sweet and savory dishes.

Sesame Seeds

Tiny and delicate, the flavor of sesame seeds increases exponentially when they are toasted. Used as a flavoring in many Asian preparations, sesame seeds are also delicious in sweet and savory baked goods.

Nut and Seed Butters

Delicious, nutritious, ultra-convenient nut and seed butters are a boon for any meal of the day, as well as for snacks, desserts and quick breads.

Delicious, nutritious, ultra-convenient nut and seed butters are a boon for any meal of the day, as well as for snacks, desserts and quick breads. They can also impart instant richness to a wide range of sauces and dressings.

A wide variety of all-natural, unsalted nut and seed butters is increasingly available at well-stocked supermarkets, co-ops and natural food stores. Seed butters, such as tahini and sunflower seed butter, are an excellent substitution for nut butters for those with tree nut allergies or sensitivities.

Below are some of the butters used in this collection. They may be used interchangeably in any recipe calling for nut butter, unless otherwise specified. Store opened jars in the refrigerator.

- Unsalted natural peanut butter
- Unsalted natural almond butter
- Unsalted natural cashew butter
- Tahini (sesame seed butter)
- Sunflower seed butter

Eggs, Dairy and Non-Dairy Milks

Eggs, dairy products and non-dairy milks are essential ingredients in any kitchen, helping you prepare everything from short-order breakfasts and dinners to countless baked goods.

Eggs

All of the recipes in this book were tested with large eggs. Select clean, fresh eggs that have been handled properly and refrigerated. Do not use dirty, cracked or leaking eggs, or eggs that have a bad odor or unnatural color when cracked open; they may have become contaminated with harmful bacteria, such as salmonella.

Decoding Egg Labels

These days, egg cartons are covered in labels ranging from "organic" to "cage-free" to "animal welfare approved." It's confusing, to say the least. Here's a quick guide to the terms you need to know, according to USDA guidelines:

- *Organic:* Chickens must be cage-free with some outdoor access (amount not defined), cannot be given antibiotics, and must be fed organic, vegetarian food. The USDA Organic seal is the only official egg label claim that's backed by federal regulations.
- *Free Range:* Chickens are out of cages, and can roam freely around a farmyard for at least part of the day, but there is no regulation in the U.S. about the amount or quality of outdoor access. There are no restrictions on what the birds can be fed.
- *Cage Free:* Chickens have continuous access to food and water and are out of cages, but do not necessarily have access to the outdoors. They may be tightly packed into a shed, with no access to a farmyard.
- *Certified Humane:* Chickens are out of cages inside barns or warehouses, but may not have access to the outdoors. There are regulations to ensure that the chickens can perform natural behaviors and to limit the density of birds. More information is available at www.certifiedhumane.com.
- *Animal Welfare Approved:* This term is given to independent family farmers with flocks of up to 500 chickens, who are free to spend unlimited time outside on pesticide-free pasture and cannot have their beaks cut (beak cutting is allowed in all the previous definitions and is very common). Eggs from these farms are most commonly found at specialty or health food stores and at farmers' markets.

The following terms are unregulated and therefore mean nothing:

- Natural
- Naturally Raised
- No Hormones
- No Antibiotics

Make Flax Eggs for Eggless Baking

Whether you have an egg allergy or sensitivity, want to make baked goods for a vegan friend or are simply out of eggs, consider substituting flax eggs (sometimes called "fleggs") in baked goods and breakfast items such as muffins, cakes, pancakes and waffles.

For each egg, combine 2 tbsp (30 mL) ground flax seeds (flaxseed meal) and 3 tbsp (45 mL) water in a blender; blend on high speed for 1 minute or until thickened and frothy. Use immediately, adding the mixture to the recipe when it calls for eggs.

Dairy

Enjoy your dairy, but choose wisely.

All dairy foods are not created equal. Although they are generally rich in calcium and protein, some higher-fat varieties can also be high in artery-clogging saturated fat and cholesterol. So enjoy your dairy, but choose wisely, using the list below as a guide.

Lower-Fat Milk

Both lower-fat and skim (nonfat) milk are used in a wide range of recipes in this book.

Buttermilk

Commercially prepared buttermilk has a delicious and distinctive tang. It is made by culturing 1% milk with bacteria. When added to baked goods, it yields a tender, moist result and a slightly buttery flavor.

If you don't have buttermilk, it's easy to make a substitute. Mix 1 tbsp (15 mL) lemon juice or white vinegar into 1 cup (250 mL) milk. Let stand for at least 15 minutes before using, to allow the milk to curdle. Any extra can be stored in the refrigerator for the same amount of time as the milk from which it was made.

Evaporated Nonfat Milk

Produced by evaporating nearly half the water from fresh skim (nonfat) milk, evaporated nonfat milk is a shelf-stable canned milk. It is an excellent option for adding richness to recipes in place of cream.

Yogurt

Yogurt, like buttermilk, is acidic and adds a distinctive tang to recipes. It tenderizes meats and baked goods, and makes an excellent substitution for sour cream in a wide range of recipes. All of the recipes in this collection call for plain (unflavored) nonfat yogurt.

Greek yogurt is a thick, creamy yogurt similar in texture to sour cream. It is made by straining the whey from yogurt and is very high in protein, not to mention incredibly delicious.

Nonfat Ricotta Cheese

Ricotta is a rich, fresh cheese with a texture that is slightly grainy but still far smoother than cottage cheese. It is white and moist and has a slightly sweet flavor. The nonfat variety is readily available and adds richness without fat to a wide range of dishes. It also has significantly fewer calories than the full-fat variety.

Nonfat Cottage Cheese

Nonfat cottage cheese is used in many recipes in this collection, from morning muffins to evening main dishes. In addition to its versatility, it has significant nutritional value (most notably in protein and calcium).

Non-Dairy Milks

Non-dairy milks are essential for vegans, as well as those who are lactose intolerant or are allergic to dairy. But they are also a delicious option for all of us, whether to use in cooking or baking, or to drink straight up. The variety and availability of non-dairy milks is greater than ever, and you cannot beat their shelf-stable convenience. Although non-dairy milks are available in a variety of flavors, opt for plain when substituting for milk in any of the recipes in this collection.

Soy Milk

Soy milk is made by combining ground soybeans with water and cooking the mixture. Finally, the liquid is pressed from the solids and then filtered.

Almond Milk

Almond milk is made from almonds, water, sea salt and typically a small amount of sweetener. It works particularly well as a substitute for dairy milk in baked good recipes.

Rice Milk

Rice milk is made from brown rice, water, sea salt and typically a small amount of oil. It is a very light, sweet beverage that can replace cow's milk in most recipes.

Hemp Milk

Hemp milk is a thick, rich milk made from hemp seeds, water and a touch of brown rice syrup. It is rich in healthy omega-3 fatty acids, protein and essential vitamins and minerals. Because of its neutral taste, it can be used in a broad range of sweet and savory dishes.

Light Coconut Milk

Typically available canned or in Tetra Paks, light coconut milk adds instant exotic flair to curries, soups and sauces; it is also fantastic in desserts, such as ice cream, that usually rely on heavy dairy products. It is readily available and very affordable at supermarkets. The light varieties have 50% to 75% less fat than regular coconut milk, but retain all of the tropical flavor and much of the lush texture.

Fats and Oils

Fats and oils can be healthy or unhealthy; it all depends on the type you use and how much you consume. Some oils, such as those that contain essential fatty acids (omega-3 and omega-6, for example), are a necessary part of your diet. And when it comes to eating healthier over the long term, you'll feel happy and satisfied when you cook your food with a healthy amount of good fats.

When it comes to eating healthier over the long term, you'll feel happy and satisfied when you cook your food with a healthy amount of good fats.

Butter

Butter is used sparingly in a small number of recipes in the Natural Sugar Sweets chapter. Fresh butter has a delicate cream flavor and a pale yellow color, and adds tremendous flavor to a wide range of recipes.

The salted butter at the supermarket may be far less fresh than the unsalted option, and has sometimes been made from cream that is less fresh too.

Butter quickly picks up off-flavors during storage and when exposed to oxygen, so once the carton or wrap is opened, place it in a sealable plastic food bag or other airtight container. Store it away from foods with strong odors, especially items such as onions or garlic.

I recommend buying and using only unsalted butter for the recipes in this collection. The obvious reason is the added salt. Different manufacturers use different amounts of salt in their butter, so it's not possible to reliably determine how much salt is in any given stick or cube. The less obvious reason is that salt is a preservative: salted butter has a longer shelf life in the refrigerator (as much as 2 or 3 months). As such, the salted butter at the supermarket may be far less fresh than the unsalted option, and has sometimes been made from cream that is less fresh too. If you are concerned about keeping unsalted butter fresh once you've purchased it, you can store it in the freezer for up to 6 months.

Substituting Margarine for Butter

Margarine may be substituted for butter, but I don't recommended doing so. Margarine is highly processed and lacks the rich flavor that butter offers. In addition, some brands contain high levels of unhealthy trans fats. If, however, you need to substitute margarine for butter because of specific dietary requirements, avoid spreads in tub form; to make them spreadable, these products have a much higher percentage of water than sticks. Using a spread will alter the liquid and fat combination of the recipe, leading to either unsatisfactory or downright disastrous results. For best results, choose high-quality margarine sticks with at least an 80% fat content.

Nonstick Cooking Spray

A number of recipes in this collection call for the use of nonstick cooking spray, which helps keep foods from sticking while simultaneously cutting back on fat and calories in a dish. While any variety of cooking spray may be used, I recommend using an organic cooking spray for two reasons: first, these sprays are typically made with higher-quality oils (in many cases expeller-pressed or cold-pressed oils) than most commercial brands; second, they are more likely to use compressed gas to expel the propellant, so no hydrocarbons are released into the environment. Read the label and choose wisely.

Vegetable Oil

"Vegetable oil" is a generic term used to describe any neutral, plant-based oil that is liquid at room temperature. You can choose from a variety of vegetable oils (e.g., safflower, sunflower, canola), but opt for those that are:

1. Expeller-pressed or cold-pressed. Expeller-pressed oils are pressed simply by crushing the seeds, while cold-pressed oils are expeller-pressed oils that are produced in a heat-controlled environment.
2. High in healthful unsaturated fats (no more than 7% saturated fat).

Extra Virgin Olive Oil

Olive oil is monounsaturated oil that is prized for its use in a wide range of dishes. Extra virgin olive oil is the cold-pressed result of the first pressing of the olives and is considered the finest and fruitiest of the olive oils. It is suitable for many types of cooking preparations because it has a relatively high smoking point, but it can be expensive. The good news is that it is used very sparingly in the recipes throughout this collection, so a little bit will go a long way.

Although extra virgin olive oil is excellent for cooking, the subtle nuances of the oil shine best when it is uncooked, whether in salad dressings or drizzled on top of soup.

Unrefined Virgin Coconut Oil

Virgin coconut oil can be used in both cooking and baking. It is semi-solid at room temperature and must be melted slowly, over low heat, to avoid burning.

Toasted Sesame Oil

Toasted sesame oil has a dark brown color and a rich, nutty flavor. It is used sparingly, mostly in Asian recipes, to add a tremendous amount of flavor.

Natural Sweeteners

Natural sweeteners are closer to their whole form than refined sweeteners, which have most or all of their natural vitamins and minerals removed during the refining process. From a flavor perspective, natural sweeteners contain a broader spectrum of flavors than refined sugar; hence, they add more than sweetness alone to sweet and savory dishes.

Natural sweeteners contain a broader spectrum of flavors than refined sugar; hence, they add more than sweetness alone to sweet and savory dishes.

Evaporated Cane Sugar

Evaporated cane sugar, also called whole cane sugar or dried cane juice, is made from the dried juice of the sugar cane plant. Many of the minerals from the plant are still present, which helps the human body digest the sugars. Dried cane juice resembles brown sugar in appearance and taste, though it is less sweet. It can be substituted cup for cup for granulated sugar in baked goods. Trade names for this type of sugar are Rapadura and Sucanat.

Turbinado Sugar

Turbinado sugar is raw sugar that has been steam-cleaned. The coarse crystals are blond in color and have a delicate molasses flavor. They are typically used for decoration and texture atop baked goods.

Brown Rice Syrup

Brown rice syrup is made from brown rice that has been soaked, sprouted and cooked with an enzyme that breaks the starches into maltose. Brown rice syrup has a light, mild flavor and a similar appearance to honey, though it is less sweet. Rice syrup can be substituted one for one for honey or maple syrup.

Honey

Honey is plant nectar that has been gathered and concentrated by honey bees. Any variety of honey may be used in the recipes in this collection. Unopened containers of honey may be stored at room temperature. After opening, store honey in the refrigerator to protect against mold. Honey will keep indefinitely when stored properly.

Maple Syrup

Maple syrup is a thick liquid sweetener made by boiling the sap from maple trees. It has a strong, pure maple flavor. Maple-flavored pancake syrup is just corn syrup with coloring and artificial maple flavoring added, and it is not recommended as a substitute for pure maple syrup. Unopened containers of maple syrup may be stored at room temperature. After opening, store maple syrup in the refrigerator to protect against mold. Maple syrup will keep indefinitely when stored properly.

Molasses

Molasses is made from the juice of sugar cane or sugar beets, which is boiled until a syrupy mixture remains. The recipes in this collection were tested using dark (cooking) molasses, but you can substitute light (fancy) molasses if you prefer. Blackstrap molasses is thick and very dark, and it has a bitter flavor; it is not recommended for the recipes in this collection. Unopened containers of molasses may be stored at room temperature. After opening, store molasses in the refrigerator to protect against mold. Molasses will keep indefinitely when stored properly.

Agave Nectar

Agave nectar (or agave syrup) is a plant-based sweetener derived from the agave cactus, native to Mexico. Used for centuries to make tequila, agave juice produces a light golden syrup.

Stevia

Stevia is about 300 times sweeter than cane sugar

Stevia is derived from the leaves of a South American shrub, *Stevia rehaudiana.* It is about 300 times sweeter than cane sugar, or sucrose. Stevia is not absorbed through the digestive tract, and therefore has no calories. Stevia comes in several forms: dried leaf, liquid extract and powdered extract. The few recipes in this collection that call for stevia use it in powdered form.

Fresh Dates

Fresh dates — the fruit of the date palm tree — are among the sweetest fruits in the world, with a flavor similar to brown sugar. They can be used in desserts, snacks, sauces and even soups, stews and chilis to add sweetness. The most commonly available dates in the United States and Canada are Medjool dates, which are plump and tender, and

Deglet Noor dates, which are semi-soft, slender and a bit chewy; both varieties have often been left on the tree for a while after they are ripe to dry a bit (and thus last longer after harvest). When choosing fresh dates, select those that are plump-looking; it is okay if they are slightly wrinkled, but they shouldn't feel hard.

Fresh Herbs

Fresh herbs add an aromatic backbone to cooked food. When added during the cooking process, they willingly surrender their flavors and aromas in minutes. Alternatively, you can add them as a final flourish for a bright note of fresh flavor and color.

Flat-leaf (Italian) parsley, cilantro and chives are readily available and inexpensive, and they store well in the produce bin of the refrigerator, so keep them on hand year-round. Basil, mint and thyme are best in the spring and summer, when they are in season in your own garden or at the farmers' market.

Flavorings

Elevating everyday dishes to exceptional levels of deliciousness can be as easy as creating a harmonious balance of simple flavorings — even if you're just adding salt and pepper. Here are my top recommendations for ingredients that will make the ordinary extraordinary.

Fine Sea Salt

Unless otherwise specified, the recipes in this collection were tested using fine-grain sea salt.

Conventional salt production uses chemicals, additives and heat processing to achieve the end product commonly called table salt. By contrast, unrefined sea salt contains an abundance of naturally occurring trace minerals.

Black Pepper

Black pepper is made by grinding black peppercorns, which have been picked when the berry is not quite ripe, then dried until it shrivels and the skin turns dark brown to black. Black pepper has a strong, slightly hot flavor, with a hint of sweetness.

Spices and Dried Herbs

Spices and dried herbs can turn the simplest of meals into masterpieces. They should be stored in light- and air-proof containers, away from direct sunlight and heat, to preserve their flavors.

Co-ops, health food stores and mail order sources that sell herbs and spices in bulk are all excellent options for purchasing very fresh, organic spices and dried herbs, often at a low cost.

With ground spices and dried herbs, freshness is everything. To determine whether a ground spice or dried herb is fresh, open the container and sniff. A strong fragrance means it is still acceptable for use.

Spices and dried herbs can turn the simplest of meals into masterpieces.

Note that ground spices, not whole, are used throughout this collection. Here are my favorite ground spices and dried herbs:

Ground Spices

- Black pepper (cracked and ground)
- Cardamom
- Cayenne pepper (also labeled "ground red pepper")
- Chili powder
- Chinese five-spice powder
- Cinnamon
- Chipotle chile powder
- Coriander
- Cumin
- Garam masala
- Ginger
- Hot pepper flakes
- Mild curry powder
- Nutmeg
- Paprika
- Smoked paprika (both hot and sweet)
- Turmeric

Dried Herbs

- Bay leaves
- Oregano
- Rosemary
- Rubbed sage
- Thyme

Citrus Zest

Zest is the name for the colored outer layer of citrus peel.

Zest is the name for the colored outer layer of citrus peel. The oils in zest are intense in flavor. Use a zester, a rasp grater, such as a Microplane, or the small holes of a box grater to grate zest. Avoid grating the white layer (pith) just below the zest; it is very bitter.

Cocoa Powder

Select natural cocoa powder rather than Dutch process for the recipes in this collection. Natural cocoa powder has a deep, true chocolate flavor. The packaging should state whether it is Dutch process or not, but you can also tell the difference by sight: if it is dark to almost black, it is Dutch process; natural cocoa powder is much lighter and is typically brownish red in color.

Vanilla Extract

Vanilla extract adds a sweet, fragrant flavor to dishes, especially baked goods. It is produced by combining an extraction from dried vanilla beans with an alcohol and water mixture. It is then aged for several months. The three most common types of vanilla beans used to make vanilla extract are Bourbon-Madagascar, Mexican and Tahitian.

Almond Extract

Almond extract is a flavoring manufactured by combining bitter almond oil with ethyl alcohol. It is used in much the same way as vanilla extract. Almond extract has a highly concentrated, intense flavor, so measure with care.

Reduced-Sodium Tamari

Tamari is a natural, aged soy sauce made from soybeans, water, sea salt and sometimes added wheat. It can be used in place of regular soy sauce. If you're avoiding gluten, look for wheat-free tamari.

Miso

Miso is a sweet, fermented soybean paste usually made with some sort of grain. It comes unpasteurized and in several varieties, from golden yellow to deep red to sweet white. It can be made into a soup or a sauce or used as a salt substitute.

Wasabi

Wasabi is a Japanese horseradish. It is dried into a pale green powder that, when mixed with water, makes a potent, fiery paste. Store it in a tightly covered glass jar, away from heat or light, to preserve its flavor.

Thai Curry Paste

Available in small jars, Thai curry paste is a blend of Thai chiles, garlic, lemongrass, galangal, ginger and wild lime leaves. It is a fast and delicious way to add Southeast Asian flavor to a broad spectrum of recipes in a single step. Panang and yellow curry pastes tend to be the mildest. Red curry paste is medium hot, and green curry paste is typically the hottest.

Dijon Mustard

Dijon mustard adds depth of flavor to a wide range of dishes. It is most commonly used in this collection for salad dressing because it facilitates the emulsification of oil and vinegar.

Vinegars

Vinegars are multipurpose flavor powerhouses. Delicious in vinaigrettes and dressings, they are also stealth ingredients for use at the end of cooking time to enhance and balance the natural flavors of dishes. Store vinegars in a dark place, away from heat or light.

Delicious in vinaigrettes and dressings, vinegars are also stealth ingredients for use at the end of cooking time to enhance and balance the natural flavors of dishes.

Cider Vinegar

Cider vinegar is made from the juice of crushed apples. After the juice is collected, it is aged in wooden barrels.

Unseasoned Rice Vinegar

Rice vinegar is made from an alcohol fermentation of mashed rice. It then undergoes another fermentation to produce vinegar. In general, rice vinegar tends to be more acidic than other vinegars. Be sure to check the label to make sure it is unseasoned; seasoned rice vinegar has added salt and sugar.

Red Wine Vinegar

Red wine vinegar is produced by fermenting red wine in wooden barrels. This produces acetic acid, which gives red wine vinegar its distinctive taste. Red wine vinegar has a characteristic dark red color and red wine flavor.

White Wine Vinegar

White wine vinegar is a moderately tangy vinegar made from a blend of white wines. The wine is fermented, aged and filtered to produce a vinegar with a slightly lower acidity level than red wine vinegar.

Sherry Vinegar

Sherry vinegar has a deep, complex flavor and a dark reddish color. It is made from three different white grape varieties grown in the Jerez region of Spain. Most of the sherry vinegar produced comes from this region, making it a popular ingredient in Spanish cooking.

Balsamic Vinegar

Balsamic vinegar is a thick, aromatic vinegar made from concentrated grape must. Grape must is the freshly pressed juice of the grape, and also contains pulp, skins, stems and seeds. The must is boiled down to a sap and aged in wooden barrels for 6 months to 12 years. Some very expensive balsamic vinegars are aged for up to 25 years.

Opt for certified organic broths that are all-natural, reduced-sodium and MSG-free.

Ready-to-Use Broths

Ready-made chicken, beef and vegetable broths are essential for many of the recipes in this collection. Opt for certified organic broths that are all-natural, reduced-sodium and MSG-free. For chicken and beef broths, look for brands that are made from chicken or cattle raised without hormones or antibiotics.

For convenience, look for broths in Tetra Paks, which typically come in 32-oz (1 L), 48-oz (1.5 L) and occasionally 16-oz (500 mL) sizes. Once opened, these can be stored in the refrigerator for up to 1 week.

Specialty Items

The following four ingredients may not be staples, but they are well worth adding to your pantry. Olives and capers add instant, intense, briny flavor to a host of healthy recipes; delicate nori contributes a toasty, subtle saltiness to salads, soups and snacks; and agar works like magic to create perfectly gelled desserts.

Olives

Olives are a fruit that must be cured before they are edible. A brine made from salt and water is typically used, though kalamata olives are cured in a salted vinegar brine. Choose olives that are made with sea salt and avoid brands that have been treated with preservatives. With their pungent flavor, olives add instant impact to countless dishes, making them a great item to keep in the pantry. Keep jars of both green and black olives on hand. Once opened, jars of olives in their brine can be stored in the refrigerator for several months.

Capers

Capers are the unripened flower buds of *Capparis spinosa*, a prickly perennial plant native to the Mediterranean and some parts of Asia.

Once the buds are harvested, they are dried in the sun, then pickled in vinegar, brine, wine or salt. The curing brings out their piquant, citrusy-salty flavor. Use them to enhance the flavor of salads, sauces, vegetables and entrées. Once opened, jars of capers can be stored in the refrigerator for several months.

Nori

Nori is made from an edible seaweed. It comes in thin sheets and is the black wrapper typical of many sushi rolls. It can also be sweetened and/or toasted for a quick snack, or added to salads and soups. Nori has a high protein content and is easily digested. It contains an enzyme that helps break down cholesterol deposits in the body.

Agar Flakes

Agar-agar, usually abbreviated to agar, is a gelatinous substance derived from red algae. Most typically available for culinary use in flake form, it is a vegetarian alternative to regular gelatin for a wide range of desserts. Agar will gel a liquid much like gelatin, though the consistency is slightly different. As a general rule of thumb, one tablespoon (15 mL) of agar flakes will gel 1 cup (250 mL) of liquid.

Measuring Ingredients

Accurate measurements are important for healthy cooking — and essential for healthy baking — to achieve consistent results time and again. So take both time and care as you measure.

Accurate measurements are important for healthy cooking — and essential for healthy baking — to achieve consistent results time and again.

Measuring Dry Ingredients

When measuring a dry ingredient, such as flour, cocoa powder, sugar, spices or salt, spoon it into the appropriate-size dry measuring cup or measuring spoon, heaping it up over the top. Slide a straight-edged utensil, such as a knife, across the top to level off the extra. Be careful not to shake or tap the cup or spoon to settle the ingredient, or you will have more than you need.

Measuring Moist Ingredients

Moist ingredients, such as brown sugar, coconut and dried fruit, must be firmly packed in a measuring cup or spoon to be measured accurately. Use a dry measuring cup or spoon for these ingredients. Fill to slightly overflowing, then pack down the ingredient firmly with the back of a spoon. Add more of the ingredient and pack down again until full and even with the top of the measure.

Measuring Liquid Ingredients

Use a clear plastic or glass measuring cup or container with lines up the sides to measure liquid ingredients. Set the container on the counter and pour the liquid to the appropriate mark. Lower your head to read the measurement at eye level.

Breakfasts

Multigrain Pancake and Waffle Mix . . . 44
Oatmeal Buttermilk Pancakes . . . 46
Cottage Cheese Pancakes with Yogurt and Jam . . . 47
Quinoa Blueberry Pancakes . . . 48
Make-Ahead Whole Wheat Crêpes . . . 49
Walnut Flax Waffles . . . 50
Pumpkin Maple Waffles . . . 51
Microwave Poached Eggs . . . 52
Baked Eggs in Marinara . . . 52
Favorite Frittata . . . 53
Tofu Scramble . . . 54
Power Pitas with Eggs and Vegetables . . . 54
Healthy Know-How: From Pyramid to Plate — Understanding the USDA MyPlate . . . 55
Avocado and Egg Breakfast Wraps . . . 56
Quinoa Kale Breakfast Casserole . . . 57
Breakfast Polenta with Cherries and Almonds . . . 57
Overnight Oatmeal . . . 58
Toasted Quinoa Porridge . . . 58
Power Granola . . . 59
Quinoa Cranberry Granola . . . 60
Toasted Oat Muesli with Dried Fruit and Pecans . . . 61

Pumpkin Yogurt with Quinoa Crunch 62
Greek Yogurt, Grain and Blackberry Parfaits 63
Chunky Applesauce 63
Spinach and Ricotta Bruschetta 64
Scandinavian Breakfast Toasts with Smoked Salmon and Avocado 64
Whole-Grain Blueberry Maple Muffins 65
Yogurt Bran Muffins 66
Banana and Toasted Millet Muffins 67
Cheese, Almond and Mushroom Muffins 68
Oats and Dried Fruit Breakfast Bars 69
Healthy Know-How: The Importance of Drinking Water 70
Sunflower Apricot Go-Bars 70
Quinoa Blueberry Breakfast Cookies 71
Multigrain Cranberry Breakfast Cookies 72
Carrot Oat Breakfast Cookies 73
Berry Protein Shake 74
Banana Buttermilk Smoothie 74
Super C Smoothie 75
Super Antioxidant Smoothie 75
Papaya Pineapple Smoothie 76
Green Machine Smoothie 76
Pumpkin Smoothie 77

Multigrain Pancake and Waffle Mix

Makes about 4½ cups (1.125 L)

✪ Great for Steps 3, 4 and 5

Leave the ready-made mixes on the supermarket shelf — this quick mix is much better and more economical by far. Moreover, the whole grains are slow to digest, meaning you'll feel satisfied for hours.

1½ cups	whole wheat pastry flour	375 mL
1½ cups	finely ground cornmeal (not corn grits or polenta)	375 mL
½ cup	quick-cooking rolled oats	125 mL
½ cup	ground flax seeds (flaxseed meal)	125 mL
½ cup	instant skim milk powder	125 mL
2 tbsp	unrefined cane sugar	30 mL
2 tbsp	baking powder	30 mL
1 tsp	fine sea salt	5 mL
¾ tsp	baking soda	3 mL

1. In a large bowl, whisk together flour, cornmeal, oats, flax seeds, milk powder, sugar, baking powder, salt and baking soda.
2. Transfer to a large airtight container and store in the refrigerator for up to 1 month.

To Prepare Multigrain Pancakes

Makes 6 pancakes

Tip

Choose a vegetable oil that is high in unsaturated fat.

1 cup	Multigrain Pancake and Waffle Mix	250 mL
1	large egg	1
½ cup	water	125 mL
1 tsp	vegetable oil	5 mL
	Nonstick cooking spray	

1. In a medium bowl, combine pancake mix, egg, water and oil until blended.
2. Heat a griddle or skillet over medium heat. Spray with cooking spray. For each pancake, pour about ¼ cup (60 mL) batter onto griddle. Cook until bubbles appear on top. Turn pancake over and cook for about 1 minute or until golden brown. Repeat with the remaining batter, spraying griddle and adjusting heat as necessary between batches.

Nutrients per Pancake	
Calories	87
Total fat	2 g
Saturated fat	0 g
Cholesterol	30 mg
Sodium	226 mg
Carbohydrate	13 g
Fiber	2 g
Protein	4 g
Calcium	58 mg
Iron	0.5 mg

Makes 4 small waffles

Tip

If you want to try making egg-free waffles, see "Make Flax Eggs for Eggless Baking" on page 31.

Nutrients per Waffle	
Calories	131
Total fat	4 g
Saturated fat	0 g
Cholesterol	45 mg
Sodium	338 mg
Carbohydrate	19 g
Fiber	3 g
Protein	5 g
Calcium	86 mg
Iron	0.8 mg

To Prepare Multigrain Waffles

- **Preheat waffle maker to medium-high**

1 cup	Multigrain Pancake and Waffle Mix	250 mL
1	large egg	1
½ cup	water	125 mL
1 tsp	vegetable oil	5 mL
	Nonstick cooking spray	

1. In a medium bowl, combine pancake mix, egg, water and oil until blended.
2. Spray preheated waffle maker with cooking spray. For each waffle, pour about ⅓ cup (75 mL) batter into waffle maker. Cook according to manufacturer's instructions until golden brown.

Oatmeal Buttermilk Pancakes

Makes 14 pancakes

✪ Great for Steps 3, 4 and 5

There's nothing like homemade pancakes, and this fluffy oats-and-buttermilk variation is a winner with kids and adults alike. The buttermilk in the batter is the key to the light-as-air texture, and is also a great source of calcium and protein.

Tip

If you don't have buttermilk, it's easy to make a substitute. Stir 2 tbsp (30 mL) lemon juice or white vinegar into 2 cups (500 mL) milk. Let stand for at least 15 minutes, to allow the milk to curdle, before using.

1 cup	quick-cooking rolled oats	250 mL
1¾ cups	1% buttermilk, divided	425 mL
¾ cup	whole wheat flour	175 mL
1½ tsp	baking powder	7 mL
¾ tsp	baking soda	3 mL
1 tsp	ground cinnamon	5 mL
½ tsp	fine sea salt	2 mL
1	large egg	1
2 tbsp	vegetable oil	30 mL
1 tbsp	brown rice syrup or liquid honey	15 mL
	Nonstick cooking spray	

1. In a small bowl, combine oats and 1 cup (250 mL) of the buttermilk. Let stand for 10 minutes.
2. In a large bowl, whisk together flour, baking powder, baking soda, cinnamon and salt. Add oat mixture, the remaining buttermilk, egg, oil and brown rice syrup, stirring until blended.
3. Heat a griddle or skillet over medium heat. Spray with cooking spray. For each pancake, pour about ¼ cup (60 mL) batter onto griddle. Cook until bubbles appear on top. Turn pancake over and cook for about 1 minute or until golden brown. Repeat with the remaining batter, spraying griddle and adjusting heat as necessary between batches.

Superfood Spotlight

Oats • Economical oats are rich in the soluble fiber beta-glucan and have been proven to help lower "bad" cholesterol, boost "good" cholesterol, maintain a healthy circulatory system and help prevent heart attacks. They also contain a range of antioxidants and plant chemicals that help keep the heart and arteries healthy, such as avenanthramides (a plant chemical with antibiotic properties), saponins and vitamin E, as well as polyphenols, plant compounds that can suppress tumor growth. They are relatively low on the glycemic index, which means they are suitable for people with insulin resistance, those with diabetes and all others interested in following a healthy eating plan.

Nutrients per Pancake	
Calories	91
Total fat	3 g
Saturated fat	1 g
Cholesterol	15 mg
Sodium	242 mg
Carbohydrate	13 g
Fiber	2 g
Protein	3 g
Calcium	56 mg
Iron	0.7 mg

Cottage Cheese Pancakes with Yogurt and Jam

Makes 12 pancakes

✪ Great for Steps 3 and 5

Much more interesting — and delicious — than plain cottage cheese with fruit, these blintz-like pancakes get an additional nutrition boost from whole wheat flour and tart yogurt, and an amazing zing from berry jam atop all.

Tip

Store whole wheat flour in the refrigerator to prevent rancidity.

Nutrients per Pancake	
Calories	108
Total fat	4 g
Saturated fat	1 g
Cholesterol	48 mg
Sodium	228 mg
Carbohydrate	12 g
Fiber	1 g
Protein	7 g
Calcium	66 mg
Iron	0.6 mg

1 cup	whole wheat flour	250 mL
½ tsp	baking soda	2 mL
¼ tsp	fine sea salt	1 mL
3	large eggs	3
2	large egg whites	2
1 cup	nonfat cottage cheese	250 mL
½ cup	skim milk	125 mL
2 tbsp	vegetable oil	30 mL
2 tbsp	liquid honey	30 mL
	Nonstick cooking spray	
1 cup	nonfat plain yogurt	250 mL
¼ cup	fruit-sweetened blackberry or raspberry jam	60 mL

1. In a large bowl, whisk together flour, baking soda and salt.
2. In a medium bowl, whisk together eggs, egg whites, cottage cheese, milk, oil and honey until blended.
3. Add the egg mixture to the flour mixture and stir until just blended.
4. Heat a griddle or skillet over medium heat. Spray with cooking spray. For each pancake, pour about ¼ cup (60 mL) batter onto griddle. Cook until bubbles appear on top. Turn pancake over and cook for about 1 minute or until golden brown. Repeat with the remaining batter, spraying griddle and adjusting heat as necessary between batches.
5. Serve pancakes topped with yogurt and jam.

▸ Health Note

Lower-fat and nonfat dairy products have just as much calcium as their full-fat counterparts.

Quinoa Blueberry Pancakes

Makes 16 pancakes

✪ Great for Steps 3, 4 and 5

Here, quinoa turns blueberry pancakes into something extra-special. You can skip the orange juice: blueberries, like all berries, contain a large amount of vitamin C.

Tip

Want to try making egg-free pancakes? See "Make Flax Eggless Baking" on page 31.

1½ cups	whole wheat pastry flour	375 mL
2 tsp	baking powder	10 mL
1 tsp	baking soda	5 mL
⅛ tsp	fine sea salt	0.5 mL
2	large eggs	2
1½ cups	1% buttermilk	375 mL
2 tbsp	vegetable oil	30 mL
1 tbsp	liquid honey or brown rice syrup	15 mL
1 cup	cooked quinoa (see page 438), cooled	250 mL
	Nonstick cooking spray	
1½ cups	blueberries	375 mL

1. In a large bowl, whisk together flour, baking powder, baking soda and salt.
2. In a medium bowl, whisk together eggs, buttermilk, oil and honey.
3. Add the egg mixture to the flour mixture and stir until just blended. Gently stir in quinoa.
4. Heat a griddle or skillet over medium heat. Spray with cooking spray. For each pancake, pour about ¼ cup (60 mL) batter onto griddle and top with 6 to 8 blueberries. Cook until bubbles appear on top. Turn pancake over and cook for about 1 minute or until golden brown. Repeat with the remaining batter, spraying griddle and adjusting heat as necessary between batches.

Superfood Spotlight

Blueberries • Deep purple blueberries are the richest of all fruits in antioxidant compounds. Multiple scientific studies indicate that the compound pterostilbene, found in the berries, helps lower cholesterol and may help prevent diabetes and some cancers. Their carotene, in the form of lutein and zeaxanthin, helps keep eyes healthy, and they are a good source of anthocyanins, which can help prevent heart disease and memory loss. They are high in vitamin C and fiber, and also appear to help urinary tract infections.

Nutrients per Pancake	
Calories	88
Total fat	3 g
Saturated fat	0 g
Cholesterol	24 mg
Sodium	172 mg
Carbohydrate	13 g
Fiber	1 g
Protein	3 g
Calcium	52 mg
Iron	0.5 mg

Make-Ahead Whole Wheat Crêpes

Makes 12 crêpes

✪ Great for Step 5

The French sure know how to do pancakes. This super-satisfying, high-fiber variation on classic crêpes can be made in advance, then reheated with just about any filling — sweet or savory — that suits your fancy.

Storage Tip

Refrigerate crêpes between sheets of waxed paper, tightly covered in plastic wrap, for up to 2 days, or freeze, enclosed in a sealable plastic bag, for up to 1 month.

Nutrients per Crêpe	
Calories	55
Total fat	2 g
Saturated fat	1 g
Cholesterol	32 mg
Sodium	78 mg
Carbohydrate	7 g
Fiber	1 g
Protein	3 g
Calcium	33 mg
Iron	0.3 mg

- **Blender**

2	large eggs	2
1 cup	2% milk	250 mL
1⁄2 cup	water	125 mL
1 1⁄2 tsp	vegetable oil	7 mL
1⁄4 tsp	fine sea salt	1 mL
1 cup	whole wheat pastry flour	250 mL
	Nonstick cooking spray	

1. In blender, combine eggs, milk, water, oil and salt. Add flour and blend until smooth. Transfer to a bowl, cover and refrigerate for 1 hour.
2. Heat a large skillet over medium-high heat. Remove from heat and lightly coat pan with cooking spray. Whisk the crêpe batter slightly. For each crêpe, pour about 1⁄4 cup (60 mL) batter into pan, quickly tilting in all directions to cover bottom of pan. Cook for about 45 seconds or until just golden at the edges. With a spatula, carefully lift edge of crêpe to test for doneness. The crêpe is ready to turn when it is golden brown on bottom and can be shaken loose from pan. Turn crêpe over and cook for about 15 to 30 seconds or until golden brown.
3. Transfer crêpe to an unfolded kitchen towel to cool completely. Repeat with the remaining batter, spraying skillet and adjusting heat as necessary between crêpes, stacking cooled crêpes between sheets of waxed paper to prevent sticking.

▶ 10 Crêpe Filling Ideas

1. Lemon juice and a drizzle of honey.
2. A thin spread of nut or seed butter and all-fruit jam.
3. Greek yogurt and fresh fruit or jam.
4. Nonfat ricotta cheese or cottage cheese and a drizzle of honey or agave nectar.
5. Grated bittersweet chocolate and (optional) toasted nuts.
6. Thinly sliced ham and shredded Gruyère (or Swiss) cheese.
7. Sautéed spinach and freshly grated Parmesan cheese.
8. Shredded sharp (old) Cheddar cheese and thinly sliced or grated tart-sweet apples.
9. Thinly sliced pears and a drizzle of pure maple syrup.
10. Scrambled eggs or egg whites, or scrambled tofu.

Walnut Flax Waffles

Makes 8 waffles

✪ Great for Steps 3, 4 and 5

You might try these waffles because of all you've heard about the benefits of flax seeds — from the omega-3s to the lignans to the fiber — but you'll fall in love with them (and make them many times over) for the flavor.

Tip

Look for packages of ready-ground flax seeds, which may be labelled "flaxseed meal," or use a spice or coffee grinder to grind whole flax seeds to a very fine meal.

Nutrients per Waffle	
Calories	114
Total fat	10 g
Saturated fat	1 g
Cholesterol	0 mg
Sodium	201 mg
Carbohydrate	5 g
Fiber	1 g
Protein	3 g
Calcium	43 mg
Iron	0.4 mg

- **Preheat waffle maker to medium-high**
- **Blender**

1½ cups	plain almond milk	375 mL
2 tbsp	vegetable oil	30 mL
1 tbsp	pure maple syrup	15 mL
2 tsp	vanilla extract	10 mL
1½ tsp	cider vinegar	7 mL
3 tbsp	ground flax seeds (flaxseed meal)	45 mL
1 cup	whole wheat flour	250 mL
1½ tsp	baking powder	7 mL
½ tsp	baking soda	2 mL
⅛ tsp	fine sea salt	0.5 mL
½ cup	chopped toasted walnuts	125 mL
	Nonstick cooking spray	

1. In blender, combine almond milk, oil, maple syrup, vanilla and vinegar. Let stand for 10 minutes. Add flax seeds and blend for 1 minute or until slightly frothy.
2. In a large bowl, whisk together flour, baking powder, baking soda and salt. Add almond milk mixture and stir until just blended. Gently stir in walnuts.
3. Spray preheated waffle maker with cooking spray. For each waffle, pour about ⅓ cup (75 mL) batter into waffle maker. Cook according to manufacturer's instructions until golden brown.

Pumpkin Maple Waffles

Makes 10 waffles

✪ Great for Steps 2, 3, 4 and 5

There's strong evidence that beta carotene — of which pumpkin has an abundance — helps protect people from a variety of health conditions, including several strains of cancer and heart disease. You can add this waffle recipe to the list of reasons for throwing a can or two of pumpkin into the shopping cart. Think of it as your new favorite pumpkin bread, made in minutes.

Nutrients per Waffle	
Calories	125
Total fat	5 g
Saturated fat	1 g
Cholesterol	20 mg
Sodium	183 mg
Carbohydrate	18 g
Fiber	3 g
Protein	4 g
Calcium	64 mg
Iron	0.9 mg

- **Preheat waffle maker to medium-high**

1¼ cups	whole wheat flour	300 mL
2 tbsp	ground flax seeds (flaxseed meal)	30 mL
2 tsp	pumpkin pie spice	10 mL
1½ tsp	baking powder	7 mL
¼ tsp	baking soda	1 mL
¼ tsp	fine sea salt	1 mL
1	large egg	1
1 cup	1% buttermilk	250 mL
1 cup	pumpkin purée (not pie filling)	250 mL
2 tbsp	vegetable oil	30 mL
2 tbsp	pure maple syrup or liquid honey	30 mL
	Nonstick cooking spray	

1. In a large bowl, whisk together flour, flax seeds, pumpkin pie spice, baking powder, baking soda and salt.
2. In a medium bowl, whisk together egg, buttermilk, pumpkin, oil and maple syrup.
3. Add the egg mixture to the flour mixture and stir until just blended.
4. Spray preheated waffle maker with cooking spray. For each waffle, pour about ⅓ cup (75 mL) batter into waffle maker. Cook according to manufacturer's instructions until golden brown.

▶ Health Note

Early American colonists apparently had a hunch that pumpkins were a superfood — they would chant the following poem in appreciation for the much-loved squash: *We have pumpkin at morning and pumpkin at noon. If it were not for pumpkin, we would soon be undoon.*

Microwave Poached Eggs

Makes 1 serving

✪ Great for Step 1

The microwave makes poached eggs easy enough to enjoy any day.

Nutrients per serving	
Calories	74
Total fat	4 g
Saturated fat	1 g
Cholesterol	180 mg
Sodium	70 mg
Carbohydrate	2 g
Fiber	0 g
Protein	6 g
Calcium	26 mg
Iron	0.9 mg

- **1-cup (250 mL) microwave-safe ramekin or mug**

1	large egg	1
1/3 cup	hot (not boiling) water	75 mL
1/2 tsp	cider vinegar or white vinegar	2 mL

1. Crack egg into ramekin. Using a pin or the tine of a fork, poke a small hole in the yolk to prevent it from bursting. Add hot water and vinegar.
2. Cover with a small microwave-safe plate and microwave on Medium-High (70%) power for 1 minute. Check egg for doneness. If necessary, microwave for 10 to 20 seconds longer for a soft-poached egg. (For a firmly set poached egg, microwave on High for 60 to 80 seconds.) Remove egg from water with a slotted spoon.

Baked Eggs in Marinara

Makes 2 servings

✪ Great for Steps 1 and 5

Nutrients per serving	
Calories	115
Total fat	5 g
Saturated fat	1 g
Cholesterol	180 mg
Sodium	312 mg
Carbohydrate	9 g
Fiber	1 g
Protein	7 g
Calcium	47 mg
Iron	2.4 mg

- **Preheat oven to 400°F (200°C)**
- **Two 1-cup (250 mL) ramekins or ovenproof cups**
- **Rimmed baking sheet**

	Nonstick cooking spray (preferably olive oil)	
1 cup	reduced-sodium marinara sauce	250 mL
2	large eggs	2
1/4 tsp	freshly ground black pepper	1 mL
Pinch	fine sea salt	Pinch

1. Spray ramekins with cooking spray and place on baking sheet.
2. Spoon 1/2 cup (125 mL) marinara sauce into each ramekin. Crack an egg into each ramekin and sprinkle with pepper and salt.
3. Bake in preheated oven for 11 to 14 minutes or until egg whites are just opaque (yolks should still be soft).

Favorite Frittata

Makes 1 serving

✪ Great for Steps 1, 2, 3 and 4

Bell peppers and spinach, plus the salty-tangy flavor of feta, give morning eggs more complexity and panache than the usual scramble, not to mention a nutrition bump — think vitamin C, iron and calcium.

Tip

It's fine to cut down on egg yolks in your frittata or morning scramble, but don't cut them out entirely. The yolk is high in protein, plus it contains vitamin B_{12}, which is necessary for muscle contraction and fat breakdown.

3	large egg whites	3
1	large egg	1
Pinch	fine sea salt	Pinch
	Nonstick cooking spray (preferably olive oil)	
1/4 cup	finely chopped red bell pepper	60 mL
1 1/2 cups	loosely packed baby spinach	375 mL
1 tsp	water	5 mL
2 tbsp	crumbled feta cheese	30 mL

1. In a small bowl, beat egg whites, egg and salt until blended.
2. Heat a small skillet over medium-high heat. Spray with cooking spray. Add red pepper and cook, stirring, for 4 to 5 minutes until softened. Add spinach and water; cook, stirring, until spinach is wilted.
3. Reduce heat to medium. Pour egg mixture over vegetables and sprinkle with feta. Cook, without stirring, for 2 to 4 minutes or until eggs are set. Remove from heat and invert onto a plate. Spray skillet with cooking spray and return frittata, browned side up, to skillet. Cook for 1 minute. Invert onto plate and serve.

▶ Health Note

Feta has a strong flavor, so you can use it sparingly and still feel you've gotten your cheese fix. It has only 4 g of saturated fat per 1-oz (30 g) serving, which is well below the American Heart Association's recommendation for keeping total saturated fat intake to below 7% of total daily calories (or 15 g for a 2,000 calorie diet). A 1-oz (30 g) serving of feta offers small amounts of a variety of vitamins and minerals, including 14% of the RDA for riboflavin, 8% for vitamin B_{12}, 9% for phosphorus, 6% for vitamin B_6, 6% for selenium and 5% for zinc.

Nutrients per serving	
Calories	126
Total fat	4 g
Saturated fat	3 g
Cholesterol	17 mg
Sodium	716 mg
Carbohydrate	8 g
Fiber	2 g
Protein	15 g
Calcium	128 mg
Iron	1.5 mg

Tofu Scramble

Makes 4 servings

✪ Great for Steps 1, 2, 3 and 4

Nutrients per serving	
Calories	151
Total fat	9 g
Saturated fat	0 g
Cholesterol	0 mg
Sodium	147 mg
Carbohydrate	7 g
Fiber	3 g
Protein	12 g
Calcium	244 mg
Iron	2.7 mg

2 tsp	extra virgin olive oil	10 mL
1	large red bell pepper, chopped	1
1 cup	chopped mushrooms	250 mL
1	package (16 oz/500 g) extra-firm or firm tofu, drained and coarsely mashed with a fork	1
¼ cup	chopped green onions	60 mL
1 tbsp	reduced-sodium tamari or soy sauce	15 mL
Pinch	freshly ground black pepper	Pinch

1. In a small skillet, heat oil over medium-high heat. Add red pepper and mushrooms; cook, stirring, for 4 to 5 minutes or until softened. Add tofu, green onions and tamari; cook, stirring, for 5 to 6 minutes or until flavors are blended and tofu is golden brown. Season with pepper.

Power Pitas with Eggs and Vegetables

Makes 2 servings

✪ Great for Steps 1, 2, 3, 4 and 5

Nutrients per serving	
Calories	251
Total fat	7 g
Saturated fat	1 g
Cholesterol	90 mg
Sodium	372 mg
Carbohydrate	29 g
Fiber	5 g
Protein	18 g
Calcium	54 mg
Iron	2.8 mg

3	large egg whites	3
1	large egg	1
½ cup	drained silken tofu, crumbled	125 mL
1 tsp	extra virgin olive oil	5 mL
½ cup	chopped fresh or thawed frozen broccoli florets	125 mL
½ cup	chopped red bell pepper	125 mL
2	6-inch (15 cm) whole wheat pitas, warmed	2
¼ cup	reduced-sodium salsa (optional)	60 mL

1. In a small bowl, beat egg whites and egg until blended. Stir in tofu.
2. In a small skillet, heat oil over medium-high heat. Add broccoli and red pepper; cook, stirring, for 4 to 5 minutes or until softened. Reduce heat to medium. Pour egg mixture over vegetables and cook, stirring gently with a spatula, for 2 to 4 minutes or until eggs are set.
3. Spoon egg mixture onto warm pitas and top with salsa, if desired. Fold in half and serve right away or wrap in foil to eat on the go.

Healthy Know-How

From Pyramid to Plate: Understanding the USDA MyPlate

In 2011, the USDA replaced the nearly 20-year-old food pyramid — a graphic launched in 1992 to help consumers make wise food choices from the main food groups — with a new solution: MyPlate. The new graphic provides a clear visual of what the proportions of each food group on your plate should look like for each meal.

The accompanying *Dietary Guidelines for Americans* — released earlier in the year — which tell consumers what they *should* be eating, can be summarized as follows:

1. **Stop overeating.** The guidelines state, "enjoy your food, but eat less," taking into consideration that many Americans are eating well beyond their daily caloric needs.
2. **Eat more fruits and vegetables.** In line with MyPlate, the message here is to "make half your plate fruits and vegetables." Fruits and vegetables are high in fiber and nutrients but low in calories, making it easier to maintain a healthy weight and lifestyle.
3. **Cut out the junk.** The guidelines say, "reduce the intake of calories from solid fats and added sugars" — in other words, the ingredients that comprise junk foods such as sugar-laden soft drinks, chips, crackers, cookies and cakes.
4. **Eat lean meats, lean protein and vegetable protein.** The guidelines recommend that we replace proteins "that are higher in solid fats with choices that are lower in solid fats and calories and/or are sources of oil and choose a variety of proteins." Research shows that making these changes can improve heart health, lower LDL cholesterol levels, extend life and lead to weight loss.
5. **Eat more whole grains.** Half of all Americans eat less than $\frac{1}{2}$ oz (15 g) of whole grains per day — the equivalent of half a slice of whole wheat bread. The guidelines recommend limiting "the consumption of foods that contain refined grains."
6. **Eat more fish.** The guidelines are fairly specific here: "Increase the amount and variety of seafood... [to] an intake of eight (or more) ounces per week." Fish is low in calories, high in protein and rich with omega-3 fatty acids.

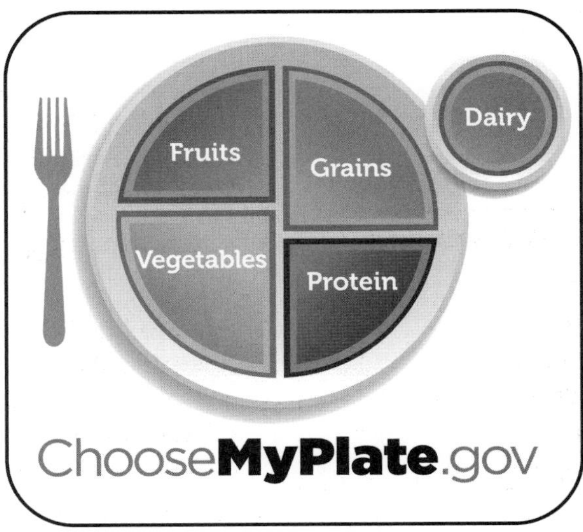

Avocado and Egg Breakfast Wraps

Makes 2 servings

✪ Great for Steps 1, 2, 3, 4 and 5

The best qualities of a healthy morning egg dish shine in this easy, colorful wrap, where earthy spinach and a sprinkle of goat cheese meld with creamy, potassium-rich avocado to form a warm, cohesive whole.

Tip

Hass avocados (sometimes called Haas avocados) are dark-skinned avocados with a nutty, buttery flesh and a longer shelf life than other varieties, making them the most popular avocado in North America. To determine whether a Hass avocado is ripe, look for purple-black skin and gently press the top — a ripe one will give slightly.

2	large eggs	2
2	large egg whites	2
Pinch	fine sea salt	Pinch
1/4 tsp	freshly ground black pepper	1 mL
1 tsp	extra virgin olive oil	5 mL
3 cups	loosely packed spinach, chopped	750 mL
2 tsp	water	10 mL
2 tbsp	crumbled soft goat cheese	30 mL
2	6-inch (15 cm) whole wheat tortillas, warmed	2
1/2	small ripe Hass avocado, sliced	1/2

1. In a small bowl, beat eggs, egg whites, salt and pepper until blended.
2. In a small skillet, heat oil over medium-high heat. Add spinach and water; cook, stirring, until leaves are wilted. Reduce heat to medium. Pour egg mixture over spinach and sprinkle with cheese. Cook, stirring gently with a spatula, for 2 to 4 minutes or until eggs are set.
3. Place half the egg mixture in the center of each warm tortilla and sprinkle each with 1 tbsp (15 mL) goat cheese. Top with avocado and fold or roll up.

▶ Health Note

A study conducted at the University of Connecticut found that men who ate three large eggs a day increased their HDL ("good") cholesterol by 20% without any effect on their LDL ("bad") cholesterol. Men who ate a cholesterol-free, fat-free substitute saw no changes.

Nutrients per serving	
Calories	391
Total fat	19 g
Saturated fat	5 g
Cholesterol	187 mg
Sodium	702 mg
Carbohydrate	37 g
Fiber	9 g
Protein	20 g
Calcium	139 mg
Iron	4.4 mg

Quinoa Kale Breakfast Casserole

Makes 8 servings

✪ Great for Steps 1, 2, 3, 4 and 5

Nutrients per serving	
Calories	144
Total fat	6 g
Saturated fat	2 g
Cholesterol	186 mg
Sodium	335 mg
Carbohydrate	11 g
Fiber	1 g
Protein	10 g
Calcium	102 mg
Iron	1.4 mg

- **Preheat oven to 350°F (180°C)**
- **9-inch (23 cm) square glass baking dish, sprayed with nonstick cooking spray (preferably olive oil)**

8	large eggs	8
1¼ cups	1% milk	300 mL
2 tsp	Asian chili-garlic sauce	10 mL
½ tsp	fine sea salt	2 mL
2½ cups	coarsely chopped kale (stems and center ribs removed)	625 mL
½ cup	quinoa, rinsed	125 mL
½ cup	finely shredded smoked Gouda cheese	125 mL

1. In a large bowl, whisk together eggs, milk, chili-garlic sauce and salt until blended. Stir in kale and quinoa. Pour into prepared baking dish and cover tightly with foil.
2. Bake in preheated oven for 40 to 45 minutes or until just set. Remove foil and sprinkle with Gouda. Bake, uncovered, for 10 to 15 minutes or until golden brown. Transfer baking dish to a wire rack and let cool for at least 10 minutes before serving.

Breakfast Polenta with Cherries and Almonds

Makes 2 servings

✪ Great for Steps 3, 4 and 5

Nutrients per serving	
Calories	350
Total fat	11 g
Saturated fat	1 g
Cholesterol	3 mg
Sodium	535 mg
Carbohydrate	54 g
Fiber	5 g
Protein	9 g
Calcium	109 mg
Iron	4.2 mg

2¼ cups	plain almond milk, skim milk or other plain non-dairy milk (soy, rice, hemp), divided	550 mL
½ cup	quick-cooking polenta	125 mL
2 tsp	liquid honey	10 mL
¼ cup	dried cherries, chopped	60 mL
2 tbsp	sliced toasted almonds	30 mL

1. In a medium saucepan, over medium heat, bring 2 cups (500 mL) of the almond milk to a boil. Gradually pour in polenta, whisking constantly. Reduce heat to low and cook, whisking, for about 2 minutes or until creamy.
2. Divide polenta between two bowls, drizzle with honey and the remaining almond milk, and sprinkle with cherries and almonds.

Overnight Oatmeal

Makes 2 servings

✪ Great for Steps 3, 4 and 5

Nutrients per serving	
Calories	232
Total fat	6 g
Saturated fat	1 g
Cholesterol	3 mg
Sodium	54 mg
Carbohydrate	35 g
Fiber	6 g
Protein	11 g
Calcium	176 mg
Iron	2.2 mg

1 cup	large-flake (old-fashioned) rolled oats	250 mL
2 tbsp	ground flax seeds (flaxseed meal)	30 mL
1 cup	skim milk or plain non-dairy milk (such as soy, almond, rice or hemp)	250 mL
1/2 tsp	vanilla extract	2 mL

Suggested Accompaniments

Warm or cold skim milk or plain non-dairy milk

Agave nectar, liquid honey or pure maple syrup

Fresh fruit, dried fruit, toasted nuts or seeds

1. In a medium bowl, combine oats, flax seeds, milk and vanilla. Cover and refrigerate overnight.
2. Serve cold or microwave on Medium (50%) for 1 to 2 minutes or until warm. Top with any of the suggested accompaniments, as desired.

Toasted Quinoa Porridge

Makes 2 servings

✪ Great for Steps 3, 4 and 5

This great power breakfast is an easy bowlful of deliciousness.

Nutrients per serving	
Calories	210
Total fat	3 g
Saturated fat	1 g
Cholesterol	3 mg
Sodium	209 mg
Carbohydrate	35 g
Fiber	3 g
Protein	11 g
Calcium	219 mg
Iron	2.2 mg

1/2 cup	quinoa, rinsed	125 mL
1 1/4 cups	skim milk or plain non-dairy milk (such as soy, almond, rice or hemp), divided	300 mL
1 cup	water	250 mL
1/2 tsp	ground cinnamon	2 mL
1/8 tsp	fine sea salt	0.5 mL

Suggested Accompaniments

Agave nectar, liquid honey, brown rice syrup or pure maple syrup

Fresh or dried fruit

1. In a small saucepan, over medium heat, toast quinoa, stirring, for 2 to 3 minutes or until golden and fragrant. Add 1 cup (250 mL) of the milk, water, cinnamon and salt; bring to a boil. Reduce heat to low, cover and simmer, stirring occasionally, for about 25 minutes or until liquid is absorbed.
2. Serve drizzled with the remaining milk and any of the suggested accompaniments, as desired.

Power Granola

Makes about 3½ cups (875 mL)

✪ Great for Steps 3, 4 and 5

Brown rice syrup, apple juice and dried berries sweeten oats, nuts and ground flax seeds in this easy stir-and-bake cereal. The high fiber content of the oats will keep you happily full until lunchtime.

- **Preheat oven to 300°F (150°C)**
- **Large rimmed baking sheet, lined with parchment paper**

2 cups	large-flake (old-fashioned) rolled oats	500 mL
½ cup	chopped pecans	125 mL
⅓ cup	ground flax seeds (flaxseed meal)	75 mL
2 tsp	ground cinnamon	10 mL
½ cup	unsweetened apple juice	125 mL
½ cup	brown rice syrup or liquid honey	125 mL
1 tbsp	vegetable oil	15 mL
2 tsp	vanilla extract	10 mL
½ cup	dried blueberries, cranberries or cherries	125 mL

1. In a large bowl, whisk together oats, pecans, flax seeds and cinnamon.
2. In a medium bowl, whisk together apple juice, brown rice syrup, oil and vanilla until well blended.
3. Add the apple juice mixture to the oats mixture and stir until well coated. Spread mixture in a single layer on prepared baking sheet.
4. Bake in preheated oven for 20 to 25 minutes or until oats are golden brown. Let cool completely on pan.
5. Transfer granola to an airtight container and stir in blueberries. Store at room temperature for up to 2 weeks.

▶ Health Note

According to Physicians' Health Study, a bowl of whole-grain cereal may help lower the risk of heart failure. Individuals who ate a bowl of high-fiber cereal two to four times per week were 22% less likely to develop heart failure than those who didn't.

Nutrients per ¼ cup (60 mL)

Calories	160
Total fat	6 g
Saturated fat	1 g
Cholesterol	1 mg
Sodium	22 mg
Carbohydrate	24 g
Fiber	3 g
Protein	3 g
Calcium	19 mg
Iron	0.9 mg

Quinoa Cranberry Granola

Makes about 4½ cups (1.125 L)

✪ Great for Steps 3, 4 and 5

The gentle sweetness of this quinoa and oats granola is accentuated by crunchy almonds and the grassy notes of olive oil. The dried cranberries are more than a tart-sweet complement: they are powerful antioxidants, able to help cut "bad" cholesterol and fight infection. Just ½ cup (125 mL) of dried cranberries provides about 13 mg of vitamin C and 4 g of fiber. Pass the bowl!

- **Preheat oven to 300°F (150°C)**
- **Large rimmed baking sheet, lined with parchment paper**

2 cups	large-flake (old-fashioned) rolled oats	500 mL
1 cup	quinoa, rinsed	250 mL
¾ cup	almonds, coarsely chopped	175 mL
¾ cup	unsweetened flaked coconut	175 mL
2 tsp	ground cinnamon	10 mL
½ cup	brown rice syrup or pure maple syrup	125 mL
½ cup	vegetable oil or warmed coconut oil	125 mL
⅔ cup	dried cranberries	150 mL

1. In a large bowl, whisk together oats, quinoa, almonds, coconut and cinnamon.
2. In a medium bowl, whisk together brown rice syrup and oil until well blended.
3. Add the syrup mixture to the oats mixture and stir until well coated. Spread mixture in a single layer on prepared baking sheet.
4. Bake in preheated oven for 20 to 25 minutes or until oats are golden brown. Let cool completely on pan.
5. Transfer granola to an airtight container and stir in cranberries. Store at room temperature for up to 2 weeks.

▶ Health Note

Quinoa is a quintessential superfood: 1 cup (250 mL) of cooked quinoa has 9 g of protein, plus it contains all 8 of the essential amino acids, making it a complete protein.

Nutrients per ¼ cup (60 mL)

Calories	223
Total fat	12 g
Saturated fat	3 g
Cholesterol	0 mg
Sodium	18 mg
Carbohydrate	26 g
Fiber	3 g
Protein	4 g
Calcium	27 mg
Iron	1.3 mg

Toasted Oat Muesli with Dried Fruit and Pecans

Makes about 6 cups (1.5 L)

✪ Great for Steps 3, 4 and 5

Weekday mornings always feel somewhat rushed, especially when it comes to breakfast, so whip up a batch of this muesli over the weekend for a healthy go-to breakfast (and snack) for the rest of the week. Traditional muesli sticks with oats, but I add bran cereal and ground flax seeds for a tasty and über-healthy twist — think extra soluble fiber and omega-3 fatty acids.

- **Preheat oven to 350°F (180°C)**
- **Large rimmed baking sheet, lined with parchment paper**

3 cups	large-flake (old-fashioned) rolled oats	750 mL
1/2 cup	chopped pecans	125 mL
1 cup	bran cereal (such as All-Bran)	250 mL
1 1/2 cups	chopped mixed dried fruit	375 mL
1/2 cup	ground flax seeds (flaxseed meal)	125 mL

Suggested Accompaniments

Skim milk, non-dairy milk or nonfat plain yogurt (regular or Greek)

Liquid honey or agave nectar

1. Spread oats and pecans in a single layer on prepared baking sheet. Bake in preheated oven for 7 to 8 minutes or until golden and fragrant. Let cool completely on pan.
2. In an airtight container, combine oat mixture, bran cereal, dried fruit and flax seeds. Store in the refrigerator for up to 1 month.
3. Serve with any of the suggested accompaniments, as desired.

Nutrients per 1/4 cup (60 mL)

Calories	97
Total fat	4 g
Saturated fat	0 g
Cholesterol	0 mg
Sodium	9 mg
Carbohydrate	16 g
Fiber	3 g
Protein	3 g
Calcium	15 mg
Iron	1.2 mg

Pumpkin Yogurt with Quinoa Crunch

Makes 1 serving

✪ Great for Steps 2, 3, 4 and 5

Nutrients per serving	
Calories	338
Total fat	3 g
Saturated fat	0 g
Cholesterol	5 mg
Sodium	175 mg
Carbohydrate	66 g
Fiber	4 g
Protein	14 g
Calcium	328 mg
Iron	1.6 mg

1 cup	nonfat plain yogurt	250 mL
1/4 cup	pumpkin purée (not pie filling)	60 mL
1 1/2 tbsp	liquid honey or agave nectar	22 mL
1 tsp	vanilla extract	5 mL
1/4 tsp	ground cinnamon	1 mL
2 tbsp	Quinoa Crunch (see recipe, below)	30 mL

1. In a small bowl, whisk together yogurt, pumpkin, honey, vanilla and cinnamon until blended and smooth. Sprinkle with Quinoa Crunch.

▶ Health Note

According to a 25-year study of the health and eating habits of more than 10,000 doctors, those who ate whole grains for breakfast had a significantly lower chance of developing heart failure than those who did not eat such cereals.

Quinoa Crunch

Makes about 1 cup (250 mL)

Quinoa is far more than a side dish: this supergrain can be transformed into a crispy-sweet topping that's heavenly sprinkled on yogurt, cereal or muffins or simply eaten out of hand.

Nutrients per 2 tbsp (30 mL)	
Calories	102
Total fat	3 g
Saturated fat	0 g
Cholesterol	0 mg
Sodium	37 mg
Carbohydrate	16 g
Fiber	2 g
Protein	3 g
Calcium	10 mg
Iron	1.0 mg

- **Preheat oven to 375°F (190°C)**
- **Rimmed baking sheet, lined with parchment paper**

1 cup	quinoa, rinsed	250 mL
1 tbsp	vegetable oil	15 mL
1 tbsp	liquid honey	15 mL
1/8 tsp	fine sea salt	0.5 mL

1. In a small bowl, combine quinoa, oil and honey. Spread in a single layer on prepared baking sheet.
2. Bake in preheated oven for 11 to 13 minutes, stirring occasionally, until quinoa is crisp. Transfer to a large plate and let cool completely.
3. Transfer quinoa crunch to an airtight container and store at room temperature for up to 1 month.

Greek Yogurt, Grain and Blackberry Parfaits

Makes 2 servings

✪ Great for Steps 1, 2, 3, 4 and 5

Nutrients per serving	
Calories	209
Total fat	1 g
Saturated fat	0 g
Cholesterol	0 mg
Sodium	188 mg
Carbohydrate	38 g
Fiber	5 g
Protein	13 g
Calcium	104 mg
Iron	1.7 mg

- 2 parfait glasses

¾ cup	cooked whole grains (such as quinoa, barley or brown rice), chilled	175 mL
2 tbsp	liquid honey, divided	30 mL
⅛ tsp	fine sea salt	0.5 mL
1 cup	nonfat plain Greek yogurt	250 mL
1 cup	blackberries, lightly crushed with a fork	250 mL

1. In a small bowl, combine grains, 1 tbsp (15 mL) of the honey and salt.
2. Spoon ¼ cup (60 mL) yogurt into each parfait glass. Top each with 3 tbsp (45 mL) grain mixture and ¼ cup (60 mL) blackberries. Repeat layers. Drizzle with the remaining honey.

Chunky Applesauce

Makes 6 servings

✪ Great for Steps 1, 2 and 4

Storage Tip

Refrigerate cooled applesauce in an airtight container for up to 3 days.

Nutrients per serving	
Calories	131
Total fat	0 g
Saturated fat	0 g
Cholesterol	0 mg
Sodium	1 mg
Carbohydrate	35 g
Fiber	3 g
Protein	1 g
Calcium	16 mg
Iron	0.3 mg

3 lbs	tart-sweet apples (such as Gala or Braeburn), peeled, cored and quartered	1.5 kg
½ cup	unsweetened apple juice	125 mL
1 tbsp	liquid honey or pure maple syrup (optional)	15 mL
1 tbsp	freshly squeezed lemon juice	15 mL
1	2-inch (5 cm) cinnamon stick	1

Suggested Accompaniments

Nonfat plain Greek yogurt

Quinoa Crunch (page 62), Power Granola (page 59) or Toasted Oat Muesli (page 61)

1. In a large saucepan, over medium heat, combine apples, apple juice, honey (if using), lemon juice and cinnamon stick. Bring to a boil, then reduce heat to low and simmer, stirring occasionally, for 30 to 35 minutes or until apples break down.
2. Remove from heat and discard cinnamon stick. Mash apples slightly with a potato masher or fork (or, for a smooth texture, run applesauce through a food mill or process in a food processor). Serve warm or at room temperature.

Spinach and Ricotta Bruschetta

Makes 2 servings

✪ Great for Steps 1, 2, 3, 4 and 5

Nutrients per serving	
Calories	168
Total fat	4 g
Saturated fat	0 g
Cholesterol	4 mg
Sodium	553 mg
Carbohydrate	30 g
Fiber	9 g
Protein	12 g
Calcium	225 mg
Iron	2.6 mg

1 tsp	extra virgin olive oil	5 mL
1	clove garlic, minced	1
4 cups	packed baby spinach	1 L
3 tbsp	water	45 mL
1 tsp	finely grated lemon zest	5 mL
2 tbsp	freshly squeezed lemon juice	30 mL
¼ tsp	fine sea salt	1 mL
	Freshly ground black pepper	
2	slices rustic whole-grain bread	2
6 tbsp	nonfat ricotta cheese	90 mL

1. In a medium skillet, heat oil over medium-high heat. Add garlic and cook, stirring, for 1 minute or until golden. Add spinach and water; cook, stirring occasionally, for about 8 minutes or until spinach is wilted and tender. Stir in lemon juice, salt, and pepper to taste.
2. Meanwhile, toast bread. Spread 3 tbsp (45 mL) ricotta over each slice. Top with spinach mixture and sprinkle with lemon zest.

Scandinavian Breakfast Toasts with Smoked Salmon and Avocado

Makes 2 servings

✪ Great for Steps 1, 2, 3, 4 and 5

Nutrients per serving	
Calories	326
Total fat	18 g
Saturated fat	3 g
Cholesterol	13 mg
Sodium	647 mg
Carbohydrate	28 g
Fiber	9 g
Protein	17 g
Calcium	77 mg
Iron	2.4 mg

1	small Hass avocado, quartered, peeled and pitted	1
2 tsp	freshly squeezed lemon juice	10 mL
2	slices dark whole-grain bread	2
4 oz	thinly sliced smoked salmon	125 g

1. On a cutting board, coarsely mash avocado. Sprinkle with lemon juice.
2. Toast bread. Spread avocado over toast and top with smoked salmon.

Whole-Grain Blueberry Maple Muffins

Makes 12 muffins

✪ Great for Steps 1, 2, 3, 4 and 5

By now you've undoubtedly heard that whole grains of all varieties are a healthy choice. But this modern spin on the blueberry muffin proves that they are a delicious choice too. The health benefits of whole grains come from the nutrients and fiber found in the entire grain kernel. Those same elements add depth of flavor and nuttiness to quick breads such as these muffins.

Storage Tip

Store cooled muffins in an airtight container in the refrigerator for up to 3 days.

Nutrients per Muffin	
Calories	233
Total fat	7 g
Saturated fat	1 g
Cholesterol	32 mg
Sodium	355 mg
Carbohydrate	38 g
Fiber	3 g
Protein	5 g
Calcium	63 mg
Iron	1.3 mg

- **Preheat oven to 400°F (200°C)**
- **Food processor**
- **12-cup muffin pan, greased**

1¾ cups	large-flake (old-fashioned) rolled oats	425 mL
1 cup	whole wheat flour	250 mL
2 tsp	ground cinnamon	10 mL
1 tsp	baking powder	5 mL
1 tsp	baking soda	5 mL
¾ tsp	fine sea salt	3 mL
2	large eggs	2
¾ cup	pure maple syrup, liquid honey or brown rice syrup	175 mL
¼ cup	vegetable oil	60 mL
2 tsp	vanilla extract	10 mL
1½ cups	1% buttermilk	375 mL
1½ cups	blueberries	375 mL

1. In food processor, pulse oats five or six times, until oats resemble coarse meal.
2. Transfer oats to a large bowl and whisk in flour, cinnamon, baking powder, baking soda and salt.
3. In a medium bowl, whisk together eggs, maple syrup, oil and vanilla until well blended. Whisk in buttermilk until blended.
4. Add the egg mixture to the flour mixture and stir until just blended. Gently fold in blueberries.
5. Divide batter equally among prepared muffin cups.
6. Bake in preheated oven for 18 to 23 minutes or until tops are golden and a toothpick inserted in the center comes out clean. Let cool in pan on a wire rack for 5 minutes, then transfer to the rack to cool.

Yogurt Bran Muffins

Makes 12 muffins

✪ Great for Steps 3 and 5

These muffins are the breakfast of champions: you get a wallop of fiber from the whole wheat flour and bran, omega-3 fatty acids from the flax seeds and a healthy dose of bone-building calcium from the yogurt.

Storage Tip

Store cooled muffins in an airtight container in the refrigerator for up to 3 days.

Nutrients per Muffin

Calories	193
Total fat	7 g
Saturated fat	1 g
Cholesterol	31 mg
Sodium	519 mg
Carbohydrate	30 g
Fiber	3 g
Protein	6 g
Calcium	65 mg
Iron	1.2 mg

- **Preheat oven to 400°F (200°C)**
- **12-cup muffin pan, greased**

1½ cups	whole wheat flour	375 mL
1 cup	natural bran	250 mL
3 tbsp	ground flax seeds (flaxseed meal)	45 mL
1¼ tsp	baking soda	6 mL
½ tsp	fine sea salt	2 mL
2	large eggs	2
½ cup	liquid honey	125 mL
¼ cup	vegetable oil	60 mL
1 tsp	vanilla extract	5 mL
1¼ cups	nonfat plain yogurt	300 mL
½ cup	raisins (optional)	125 mL

1. In a large bowl, whisk together flour, bran, flax seeds, baking soda and salt.
2. In a medium bowl, whisk together eggs, honey, oil and vanilla until well blended. Whisk in yogurt until blended.
3. Add the egg mixture to the flour mixture and stir until just blended. Gently fold in raisins (if using).
4. Divide batter equally among prepared muffin cups.
5. Bake in preheated oven for 18 to 23 minutes or until tops are light golden brown and a toothpick inserted in the center comes out clean. Let cool in pan on a wire rack for 3 minutes, then transfer to the rack to cool.

Banana and Toasted Millet Muffins

Makes 12 muffins

✪ Great for Steps 1, 2, 3, 4 and 5

Millet may be a common ingredient in bird seed blends, but when it comes to great health, flavor and versatility, this mighty seed is by no means for the birds. In addition to being a good source of manganese, magnesium and tryptophan, millet is rich in lignans, a group of phytonutrients that studies indicate is widely beneficial in promoting good health and preventing disease.

Storage Tip

Store cooled muffins in an airtight container in the refrigerator for up to 3 days.

- **12-cup muffin pan, greased**

1/2 cup	millet	125 mL
2 cups	whole wheat flour	500 mL
1/4 cup	ground flax seeds (flaxseed meal)	60 mL
1 tbsp	ground cinnamon	15 mL
1 tsp	baking soda	5 mL
1 tsp	fine sea salt	5 mL
2	large eggs	2
1 1/2 cups	mashed ripe bananas	375 mL
2/3 cup	1% plain yogurt	150 mL
1/2 cup	liquid honey or agave nectar	125 mL
3 tbsp	vegetable oil	45 mL
2 tsp	vanilla extract	10 mL

1. Heat a large skillet over medium-high heat. Toast millet, stirring occasionally, for 3 to 4 minutes or until golden brown and just beginning to pop. Transfer to a large bowl and let cool.
2. Preheat oven to 350°F (180°C).
3. Whisk flour, flax seeds, cinnamon, baking soda and salt into cooled millet.
4. In a medium bowl, whisk together eggs, bananas, yogurt, honey, oil and vanilla until well blended.
5. Add the egg mixture to the flour mixture and stir until just blended.
6. Divide batter equally among prepared muffin cups.
7. Bake in preheated oven for 23 to 28 minutes or until tops are golden and a toothpick inserted in the center comes out clean. Let cool in pan on a wire rack for 3 minutes, then transfer to the rack to cool.

Nutrients per Muffin	
Calories	237
Total fat	6 g
Saturated fat	1 g
Cholesterol	31 mg
Sodium	361 mg
Carbohydrate	41 g
Fiber	4 g
Protein	6 g
Calcium	42 mg
Iron	1.4 mg

Cheese, Almond and Mushroom Muffins

Makes 9 muffins

✪ Great for Steps 1, 2 and 4

Savory breakfast lovers, rejoice! These cheese- and almond-packed muffins — which taste like a cross between a quick bread and a quiche — will mollify any cravings for a fast-food muffin sandwich. The secret is more than the satisfying flavor: the cottage cheese and almond flour pack a significant amount of good-for-you protein that keeps you feeling full for hours. Additionally, research indicates that the fiber in almonds may prevent the body from absorbing some fat.

Storage Tip

Store cooled muffins in an airtight container in the refrigerator for up to 3 days.

Nutrients per Muffin	
Calories	158
Total fat	11 g
Saturated fat	3 g
Cholesterol	92 mg
Sodium	308 mg
Carbohydrate	6 g
Fiber	2 g
Protein	10 g
Calcium	129 mg
Iron	1.2 mg

- **12-cup muffin pan, 9 cups greased**

1 tsp	olive oil	5 mL
8 oz	cremini or button mushrooms, coarsely chopped	250 g
1 cup	almond flour	250 mL
1 tsp	baking powder	5 mL
1/4 tsp	fine sea salt	1 mL
1/4 tsp	freshly ground black pepper	1 mL
4	large eggs	4
2/3 cup	small-curd cottage cheese	150 mL
2 tbsp	freshly grated Parmesan cheese	30 mL
1/2 cup	crumbled feta cheese	125 mL
1/4 cup	chopped green onions	60 mL

1. In a large skillet, heat oil over medium-high heat. Add mushrooms and cook, stirring, for 4 to 5 minutes or until starting to brown and liquid has evaporated. Remove from heat and let cool.
2. Preheat oven to 400°F (200°C).
3. In a large bowl, whisk together flour, baking powder, salt and pepper. Stir in eggs, cottage cheese and Parmesan until just blended. Fold in sautéed mushrooms, feta and green onions.
4. Divide batter equally among prepared muffin cups.
5. Bake for 23 to 25 minutes or until tops are golden and a toothpick inserted in the center comes out clean. Let cool in pan on a wire rack for 5 minutes, then transfer to the rack to cool slightly. Serve warm or let cool to room temperature.

Oats and Dried Fruit Breakfast Bars

Makes 16 bars

✪ Great for Steps 2, 3, 4 and 5

Oats are a perfect food for the beginning of the day: high in protein, they also contain essential fats and are rich in minerals including zinc, calcium, magnesium and iron. Vitamin C assists in the absorption of iron, so one of these bars and some orange juice in a travel mug is an ideal meal on the go.

Storage Tip

Wrap bars individually and refrigerate for up to 2 weeks.

- **Preheat oven to 350°F (180°C)**
- **Large rimmed baking sheet, lined with parchment paper**
- **Food processor**
- **9-inch (23 cm) square metal baking pan, lined with foil (see tip, page 518)**

2½ cups	large-flake (old-fashioned) rolled oats	625 mL
½ cup	chopped pecans or walnuts	125 mL
½ cup	brown rice syrup or liquid honey	125 mL
¾ cup	pitted dates, chopped	175 mL
¼ cup	ground flax seeds (flaxseed meal)	60 mL
1 tsp	ground cinnamon	5 mL
⅛ tsp	fine sea salt	0.5 mL
½ cup	dried cranberries	125 mL
½ cup	chopped dried apricots	125 mL

1. Spread oats and pecans on prepared baking sheet. Bake in preheated oven for 7 to 8 minutes or until fragrant and light golden.
2. In a small saucepan, over medium-low heat, warm brown rice syrup.
3. In food processor, pulse oat mixture, warmed syrup, dates, flax seeds, cinnamon and salt until mixture begins to hold together as a dough.
4. Scrape mixture into a medium bowl. Break up any clumps of dates and, if needed, chop any large date chunks. Stir in cranberries and apricots.
5. Transfer mixture to prepared pan and press flat with a square of waxed paper. Freeze for 30 minutes. Using foil liner, lift mixture from pan and invert onto a cutting board; peel off foil and cut into 16 bars.

Nutrients per Bar	
Calories	161
Total fat	4 g
Saturated fat	0 g
Cholesterol	0 mg
Sodium	35 mg
Carbohydrate	30 g
Fiber	3 g
Protein	3 g
Calcium	13 mg
Iron	0.9 mg

Healthy Know-How

The Importance of Drinking Water

Water makes up roughly 60% of the human body, and every system in the body depends on it. For example, water flushes toxins out of vital organs, carries nutrients to cells and provides a moist environment for ear, nose and throat tissues.

Lack of water can lead to dehydration, a condition that occurs when you don't have enough water in your body to carry out normal functions. Even mild dehydration can drain your energy and make you tired. Thirst is also commonly mistaken for hunger, which can lead to overeating.

How Much Water Do You Need?

Every day you lose water through your breath, perspiration, urine and bowel movements. For your body to function properly, you must replenish its water supply by consuming beverages and foods that contain water.

So how much water does an average, healthy adult living in a temperate climate need? The average urine output for adults is about 6 cups (1.5 L) a day. You lose an additional 4 cups (1 L) or so through breathing, sweating and bowel movements. Food usually accounts for 20% of your total fluid intake, so if you consume 8 cups (2 L) of water or other beverages a day along with your normal diet, you will typically replace your lost fluids.

Sunflower Apricot Go-Bars

Makes 16 bars

✪ Great for Steps 2, 3, 4 and 5

Nutrients per Bar	
Calories	308
Total fat	15 g
Saturated fat	2 g
Cholesterol	0 mg
Sodium	132 mg
Carbohydrate	37 g
Fiber	5 g
Protein	8 g
Calcium	27 mg
Iron	2.3 mg

- **9-inch (23 cm) square metal baking pan, lined with foil (see tip, page 518)**

4 cups	large-flake (old-fashioned) rolled oats	1 L
1 cup	roasted lightly salted sunflower seeds	250 mL
3/4 cup	pitted dates, chopped	175 mL
3/4 cup	chopped dried apricots	175 mL
1/8 tsp	fine sea salt	0.5 mL
1 cup	sunflower seed butter	250 mL
1/2 cup	brown rice syrup or liquid honey	125 mL
1 tbsp	finely grated orange zest	15 mL

1. In a large bowl, combine oats, sunflower seeds, dates, apricots and salt. Stir in sunflower seed butter, brown rice syrup and orange zest.
2. Press mixture into prepared pan and refrigerate for at least 30 minutes, until firm. Using foil liner, lift mixture from pan and invert onto a cutting board; peel off foil and cut into 16 bars.

Quinoa Blueberry Breakfast Cookies

Makes 3 dozen large cookies

✪ Great for Steps 2, 4 and 5

Loaded with all of the essential amino acids as well as vitamins and minerals, quinoa is a perfect way to start the day. It also makes a delicious addition to these tender breakfast cookies. And dried blueberries are a smart way to enjoy this superfruit — in baked goods or out of hand — year-round.

Storage Tip

Store cooled cookies in an airtight container in the refrigerator for up to 5 days.

Nutrients per Cookie	
Calories	69
Total fat	2 g
Saturated fat	0 g
Cholesterol	5 mg
Sodium	114 mg
Carbohydrate	11 g
Fiber	1 g
Protein	1 g
Calcium	15 mg
Iron	0.2 mg

- **Preheat oven to 350°F (180°C)**
- **Baking sheets, lined with parchment paper**

1/2 cup	quinoa, rinsed	125 mL
3/4 cup	water	175 mL
2 cups	whole wheat pastry flour	500 mL
1 1/2 tsp	baking powder	7 mL
1 tsp	fine sea salt	5 mL
1/2 tsp	baking soda	2 mL
1	large egg, lightly beaten	1
1/2 cup	liquid honey	125 mL
1/3 cup	nonfat plain yogurt	75 mL
1/4 cup	vegetable oil	60 mL
1 tsp	vanilla extract	5 mL
2/3 cup	dried blueberries	150 mL

1. In a small saucepan, combine quinoa and water. Bring to a boil over medium-high heat. Reduce heat to low, cover and simmer for 15 minutes or until water is absorbed (quinoa will still be slightly chewy). Fluff with a fork and let cool.
2. In a large bowl, whisk together flour, baking powder, salt and baking soda. Stir in egg, honey, yogurt, oil and vanilla until just blended. Gently fold in quinoa and blueberries.
3. Drop batter by 2 tbsp (30 mL) onto prepared baking sheets, spacing cookies 2 inches (5 cm) apart.
4. Bake one sheet at a time in preheated oven for 12 to 15 minutes or until just set at the center. Let cool in pan on a wire rack for 5 minutes, then transfer to the rack to cool.

Multigrain Cranberry Breakfast Cookies

Makes 2½ dozen cookies

✪ Great for Steps 2, 3, 4 and 5

There's nothing quite like beginning the day with a cookie, especially when the cookie in question is equally delicious and nutritious. It's also endlessly variable: change the type of nut or seed butter, dried fruit or sweetener, or swap pumpkin purée, frozen squash purée or baby food carrots for the banana. While the possibilities are endless, I love this maple-sweetened variation with barley flakes and berries.

Storage Tip

Store cooled cookies in an airtight container in the refrigerator for up to 5 days.

Nutrients per Cookie	
Calories	78
Total fat	3 g
Saturated fat	0 g
Cholesterol	1 mg
Sodium	49 mg
Carbohydrate	12 g
Fiber	2 g
Protein	2 g
Calcium	15 mg
Iron	0.3 mg

- **Preheat oven to 350°F (180°C)**
- **Baking sheets, lined with parchment paper**

1 cup	rolled barley flakes or large-flake (old-fashioned) rolled oats	250 mL
½ cup	whole wheat flour	125 mL
¼ cup	instant skim milk powder	60 mL
2 tsp	ground cinnamon	10 mL
¼ tsp	baking soda	1 mL
¼ tsp	fine sea salt	1 mL
½ cup	mashed ripe banana	125 mL
½ cup	unsweetened natural peanut butter or other nut butter	125 mL
½ cup	pure maple syrup	125 mL
1 tsp	vanilla extract	5 mL
¾ cup	dried cranberries, blueberries or cherries	175 mL

1. In a large bowl, whisk together barley, flour, milk powder, cinnamon, baking soda and salt. Stir in banana, peanut butter, maple syrup and vanilla until just blended. Gently fold in cranberries.
2. Drop batter by 2 tbsp (30 mL) onto prepared baking sheets, spacing cookies 2 inches (5 cm) apart. With a metal spatula, flatten each mound to ½-inch (1 cm) thickness.
3. Bake one sheet at a time in preheated oven for 12 to 15 minutes or until just set at the center. Let cool in pan on a wire rack for 5 minutes, then transfer to the rack to cool.

Carrot Oat Breakfast Cookies

Makes 3 dozen cookies

✪ Great for Steps 1, 2, 3, 4 and 5

Cookies for breakfast? Absolutely, when they're made with a host of energizing ingredients that can sustain you through the busiest of mornings. I strongly suggest eating two, not one, of these cookies!

Storage Tip

Store cooled cookies in an airtight container in the refrigerator for up to 5 days.

Nutrients per Cookie

Calories	86
Total fat	4 g
Saturated fat	0 g
Cholesterol	10 mg
Sodium	68 mg
Carbohydrate	12 g
Fiber	1 g
Protein	2 g
Calcium	10 mg
Iron	0.5 mg

- **Preheat oven to 375°F (190°C)**
- **Baking sheets, lined with parchment paper**

1½ cups	large-flake (old-fashioned) rolled oats	375 mL
1 cup	whole wheat flour	250 mL
¼ cup	ground flax seeds (flaxseed meal)	60 mL
2 tsp	ground cinnamon	10 mL
1 tsp	baking soda	5 mL
¼ tsp	fine sea salt	1 mL
2	large eggs, lightly beaten	2
½ cup	unsweetened applesauce	125 mL
½ cup	brown rice syrup or liquid honey	125 mL
¼ cup	vegetable oil	60 mL
2 cups	shredded carrots	500 mL
⅔ cup	raisins	150 mL
½ cup	chopped toasted walnuts	125 mL

1. In a large bowl, whisk together oats, flour, flax seeds, cinnamon, baking soda and salt. Stir in eggs, applesauce, brown rice syrup and oil until just blended. Gently fold in carrots, raisins and walnuts.
2. Drop batter by 2 tbsp (30 mL) onto prepared baking sheets, spacing cookies 2 inches (5 cm) apart.
3. Bake one sheet at a time in preheated oven for 12 to 15 minutes or until just set at the center. Let cool in pan on a wire rack for 5 minutes, then transfer to the rack to cool.

▸ Health Note

Falcarinol, a compound found in carrots, may help lower the risk of breast cancer, lung cancer and colon cancer.

Berry Protein Shake

Makes 2 servings

✪ Great for Steps 1, 2, 3 and 4

Nutrients per serving	
Calories	313
Total fat	13 g
Saturated fat	1 g
Cholesterol	0 mg
Sodium	19 mg
Carbohydrate	35 g
Fiber	5 g
Protein	23 g
Calcium	118 mg
Iron	3.0 mg

- **Blender**

1 cup	frozen berries (such as strawberries, blueberries, blackberries and/or raspberries)	250 mL
1 cup	sliced frozen ripe banana	250 mL
1 cup	drained soft silken tofu	250 mL
¾ cup	cold water	175 mL
1 tbsp	ground flax seeds (flaxseed meal)	15 mL
1 tbsp	agave nectar or liquid honey (optional)	15 mL

1. In blender, purée berries, banana, tofu, cold water, flax seeds and agave nectar (if using) until smooth. Pour into two glasses and serve immediately.

Banana Buttermilk Smoothie

Makes 2 servings

✪ Great for Steps 1, 2, 3, 4 and 5

For a thick, milkshake-like smoothie, look no further. The handful of oats increases the creaminess.

Nutrients per serving	
Calories	165
Total fat	2 g
Saturated fat	1 g
Cholesterol	4 mg
Sodium	69 mg
Carbohydrate	36 g
Fiber	4 g
Protein	5 g
Calcium	70 mg
Iron	0.8 mg

- **Blender**

¼ cup	large-flake (old-fashioned) rolled oats	60 mL
⅛ tsp	ground cinnamon	0.5 mL
1 cup	sliced frozen ripe banana	250 mL
½ cup	1% buttermilk	125 mL
½ cup	cold water	125 mL

1. In blender, purée oats, cinnamon, banana, buttermilk and cold water until smooth. Pour into two glasses and serve immediately.

Variation

For a non-dairy alternative, substitute ½ cup (125 mL) plain cultured soy yogurt for the buttermilk.

Super C Smoothie

Makes 2 servings

✪ Great for Steps 1, 2 and 4

This refreshing, tart-sweet smoothie is a drinkable wake-up call.

Nutrients per serving	
Calories	117
Total fat	1 g
Saturated fat	0 g
Cholesterol	0 mg
Sodium	1 mg
Carbohydrate	34 g
Fiber	5 g
Protein	2 g
Calcium	54 mg
Iron	0.4 mg

- **Blender**

2	oranges, peel and pith removed, flesh cut into chunks	2
1 cup	frozen raspberries	250 mL
1 cup	frozen blueberries	250 mL
½ cup	cold water	125 mL

1. In blender, purée oranges, raspberries, blueberries and cold water until smooth. Pour into two glasses and serve immediately.

▶ Health Note

One medium orange supplies nearly 100% of the recommended daily dietary intake of vitamin C.

Super Antioxidant Smoothie

Makes 2 servings

✪ Great for Steps 1, 2, 3 and 4

Nutrients per serving	
Calories	69
Total fat	2 g
Saturated fat	0 g
Cholesterol	0 mg
Sodium	93 mg
Carbohydrate	14 g
Fiber	3 g
Protein	1 g
Calcium	12 mg
Iron	0.4 mg

- **Blender**

1 cup	loosely packed baby spinach	250 mL
1 cup	frozen cherries, blueberries or blackberries	250 mL
1 cup	plain almond milk	250 mL

1. In blender, purée spinach, cherries and almond milk until smooth. Pour into two glasses and serve immediately.

▶ Health Note

In addition to being high in protein, almond milk is an excellent source of vitamin E, an important antioxidant that plays a role in supporting normal heart and brain function, as well as in promoting a healthy complexion.

Papaya Pineapple Smoothie

Makes 2 servings

✪ Great for Steps 1, 2, 3 and 4

Variation

Substitute vanilla-flavored cultured soy yogurt for the yogurt.

Nutrients per serving	
Calories	316
Total fat	0 g
Saturated fat	0 g
Cholesterol	1 mg
Sodium	44 mg
Carbohydrate	77 g
Fiber	2 g
Protein	5 g
Calcium	146 mg
Iron	1.5 mg

- **Blender**

1 cup	frozen papaya chunks	250 mL
1 cup	unsweetened pineapple juice	250 mL
$\frac{1}{2}$ cup	nonfat plain yogurt	125 mL
$\frac{3}{4}$ tsp	ground ginger	3 mL

1. In blender, purée papaya, pineapple juice, yogurt and ginger until smooth. Pour into two glasses and serve immediately.

Superfood Spotlight

Papaya • The tropical papaya is extremely high in beta carotene, which can help prevent prostate cancer. Papayas are also a good source of the carotenes lutein and zeaxanthin, which can help protect eyes from macular degeneration, and are rich in beta-cryptoxanthin, which can help maintain healthy lungs and may help prevent arthritis. Papayas have a high soluble fiber content. They are one of the richest fruits in potassium and calcium, extremely high in vitamin C (a serving of papaya has 250% of the RDA of vitamin C) and a good source of magnesium and vitamin E. In addition, they contain the enzyme papain, which aids digestion.

Green Machine Smoothie

Makes 2 servings

✪ Great for Steps 1, 2 and 4

Nutrients per serving	
Calories	140
Total fat	1 g
Saturated fat	0 g
Cholesterol	0 mg
Sodium	42 mg
Carbohydrate	36 g
Fiber	5 g
Protein	2 g
Calcium	43 mg
Iron	1.3 mg

- **Blender**

2 cups	loosely packed spinach leaves or trimmed kale leaves	500 mL
1 cup	green grapes	250 mL
$\frac{1}{2}$ cup	chopped kiwifruit	125 mL
$\frac{1}{2}$ cup	sliced frozen ripe banana	125 mL
$\frac{1}{2}$ cup	cold water	125 mL

1. In blender, purée spinach, grapes, kiwi, banana and cold water until smooth. Pour into two glasses and serve immediately.

Pumpkin Smoothie

Makes 2 servings

✪ Great for Steps 1, 2, 3 and 4

Pumpkin may sound like an unusual addition to a smoothie, but tasting is believing: its natural sweetness and silken texture coalesce with the tangy yogurt and tart-sweet orange juice, resulting in an indulgent-tasting morning potable. Need additional reasons to imbibe? Pumpkin is high in fiber (to keep you feeling full through the morning) and rich in disease-fighting nutrients such as alpha carotene, beta carotene, vitamins C and E, potassium and magnesium.

Variation

For a non-dairy alternative, substitute plain cultured soy yogurt for the yogurt.

Nutrients per serving	
Calories	199
Total fat	1 g
Saturated fat	0 g
Cholesterol	3 mg
Sodium	73 mg
Carbohydrate	46 g
Fiber	7 g
Protein	8 g
Calcium	182 mg
Iron	1.1 mg

- **Blender**

1 cup	sliced frozen ripe banana	250 mL
1 cup	nonfat plain yogurt	250 mL
3/4 cup	pumpkin purée (not pie filling)	175 mL
1/2 cup	ice cubes	125 mL
1/3 cup	freshly squeezed orange juice	75 mL
1/2 tsp	ground cinnamon	2 mL

1. In blender, purée banana, yogurt, pumpkin, ice cubes, orange juice and cinnamon until smooth. Pour into two glasses and serve immediately.

Superfood Spotlight

Cinnamon • Cinnamon contains several volatile oils and compounds, including cinnamaldehyde, cinnamyl acetate and cinnamyl alcohol, that have a variety of benefits. Cinnamaldehyde acts as an anticoagulant, meaning it can help protect against strokes, and is anti-inflammatory, relieving the symptoms of arthritis and asthma. The spice is a digestive aid, relieving bloating and flatulence, and can reduce the discomfort of heartburn. Cinnamon has antibacterial action that can block the yeast fungus *Candida* and bugs that can cause food poisoning. In one study, cinnamon was shown to lower blood sugar and blood cholesterol.

Power Snacks, Spreads and Nibbles

Crunchy Vanilla Granola Bars 80
Chewy Cherry Granola Bars 81
Fruit and Nut Raw Energy Bars 82
Walnut Quinoa Power Bars 83
Almond Flax Seed Energy Cookies 84
Quinoa Cashew Power Balls 85
PB&J Energy Balls 86
Carob Energy Nuggets 87
Sweet and Spicy Nuts and Seeds 88
Tamari Seed and Nut Mix 88
Spicy, Crispy Roasted Chickpeas 89
Roasted Salt and Pepper Edamame 89
Garlic Pita Chips 90
Oven Tortilla Chips 90
Crispy Kale Chips 91
Sweet Potato Chips 91
Cinnamon Apple Chips 92
Healthy Know-How: Smart Snacking 93
Oven-Baked Tofu "Fries" 94

Quick Whole Wheat Breadsticks 95
Roasted Vegetable Salsa 96
Pineapple Salsa 97
Black Bean Avocado Salsa 98
White Bean Garlic Spread 98
Red Lentil Dal Spread 99
Lentil, Walnut and Arugula Spread 100
Healthy Know-How: Non-Perishable Healthy Snacks 101
Edamame Basil Spread 102
Muhammara (Syrian Red Pepper Walnut Spread) 103
Middle Eastern Eggplant Spread 104
Fresh Herb Goat Cheese Spread 105
Traditional Hummus 105
Pumpkin Pepita Hummus 106
Greek Yogurt Dip with Fresh Squash "Chips" 107
Creamy Cashew Maple Dip with Apples 108
Swiss Chard Spring Rolls with Sesame Lime Dipping Sauce 109
Spinach-Stuffed Mushrooms 110
Herbed Deviled Eggs 111

Crunchy Vanilla Granola Bars

Makes 24 bars

✪ Great for Steps 4 and 5

These bars will soon become your favorite form of portable energy. Vary them with spices, dried fruits, nuts or different sweeteners.

Tip

Measure the oil in a glass measuring cup, then measure the honey in the same cup; the residue from the oil will allow the honey to slide right out without sticking.

Storage Tip

Store cooled granola bars in an airtight container at room temperature for up to 1 week. Or wrap them in plastic wrap, then foil, completely enclosing them, and freeze for up to 6 months. Let thaw at room temperature for 1 hour before serving.

Nutrients per Bar	
Calories	108
Total fat	4 g
Saturated fat	0 g
Cholesterol	0 mg
Sodium	62 mg
Carbohydrate	17 g
Fiber	2 g
Protein	2 g
Calcium	2 mg
Iron	0.6 mg

- **Preheat oven to 350°F (180°C)**
- **Large baking sheet, lined with parchment paper**
- **13- by 9-inch (33 by 23 cm) metal baking pan, lined with foil (see tip, page 518), foil sprayed with nonstick cooking spray**

4 cups	quick-cooking rolled oats	1 L
1⁄3 cup	vegetable oil	75 mL
2⁄3 cup	liquid honey or brown rice syrup	150 mL
1 tbsp	vanilla extract	15 mL
1⁄2 tsp	fine sea salt	2 mL

1. Spread oats on prepared baking sheet. Bake in preheated oven for 13 to 15 minutes, stirring once or twice, until golden brown. Remove from oven, leaving oven on, and let cool in pan for 5 minutes.
2. In a large bowl, whisk together oil, honey, vanilla and salt. Stir in cooled oats. Spread mixture in prepared pan.
3. Bake for 25 to 30 minutes or until deep golden at edges. Let cool in pan on a wire rack for 5 minutes. Using foil liner, lift mixture from pan and transfer to a cutting board. Peel off foil and cut into 24 bars while still warm. Let cool completely.

Chewy Cherry Granola Bars

Makes 15 bars

✪ Great for Steps 2, 3, 4 and 5

How could something that tastes so good also be good for you? Eating is believing.

Tips

Use a square of plastic wrap or waxed paper to press the sticky oat mixture into the prepared pan.

If the bars crumble while you're cutting them, refrigerate for 15 to 30 minutes, until they are more firm.

Storage Tip

Store cooled granola bars in an airtight container at room temperature for up to 5 days. Or wrap them in plastic wrap, then foil, completely enclosing them, and freeze for up to 6 months. Let thaw at room temperature for 1 hour before serving.

Nutrients per Bar	
Calories	238
Total fat	13 g
Saturated fat	8 g
Cholesterol	0 mg
Sodium	125 mg
Carbohydrate	31 g
Fiber	3 g
Protein	3 g
Calcium	8 mg
Iron	0.9 mg

- **Preheat oven to 350°F (180°C)**
- **8-inch (20 cm) square metal baking pan, lined with foil (see tip, page 518), foil sprayed with nonstick cooking spray**

1¾ cups	quick-cooking rolled oats	425 mL
1 cup	dried cherries or dried cranberries	250 mL
1 cup	unsweetened flaked coconut	250 mL
¼ cup	oat bran	60 mL
½ tsp	fine sea salt	2 mL
½ tsp	ground cinnamon	2 mL
¾ cup	brown rice syrup or liquid honey	175 mL
6 tbsp	coconut oil, warmed, or vegetable oil	90 mL
⅓ cup	unsweetened natural peanut butter	75 mL

1. In a large bowl, stir together oats, cherries, coconut, oat bran, salt and cinnamon.
2. In a medium bowl, whisk together brown rice syrup, oil and peanut butter until blended.
3. Add the syrup mixture to the oats mixture and stir until evenly coated. Firmly press mixture into prepared pan.
4. Bake in preheated oven for 30 to 40 minutes or until browned at the edges but still slightly soft at the center. Let cool completely in pan on a wire rack. Using foil liner, lift mixture from pan and transfer to a cutting board. Peel off foil and cut into 15 bars.

Superfood Spotlight

Cherries • Cherries are one of the best fruit sources of antioxidants, which help prevent many diseases associated with aging. They are rich in several plant compounds that have definite health benefits, including quercetin, a flavonoid that has anticancer and heart-protecting qualities. The soluble fiber contained in cherries helps keep LDL cholesterol levels low.

Fruit and Nut Raw Energy Bars

Makes 6 bars

✪ Great for Steps 2, 3 and 4

These bars taste like the best candy you've never had before.

Tips

Place a square of plastic wrap or waxed paper on top of the sticky fruit-nut mixture to help press it into the prepared pan.

You can also roll the fruit-nut mixture into 1-inch (2.5 cm) balls instead of making bars.

Storage Tip

Store bars in an airtight container at room temperature for up to 1 week or in the refrigerator for up to 3 weeks. Or wrap them in plastic wrap, then foil, completely enclosing them, and freeze for up to 6 months. Let thaw at room temperature for 1 hour.

Nutrients per Bar	
Calories	185
Total fat	13 g
Saturated fat	1 g
Cholesterol	0 mg
Sodium	0 mg
Carbohydrate	19 g
Fiber	3 g
Protein	2 g
Calcium	17 mg
Iron	0.5 mg

- **Food processor**
- **9- by 5-inch (23 by 12.5 cm) metal loaf pan, lined with foil (see tip, page 518), foil sprayed with nonstick cooking spray**

3/4 cup	packed pitted Medjool dates	175 mL
3/4 cup	dried cranberries or dried cherries	175 mL
1 cup	pecan halves	250 mL
1/4 tsp	ground cinnamon	1 mL

1. In food processor, pulse dates and cranberries until mixture resembles a thick paste. Transfer to a medium bowl.
2. In the same food processor bowl (no need to clean it), pulse pecans until finely chopped. Add pecans and cinnamon to fruit paste and, using your fingers or a wooden spoon, combine well.
3. Firmly press mixture into prepared pan. Refrigerate for 15 minutes. Using foil liner, lift mixture from pan and transfer to a cutting board. Peel off foil and cut into 6 bars.

Variations

Apricot Almond Energy Bars: Reduce the dates to 1/2 cup (125 mL) and replace the cranberries with 1 cup (250 mL) packed soft dried apricots. Substitute almonds for the pecans and omit the cinnamon.

PB&J Energy Bars: Replace the pecans with raw peanuts and omit the cinnamon.

Cashew "Cookie Dough" Energy Bars: Increase the dates to 1 cup (250 mL) and omit the cranberries. Substitute 1 1/2 cups (375 mL) cashews for the pecans and omit the cinnamon.

Chocolate Chip "Cookie Dough" Energy Bars: Increase the dates to 1 cup (250 mL) and omit the cranberries. Substitute 1 1/2 cups (375 mL) cashews for the pecans. Add 2 oz (60 g) very finely chopped semisweet or bittersweet chocolate and 1 tsp (5 mL) vanilla extract. Decrease the cinnamon to 1/8 tsp (0.5 mL).

Pistachio Energy Bars: Increase the dates to 1 cup (250 mL) and omit the cranberries. Substitute 1 1/2 cups (375 mL) pistachios for the pecans, add 1/4 tsp (1 mL) almond extract and omit the cinnamon.

Walnut Quinoa Power Bars

Makes 8 bars

✪ Great for Steps 3, 4 and 5

Much like rolled oats, quinoa flakes are steamed and rolled; together with walnuts and almond butter, they give these bars a major punch of protein power.

Tip

You can also roll the mixture into 1-inch (2.5 cm) balls instead of making bars.

Storage Tip

Store bars in an airtight container at room temperature for up to 1 week or in the refrigerator for up to 3 weeks. Or wrap them in plastic wrap, then foil, completely enclosing them, and freeze for up to 6 months. Let thaw at room temperature for 1 hour before serving.

Nutrients per Bar	
Calories	341
Total fat	13 g
Saturated fat	1 g
Cholesterol	0 mg
Sodium	94 mg
Carbohydrate	48 g
Fiber	5 g
Protein	10 g
Calcium	67 mg
Iron	2.6 mg

- **8-inch (20 cm) metal baking pan, lined with foil (see tip, page 518), sprayed with nonstick cooking spray**

½ cup	brown rice syrup or liquid honey	125 mL
⅓ cup	unsweetened natural almond butter	75 mL
½ tsp	ground cinnamon	2 mL
⅛ tsp	fine sea salt	0.5 mL
½ tsp	almond extract	2 mL
2 cups	quinoa flakes	500 mL
½ cup	coarsely chopped toasted walnuts	125 mL

1. In a large bowl, whisk together brown rice syrup, almond butter, cinnamon, salt and almond extract until well blended. Stir in quinoa flakes and walnuts until just combined.
2. Press mixture into prepared pan. Refrigerate for 30 minutes. Using foil liner, lift mixture from pan and transfer to a cutting board. Peel off foil and cut into 8 bars.

Variations

Replace the quinoa flakes with quick-cooking rolled oats.

Any other nuts, or sunflower seeds, can be substituted for the walnuts.

Almond Flax Seed Energy Cookies

Makes 12 cookies

✪ Great for Steps 3 and 4

Almonds not only make these cookies delicious, but also deliver a significant nutritional boost.

Tip

Look for roasted almonds lightly seasoned with sea salt. If using unsalted roasted almonds (or toasted almonds), add 1⁄8 tsp (0.5 mL) fine sea salt to the recipe.

Storage Tip

Store cooled cookies in an airtight container at room temperature for up to 5 days. Or wrap them in plastic wrap, then foil, completely enclosing them, and freeze for up to 6 months. Let thaw at room temperature for 2 to 3 hours before serving.

Nutrients per Cookie	
Calories	202
Total fat	12 g
Saturated fat	1 g
Cholesterol	0 mg
Sodium	44 mg
Carbohydrate	20 g
Fiber	3 g
Protein	5 g
Calcium	64 mg
Iron	1.0 mg

- **Preheat oven to 325°F (160°C)**
- **12-cup muffin pan, sprayed with nonstick cooking spray**

2⁄3 cup	ground flax seeds (flaxseed meal)	150 mL
1⁄2 cup	unsweetened natural almond or peanut butter	125 mL
1⁄3 cup	liquid honey or brown rice syrup	75 mL
1⁄3 cup	plain almond milk	75 mL
2⁄3 cup	raisins	150 mL
2⁄3 cup	lightly salted roasted almonds, chopped	150 mL

1. In a large bowl, whisk together ground flax seeds, almond butter, honey and milk until well combined. Stir in raisins and almonds until just combined.
2. Roll dough into 12 balls of equal size. Press each ball into a prepared muffin cup.
3. Bake in preheated oven for 25 to 30 minutes or until edges are golden brown and tops appear somewhat dry. Let cool in pan on a wire rack for 5 minutes, then transfer to the rack to cool.

Superfood Spotlight

Almonds • Almonds are the seeds of the drupe fruit, related to peaches and plums. They are rich in monounsaturated fats and, due to their high fat content, take a long time for the body to digest. This can help keep hunger at bay and help people who are watching their weight. Almonds are extremely high in vitamin E, which may help protect against cancer and cardiovascular diseases, helps reduce the pain of osteoarthritis and keeps skin healthy. Almonds are higher in calcium than almost any other plant food and are therefore an excellent choice for anyone who does not or cannot eat dairy products.

Quinoa Cashew Power Balls

Makes 16 balls

✪ Great for Steps 3, 4 and 5

You may have purchased a bag of quinoa for health reasons, but you'll want to make these delicately sweet power balls for flavor alone. Cashews add to the subtle sweetness.

Tip

Look for roasted cashews lightly seasoned with sea salt.

Storage Tip

Store cooled power balls in an airtight container at room temperature for up to 3 days. Or wrap them in plastic wrap, then foil, completely enclosing them, and freeze for up to 6 months. Let thaw at room temperature for 2 to 3 hours before serving.

Nutrients per Ball	
Calories	110
Total fat	6 g
Saturated fat	1 g
Cholesterol	0 mg
Sodium	84 mg
Carbohydrate	12 g
Fiber	1 g
Protein	3 g
Calcium	18 mg
Iron	1.3 mg

- **Baking sheet**
- **Food processor**
- **Rimmed baking sheet, lined with parchment paper**

2/3 cup	quinoa, rinsed	150 mL
1 1/3 cups	water	325 mL
1 1/2 cups	lightly salted roasted cashews	375 mL
1 tsp	ground cinnamon	5 mL
3 tbsp	dark (cooking) molasses or pure maple syrup	45 mL
1 tsp	vanilla extract	5 mL

1. In a large saucepan, combine quinoa and water. Bring to a boil over medium-high heat. Reduce heat to low, cover and simmer for 14 to 16 minutes or until water is absorbed. Fluff with a fork. Spread quinoa on unlined baking sheet and refrigerate until completely cooled.
2. Preheat oven to 375°F (190°C).
3. In food processor, pulse cashews until finely chopped. Add cooled quinoa, cinnamon, molasses and vanilla; pulse until mixture forms a dough.
4. Roll dough into 16 balls of equal size. Place on prepared baking sheet.
5. Bake in preheated oven for 20 to 25 minutes or until golden brown. Let cool in pan on a wire rack for 10 minutes, then transfer to the rack to cool.

▶ Health Note

Recent research indicates that, because cashews have a low glycemic index score, they are ideal for gradually increasing blood sugar levels without spiking them.

PB&J Energy Balls

Makes 24 balls

✪ Great for Steps 2, 3, 4 and 5

Peanuts and dried blueberries share more than an affinity for each other in this delicious snack: they both contain a naturally occurring compound called resveratrol. According to recent studies, resveratrol appears to reduce fat stores in the human body.

Tip

Look for roasted peanuts lightly seasoned with sea salt.

Storage Tip

Store power balls in an airtight container in the refrigerator for up to 1 week. Or wrap them in plastic wrap, then foil, completely enclosing them, and freeze for up to 6 months. Let thaw at room temperature for 1 hour before serving.

Nutrients per Ball	
Calories	107
Total fat	5 g
Saturated fat	1 g
Cholesterol	1 mg
Sodium	40 mg
Carbohydrate	12 g
Fiber	2 g
Protein	3 g
Calcium	2 mg
Iron	0.5 mg

- **Food processor**

2½ cups	large-flake (old-fashioned) rolled oats, divided	625 mL
⅔ cup	dried blueberries, cranberries or cherries	150 mL
Pinch	fine sea salt	Pinch
½ cup	unsweetened natural peanut butter	125 mL
3 tbsp	brown rice syrup or liquid honey	45 mL
1 tsp	vanilla extract	5 mL
½ cup	lightly salted roasted peanuts, chopped	125 mL

1. In food processor, pulse ½ cup (125 mL) of the oats until powdery. Transfer to a small dish.
2. In the same food processor bowl (no need to clean it), pulse the remaining oats until finely chopped. Add blueberries, salt, peanut butter, brown rice syrup and vanilla; pulse until mixture forms a dough.
3. Transfer dough to a medium bowl and knead in peanuts.
4. Roll dough into 24 balls of equal size. Roll balls in ground oats to coat. Transfer to an airtight container and refrigerate for 1 hour.

Superfood Spotlight

Peanuts • The antioxidant content of peanuts rivals that of blackberries and strawberries. They are rich in polyphenols, including resveratrol, which may protect against hardened arteries and help thin the blood. Peanuts have particularly high levels of a polyphenol compound called p-coumaric acid; roasting the peanuts increases the levels of this compound, boosting overall antioxidant levels by as much as 22%. Peanuts also contain high levels of calcium, for bone health; niacin, which may help protect against Alzheimer's disease and age-related cognitive problems; and vitamin E, an antioxidant linked with heart and arterial health, and protection from strokes, heart attacks and cancer. Peanuts contain mostly monounsaturated fat, which has a better effect on blood cholesterol levels than polyunsaturates. They are a good source of the amino acids tryptophan (which helps boost mood) and l-tyrosine (which is linked with increased mental alertness).

Carob Energy Nuggets

Makes 24 nuggets

✪ Great for Steps 3 and 4

Carob may have had its heyday in the 1970s, but this chocolate taste-alike is worth rediscovering: it's high in calcium, rich in antioxidants and caffeine-free.

- **Food processor**
- **9-inch (23 cm) square metal baking pan, lined with foil (see tip, page 518)**

2 cups	cashews	500 mL
1 cup	unsweetened flaked coconut	250 mL
1/2 cup	unsweetened carob powder	125 mL
1/2 tsp	fine sea salt	2 mL
1/2 cup	brown rice syrup or liquid honey	125 mL
1 tbsp	vanilla extract	15 mL

1. In food processor, pulse cashews and coconut until finely chopped. Add carob powder, salt, brown rice syrup and vanilla; pulse until mixture forms a dough.
2. Press dough into prepared pan. Refrigerate for 1 hour. Using foil liner, lift dough from pan and transfer to a cutting board. Peel off foil and cut into small squares.

▶ Health Note

In a 2001 study at the University of Potsdam in Germany, participants were able to lower their LDL ("bad") cholesterol by 7% in just 8 weeks after eating 15 g of carob daily.

Storage Tip

Store nuggets in an airtight container in the refrigerator for up to 1 week. Or wrap them in plastic wrap, then foil, completely enclosing them, and freeze for up to 6 months. Let thaw at room temperature for 1 hour before serving.

Variation

Cocoa Energy Nuggets: Use unsweetened cocoa powder (not Dutch process) in place of the carob powder.

Nutrients per Nugget	
Calories	120
Total fat	8 g
Saturated fat	3 g
Cholesterol	0 mg
Sodium	73 mg
Carbohydrate	12 g
Fiber	1 g
Protein	2 g
Calcium	8 mg
Iron	0.8 mg

Sweet and Spicy Nuts and Seeds

Makes about 4 cups (1 L)

✪ Great for Steps 3 and 4

Nutrients per ¼ cup (60 mL)	
Calories	217
Total fat	18 g
Saturated fat	2 g
Cholesterol	0 mg
Sodium	95 mg
Carbohydrate	12 g
Fiber	3 g
Protein	6 g
Calcium	29 mg
Iron	1.6 mg

- **Preheat oven to 300°F (150°C)**
- **Rimmed baking sheet, lined with parchment paper**

¼ cup	unrefined cane sugar	60 mL
2 tsp	ground cinnamon	10 mL
1½ tsp	chili powder	7 mL
½ tsp	fine sea salt	2 mL
⅛ tsp	cayenne pepper	0.5 mL
1	large egg white, at room temperature	1
4 cups	mixed nuts and/or seeds	1 L

1. In a small bowl, whisk together sugar, cinnamon, chili powder, salt and cayenne.
2. In a large bowl, whisk egg white until light and frothy. Add nuts and toss to coat. Add sugar mixture and toss to coat. Spread in a single layer on prepared baking sheet.
3. Bake in preheated oven for 30 to 35 minutes, stirring once or twice, until deep golden brown and dry-looking. Let cool completely in pan. Store in an airtight container at room temperature for up to 2 weeks.

Tamari Seed and Nut Mix

Makes about 3½ cups (875 mL)

✪ Great for Steps 3 and 4

Nutrients per ¼ cup (60 mL)	
Calories	207
Total fat	18 g
Saturated fat	2 g
Cholesterol	0 mg
Sodium	75 mg
Carbohydrate	6 g
Fiber	2 g
Protein	7 g
Calcium	29 mg
Iron	1.7 mg

- **Large rimmed baking sheet, lined with parchment paper or foil**

2 tsp	vegetable oil	10 mL
1 cup	green pumpkin seeds (pepitas)	250 mL
¾ cup	peanuts	175 mL
¾ cup	almonds	175 mL
¾ cup	pecan halves	175 mL
⅛ tsp	cayenne pepper	0.5 mL
1 tbsp	tamari	15 mL
1 tsp	freshly squeezed lime juice	5 mL

1. In a large skillet, heat oil over medium heat. Add pumpkin seeds, peanuts, almonds and pecans; cook, stirring, for 4 to 7 minutes or until golden brown. Add cayenne, tamari and lime juice; cook, stirring, for 2 minutes or until dry.
2. Spread mixture on prepared baking sheet and let cool completely. Store in an airtight container at room temperature for up to 2 weeks.

Spicy, Crispy Roasted Chickpeas

Makes 8 servings

✪ Great for Steps 2, 3 and 4

Chickpeas sprinkled with cayenne and lemon, then roasted until crispy, are a habit-forming snack. They're also great tossed into salads.

Nutrients per serving	
Calories	52
Total fat	2 g
Saturated fat	0 g
Cholesterol	0 mg
Sodium	331 mg
Carbohydrate	7 g
Fiber	2 g
Protein	2 g
Calcium	9 mg
Iron	0.5 mg

- **Preheat oven to 425°F (220°C)**
- **Large rimmed baking sheet, lined with parchment paper**

1	can (14 to 19 oz/398 to 540 mL) chickpeas, drained, rinsed and patted dry	1
3/4 tsp	fine sea salt	3 mL
1/8 tsp	cayenne pepper	0.5 mL
2 tsp	extra virgin olive oil	10 mL
1 tsp	freshly squeezed lemon juice	5 mL

1. In a large bowl, combine chickpeas, salt, cayenne, oil and lemon juice. Spread in a single layer on prepared baking sheet.
2. Bake in preheated oven for 32 to 38 minutes or until crisp and dry. Let cool completely in pan. Store in an airtight container at room temperature for up to 2 weeks.

Variation

You can use any ground spice or dried herb in place of, or in addition to, the cayenne.

Roasted Salt and Pepper Edamame

Makes 12 servings

✪ Great for Steps 2, 3 and 4

Nutrients per serving	
Calories	56
Total fat	3 g
Saturated fat	0 g
Cholesterol	0 mg
Sodium	97 mg
Carbohydrate	4 g
Fiber	2 g
Protein	5 g
Calcium	27 mg
Iron	1.0 mg

- **Preheat oven to 400°F (200°C)**
- **Large rimmed baking sheet, lined with parchment paper**

1 lb	frozen shelled edamame, thawed	500 g
1/2 tsp	fine sea salt	2 mL
1/2 tsp	cracked black pepper	2 mL
1 1/2 tsp	extra virgin olive oil	7 mL

1. In a large bowl, combine edamame, salt, pepper and oil. Spread in a single layer on prepared baking sheet.
2. Bake in preheated oven for 35 to 40 minutes or until crisp and dry. Let cool completely in pan. Store in an airtight container at room temperature for up to 2 weeks.

Garlic Pita Chips

Makes 8 servings

✪ Great for Step 5

Nutrients per serving	
Calories	129
Total fat	1 g
Saturated fat	0 g
Cholesterol	0 mg
Sodium	343 mg
Carbohydrate	27 g
Fiber	4 g
Protein	5 g
Calcium	8 mg
Iron	1.5 mg

- **Preheat oven to 425°F (220°C)**
- **2 rimmed baking sheets, lined with parchment paper**

6	6-inch (15 cm) whole wheat pitas	6
	Nonstick cooking spray (preferably olive oil)	
1 tsp	garlic powder	5 mL
1/4 tsp	fine sea salt	1 mL

1. Spray one side of each pita with cooking spray. Sprinkle with garlic powder and salt. Cut each pita into 8 wedges of equal size. Arrange in a single layer on prepared baking sheets.
2. Bake in preheated oven for 5 to 8 minutes or until golden. Let cool completely in pans. Store in an airtight container at room temperature for up to 2 weeks.

Oven Tortilla Chips

Makes 12 servings

✪ Great for Step 5

Making chips from scratch allows you to control the fat, salt and other seasonings.

Nutrients per serving	
Calories	70
Total fat	1 g
Saturated fat	0 g
Cholesterol	0 mg
Sodium	93 mg
Carbohydrate	14 g
Fiber	1 g
Protein	1 g
Calcium	0 mg
Iron	0.0 mg

- **Preheat oven to 350°F (180°C)**
- **2 rimmed baking sheets, lined with parchment paper**

12	6-inch (15 cm) corn tortillas	12
	Nonstick cooking spray (preferably olive oil)	
1 tsp	chili powder (optional)	5 mL
1/4 tsp	fine sea salt	1 mL

1. Spray one side of each tortilla with cooking spray. Sprinkle with chili powder (if using) and salt. Cut each tortilla into 8 wedges of equal size. Arrange in a single layer on prepared baking sheets.
2. Bake in preheated oven for 12 to 15 minutes or until golden brown. Let cool completely in pans. Store in an airtight container at room temperature for up to 2 weeks.

Crispy Kale Chips

Makes 6 servings

✪ Great for Steps 1, 2 and 4

Nutrients per serving	
Calories	32
Total fat	1 g
Saturated fat	0 g
Cholesterol	0 mg
Sodium	170 mg
Carbohydrate	6 g
Fiber	1 g
Protein	2 g
Calcium	155 mg
Iron	2.3 mg

- **Preheat oven to 325°F (160°C)**
- **2 rimmed baking sheets, lined with parchment paper**

1 lb	kale, rinsed and patted dry	500 g
	Nonstick cooking spray (preferably olive oil)	
1⁄4 tsp	fine sea salt	1 mL

1. Remove tough stems and center ribs from kale, then tear leaves into approximately 3-inch (7.5 cm) pieces. Arrange leaves in a single layer on prepared baking sheets. Spray with cooking spray and sprinkle with salt.
2. Bake in preheated oven for 12 to 15 minutes or until edges are browned and leaves are crispy. Serve warm or let cool completely in pans.

Sweet Potato Chips

Makes 8 servings

✪ Great for Steps 1 and 2

Storage Tip

Store chips in an airtight container at room temperature for up to 1 week.

Nutrients per serving	
Calories	25
Total fat	0 g
Saturated fat	0 g
Cholesterol	0 mg
Sodium	105 mg
Carbohydrate	6 g
Fiber	1 g
Protein	1 g
Calcium	5 mg
Iron	0.2 mg

- **Preheat oven to 375°F (190°C)**
- **2 rimmed baking sheets, lined with parchment paper**

2	medium-large sweet potatoes	2
	Nonstick cooking spray (preferably olive oil)	
1⁄4 tsp	fine sea salt	1 mL

1. Using a very sharp knife or a mandoline, cut sweet potatoes into 1⁄16-inch (2 mm) thick slices. Arrange in a single layer on prepared baking sheets. Spray with cooking spray and sprinkle with salt.
2. Bake in preheated oven for 11 to 16 minutes or until edges are golden brown. Transfer chips to a wire rack and let cool completely (they will crisp more as they cool).

▸ Health Note

Snacking on sweet potatoes can help your skin stay clear, smooth and young-looking. The reason is the beta carotene that gives sweet potatoes their vibrant orange hue. When the antioxidant converts to vitamin A in your body, it switches on DNA that's in charge of producing new skin cells and shedding old ones.

Cinnamon Apple Chips

Makes 8 servings

✪ Great for Steps 1, 2 and 4

Eating some of these apple chips each day might keep the doctor away, but the cinnamon would share the credit: recent studies indicate that eating as little as 1/2 tsp (2 mL) of ground cinnamon per day can lower LDL ("bad") cholesterol levels, boost cognitive function and memory, and even have a regulatory effect on blood sugar levels.

Tip

Be sure to transfer the chips from the parchment paper to a wire rack while still warm, or they will stick.

Nutrients per serving	
Calories	58
Total fat	0 g
Saturated fat	0 g
Cholesterol	0 mg
Sodium	0 mg
Carbohydrate	15 g
Fiber	2 g
Protein	0 g
Calcium	7 mg
Iron	0.1 mg

- **Preheat oven to 325°F (160°C)**
- **2 rimmed baking sheets, lined with parchment paper**

4	large tart-sweet apples (such as Braeburn, Gala or Pippin), halved and cored	4
4 tsp	stevia powder	20 mL
1/2 tsp	ground cinnamon	2 mL
	Nonstick cooking spray (preferably olive oil)	

1. Using a very sharp knife or a mandoline, cut apples into 1/8-inch (3 mm) thick slices.
2. In a small bowl, combine stevia and cinnamon.
3. Arrange apple slices in a single layer on prepared baking sheets. Spray with cooking spray and sprinkle with stevia mixture.
4. Bake in preheated oven for 35 to 40 minutes or until edges are browned and slices are dry and crispy. Transfer chips to a wire rack and let cool completely (they will crisp more as they cool). Store in an airtight container at room temperature for up to 1 week.

Variation

Pear Chips: Use 4 medium Bosc pears, halved and cored, in place of the apples.

Healthy Know-How

Smart Snacking

Well-chosen snacks can be an important part of a healthful diet, helping you manage your weight, hunger, health and energy.

Whether you want to gain or lose weight, snacks can help. For weight gain, eat energy-dense snacks throughout the day. For weight loss, eat several small, healthy snacks between meals to keep cravings down and prevent excessive hunger that may lead to overeating.

Snacks can also help you meet guidelines for grain, vegetable, fruit, calcium and protein intake, and can help sustain your energy throughout the day. The following tips will make snacks a nutritious, enjoyable part of healthy eating:

- **Work snacks into your diet plan.** Rather than considering them "extras," opt for snacks that contribute to your overall calorie and nutrient needs. Snack on foods that complement your meals and add variety to your diet.
- **Match snacks to your calorie needs and weight goals.** If your goal is weight loss or maintenance, try to consume nutrient-dense snacks that are between 100 and 200 calories. If you are physically active or trying to gain weight, consume nutrient-dense snacks that are between 200 and 400 calories.
- **Be mindful of portion size.** Snack portions are smaller than meal portions. They shouldn't fill you up but rather should help you to not be hungry. Although appropriate caloric content for snacks depends on your activity level and weight goals, they should generally not have more than 500 calories (this would be similar to a meal).
- **Snack only when you're hungry.** Fight the urge to nibble in response to non-hunger eating impulses such as boredom, frustration or stress.
- **Snack consciously.** Don't mix snacking with other activities. Snacking absentmindedly — while reading or watching TV, for example — leads to overeating.
- **Plan ahead for smart snacking.** Keep a variety of tasty, nutritious, ready-to-eat snacks on hand at home, at work or wherever you need a light bite to take the edge off hunger. That way, you won't be limited to snacks from vending machines, fast-food restaurants or convenience stores. See page 101 for some non-perishable snack suggestions.

Oven-Baked Tofu "Fries"

Makes 6 servings

✪ Great for Step 3

Fast food, meet your match. Crispy and undeniably dippable, these superfood fries are rich in nutrients, including protein, iron and omega-3 fatty acids. Serve with warmed marinara sauce for dipping.

Storage Tip

The pressed tofu sticks can be stored in an airtight container in the refrigerator for up to 2 days.

- **2 rimmed baking sheets**

1 lb	extra-firm tofu, drained and patted dry	500 g
	Nonstick cooking spray	
1⁄4 tsp	fine sea salt	1 mL
1⁄4 tsp	freshly ground black pepper	1 mL

1. Line one of the baking sheets with a kitchen towel or a double layer of paper towels.
2. Cut tofu crosswise into 8 rectangles. Cut each rectangle lengthwise into 3 sticks. Arrange in a single layer on towel-lined baking sheet. Place second baking sheet on top and weigh down with 6 to 8 heavy cans. Let stand for 1 hour to drain liquid from tofu.
3. Preheat oven to 375°F (190°C).
4. Remove weights and lift top baking sheet off tofu. Wipe any dampness from bottom. Spray top of baking sheet with cooking spray. Remove tofu sticks from towel-lined baking sheet and arrange in single layer on sprayed baking sheet. Lightly spray tofu sticks with cooking spray. Sprinkle with salt and pepper.
5. Bake in preheated oven for 8 minutes. Carefully turn tofu sticks over. Bake for 6 to 8 minutes or until tofu is crispy and golden. Serve warm or let cool completely in pan.

Nutrients per serving	
Calories	67
Total fat	4 g
Saturated fat	0 g
Cholesterol	0 mg
Sodium	117 mg
Carbohydrate	2 g
Fiber	1 g
Protein	7 g
Calcium	144 mg
Iron	1.4 mg

Quick Whole Wheat Breadsticks

Makes 18 breadsticks

✪ Great for Step 5

This play of crispy and tender goes perfectly with a bit of warmed marinara sauce. And because these breadsticks are made with nutrient-rich whole wheat flour, you can definitely snack on more than one.

Storage Tip

Store breadsticks in an airtight container in the refrigerator for up to 3 days.

Nutrients per breadstick	
Calories	54
Total fat	2 g
Saturated fat	1 g
Cholesterol	5 mg
Sodium	102 mg
Carbohydrate	8 g
Fiber	1 g
Protein	1 g
Calcium	10 mg
Iron	0.1 mg

- **Preheat oven to 375°F (190°C)**
- **Food processor**
- **Large rimmed baking sheet, lined with parchment paper**

2 cups	whole wheat pastry flour	500 mL
3/4 tsp	fine sea salt	3 mL
1/2 tsp	baking powder	2 mL
3 tbsp	cold unsalted butter or virgin coconut oil	45 mL
2/3 cup	ice water	150 mL
	Nonstick cooking spray (preferably olive oil)	

1. In food processor, pulse flour, salt and baking powder to combine. Add butter and pulse until mixture resembles fresh, moist bread crumbs. With the motor running, through the feed tube, add ice water and process just until dough comes together.
2. Transfer dough to a lightly floured work surface and pat into a 1-inch (2.5 cm) thick rectangle. Roll out to a 12- by 10-inch (30 by 25 cm) rectangle about 1/4 inch (0.5 cm) thick. Using a sharp knife or pizza cutter, cut dough crosswise into 1/4-inch (0.5 cm) thick strips.
3. Gently roll each strip into a 14-inch (35 cm) long stick. Brush 1 stick with water and twist it with another stick, pressing at the top and the bottom. Repeat with remaining sticks. Arrange twists at least 1 inch (2.5 cm) apart on prepared baking sheet. Spray twists lightly with cooking spray.
4. Bake in preheated oven for 20 to 25 minutes or until golden brown. Let cool in pan on a wire rack for 5 minutes, then transfer to the rack to cool.

Roasted Vegetable Salsa

Makes about 2 cups (500 mL)

✪ Great for Steps 1, 2 and 4

Red, purple, yellow, green — this stylish symphony of vegetables makes it easy to heed the advice "eat the rainbow." The tart tomatoes and meaty eggplants are the stars, but the supporting players, squash and parsley, add plenty of intrigue, as well as vitamins A and C.

Tip

Toss leftover salsa with hot or cold cooked whole-grain pasta (small shapes) for a quick and simple meal.

Storage Tip

This salsa can be stored in an airtight container in the refrigerator for up to 2 days.

Nutrients per 1 tbsp (15 mL)	
Calories	11
Total fat	0 g
Saturated fat	0 g
Cholesterol	0 mg
Sodium	45 mg
Carbohydrate	2 g
Fiber	1 g
Protein	0 g
Calcium	6 mg
Iron	0.2 mg

- **Preheat broiler, with rack set 4 to 6 inches (10 to 15 cm) from heat source**
- **2 large rimmed baking sheets, lined with parchment paper**

3	red or yellow tomatoes, cut into 1-inch (2.5 cm) chunks	3
2	Japanese eggplants, cut into 1⁄4-inch (0.5 cm) thick slices	2
	Nonstick cooking spray (preferably olive oil)	
2 tsp	ground cumin, divided	10 mL
1⁄2 tsp	fine sea salt, divided	2 mL
2	zucchini or yellow summer squash (yellow zucchini), cut into 1⁄4-inch (0.5 cm) thick slices	2
1	clove garlic, minced	1
1⁄4 cup	packed fresh flat-leaf (Italian) parsley, chopped	60 mL
1 tbsp	freshly squeezed lemon juice	15 mL
2 tsp	extra virgin olive oil	10 mL

1. Arrange tomatoes and eggplants in a single layer on one of the baking sheets. Lightly spray with cooking spray and sprinkle with half the cumin and half the salt. Broil for 4 to 7 minutes or until deep golden brown. Let cool completely.
2. Arrange zucchini in a single layer on the other baking sheet. Lightly spray with cooking spray and sprinkle with the remaining cumin and salt. Broil for 4 to 7 minutes or until deep golden brown. Let cool completely.
3. Chop cooled tomatoes, eggplants and zucchini into small pieces and place in a large bowl. Add garlic, parsley, lemon juice and oil. Cover and refrigerate for about 30 minutes or until chilled.

Pineapple Salsa

Makes about 2¼ cups (550 mL)

✪ Great for Steps 1, 2 and 4

Delivering a lot of tropical glamour for minimal work, this gorgeous salsa balances the sweetness of fresh pineapple with the acidity of lime and the heat of jalapeños. Pineapple is a vitamin C jackpot with a bonus: it has an enzyme that helps relieve indigestion, making it a snack your stomach will welcome.

Tip

For the best results, make this salsa at least 30 minutes ahead of time to allow the flavors to mingle.

Storage Tip

This salsa can be stored in an airtight container in the refrigerator for up to 2 days.

Nutrients per 1 tbsp (15 mL)	
Calories	5
Total fat	0 g
Saturated fat	0 g
Cholesterol	0 mg
Sodium	0 mg
Carbohydrate	1 g
Fiber	0 g
Protein	0 g
Calcium	2 mg
Iron	0.0 mg

1	small jalapeño pepper, seeded and minced	1
2 cups	diced fresh pineapple (see tip, page 313)	500 mL
¾ cup	packed fresh cilantro leaves, chopped	175 mL
¼ cup	finely chopped red onion	60 mL
1 tsp	finely grated lime zest	5 mL
1 tbsp	freshly squeezed lime juice	15 mL
⅛ tsp	fine sea salt	0.5 mL

1. In a medium bowl, combine jalapeño, pineapple, cilantro, red onion, lime zest, lime juice and salt.

Superfood Spotlight

Pineapple • Pineapples have long been used as a medicinal plant in various parts of the world, particularly the Americas. Apart from being a good source of vitamin C and other vitamins and minerals, including magnesium, pineapple contains an active substance known as bromelain. This protein has been proven to ease the inflammation associated with arthritis and joint pain, and may also help to reduce the incidence of blood clots, which can lead to heart attack and strokes. Pineapple is also a good source of ferulic acid, which can help prevent cancer.

Black Bean Avocado Salsa

Makes about 3½ cups (875 mL)

✪ Great for Steps 1, 2, 3 and 4

Nutrients per 2 tbsp (30 mL)	
Calories	35
Total fat	2 g
Saturated fat	0 g
Cholesterol	0 mg
Sodium	109 mg
Carbohydrate	5 g
Fiber	1 g
Protein	1 g
Calcium	9 mg
Iron	0.3 mg

2	cloves garlic, minced	2
1	can (14 to 19 oz/398 to 540 mL) black beans, drained and rinsed	1
1	can (14 to 15 oz/398 to 425 mL) fire-roasted diced tomatoes, with juice	1
1 cup	fresh or thawed frozen corn kernels	250 mL
¼ cup	packed fresh cilantro leaves, chopped	60 mL
1 tsp	ground cumin	5 mL
½ tsp	chipotle chile powder	2 mL
¼ tsp	fine sea salt	1 mL
3 tbsp	freshly squeezed lime juice	45 mL
2 tsp	extra virgin olive oil	10 mL
1	avocado, diced	1

1. In a medium bowl, combine garlic, beans, tomatoes with juice, corn, cilantro, cumin, chipotle powder, salt, lime juice and oil. Gently fold in avocado.

White Bean Garlic Spread

Makes about 2 cups (500 mL)

✪ Great for Steps 2, 3 and 4

Nutrients per 1 tbsp (15 mL)	
Calories	22
Total fat	1 g
Saturated fat	0 g
Cholesterol	0 mg
Sodium	80 mg
Carbohydrate	2 g
Fiber	1 g
Protein	2 g
Calcium	10 mg
Iron	0.3 mg

- **Food processor**

3	cloves garlic, minced	3
1	can (14 to 19 oz/398 to 540 mL) cannellini (white kidney) beans, drained and rinsed	1
½ cup	drained soft silken tofu	125 mL
2 tsp	dried Italian seasoning	10 mL
½ tsp	fine sea salt	2 mL
¼ cup	freshly squeezed lemon juice	60 mL
1 tbsp	extra virgin olive oil	15 mL

1. In food processor, combine garlic, beans, tofu, Italian seasoning, salt, lemon juice and olive oil; process until smooth. Transfer to a serving dish.

Red Lentil Dal Spread

Makes about 2¼ cups (560 mL)

✪ Great for Steps 2, 3 and 4

Distinctive flavors of India — cumin, mustard seed, turmeric and coriander — combine with velvety red lentils and creamy coconut in this sensational spread. Serve with pita bread or pita chips.

Storage Tip

This spread can be stored in an airtight container in the refrigerator for up to 3 days.

Nutrients per 1 tbsp (15 mL)	
Calories	27
Total fat	0 g
Saturated fat	0 g
Cholesterol	0 mg
Sodium	42 mg
Carbohydrate	4 g
Fiber	1 g
Protein	2 g
Calcium	7 mg
Iron	0.4 mg

1 cup	dried red lentils	250 mL
2 cups	reduced-sodium ready-to-use vegetable broth	500 mL
1 tbsp	vegetable oil	15 mL
2	cloves garlic, minced	2
1½ cups	chopped onions	375 mL
1½ tsp	ground cumin	7 mL
1 tsp	yellow mustard seeds	5 mL
1 tsp	ground turmeric	5 mL
½ tsp	ground coriander	2 mL
⅛ tsp	cayenne pepper	0.5 mL
½ tsp	fine sea salt	2 mL
½ cup	light coconut milk	125 mL
1 tbsp	tomato paste	15 mL
2 tbsp	freshly squeezed lime juice	30 mL

1. In a medium saucepan, combine lentils and broth. Bring to a boil over medium-high heat. Reduce heat to low, cover, leaving lid ajar, and simmer for 15 to 20 minutes or until lentils are tender. Remove from heat.
2. Meanwhile, in a large skillet, heat oil over medium heat. Add garlic, onions, cumin, mustard seeds, turmeric, coriander and cayenne; cook, stirring, for 8 to 10 minutes or until onions are softened. Add lentils and cooking liquid, salt, coconut milk and tomato paste; cook, stirring, for 5 to 8 minutes or until lentils are broken down. Remove from heat and stir in lime juice. Let cool to room temperature.

▸ Health Note

The high levels of fiber found in lentils may help reduce cholesterol levels and maintain blood sugar, while the folate helps to regulate homocysteine levels, protecting the heart from disease.

Lentil, Walnut and Arugula Spread

Makes about 2 cups (500 mL)

✪ Great for Steps 1, 2, 3 and 4

Favorite Mediterranean ingredients come together in this vibrant dip. The lentils are packed with protein, not to mention B vitamins and zinc, and the walnuts offer ALA, the plant-based source of omega-3 fatty acids.

Storage Tip

This spread can be stored in an airtight container in the refrigerator for up to 4 days.

- **Food processor**

3⁄4 cup	dried brown lentils	175 mL
1 1⁄2 cups	water	375 mL
1	clove garlic	1
3 cups	packed arugula	750 mL
1⁄4 cup	chopped toasted walnuts	60 mL
1⁄2 tsp	fine sea salt	2 mL
1 tbsp	extra virgin olive oil	15 mL
2 tsp	ground cumin	10 mL
3 tbsp	reduced-sodium ready-to-use vegetable broth	45 mL
1 tbsp	sherry vinegar or white wine vinegar	15 mL

1. In a medium saucepan, combine lentils and water. Bring to a boil over medium-high heat. Reduce heat to low, cover, leaving lid ajar, and simmer for 35 to 40 minutes or until lentils are tender and most of the water has been absorbed. Drain and let cool to room temperature.
2. In food processor, combine garlic, arugula, walnuts, salt and oil; process until finely chopped. Add cooled lentils, cumin, broth and vinegar; pulse until combined but not completely smooth.
3. Transfer spread to a serving dish, cover and refrigerate for at least 30 minutes to blend the flavors.

Nutrients per 1 tbsp (15 mL)

Calories	26
Total fat	1 g
Saturated fat	0 g
Cholesterol	0 mg
Sodium	37 mg
Carbohydrate	3 g
Fiber	1 g
Protein	1 g
Calcium	7 mg
Iron	0.4 mg

Healthy Know-How

Non-Perishable Healthy Snacks

Whether for bag lunches, travel, weight loss, refueling mid-day or post-workout, or healthy snacking in general, it pays to plan ahead and keep some non-perishable, healthy snacks on hand.

- Unsweetened dried fruit: apricots, apples, blueberries, cherries, cranberries, dates, papaya, peaches, pears, pineapple, prunes, raisins
- Lightly salted or unsalted nuts: almonds, brazil nuts, cashews, macadamia nuts, peanuts, pecans, pistachios, soy nuts, walnuts
- Lightly salted or unsalted seeds: chia seeds, hemp seeds, green pumpkin seeds (pepitas), sunflower seeds (shelled or unshelled)
- Unsweetened natural nut and seed butters: almond, cashew, peanut, soy nut, hemp seed, sunflower seed
- Dried vegetables: dry-packed sun-dried tomatoes (look for moist varieties that have the texture of dried fruit), wasabi peas, freeze-dried vegetables
- Whole-grain, low-sugar cookies: graham crackers, fruit newtons, hard gingersnaps, oatmeal cookies
- Low-sodium baked snacks: pretzels, vegetable chips, air-popped popcorn, soy chips, apple chips, pita chips
- All-natural energy bars or granola bars
- Whole-grain and/or nut crackers
- Whole-grain cereal, granola or trail mix
- Low-sodium soup-in-a-cup
- Shelf-stable dairy or non-dairy individual milk boxes
- Preservative-free, no-sugar-added applesauce and fruit cups

Edamame Basil Spread

Makes about 1⅔ cups (400 mL)

✪ Great for Steps 2, 3 and 4

The bliss you experience snacking on this gorgeous green dip may be based on the edamame's high levels of folate as much as the fantastic flavor: in a few small studies, people with higher levels of folate in their systems reported less mood variability. Dig in!

Storage Tip

This spread can be stored in an airtight container in the refrigerator for up to 3 days.

Nutrients per 1 tbsp (15 mL)	
Calories	35
Total fat	2 g
Saturated fat	0 g
Cholesterol	0 mg
Sodium	50 mg
Carbohydrate	2 g
Fiber	1 g
Protein	2 g
Calcium	14 mg
Iron	0.4 mg

- **Food processor**

6	cloves garlic	6
12 oz	frozen shelled edamame	375 g
1 cup	packed fresh basil leaves	250 mL
½ tsp	fine sea salt	2 mL
3 tbsp	extra virgin olive oil	45 mL
3 tbsp	freshly squeezed lemon juice	45 mL

1. In a medium saucepan of boiling water, cook garlic and edamame for 7 to 10 minutes or until edamame are very tender. Drain, reserving ½ cup (125 mL) of the cooking liquid. Let cool.
2. In food processor, combine cooled garlic and edamame, basil, salt, half the reserved cooking liquid, oil and lemon juice; process until smooth. Add more reserved liquid, 1 tbsp (15 mL) at a time, until mixture is creamy. Transfer to a serving dish, cover and refrigerate for 30 minutes or until chilled.

Superfood Spotlight

Garlic • Valued as a contributor to good health for thousands of years, garlic is a useful antibiotic and inhibits fungal infections such as athlete's foot. Its powerful sulfur compounds are the cause of its strong odor but are also the main source of its health benefits. Eating garlic appears to boost our natural supply of hydrogen sulfide, which acts as an antioxidant and transmits cellular signals that relax blood vessels and increase blood flow. The human body already produces hydrogen sulfide, but boosted production could help explain why a garlic-rich diet may protect against various cancers, including breast, prostate and colon cancer. Additional research suggest that higher hydrogen sulfide might also protect the heart, preventing formation of blood clots and arterial plaque. Garlic also appears to minimize stomach ulcers. Eaten in reasonable quantity, it is a good source of vitamin C, selenium, potassium and calcium.

Muhammara (Syrian Red Pepper Walnut Spread)

Makes about 2⅓ cups (575 mL)

✪ Great for Steps 2, 3 and 4

This spread is spicy, nutty and mildly sweet. Think of muhammara as the Middle East in a bowl. Be sure to keep a jar (or two) of roasted red bell peppers on hand in case a sudden urge to make this spectacular spread occurs; in addition to their convenience, they, like their raw counterparts, are a terrific source of vitamins A and C.

Storage Tip

This spread can be stored in an airtight container in the refrigerator for up to 3 days.

Nutrients per 1 tbsp (15 mL)	
Calories	33
Total fat	3 g
Saturated fat	0 g
Cholesterol	0 mg
Sodium	12 mg
Carbohydrate	2 g
Fiber	0 g
Protein	1 g
Calcium	4 mg
Iron	0.2 mg

- **Food processor**

3	cloves garlic, minced	3
1	jar (12 oz/341 mL) roasted red bell peppers, drained	1
1 cup	chopped walnuts	250 mL
⅓ cup	fresh whole wheat bread crumbs	75 mL
1 tsp	ground cumin	5 mL
¼ tsp	cayenne pepper	1 mL
2 tbsp	extra virgin olive oil	30 mL
1 tbsp	freshly squeezed lemon juice	15 mL
2 tsp	liquid honey, agave nectar or brown rice syrup	10 mL

1. In food processor, combine garlic, roasted peppers, walnuts, bread crumbs, cumin, cayenne, oil, lemon juice and honey; process until smooth. Transfer to a serving dish.

Middle Eastern Eggplant Spread

Makes about 2⅔ cups (650 mL)

✪ Great for Steps 1, 2, 3 and 4

Melt-in-your-mouth roasted eggplant gets a stealthy boost of protein from white beans in this impressive snack; roasted peppers and lemon juice brighten everything.

Storage Tip

This spread can be stored in an airtight container in the refrigerator for up to 3 days.

- **Preheat oven to 450°F (230°C)**
- **Large rimmed baking sheet, lined with foil and sprayed with nonstick cooking spray (preferably olive oil)**
- **Food processor**

1	large eggplant (about 1 lb/500 g), trimmed and halved lengthwise	1
½ cup	loosely packed fresh parsley leaves, chopped, divided	125 mL
1	clove garlic, roughly chopped	1
1 cup	drained and rinsed canned white beans	250 mL
¾ cup	drained roasted red bell peppers	175 mL
3 tbsp	tahini	45 mL
1 tbsp	freshly squeezed lemon juice	15 mL

1. Place eggplant cut side down on prepared baking sheet. Prick all over with a fork. Bake in preheated oven for 40 to 45 minutes or until soft and collapsed. Let cool completely.
2. Scoop eggplant flesh into food processor bowl, discarding skin. Set aside 1 tbsp (15 mL) of the parsley. Add the remaining parsley, garlic, beans, red peppers, tahini and lemon juice to the food processor and process until smooth.
3. Transfer spread to a serving bowl and garnish with the reserved parsley.

Nutrients per 2 tbsp (30 mL)	
Calories	32
Total fat	1 g
Saturated fat	0 g
Cholesterol	0 mg
Sodium	48 mg
Carbohydrate	4 g
Fiber	2 g
Protein	2 g
Calcium	15 mg
Iron	0.5 mg

Fresh Herb Goat Cheese Spread

Makes about 1¼ cups (300 mL)

✪ Great for Steps 3 and 4

Nutrients per 1 tbsp (15 mL)	
Calories	23
Total fat	1 g
Saturated fat	0 g
Cholesterol	3 mg
Sodium	52 mg
Carbohydrate	1 g
Fiber	0 g
Protein	2 g
Calcium	16 mg
Iron	0.2 mg

- **Food processor**

1	clove garlic, chopped	1
4 oz	soft mild goat cheese	125 g
⅔ cup	nonfat cottage cheese	150 mL
3 tbsp	minced fresh chives	45 mL
1 tbsp	chopped fresh parsley	15 mL
1 tbsp	chopped fresh basil	15 mL

1. In food processor, combine garlic, goat cheese and cottage cheese; process until smooth.
2. Transfer spread to a serving bowl and stir in chives, parsley and basil. Cover and refrigerate for at least 30 minutes to blend the flavors.

Traditional Hummus

Makes about 2½ cups (625 mL)

✪ Great for Steps 2, 3 and 4

Nutrients per 2 tbsp (30 mL)	
Calories	31
Total fat	2 g
Saturated fat	0 g
Cholesterol	0 mg
Sodium	77 mg
Carbohydrate	4 g
Fiber	1 g
Protein	1 g
Calcium	8 mg
Iron	0.3 mg

- **Food processor**

2	cloves garlic, coarsely chopped	2
1	can (14 to 19 oz/398 to 540 mL) chickpeas, drained and rinsed	1
1 tsp	ground cumin	5 mL
¼ tsp	fine sea salt	1 mL
Pinch	cayenne pepper	Pinch
¼ cup	warm water	60 mL
3 tbsp	tahini	45 mL
2 tbsp	freshly squeezed lemon juice	30 mL

1. In food processor, combine garlic and chickpeas; process until finely chopped. Add cumin, salt, cayenne, warm water, tahini and lemon juice; process until smooth, stopping to scrape down the sides of the bowl as needed. Transfer to a serving dish.

Pumpkin Pepita Hummus

Makes about 2 cups (500 mL)

✪ Great for Steps 2, 3 and 4

You'll love the contrasts at play in this dish, from its earthy and sweet flavors to its velvety and crisp textures. It proves that pumpkin is far more than pie filling.

Tips

If you use homemade pumpkin purée instead of canned, you'll need about 1¾ cups (425 mL).

Look for roasted green pumpkin seeds that are lightly seasoned with sea salt.

Storage Tip

This spread can be stored in an airtight container in the refrigerator for up to 3 days.

Nutrients per 2 tbsp (30 mL)	
Calories	36
Total fat	2 g
Saturated fat	0 g
Cholesterol	0 mg
Sodium	74 mg
Carbohydrate	3 g
Fiber	1 g
Protein	1 g
Calcium	12 mg
Iron	0.5 mg

- **Food processor**

2	cloves garlic, coarsely chopped	2
1	can (15 oz/425 mL) pumpkin purée (not pie filling)	1
2 tsp	ground cumin	10 mL
¾ tsp	fine sea salt	3 mL
⅛ tsp	cayenne pepper	0.5 mL
3 tbsp	tahini	45 mL
2 tbsp	freshly squeezed lemon juice	30 mL
2 tbsp	lightly salted roasted green pumpkin seeds (pepitas), chopped	30 mL
1 tbsp	chopped fresh flat-leaf (Italian) parsley	15 mL

1. In food processor, combine garlic, pumpkin, cumin, salt, cayenne, tahini and lemon juice; process until smooth. Transfer to a serving dish and sprinkle with pumpkin seeds and parsley.

Superfood Spotlight

Green Pumpkin Seeds (Pepitas) • Green pumpkin seeds, also called pepitas, are a nutritious snack. Even in small servings, they provide a significant amount of zinc and iron. Zinc is an antioxidant mineral that boosts the immune system and, for men, improves fertility and protects against prostate enlargement and cancer. Iron is important for healthy blood cells and energy levels. Their high iron and zinc content make pumpkin seeds a particularly significant food for vegetarians. The seeds also contain sterols, which can help remove LDL ("bad") cholesterol from the body and inhibit the development of breast, colon and prostate cancer cells. In addition, pumpkin seeds contain omega-3 fats, vitamin E, folate and magnesium, all of which can help maintain heart health.

Greek Yogurt Dip with Fresh Squash "Chips"

Makes 20 servings

✪ Great for Steps 1, 2, 3 and 4

Thick, creamy nonfat Greek yogurt tastes every bit as rich and decadent as sour cream, with a fraction of the calories and zero fat. Case in point, this mint and cucumber dip, which finds harmony with zucchini and yellow squash "chips." Adding further appeal, Greek yogurt has double the protein of most yogurts and far less sugar. The lower carbohydrate levels help keep blood sugar on an even keel, making it an ideal between-meals snack.

Storage Tip

The dip can be stored in an airtight container in the refrigerator for up to 3 days. Prepare the vegetable chips the day you plan to eat them.

Nutrients per serving	
Calories	13
Total fat	0 g
Saturated fat	0 g
Cholesterol	0 mg
Sodium	6 mg
Carbohydrate	2 g
Fiber	1 g
Protein	2 g
Calcium	16 mg
Iron	0.1 mg

2	zucchini, cut into 1⁄4-inch (0.5 cm) thick rounds	2
2	yellow summer squash (yellow zucchini), cut into 1⁄4-inch (0.5 cm) thick rounds	2
	Ice water	
	Fine sea salt	
1 cup	finely chopped peeled seeded cucumber	250 mL
1⁄2 cup	packed mint leaves, finely chopped	125 mL
1⁄4 tsp	cracked black pepper	1 mL
1 1⁄4 cups	nonfat plain Greek yogurt	300 mL
1 tsp	finely grated lemon zest	5 mL
2 tsp	freshly squeezed lemon juice	10 mL

1. In a large bowl, combine zucchini and squash. Add enough ice water to cover. Refrigerate for at least 30 minutes or until vegetables are very crisp. Drain and pat dry with paper towels. Sprinkle with 1⁄4 tsp (1 mL) salt.
2. In a medium bowl, combine cucumber, mint, pepper, 1⁄8 tsp (0.5 mL) salt, yogurt, lemon zest and lemon juice. Serve with zucchini and squash "chips" for dipping.

Creamy Cashew Maple Dip with Apples

Makes 8 servings

✪ Great for Steps 1, 2, 3 and 4

Newsflash: eating this creamy, dreamy dip could help lower the risk of weight gain. Although nuts are known to provide a variety of cardio-protective benefits, many people eschew them for fear of weight gain. A study published in the journal Obesity, *however, shows that such fears are groundless. In fact, people who eat nuts, including cashews, at least twice a week are much less likely to gain weight than those who almost never eat nuts. Dippity-do-da!*

Storage Tip

This dip can be stored in an airtight container in the refrigerator for up to 1 week. The apples are best prepared just before serving.

Nutrients per serving	
Calories	92
Total fat	4 g
Saturated fat	1 g
Cholesterol	0 mg
Sodium	91 mg
Carbohydrate	14 g
Fiber	2 g
Protein	2 g
Calcium	11 mg
Iron	0.6 mg

- **Blender or food processor**

3	tart-sweet apples (such as Gala, Braeburn or Honeycrisp), cored and each cut into 8 slices	3
	Ice water	
½ cup	cashews	125 mL
Pinch	fine sea salt	Pinch
½ cup	water	125 mL
1 tbsp	pure maple syrup	15 mL
½ tsp	vanilla extract	2 mL

1. Place apple slices in a large bowl and add enough ice water to cover. Refrigerate for at least 30 minutes or until apples are very crisp. Drain and pat dry with paper towels.
2. In blender, combine cashews, salt, water, maple syrup and vanilla; blend until very smooth and creamy.
3. Transfer dip to a serving dish. Serve with apple slices for dipping.

Swiss Chard Spring Rolls with Sesame Lime Dipping Sauce

Makes 8 rolls

✪ Great for Steps 1, 2 and 4

Workaday Swiss chard leaves are transformed into elegant spring rolls stuffed with gorgeous ingredients from the garden. A tamari and lime dipping sauce makes an easy accompaniment.

Tip

Use the coarse side of a box cheese grater to shred the carrots and beets. Or, to make quick work of the task, use the shredding disk on a food processor. To prevent the carrots from turning purple, shred them first, then measure them, then shred the beets.

Nutrients per roll

Calories	42
Total fat	1 g
Saturated fat	0 g
Cholesterol	0 mg
Sodium	625 mg
Carbohydrate	7 g
Fiber	2 g
Protein	2 g
Calcium	37 mg
Iron	1.3 mg

Dipping Sauce

1/4 cup	reduced-sodium tamari or soy sauce	60 mL
2 tbsp	freshly squeezed lime juice	30 mL
2 tsp	toasted sesame oil	10 mL
2 tsp	brown rice syrup or liquid honey	10 mL
1/4 tsp	ground ginger	1 mL

Rolls

8	Swiss chard leaves, tough stems trimmed off	8
3/4 cup	shredded carrots	175 mL
3/4 cup	shredded peeled beets	175 mL
3/4 cup	mung bean sprouts or sunflower sprouts	175 mL
1/2 cup	packed fresh basil leaves	125 mL

1. *Sauce:* In a small bowl, whisk together tamari, lime juice, oil, brown rice syrup and ginger.
2. *Spring Rolls:* Place Swiss chard leaves on a work surface. Fill each with an equal amount of carrots, beets, sprouts and basil. Roll leaves around filling, tucking in edges. Serve immediately, with sauce, or store loosely covered in the refrigerator for up to 4 hours.

▸ Health Note

Tamari provides niacin (vitamin B_3), manganese and tryptophan. The latter is an amino acid responsible for a variety of health functions, including nitrogen balance in adults and the production of serotonin, which is thought to improve both mood and sleep patterns.

Spinach-Stuffed Mushrooms

Makes 6 servings

✪ Great for Steps 1, 2 and 4

Spinach and mushrooms go hand in hand, especially when cheese is added to the mix.

Tip

When selecting mushrooms, choose those with a fresh, smooth appearance, free from major blemishes and with a dry surface. Once home, keep mushrooms refrigerated; they're best when used within several days of purchase. When ready to use, gently wipe mushrooms with a damp cloth or soft brush to remove dirt. Alternatively, rinse them quickly with cold water, then immediately pat dry with paper towels.

Nutrients per serving	
Calories	127
Total fat	7 g
Saturated fat	4 g
Cholesterol	19 mg
Sodium	414 mg
Carbohydrate	12 g
Fiber	4 g
Protein	9 g
Calcium	253 mg
Iron	2.2 mg

- **Preheat oven to 350°F (180°C)**
- **Rimmed baking sheet, lined with parchment paper**

2 tsp	extra virgin olive oil	10 mL
1 lb	cremini mushrooms, stems removed and finely chopped, caps left intact	500 g
1¼ cups	chopped onions	300 mL
¼ tsp	fine sea salt	1 mL
⅛ tsp	freshly ground black pepper	0.5 mL
1 lb	frozen spinach, thawed and excess water squeezed out	500 g
4 oz	feta cheese, crumbled	125 g

1. In a large skillet, heat oil over medium-high heat. Add mushroom stems, onions, salt and pepper; cook, stirring occasionally, for 8 to 10 minutes or until vegetables are softened. Transfer to a large bowl and let cool.
2. Add spinach and feta to onion mixture and stir until combined.
3. Arrange mushroom caps, hollow side up, in a single layer on prepared baking sheet. Divide spinach mixture evenly among mushrooms, mounding it in the center of each.
4. Bake in preheated oven for 18 to 22 minutes or until mushrooms are browned. Let cool in pan on a wire rack for 5 minutes before serving.

Herbed Deviled Eggs

Makes 8 servings

✪ Great for Step 4

Mayonnaise is a traditional component of deviled egg fillings, but replacing it with Greek yogurt lightens this into a healthy snack and adds another layer of flavor.

Variation

Southern Deviled Eggs: Omit the basil and add 1 tbsp (15 mL) sweet pickle relish to the egg yolk mixture. Garnish tops of eggs with 1/4 tsp (1 mL) sweet paprika.

4	large eggs	4
	Cold water	
	Ice water	
1 tbsp	finely chopped fresh basil, parsley or dill	15 mL
1/4 tsp	fine sea salt	1 mL
1/4 tsp	freshly ground black pepper	1 mL
3 tbsp	nonfat plain Greek yogurt	45 mL
1 tsp	Dijon mustard	5 mL

1. Place eggs in a medium saucepan and add enough cold water to cover by 1 inch (2.5 cm). Bring to a boil over medium-high heat. Remove from heat, cover and let stand for 13 minutes. Drain and transfer eggs to a bowl of ice water. Let stand until cool.
2. Peel eggs and cut in half lengthwise. Transfer yolks to a medium bowl and mash with a fork until smooth. Stir in basil, salt, pepper, yogurt and mustard.
3. Place egg whites, hollow side up, on a serving plate. Spoon yolk mixture into egg whites, dividing evenly. Cover and refrigerate for at least 15 minutes, until filling is set, or for up to 24 hours.

Nutrients per serving	
Calories	41
Total fat	2 g
Saturated fat	1 g
Cholesterol	90 mg
Sodium	123 mg
Carbohydrate	1 g
Fiber	0 g
Protein	4 g
Calcium	17 mg
Iron	0.5 mg

Salads

Waldorf Salad . . . 114
Swiss Chard, Cherry and Pecan Salad . . . 115
Spinach, Avocado and Orange Salad . . . 115
Fennel, Orange and Olive Salad . . . 116
Arugula, Watermelon and Feta Salad . . . 117
Mesclun Salad with Dates and Goat Cheese . . . 117
Roasted Beet and Beet Greens Salad . . . 118
Bok Choy Salad with Miso Ginger Dressing . . . 119
Chopped Greek Salad . . . 119
Brussels Sprouts Salad with Maple Mustard Dressing . . . 120
Warm Cauliflower and Parsley Salad . . . 121
Roasted Cauliflower and Radicchio Salad . . . 122
Chard and Red Pepper Salad with Tahini Yogurt Dressing . . . 123
Edamame and Corn Salad . . . 124
Green Pea and Radish Salad . . . 124
Green Bean Salad with Toasted Hazelnuts . . . 125
Turkish Tomato, Pepper and Herb Salad . . . 126
Napa Cabbage and Ginger Slaw . . . 127
Winter Red Cabbage Slaw . . . 127
Kale, Apple and Walnut Slaw . . . 128
Lemony Brussels Sprouts Slaw . . . 128
Broccoli Carrot Slaw with Cranberries and Sunflower Seeds . . . 129
Shredded Beet, Carrot and Mint Salad . . . 129
Moroccan Carrot Salad . . . 130
Healthy Know-How: The Raw Food Diet . . . 131
Shaved Beet Salad with Pistachios and Goat Cheese . . . 132
Minted Sprout Salad . . . 132
Mustard Dill Red Potato Salad . . . 133
Southwestern Sweet Potato Salad . . . 133
Sweet Potato, Lentil and Arugula Salad . . . 134
Winter White Bean, Cauliflower and Arugula Salad . . . 135

Spicy Three-Bean Salad 136
Zucchini and Chickpea Salad 136
Persian Brown Rice and Cashew Salad 137
California Sushi Roll Salad 138
French Green Bean, Barley and Tomato Salad 139
Barley, Parsley and Walnut Salad 140
Tabbouleh 141
Bulgur Salad with Oranges, Cashews and Fresh Mint 142
Lentil and Bulgur Salad with Grapes and Mint 143
Pistachio and Citrus Couscous Salad 144
Middle Eastern Couscous, Date and Chickpea Salad 145
Farro Salad with Arugula and Tomatoes 146
Quinoa and Black Bean Salad 147
Lemony Lentil and Quinoa Salad 148
Pomegranate and Quinoa Salad with Sunflower Seeds 149
Indian-Spiced Quinoa, Watercress and Chickpea Salad 150
Wheat Berry, Pecan and Cherry Salad 151
Soba and Tofu Salad with Carrot Miso Dressing 152
Sesame Peanut Vegetable Noodle Salad 153
Garden Pasta Salad 154
Orzo Salad with Fennel, Radishes and Goat Cheese 155
Healthy Know-How: Organic Vs. Natural 156
Provençal Chicken and Orzo Salad 157
Thai Chicken Salad 158
Summer Salmon Panzanella 159
Balsamic Tuna Salad in Avocado Halves 160
Tuna and White Bean Salad 160
Sicilian Tuna and Rice Salad 161
Crab and Papaya Salad with Mint Dressing 162
Shrimp, Grapefruit and Watercress Salad 163

Waldorf Salad

Makes 6 side-dish servings

✪ Great for Steps 1, 2, 3 and 4

A mustard-enhanced, creamy dressing and the earthy crunch of sunflower seeds are wonderful foils for apples, grapes and dried cherries in this updated version of classic Waldorf salad. The skin of red grapes contains the protective chemical resveratrol, which may sharpen your brain and reduce your risk for both heart disease and cancer.

1/2 cup	nonfat plain Greek yogurt	125 mL
2 tbsp	mayonnaise	30 mL
2 tsp	Dijon mustard	10 mL
2 tsp	liquid honey	10 mL
4	Granny Smith or other tart apples, peeled and diced	4
1 1/2 cups	thinly sliced celery	375 mL
1 1/2 cups	red seedless grapes, halved	375 mL
3 tbsp	dried cherries, chopped	45 mL
2	small heads Belgian endive, leaves separated (optional)	2
3 tbsp	roasted sunflower seeds (optional)	45 mL

1. In a small bowl, whisk together yogurt, mayonnaise, mustard and honey.
2. In a large bowl, combine apples, celery, grapes and cherries. Add dressing and gently toss to coat. Cover and refrigerate for at least 30 minutes, until chilled, or for up to 2 hours.
3. If desired, serve on endive leaves, sprinkled with sunflower seeds.

Superfood Spotlight

Belgian Endive • Endive leaves, with their slightly bitter, distinctive flavor, make an ideal addition to a salad. Belgian endive is protected from light as it grows, because keeping it in the dark prohibits chlorophyll production, making it more palatable; otherwise, it would be almost too bitter to eat. But bitterness has its benefits: in this case, the bitter flavor comes from coumarin and lactucin, anti-inflammatory chemicals that can relieve gout and arthritis and are said to be sedative. In addition, endive contains a type of fiber called inulin, which acts as a prebiotic in the digestive system, stimulating the "good" bacteria essential for gut health. Inulin also helps regulate blood sugar levels, boosts the immune system and can increase HDL ("good") cholesterol and reduce LDL ("bad") cholesterol.

Nutrients per serving

Calories	92
Total fat	2 g
Saturated fat	0 g
Cholesterol	1 mg
Sodium	84 mg
Carbohydrate	18 g
Fiber	2 g
Protein	2 g
Calcium	29 mg
Iron	0.1 mg

Swiss Chard, Cherry and Pecan Salad

Makes 4 side-dish servings

✪ Great for Steps 1, 2, 3 and 4

Nutrients per serving	
Calories	100
Total fat	7 g
Saturated fat	1 g
Cholesterol	0 mg
Sodium	272 mg
Carbohydrate	9 g
Fiber	2 g
Protein	1 g
Calcium	34 mg
Iron	1.1 mg

1 tbsp	extra virgin olive oil	15 mL
1 tbsp	pure maple syrup	15 mL
1 tbsp	sherry vinegar or white wine vinegar	15 mL
1/4 tsp	fine sea salt	1 mL
1	large bunch red Swiss chard, ribs removed, leaves thinly sliced crosswise (about 5 cups/1.25 L)	1
2 tbsp	dried tart or sweet cherries, chopped	30 mL
3 tbsp	chopped toasted pecans	45 mL

1. In a small bowl, whisk together oil, maple syrup, vinegar and salt.
2. In a large bowl, combine Swiss chard and cherries. Add dressing and gently toss to coat. Let stand for 10 minutes to blend the flavors. Sprinkle with pecans.

Spinach, Avocado and Orange Salad

Makes 6 side-dish servings

✪ Great for Steps 1, 2, 3 and 4

Nutrients per serving	
Calories	169
Total fat	12 g
Saturated fat	2 g
Cholesterol	0 mg
Sodium	152 mg
Carbohydrate	17 g
Fiber	4 g
Protein	2 g
Calcium	43 mg
Iron	1.2 mg

1/2 tsp	ground cumin	2 mL
1/8 tsp	fine sea salt	0.5 mL
3 tbsp	extra virgin olive oil	45 mL
2 tbsp	freshly squeezed lime juice	30 mL
1 tbsp	liquid honey or agave nectar	15 mL
1/2 tsp	Dijon mustard	2 mL
2	large oranges	2
1	package (6 oz/175 g) baby spinach	1
1	small firm-ripe Hass avocado, diced	1
1 cup	matchstick-size strips peeled jicama	250 mL
1/4 cup	chopped red onion	60 mL
2 tbsp	chopped fresh mint	30 mL

1. In a small bowl, whisk together cumin, salt, oil, lime juice, honey and mustard.
2. Using a sharp knife, cut peel and pith from oranges. Quarter oranges and cut crosswise into thin slices.
3. In a large bowl, combine orange slices, spinach, avocado, jicama, red onion and mint. Add dressing and gently toss to coat.

Fennel, Orange and Olive Salad

Makes 6 side-dish servings

✪ Great for Steps 1, 2 and 4

Unmistakable for its delicate crunch and licorice undertones, fresh fennel becomes even more enticing when paired with fresh oranges and topped with sweet-hot red onion, cooling mint and briny olives.

Tip

To prepare the fennel bulb, trim off the tough stalks from the top and the bottom root end before cutting the bulb in half. Chop any feathery fronds from the stalks and sprinkle on top of the salad with the olives, if desired. If the outer layers of the bulb are tough and stringy, you can discard them or peel off the outer layer with a sharp vegetable peeler.

Nutrients per serving	
Calories	100
Total fat	6 g
Saturated fat	1 g
Cholesterol	0 mg
Sodium	151 mg
Carbohydrate	12 g
Fiber	3 g
Protein	1 g
Calcium	60 mg
Iron	0.8 mg

2	large oranges	2
1	large bulb fennel, halved lengthwise, cored and very thinly sliced crosswise	1
1/2 cup	very thinly sliced red onion	125 mL
1/3 cup	packed fresh mint leaves, torn	75 mL
1/8 tsp	fine sea salt	0.5 mL
1/8 tsp	cracked black pepper	0.5 mL
2 tbsp	extra virgin olive oil	30 mL
1/2 cup	pitted brine-cured black olives (such as kalamata), quartered	125 mL

1. Using a sharp knife, cut peel and pith from oranges. Working over a large bowl, cut between membranes to release segments. Squeeze the membranes to release any remaining juice into the bowl.
2. To the oranges, add fennel, red onion, mint, salt, pepper and oil, gently tossing to combine. Sprinkle with olives.

Superfood Spotlight

Oranges • Oranges are one of the least expensive and most readily available sources of vitamin C, which boosts the immune system and protects against cell damage, aging and disease. They are also a good source of fiber, folate and potassium, as well as calcium, which is vital for bone maintenance. They contain the carotenes zeaxanthin and lutein, which can help maintain eye health and protect against macular degeneration; rutin, a flavonoid that can help slow down or prevent the growth of tumors; and nobiletin, an anti-inflammatory compound. All of these plant compounds also help vitamin C to work more effectively.

Arugula, Watermelon and Feta Salad

Makes 6 side-dish servings

✪ Great for Steps 1, 2 and 4

Nutrients per serving	
Calories	64
Total fat	2 g
Saturated fat	1 g
Cholesterol	6 mg
Sodium	130 mg
Carbohydrate	14 g
Fiber	1 g
Protein	2 g
Calcium	86 mg
Iron	0.9 mg

2 tbsp	balsamic vinegar	30 mL
1 tbsp	dark (cooking) molasses	15 mL
1⁄8 tsp	fine sea salt	0.5 mL
1⁄8 tsp	cracked black pepper	0.5 mL
8 cups	packed baby arugula (about 5 oz/150 g)	2 L
4 cups	cubed seedless watermelon (3⁄4-inch/2 cm cubes)	1 L
1⁄4 cup	crumbled feta cheese	60 mL

1. In a small bowl, whisk together vinegar, molasses, salt and pepper.
2. Arrange arugula on a large platter. Scatter watermelon over top, then feta. Drizzle with dressing.

Mesclun Salad with Dates and Goat Cheese

Makes 4 side-dish servings

✪ Great for Steps 1, 2 and 4

Nutrients per serving	
Calories	118
Total fat	9 g
Saturated fat	2 g
Cholesterol	3 mg
Sodium	75 mg
Carbohydrate	10 g
Fiber	2 g
Protein	3 g
Calcium	46 mg
Iron	1.3 mg

2 tbsp	extra virgin olive oil	30 mL
1 tbsp	red wine vinegar	15 mL
1 tsp	reduced-sodium tamari or soy sauce	5 mL
1⁄8 tsp	freshly ground black pepper	0.5 mL
6 cups	mesclun (mixed baby lettuce)	1.5 L
1⁄2 cup	pitted Medjool dates (or other soft, fresh dates), quartered lengthwise	125 mL
3 tbsp	crumbled soft goat cheese	45 mL

1. In a small bowl, whisk together oil, vinegar, tamari and pepper.
2. Place mesclun in a large bowl. Add dressing and gently toss to coat. Add dates and goat cheese; gently toss to combine.

Roasted Beet and Beet Greens Salad

Makes 4 side-dish servings

✪ Great for Steps 1, 2 and 4

Sweet oranges balance the earthiness of beet greens and roasted beets. A garlicky dressing lends a slight Mediterranean edge.

Tip

Any type of beet (red, golden or red-and-white-striped Chioggia) would be great in this salad. To avoid stained hands, wear plastic gloves when peeling dark-colored beets.

Nutrients per serving

Calories	137
Total fat	7 g
Saturated fat	1 g
Cholesterol	0 mg
Sodium	350 mg
Carbohydrate	18 g
Fiber	4 g
Protein	2 g
Calcium	43 mg
Iron	0.8 mg

- **Preheat oven to 400°F (200°C)**
- **Large rimmed baking sheet**

4	beets, with greens attached (about 1½ lbs/750 g)	4
2	oranges	2
2	cloves garlic, minced	2
½ cup	thinly sliced red onion	125 mL
½ tsp	fine sea salt	2 mL
2 tbsp	extra virgin olive oil	30 mL
1 tbsp	red wine vinegar	15 mL

1. Trim greens from beets. Cut off and discard stems, then coarsely chop leaves. Set beet greens aside.
2. Tightly wrap each beet in foil and place on baking sheet. Roast in preheated oven for about 90 minutes or until tender when pierced with a fork. Let cool completely in foil on baking sheet.
3. Meanwhile, in a large saucepan of boiling water, cook beet greens for 2 to 3 minutes or until tender. Drain, then let cool completely.
4. Peel beets and cut each into 8 wedges. Place beets in a medium bowl.
5. Squeeze beet greens to remove any excess water, then add to beets.
6. Grate 1 tsp (5 mL) zest from oranges. Add to beet mixture, along with garlic, red onion, salt, oil and vinegar.
7. Using a sharp knife, cut peel and pith from oranges. Working over the beet mixture, cut between membranes to release segments. Squeeze the membranes to release any remaining juice. Gently toss to coat. Let stand for at least 30 minutes or overnight to blend the flavors.

Bok Choy Salad with Miso Ginger Dressing

Makes 4 side-dish servings

✪ Great for Steps 1, 2 and 4

Nutrients per serving	
Calories	45
Total fat	4 g
Saturated fat	0 g
Cholesterol	0 mg
Sodium	113 mg
Carbohydrate	3 g
Fiber	0 g
Protein	1 g
Calcium	13 mg
Iron	0.2 mg

2 tsp	minced gingerroot	10 mL
1½ tbsp	unseasoned rice vinegar	22 mL
2 tsp	white or yellow miso	10 mL
2 tsp	vegetable oil	10 mL
1 tsp	liquid honey or agave nectar	5 mL
6 cups	sliced bok choy (about 1 large)	1.5 L
1 tbsp	toasted sesame seeds (see tip, page 426)	15 mL

1. In a small bowl, whisk together ginger, vinegar, miso, oil and honey.
2. Place bok choy in a large bowl. Add dressing and gently toss to coat. Sprinkle with sesame seeds.

Chopped Greek Salad

Makes 6 side-dish servings

✪ Great for Steps 1, 2, 3 and 4

Nutrients per serving	
Calories	167
Total fat	10 g
Saturated fat	3 g
Cholesterol	12 mg
Sodium	431 mg
Carbohydrate	16 g
Fiber	4 g
Protein	6 g
Calcium	102 mg
Iron	1.5 mg

2 tbsp	freshly squeezed lemon juice	30 mL
2 tbsp	extra virgin olive oil	30 mL
¼ tsp	freshly cracked black pepper	1 mL
⅛ tsp	fine sea salt	0.5 mL
1	can (14 to 19 oz/398 to 540 mL) chickpeas, drained and rinsed	1
1	cucumber, peeled, seeded and cubed	1
1	small red bell pepper, chopped	1
2 cups	coarsely chopped romaine lettuce	500 mL
1 cup	halved grape tomatoes	250 mL
½ cup	finely chopped red onion	125 mL
½ cup	pitted brine-cured black olives (such as kalamata), roughly chopped	125 mL
½ cup	coarsely crumbled feta cheese	125 mL

1. In a small bowl, whisk together lemon juice, oil, pepper and salt.
2. In a large bowl, combine chickpeas, cucumber, red pepper, romaine, tomatoes, red onion and olives. Add dressing and gently toss to coat. Sprinkle with feta.

Brussels Sprouts Salad with Maple Mustard Dressing

Makes 6 side-dish servings

✪ Great for Steps 1, 2, 3 and 4

Mustard's tangy flavor is unmistakable. Here, a generous spoonful mingles with maple syrup to cast a spell over lightly steamed Brussels sprouts, resulting in a simply perfect side dish for a winter night.

Tip

Trim the root end from Brussels sprouts and cut off any loose, thick outer leaves, then rinse well to remove any grit that may have gathered under loose leaves.

Nutrients per serving	
Calories	120
Total fat	6 g
Saturated fat	1 g
Cholesterol	0 mg
Sodium	184 mg
Carbohydrate	16 g
Fiber	5 g
Protein	4 g
Calcium	58 mg
Iron	1.7 mg

- **Steamer basket**

1½ lbs	Brussels sprouts, trimmed	750 g
	Ice water	
2 tbsp	pure maple syrup	30 mL
1 tbsp	whole-grain Dijon mustard	15 mL
1 tbsp	cider vinegar	15 mL
1 tbsp	extra virgin olive oil	15 mL
¼ tsp	fine sea salt	1 mL
⅛ tsp	freshly cracked black pepper	0.5 mL
¼ cup	chopped toasted pecans	60 mL

1. Place Brussels sprouts in a steamer basket set over a large pot of boiling water. Cover and steam for 5 to 6 minutes or until tender-crisp but still bright green. Transfer to a large bowl of ice water to stop the cooking. Drain and pat dry with paper towels.
2. In a small bowl, whisk together maple syrup, mustard, vinegar, oil, salt and pepper.
3. Using a very sharp knife or a mandoline, thinly slice Brussels sprouts lengthwise. Transfer to a large bowl, add dressing and gently toss to coat. Cover and refrigerate for at least 30 minutes, until chilled, or for up to 2 hours. Just before serving, sprinkle with pecans.

▶ Health Note

Mustard is a very good source of selenium, a nutrient that has been shown to reduce the severity of asthma, decrease some of the symptoms of rheumatoid arthritis and help prevent cancer.

Warm Cauliflower and Parsley Salad

Makes 6 side-dish servings

✪ Great for Steps 1, 2 and 4

Steamed cauliflower gets jazzed up with golden raisins, fresh parsley and a piquant caper vinaigrette.

Tip

To mash garlic, working with one clove at a time, place the side of a chef's knife flat against the clove. Place the heel of your hand on the side of the knife and apply pressure so that the clove flattens slightly (this will loosen the peel). Remove and discard the peel, then roughly chop the garlic. Sprinkle a pinch of coarse salt over the garlic. Use the flat part of the knife as before to press the garlic against the cutting board. Repeat until the garlic turns into a fine paste.

Nutrients per serving	
Calories	45
Total fat	0 g
Saturated fat	0 g
Cholesterol	0 mg
Sodium	111 mg
Carbohydrate	10 g
Fiber	2 g
Protein	2 g
Calcium	30 mg
Iron	0.9 mg

- **Steamer basket**

4 cups	small cauliflower florets (about 1 medium head)	1 L
2	cloves garlic, mashed (see tip, at left)	2
1/4 tsp	freshly cracked black pepper	1 mL
2 tbsp	drained capers, minced	30 mL
2 tbsp	extra virgin olive oil	30 mL
2 tbsp	freshly squeezed lemon juice	30 mL
1/4 cup	golden raisins	60 mL
1/2 cup	firmly packed fresh flat-leaf (Italian) parsley leaves, roughly chopped	125 mL

1. Place cauliflower in a steamer basket set over a large pot of boiling water. Cover and steam for 4 to 5 minutes or until tender-crisp. Drain and pat dry with paper towels.
2. In a small bowl, whisk together garlic, pepper, capers, oil and lemon juice.
3. In a large bowl, combine cauliflower and raisins. Add dressing and gently toss to coat. Let cool for 15 minutes. Add parsley and gently toss to combine. Serve immediately.

Variation

Instead of steaming the cauliflower, roast it (see step 1 on page 122).

Roasted Cauliflower and Radicchio Salad

Makes 6 side-dish servings

✪ Great for Steps 1, 2, 3 and 4

A zesty sherry vinegar and mustard dressing brings out the best in nutty roasted cauliflower and bitter radicchio.

Tip

See page 29 for instructions on toasting nuts.

Nutrients per serving	
Calories	86
Total fat	7 g
Saturated fat	1 g
Cholesterol	0 mg
Sodium	261 mg
Carbohydrate	5 g
Fiber	2 g
Protein	3 g
Calcium	33 mg
Iron	1.1 mg

- **Preheat oven to 450°F (230°C)**
- **Large rimmed baking sheet, lined with parchment paper or foil**

4 cups	small cauliflower florets (about 1 medium head)	1 L
½ tsp	fine sea salt, divided	2 mL
¼ tsp	freshly ground black pepper	1 mL
2 tbsp	extra virgin olive oil, divided	30 mL
1 tbsp	sherry vinegar	15 mL
½ tsp	whole-grain Dijon mustard	2 mL
1	large head radicchio, cut crosswise into ¼-inch (0.5 cm) wide strips	1
1 cup	packed fresh flat-leaf (Italian) parsley leaves, roughly chopped	250 mL
3 tbsp	chopped toasted walnuts	45 mL

1. In a large bowl, toss cauliflower with half the salt, pepper and half the oil. Spread in a single layer on prepared baking sheet. Roast in preheated oven for 35 to 40 minutes, stirring once or twice, until tender and golden brown. Let cool slightly in pan on a wire rack.
2. In a small bowl, whisk together the remaining salt, the remaining oil, vinegar and mustard.
3. In a large bowl, combine warm cauliflower, radicchio and parsley. Add dressing and gently toss to coat. Sprinkle with walnuts.

Superfood Spotlight

Radicchio • Radicchio (sometimes called Italian chicory) has a strong, slightly bitter flavor. The astringent taste awakens the palate and promotes the secretion of hydrochloric acid, which aids digestion. Radicchio is rich in phenolic compounds, including quercetin glycosides (which help prevent precancerous substances from damaging the body) and anthocyanins (which protect against cancer and heart disease). The total phenolic content in red varieties of radicchio is about four to five times higher than in green varieties. Radicchio also contains good amounts of vitamin C, potassium and folate.

Chard and Red Pepper Salad with Tahini Yogurt Dressing

Makes 6 side-dish servings

✪ Great for Steps 1, 2, 3 and 4

A salad enriched with Swiss chard, roasted red peppers and a tangy dressing is wonderful for welcoming the cooler fall weather.

1 tbsp	extra virgin olive oil	15 mL
3	cloves garlic, minced	3
1	large bunch red Swiss chard, ribs removed, leaves thinly sliced crosswise (about 5 cups/1.25 L)	1
¼ tsp	fine sea salt, divided	1 mL
1 cup	finely chopped drained roasted red bell peppers	250 mL
½ cup	nonfat plain yogurt	125 mL
2 tbsp	tahini	30 mL
1 tbsp	freshly squeezed lemon juice	15 mL
⅛ tsp	cayenne pepper	0.5 mL

1. In a large skillet, heat oil over medium heat. Add garlic and cook, stirring, for 1 minute or until golden and fragrant. Add Swiss chard and half the salt; cook, stirring, for 6 to 8 minutes or until tender Add roasted peppers and cook, stirring, for 1 minute. Transfer vegetables to a platter, spread in a single layer and let cool completely.
2. In a small bowl, whisk together yogurt, tahini, lemon juice, cayenne and the remaining salt. Spoon dressing over salad.

Nutrients per serving	
Calories	75
Total fat	5 g
Saturated fat	1 g
Cholesterol	0 mg
Sodium	176 mg
Carbohydrate	6 g
Fiber	1 g
Protein	3 g
Calcium	65 mg
Iron	0.9 mg

Edamame and Corn Salad

Makes 8 side-dish servings

✪ Great for Steps 1, 2, 3 and 4

Nutrients per serving	
Calories	114
Total fat	5 g
Saturated fat	1 g
Cholesterol	0 mg
Sodium	78 mg
Carbohydrate	14 g
Fiber	3 g
Protein	5 g
Calcium	31 mg
Iron	1.5 mg

1½ cups	frozen shelled edamame	375 mL
2 tsp	dried oregano	10 mL
¼ tsp	fine sea salt	1 mL
¼ tsp	cracked black pepper	1 mL
2 tbsp	extra virgin olive oil	30 mL
2 tbsp	cider vinegar	30 mL
1	red bell pepper, coarsely chopped	1
2 cups	fresh or thawed frozen corn kernels	500 mL
½ cup	chopped green onions	125 mL
½ cup	packed fresh parsley leaves, chopped	125 mL

1. In a medium saucepan of boiling water, cook edamame over medium-high heat for 4 to 6 minutes or until bright green and tender. Drain and rinse under cold water.
2. In a small bowl, whisk together oregano, salt, pepper, oil and vinegar.
3. In a large bowl, combine edamame, red pepper, corn and green onions. Add dressing and gently toss to coat. Cover and refrigerate for 1 to 4 hours, until chilled. Just before serving, add parsley and toss to combine.

Green Pea and Radish Salad

Makes 4 side-dish servings

✪ Great for Steps 1, 2 and 4

Nutrients per serving	
Calories	97
Total fat	4 g
Saturated fat	1 g
Cholesterol	0 mg
Sodium	205 mg
Carbohydrate	12 g
Fiber	5 g
Protein	4 g
Calcium	25 mg
Iron	1.5 mg

2 tsp	minced fresh tarragon	10 mL
¼ tsp	fine sea salt	1 mL
1 tbsp	extra virgin olive oil	15 mL
2 tsp	white wine vinegar	10 mL
2 cups	frozen petite peas, thawed	500 mL
½ cup	chopped red radishes	125 mL
¼ cup	thinly sliced green onions	60 mL

1. In a small bowl, whisk together tarragon, salt, oil and vinegar.
2. In a large bowl, combine peas, radishes and green onions. Add dressing and gently toss to coat.

Green Bean Salad with Toasted Hazelnuts

Makes 6 side-dish servings

✪ Great for Steps 1, 2, 3 and 4

Simply prepared with a short list of ingredients, this salad is a case study in understated elegance.

- **Steamer basket**

12 oz	green beans, trimmed and halved crosswise	375 g
	Ice water	
1 tbsp	extra virgin olive oil	15 mL
1 tsp	whole-grain Dijon mustard	5 mL
1 tsp	sherry vinegar or white wine vinegar	5 mL
1⁄8 tsp	fine sea salt	0.5 mL
1⁄4 cup	finely chopped red onion	60 mL
2 tbsp	chopped toasted hazelnuts	30 mL

1. Place green beans in a steamer basket set over a large pot of boiling water. Cover and steam for 4 to 6 minutes or until tender. Transfer to a large bowl of ice water to stop the cooking. Drain and pat dry with paper towels.
2. In a small bowl, whisk together oil, mustard, vinegar and salt.
3. In a large bowl, combine green beans and red onion. Add dressing and gently toss to coat. Cover and refrigerate for at least 30 minutes, until chilled, or for up to 2 hours. Sprinkle with hazelnuts just before serving.

Superfood Spotlight

Hazelnuts • Hazelnuts are a good source of protein and monounsaturated fats, which have been shown to reduce "bad" cholesterol in the blood and even slightly raise "good" cholesterol. They are high in beta-sitosterol, a plant fat that can help reduce an enlarged prostate and lower cholesterol. Hazelnuts are also very high in vitamin E, an antioxidant that plays a role in maintaining skin and heart health and can boost the immune system. Their potassium helps control blood pressure and is a diuretic, and their magnesium contributes to heart health and bone strength.

Nutrients per serving

Calories	52
Total fat	4 g
Saturated fat	1 g
Cholesterol	0 mg
Sodium	74 mg
Carbohydrate	4 g
Fiber	2 g
Protein	2 g
Calcium	5 mg
Iron	0.1 mg

Turkish Tomato, Pepper and Herb Salad

Makes 6 side-dish servings

✪ Great for Steps 1, 2 and 4

A familiar offering at Turkish cafés and street vendors, this lively play of fresh, smoky, citrusy and peppery is a celebration of summer produce.

1/2 tsp	hot smoked paprika	2 mL
1/4 tsp	fine sea salt	1 mL
2 tbsp	extra virgin olive oil	30 mL
2 tsp	finely grated lemon zest	10 mL
2 tbsp	freshly squeezed lemon juice	30 mL
1	cucumber, peeled, seeded and thinly sliced	1
2 cups	halved cherry or grape tomatoes	500 mL
1 cup	packed arugula, roughly chopped	250 mL
1 cup	packed fresh flat-leaf (Italian) parsley leaves, roughly chopped	250 mL
1/2 cup	roughly chopped drained roasted red bell peppers	125 mL
1/2 cup	chopped green onions	125 mL
1/4 cup	packed fresh mint leaves, roughly chopped	60 mL
2 tbsp	drained capers (optional)	30 mL

1. In a small bowl, whisk together paprika, salt, oil, lemon zest and lemon juice.
2. In a large bowl, combine cucumber, tomatoes, arugula, parsley, roasted peppers, green onions, mint and capers (if using). Add dressing and gently toss to coat. Cover and refrigerate for at least 30 minutes, until chilled, or for up to 2 hours.

Nutrients per serving

Calories	64
Total fat	5 g
Saturated fat	1 g
Cholesterol	0 mg
Sodium	127 mg
Carbohydrate	5 g
Fiber	2 g
Protein	1 g
Calcium	33 mg
Iron	1.3 mg

Napa Cabbage and Ginger Slaw

Makes 6 side-dish servings

✪ Great for Steps 1, 2 and 4

Nutrients per serving	
Calories	64
Total fat	4 g
Saturated fat	0 g
Cholesterol	0 mg
Sodium	70 mg
Carbohydrate	7 g
Fiber	2 g
Protein	1 g
Calcium	46 mg
Iron	0.6 mg

2 tsp	grated gingerroot	10 mL
1 tsp	minced serrano chile pepper	5 mL
1⁄8 tsp	fine sea salt	0.5 mL
3 tbsp	unseasoned rice vinegar	45 mL
1 1⁄2 tbsp	vegetable oil	22 mL
2 tsp	agave nectar or liquid honey	10 mL
6 cups	sliced napa cabbage (about 1 small head)	1.5 L
1 cup	shredded carrots	250 mL
1 cup	thinly sliced green onions	250 mL
1 cup	packed fresh cilantro leaves (or half cilantro and half mint), chopped	250 mL

1. In a small bowl, whisk together ginger, serrano pepper, salt, vinegar, oil and agave nectar.
2. In a large bowl, combine cabbage, carrots, green onions and cilantro. Add dressing and gently toss to coat. Cover and refrigerate for at least 30 minutes, until chilled, or for up to 2 hours.

Winter Red Cabbage Slaw

Makes 6 side-dish servings

✪ Great for Steps 1, 2, 3 and 4

Nutrients per serving	
Calories	176
Total fat	6 g
Saturated fat	1 g
Cholesterol	0 mg
Sodium	127 mg
Carbohydrate	32 g
Fiber	4 g
Protein	2 g
Calcium	61 mg
Iron	1.1 mg

3 tbsp	red wine vinegar	45 mL
1 tbsp	extra virgin olive oil	15 mL
3 tbsp	liquid honey or agave nectar	45 mL
1⁄4 tsp	fine sea salt	1 mL
1⁄4 tsp	cracked black pepper	1 mL
8 cups	thinly sliced red cabbage	2 L
1⁄3 cup	dried cranberries, chopped	75 mL
2	Granny Smith or other tart apples, peeled and coarsely chopped	2
1⁄4 cup	chopped toasted pecans	60 mL

1. In a small bowl, whisk together vinegar, oil, honey, salt and pepper.
2. In a large bowl, combine cabbage and cranberries. Add dressing and gently toss to coat. Cover and refrigerate for at least 1 hour, until chilled, or for up to 2 hours. Just before serving, add apples and gently toss to combine. Sprinkle with pecans.

Kale, Apple and Walnut Slaw

Makes 4 side-dish servings

✪ Great for Steps 1, 2, 3 and 4

Nutrients per serving	
Calories	145
Total fat	9 g
Saturated fat	1 g
Cholesterol	0 mg
Sodium	216 mg
Carbohydrate	15 g
Fiber	3 g
Protein	3 g
Calcium	180 mg
Iron	3.1 mg

1½ tbsp	extra virgin olive oil	22 mL
2 tsp	sherry vinegar	10 mL
½ tsp	Dijon mustard	2 mL
¼ tsp	fine sea salt	1 mL
1	large bunch kale, stems and ribs removed, leaves very thinly sliced crosswise (about 5 cups/1.25 L)	1
1	large tart-sweet apple (such as Gala, Braeburn or Golden Delicious), halved, cored and very thinly sliced crosswise	1
½ cup	thinly sliced green onions	125 mL
3 tbsp	chopped toasted walnuts	45 mL

1. In a small bowl, whisk together oil, vinegar, mustard and salt.
2. In a large bowl, combine kale, apple and green onions. Add dressing and gently toss to coat. Sprinkle with walnuts.

Lemony Brussels Sprouts Slaw

Makes 6 side-dish servings

✪ Great for Steps 1, 2, 3 and 4

1½ lbs	Brussels sprouts, trimmed	750 g
1½ tbsp	extra virgin olive oil	22 mL
1½ tbsp	freshly squeezed lemon juice	22 mL
½ tsp	Dijon mustard	2 mL
⅛ tsp	fine sea salt	0.5 mL
⅛ tsp	freshly cracked black pepper	0.5 mL
¼ cup	chopped toasted walnuts	60 mL
¼ cup	freshly grated Parmesan cheese	60 mL

1. Using a very sharp knife or a mandoline, very thinly slice Brussels sprouts lengthwise. Use your fingers to separate the leaves.
2. In a small bowl, whisk together oil, lemon juice, mustard, salt and pepper.
3. In a large bowl, combine Brussels sprouts, walnuts and Parmesan. Add dressing and gently toss to coat.

Nutrients per serving	
Calories	136
Total fat	9 g
Saturated fat	2 g
Cholesterol	7 mg
Sodium	156 mg
Carbohydrate	11 g
Fiber	5 g
Protein	6 g
Calcium	118 mg
Iron	1.8 mg

Broccoli Carrot Slaw with Cranberries and Sunflower Seeds

Makes 6 side-dish servings

✪ Great for Steps 1, 2, 3 and 4

Nutrients per serving	
Calories	97
Total fat	3 g
Saturated fat	1 g
Cholesterol	0 mg
Sodium	148 mg
Carbohydrate	14 g
Fiber	2 g
Protein	3 g
Calcium	33 mg
Iron	0.9 mg

1/4 cup	nonfat plain Greek yogurt	60 mL
2 tbsp	freshly squeezed lemon juice	30 mL
1 tbsp	agave nectar or liquid honey	15 mL
2 tsp	Dijon mustard	10 mL
1/8 tsp	fine sea salt	0.5 mL
3 cups	shredded peeled broccoli stems (from 1 large bunch)	750 mL
2 cups	shredded peeled carrots	500 mL
1/2 cup	chopped green onions	125 mL
1/3 cup	dried cranberries, chopped	75 mL
1/4 cup	lightly salted roasted sunflower seeds	60 mL

1. In a small bowl, whisk together yogurt, lemon juice, agave nectar, mustard and salt.
2. In a large bowl, combine broccoli, carrots, green onions and cranberries. Add dressing and gently toss to coat. Cover and refrigerate for at least 30 minutes, until chilled, or for up to 2 hours. Just before serving, sprinkle with sunflower seeds.

Shredded Beet, Carrot and Mint Salad

Makes 4 side-dish servings

✪ Great for Steps 1, 2 and 4

Nutrients per serving	
Calories	132
Total fat	9 g
Saturated fat	1 g
Cholesterol	0 mg
Sodium	222 mg
Carbohydrate	12 g
Fiber	4 g
Protein	2 g
Calcium	49 mg
Iron	1.0 mg

1 tsp	finely grated orange zest	5 mL
2 tbsp	freshly squeezed orange juice	30 mL
2 tbsp	extra virgin olive oil	30 mL
1 tbsp	cider vinegar	15 mL
1/4 tsp	fine sea salt	1 mL
2 cups	coarsely shredded carrots	500 mL
2	beets, peeled and coarsely shredded	2
1/2 cup	packed fresh mint leaves, chopped	125 mL
2 tbsp	toasted sesame seeds (see tip, page 426)	30 mL

1. In a small bowl, whisk together orange zest, orange juice, oil, vinegar and salt.
2. In a large bowl, combine carrots, beets and mint. Add dressing and gently toss to coat. Cover and refrigerate for at least 30 minutes, until chilled, or for up to 4 hours. Just before serving, sprinkle with sesame seeds.

Moroccan Carrot Salad

Makes 6 side-dish servings

✪ Great for Steps 1, 2 and 4

Who knew carrots could be bewitching? They are that and so much more in this classic Moroccan salad made with everyday ingredients.

Variations

Moroccan Carrot, Orange and Mint Salad: Omit the cumin and paprika and increase the cinnamon to 1 tsp (5 mL). Add 1 tbsp (15 mL) finely grated orange zest and 1 tbsp (15 mL) liquid honey to the dressing. Replace the lemon juice with orange juice. In the salad, replace the cilantro with mint.

Turkish Carrot Yogurt Salad: Reduce the lemon juice to 1 tbsp (15 mL) and add 1 cup (250 mL) nonfat plain yogurt to the dressing.

Nutrients per serving	
Calories	104
Total fat	5 g
Saturated fat	1 g
Cholesterol	0 mg
Sodium	171 mg
Carbohydrate	15 g
Fiber	3 g
Protein	1 g
Calcium	36 mg
Iron	0.7 mg

3	cloves garlic, mashed or minced	3
1 tsp	ground cumin	5 mL
1 tsp	sweet paprika	5 mL
1⁄4 tsp	ground cinnamon	1 mL
1⁄4 tsp	fine sea salt	1 mL
1⁄8 tsp	cayenne pepper (optional)	0.5 mL
2 tbsp	extra virgin olive oil	30 mL
2 tbsp	freshly squeezed lemon juice	30 mL
4 cups	coarsely shredded carrots (about 1 lb/500 g)	1 L
3⁄4 cup	packed fresh cilantro or flat-leaf (Italian) parsley leaves, chopped	175 mL
1⁄3 cup	dried currants or raisins	75 mL

1. In a small bowl, whisk together garlic, cumin, paprika, cinnamon, salt, cayenne (if using), oil and lemon juice.
2. In a large bowl, combine carrots, cilantro and currants. Add dressing and gently toss to coat. Cover and refrigerate for at least 1 hour, until chilled, or for up to 4 hours.

Healthy Know-How

The Raw Food Diet

A raw food diet consists of unprocessed, raw, vegan foods that have not been heated above 115°F (46°C). "Raw foodists" believe that foods cooked above this temperature lose their enzymes and thus a significant amount of their nutritional value and are harmful to the body, whereas uncooked foods provide living enzymes and proper nutrition. Proponents of the raw food diet report many benefits, including weight loss, more energy, clear skin, improved digestion and better overall health. Many people eat a "high raw diet" or a diet with a certain percentage of raw foods, such as "75% raw diet." A few people include unprocessed dairy products in their diet, but most raw foodists follow a raw vegan diet.

A raw food diet typically includes raw fruits and vegetables, sprouts, seaweeds, nuts, seeds, fresh herbs and raw spices. Raw foodists also drink fresh fruit and vegetable juices, and most consume a limited amount of foods that have undergone some processing, as long as the processing does not involve heating the foods over 115°F (46°C). Some of these processed raw foods include cold-pressed oils, minimally processed olives (e.g., sun-dried olives), raw nut butters, raw nut "milks," fermented foods such as miso, kimchi and sauerkraut, pure maple syrup, unpasteurized raw soy sauce (*nama shoyu*), dried fruits and vegetables, vinegars and foods cured in vinegar, and unprocessed raw cacao (raw chocolate).

Raw food preparation is often called "uncooking" and relies on dehydrating, juicing or blending foods.

Shaved Beet Salad with Pistachios and Goat Cheese

Makes 4 side-dish servings

✪ Great for Steps 1, 2, 3 and 4

Nutrients per serving	
Calories	161
Total fat	11 g
Saturated fat	3 g
Cholesterol	4 mg
Sodium	246 mg
Carbohydrate	13 g
Fiber	3 g
Protein	4 g
Calcium	63 mg
Iron	1.3 mg

2 tbsp	freshly squeezed lemon juice	30 mL
2 tbsp	extra virgin olive oil	30 mL
2 tsp	agave nectar or liquid honey	10 mL
1/4 tsp	fine sea salt	1 mL
4	orange, yellow or red beets	4
4 cups	packed arugula	1 L
1/4 cup	crumbled soft goat cheese	60 mL
2 tbsp	chopped toasted pistachios	30 mL

1. In a small bowl, whisk together lemon juice, oil, agave nectar and salt.
2. Using a vegetable peeler, peel beets, then shave them into ribbons.
3. Arrange arugula on a large platter. Top with beets, goat cheese and pistachios. Drizzle with dressing.

Minted Sprout Salad

Makes 6 side-dish servings

✪ Great for Steps 1, 2 and 4

Nutrients per serving	
Calories	65
Total fat	3 g
Saturated fat	0 g
Cholesterol	0 mg
Sodium	85 mg
Carbohydrate	9 g
Fiber	2 g
Protein	2 g
Calcium	39 mg
Iron	0.7 mg

1 tbsp	toasted sesame oil	15 mL
1 tbsp	unseasoned rice vinegar	15 mL
2 tsp	agave nectar or liquid honey	10 mL
1/8 tsp	fine sea salt	0.5 mL
2 cups	shredded purple cabbage	500 mL
2 cups	shredded carrots	500 mL
2 cups	alfalfa or sunflower sprouts	500 mL
1/2 cup	packed fresh mint leaves, thinly sliced	125 mL
1 tbsp	toasted sesame seeds (see tip, page 426)	15 mL

1. In a small bowl, whisk together oil, vinegar, agave nectar and salt.
2. In a large bowl, combine cabbage, carrots, alfalfa sprouts and mint. Add dressing and gently toss to coat. Sprinkle with sesame seeds.

Mustard Dill Red Potato Salad

Makes 8 side-dish servings

✪ Great for Steps 1, 2 and 4

Nutrients per serving	
Calories	154
Total fat	6 g
Saturated fat	1 g
Cholesterol	0 mg
Sodium	325 mg
Carbohydrate	25 g
Fiber	3 g
Protein	3 g
Calcium	47 mg
Iron	2.1 mg

2½ lbs	red-skinned potatoes (unpeeled), cut into ¼-inch (0.5 cm) thick rounds	1.25 kg
3	cloves garlic, minced	3
¾ tsp	fine sea salt	3 mL
¼ tsp	freshly cracked black pepper	1 mL
3 tbsp	extra virgin olive oil	45 mL
3 tbsp	cider vinegar	45 mL
2 tsp	whole-grain Dijon mustard	10 mL
1 cup	packed fresh flat-leaf (Italian) parsley leaves, chopped	250 mL
3 tbsp	chopped fresh dill	45 mL

1. Place potatoes in a large pot and cover with cold water. Bring to a boil over medium-high heat. Boil for 9 to 11 minutes or until tender. Drain and let cool completely.
2. In a small bowl, whisk together garlic, salt, pepper, oil, vinegar and mustard.
3. In a large bowl, combine cooled potatoes, parsley and dill. Add dressing and gently toss to coat.

Southwestern Sweet Potato Salad

Makes 8 side-dish servings

✪ Great for Steps 1, 2 and 4

Nutrients per serving	
Calories	128
Total fat	4 g
Saturated fat	1 g
Cholesterol	0 mg
Sodium	138 mg
Carbohydrate	22 g
Fiber	4 g
Protein	2 g
Calcium	25 mg
Iron	1.3 mg

2 lbs	sweet potatoes, peeled and cut into 1-inch (2.5 cm) pieces	1 kg
2 tsp	ground cumin	10 mL
¼ tsp	fine sea salt	1 mL
2 tbsp	extra virgin olive oil	30 mL
2 tbsp	freshly squeezed lime juice	30 mL
¼ tsp	hot pepper sauce	1 mL
1	red bell pepper, finely chopped	1
¾ cup	packed fresh cilantro leaves, chopped	175 mL
½ cup	thinly sliced green onions	125 mL

1. Place potatoes in a large pot and cover with cold water. Bring to a boil over medium-high heat. Boil for 9 to 11 minutes or until tender. Drain and let cool completely.
2. In a small bowl, whisk together cumin, salt, oil, lime juice and hot pepper sauce.
3. In a large bowl, combine cooled sweet potatoes, red pepper, cilantro and green onions. Add dressing and gently toss to coat.

Sweet Potato, Lentil and Arugula Salad

Makes 8 side-dish servings

✪ Great for Steps 1, 2, 3 and 4

A slightly sweet, Andalucía-inspired dressing of smoked paprika, sherry vinegar and garlic makes this salad of lentils and sweet potatoes a sure-fire hit.

- **Preheat oven to 400°F (200°C)**
- **Large rimmed baking sheet, lined with foil and sprayed with nonstick cooking spray (preferably olive oil)**

2 cups	water	500 mL
1/2 cup	dried green lentils, rinsed	125 mL
2	large sweet potatoes (about 2 lbs/1 kg), peeled and cut into 1-inch (2.5 cm) cubes	2
	Nonstick cooking spray (preferably olive oil)	
2 tbsp	reduced-sodium tamari or soy sauce, divided	30 mL
2	cloves garlic, minced	2
1 tsp	hot smoked paprika	5 mL
2 tbsp	extra virgin olive oil	30 mL
1 tbsp	sherry vinegar	15 mL
2 tsp	liquid honey	10 mL
4 cups	packed arugula	1 L

1. In a medium saucepan, bring water to a boil over high heat. Add lentils, reduce heat and simmer for about 30 minutes or until tender but not mushy. Drain and let cool to room temperature.
2. While lentils cook, arrange sweet potatoes in a single layer on prepared baking sheet. Lightly spray with cooking spray and sprinkle with half the tamari. Gently toss to coat. Roast in preheated oven for 20 to 25 minutes or until golden brown and tender. Let cool to room temperature in pan.
3. In a small bowl, whisk together garlic, paprika, oil, the remaining tamari, vinegar and honey.
4. Arrange arugula on a large platter. Top with lentils and sweet potatoes. Drizzle dressing over top.

Nutrients per serving	
Calories	110
Total fat	4 g
Saturated fat	1 g
Cholesterol	0 mg
Sodium	155 mg
Carbohydrate	15 g
Fiber	3 g
Protein	4 g
Calcium	29 mg
Iron	1.2 mg

Winter White Bean, Cauliflower and Arugula Salad

Makes 8 side-dish servings

✪ Great for Steps 1, 2, 3 and 4

Multiple shades of white and green make for a dramatic salad in the depths of winter.

Tip

For the white beans, you could use Great Northern beans, cannellini (white kidney) beans or white pea (navy) beans.

2 tbsp	extra virgin olive oil	30 mL
4 cups	small cauliflower florets (about 1 medium head)	1 L
½ tsp	fine sea salt	2 mL
3	cloves garlic, minced	3
1 tsp	minced fresh rosemary	5 mL
1	can (14 to 19 oz/398 to 540 mL) white beans, drained and rinsed	1
1 tbsp	finely grated lemon zest	15 mL
3 tbsp	freshly squeezed lemon juice	45 mL
4 cups	packed arugula, roughly chopped	1 L
½ cup	crumbled feta cheese	125 mL

1. In a large skillet, heat oil over medium-high heat. Add cauliflower and salt, stirring until florets are coated. Cook for 3 to 4 minutes, without stirring, to brown the cauliflower. Cook, stirring, for 2 to 3 minutes to further brown cauliflower, adding garlic and rosemary in the last 30 seconds of cooking time.
2. Transfer cauliflower mixture to a large bowl. Add beans, lemon zest and lemon juice, gently tossing to combine. Let cool completely. Just before serving, add arugula and feta, gently tossing to combine.

Superfood Spotlight

Olive Oil • The main type of fat in olive oil is monounsaturated fat, which helps prevent cholesterol from being deposited on artery walls and therefore protects against cardiovascular disease and strokes. In addition, early pressings of the olives (as in extra virgin olive oil, particularly "cold pressed" oil) produce an oil that is rich in beneficial plant compounds that can lower cholesterol and protect against cancer and high blood pressure. One of its compounds, oleocanthal, is an anti-inflammatory with action similar to that of ibuprofen. Finally, olive oil is a good source of vitamin E.

Nutrients per serving	
Calories	121
Total fat	6 g
Saturated fat	2 g
Cholesterol	9 mg
Sodium	442 mg
Carbohydrate	13 g
Fiber	4 g
Protein	6 g
Calcium	103 mg
Iron	1.2 mg

Spicy Three-Bean Salad

Makes 10 side-dish servings

✪ Great for Steps 1, 2, 3 and 4

Here's a guaranteed crowd-pleaser.

Nutrients per serving	
Calories	148
Total fat	4 g
Saturated fat	0 g
Cholesterol	0 mg
Sodium	471 mg
Carbohydrate	22 g
Fiber	7 g
Protein	6 g
Calcium	46 mg
Iron	1.7 mg

1 tbsp	minced seeded jalapeño pepper	15 mL
1 tbsp	ground cumin	15 mL
$\frac{1}{4}$ tsp	fine sea salt	1 mL
2 tbsp	extra virgin olive oil	30 mL
1$\frac{1}{2}$ tbsp	balsamic vinegar	22 mL
1 tbsp	liquid honey or brown rice syrup	15 mL
1	can (14 to 19 oz/398 to 540 mL) chickpeas, drained and rinsed	1
1	can (14 to 19 oz/398 to 540 mL) black beans, drained and rinsed	1
1	can (14 to 19 oz/398 to 540 mL) dark red kidney beans, drained and rinsed	1
1	red bell pepper, chopped	1
2 cups	chopped celery	500 mL

1. In a small bowl, whisk together jalapeño, cumin, salt, oil, vinegar and honey.
2. In a large bowl, combine chickpeas, black beans, kidney beans, red pepper and celery. Add dressing and gently toss to coat. Cover and refrigerate for at least 1 hour, until chilled, or for up to 24 hours.

Zucchini and Chickpea Salad

Makes 8 side-dish servings

✪ Great for Steps 1, 2, 3 and 4

Nutrients per serving	
Calories	107
Total fat	6 g
Saturated fat	2 g
Cholesterol	9 mg
Sodium	401 mg
Carbohydrate	10 g
Fiber	2 g
Protein	4 g
Calcium	68 mg
Iron	0.8 mg

$\frac{1}{2}$ tsp	fine sea salt	2 mL
$\frac{1}{2}$ tsp	freshly ground black pepper	2 mL
1 tbsp	finely grated lemon zest	15 mL
3 tbsp	freshly squeezed lemon juice	45 mL
2 tbsp	extra virgin olive oil	30 mL
3	small zucchini, trimmed, quartered lengthwise and diced	3
2	cans (14 to 19 oz/398 to 540 mL) chickpeas, drained and rinsed	2
$\frac{1}{2}$ cup	fresh basil leaves, chopped	125 mL
$\frac{1}{2}$ cup	crumbled feta cheese	125 mL

1. In a small bowl, whisk together salt, pepper, lemon zest, lemon juice and oil.
2. In a medium bowl, combine zucchini, chickpeas, basil and feta. Add dressing and gently toss to coat.

Persian Brown Rice and Cashew Salad

Makes 6 side-dish servings

✪ Great for Steps 1, 2, 3, 4 and 5

In this exotic yet familiar salad, lime and cinnamon imbue brown rice with tremendous flavor. Mint adds color and freshness; cashews contribute a buttery crunch.

Tip

Look for roasted cashews lightly seasoned with sea salt.

1 tsp	ground cinnamon	5 mL
1/4 tsp	fine sea salt	1 mL
1 tsp	finely grated lime zest	5 mL
3 tbsp	freshly squeezed lime juice	45 mL
3 tbsp	extra virgin olive oil	45 mL
1 tbsp	liquid honey or brown rice syrup	15 mL
3 cups	cooked brown basmati rice or other long-grain brown rice (see page 438), cooled	750 mL
1/2 cup	chopped pitted dates	125 mL
3/4 cup	thinly sliced green onions	175 mL
3/4 cup	packed fresh mint leaves, chopped	175 mL
1/2 cup	lightly salted roasted cashews, coarsely chopped	125 mL

1. In a small bowl, whisk together cinnamon, salt, lime zest, lime juice, oil and honey.
2. In a large bowl, combine rice and dates. Add dressing and gently toss to coat. Cover and refrigerate for at least 30 minutes, until chilled, or for up to 24 hours. Just before serving, add green onions, mint and cashews, gently tossing to combine.

Nutrients per serving	
Calories	284
Total fat	13 g
Saturated fat	2 g
Cholesterol	0 mg
Sodium	197 mg
Carbohydrate	33 g
Fiber	6 g
Protein	4 g
Calcium	37 mg
Iron	2.0 mg

California Sushi Roll Salad

Makes 10 side-dish servings

✪ Great for Steps 1, 2, 3, 4 and 5

Sushi deconstructed: this fabulous salad has all the distinctive flavors of California rolls with minimum effort.

Tips

The brown rice can be cooked up to 1 day ahead and refrigerated in an airtight container. Alternatively, use thawed frozen brown rice from two 12-oz (340 g) packages.

Two cups (500 mL) uncooked brown rice will yield about 6 cups (1.5 L) cooked rice.

Use a very sharp knife or kitchen shears to cut the nori into strips (its dryness can make it somewhat tough to cut).

Nutrients per serving	
Calories	213
Total fat	7 g
Saturated fat	1 g
Cholesterol	0 mg
Sodium	367 mg
Carbohydrate	43 g
Fiber	4 g
Protein	4 g
Calcium	28 mg
Iron	1.2 mg

1/4 cup	unseasoned rice vinegar	60 mL
2 tbsp	agave nectar	30 mL
1 tsp	fine sea salt	5 mL
6 cups	cooked long-grain brown rice (see page 438), cooled	1.5 L
1 1/2 tbsp	vegetable oil	22 mL
1 1/2 tbsp	water	22 mL
1 1/4 tsp	wasabi paste	6 mL
2 cups	diced seeded peeled cucumber	500 mL
1 cup	coarsely shredded carrots	250 mL
1 cup	thinly sliced green onions	250 mL
3 tbsp	chopped drained pickled ginger	45 mL
1 tbsp	toasted sesame seeds (see tip, page 426)	15 mL
1	firm-ripe Hass avocado	1
1	6-inch (15 cm) square toasted nori, cut into very thin strips	1

1. In a small saucepan, combine vinegar, agave nectar and salt. Bring just to a boil over medium heat. Remove from heat.
2. Place rice in a large bowl and pour vinegar mixture over top. Gently stir to combine, then let cool completely.
3. In a small cup, whisk together oil, water and wasabi paste.
4. To the rice mixture, add cucumber, carrots, green onions, ginger and sesame seeds. Drizzle with wasabi mixture and gently toss to coat. Cover and refrigerate for at least 1 hour, until chilled, or for up to 2 hours. Just before serving, dice avocado and sprinkle over salad, along with nori strips.

Superfood Spotlight

Avocados • Avocados are very high in fat, but it is mostly heart-healthy, monounsaturated fat. The oleic acid contained in monounsaturated fats can lower the risk of breast cancer; further, these fats can help to reduce "bad" blood cholesterol levels. Avocados are rich in nutrients, including vitamins C, E and B_6, folate, iron, magnesium and potassium, and the antioxidant plant chemicals beta-sitosterol (which can also help lower blood cholesterol) and glutathione (which protects against cancer).

French Green Bean, Barley and Tomato Salad

Makes 8 side-dish servings

✪ Great for Steps 1, 2, 4 and 5

With a hint of Dijon mustard, toothsome barley and the mingling flavors of fresh garden produce, this French-inspired yet newly styled salad isn't missing a thing.

- **Steamer basket**

1 cup	pearl barley	250 mL
4 cups	water	1 L
1 lb	green beans, trimmed and cut into 2-inch (5 cm) pieces	500 g
	Ice water	
1/2 tsp	fine sea salt	2 mL
1/4 tsp	freshly cracked black pepper	1 mL
2 tbsp	white wine vinegar	30 mL
2 tbsp	extra virgin olive oil	30 mL
1 tbsp	liquid honey or brown rice syrup	15 mL
1/2 tsp	Dijon mustard	2 mL
2 cups	halved grape or cherry tomatoes	500 mL
3/4 cup	packed fresh flat-leaf (Italian) parsley leaves, chopped	175 mL
1/2 cup	thinly sliced red onion	125 mL

1. In a medium saucepan, combine barley and water. Bring to a boil over high heat. Reduce heat to low, cover and simmer for about 40 minutes or until most of the water is absorbed and barley is tender. Remove from heat and let cool completely.
2. Meanwhile, place green beans in a steamer basket set over a large pot of boiling water. Cover and steam for 4 to 6 minutes or until tender. Transfer to a large bowl of ice water to stop the cooking. Drain and pat dry with paper towels.
3. In a small bowl, whisk together salt, pepper, vinegar, oil, honey and mustard.
4. In a large bowl, combine cooled barley, green beans, tomatoes, parsley and red onion. Add dressing and gently toss to coat. Serve immediately or cover and refrigerate for at least 1 hour, until chilled, or for up to 4 hours.

Nutrients per serving

Calories	153
Total fat	4 g
Saturated fat	1 g
Cholesterol	0 mg
Sodium	196 mg
Carbohydrate	27 g
Fiber	6 g
Protein	4 g
Calcium	19 mg
Iron	1.0 mg

Barley, Parsley and Walnut Salad

Makes 8 side-dish servings

✪ Great for Steps 1, 3, 4 and 5

This salad is everything you want from a side dish: a pleasing variety of textures and flavors. Barley is terrific here, and is a great option for replacing rice — even brown rice — in a broad range of recipes.

1¼ cups	pearl barley	300 mL
5 cups	water	1.25 L
2	cloves garlic, minced	2
½ tsp	fine sea salt	2 mL
¼ tsp	freshly cracked black pepper	1 mL
2 tsp	finely grated lemon zest	10 mL
2 tbsp	freshly squeezed lemon juice	30 mL
2 tbsp	extra virgin olive oil	30 mL
½ tsp	Dijon mustard	2 mL
1 cup	packed fresh flat-leaf (Italian) parsley leaves	250 mL
½ cup	crumbled feta cheese	125 mL
¼ cup	chopped toasted walnuts	60 mL

1. In a medium saucepan, combine barley and water. Bring to a boil over high heat. Reduce heat to low, cover and simmer for about 40 minutes or until most of the water is absorbed and barley is tender. Remove from heat and let cool completely.
2. In a small bowl, whisk together garlic, salt, pepper, lemon zest, lemon juice, oil and mustard.
3. Drizzle dressing over barley and gently toss to coat. Cover and refrigerate for at least 1 hour, until chilled, or for up to 4 hours. Just before serving, add parsley, feta and walnuts, gently tossing to combine.

▶ Health Note

Barley contains almost twice as much fiber as brown rice, as well as cancer-fighting selenium. Beta-glucan, a form of fiber found in barley, helps lower cholesterol and reduces the body's rate of fat absorption.

Nutrients per serving

Calories	197
Total fat	9 g
Saturated fat	2 g
Cholesterol	9 mg
Sodium	294 mg
Carbohydrate	26 g
Fiber	6 g
Protein	6 g
Calcium	68 mg
Iron	1.4 mg

Tabbouleh

Makes 8 side-dish servings

✪ Great for Steps 1, 2, 4 and 5

Gorgeous, easy to make and utterly sublime (especially when summer tomatoes hit their peak) — is it any wonder tabbouleh is a classic?

Variations

Quinoa Tabbouleh: Use 3 cups (750 mL) cooled cooked quinoa in place of the soaked bulgur. Add the full 3⁄4 tsp (3 mL) salt in step 2.

Ancient Grain Tabbouleh: Use 3 cups (750 mL) cooled cooked farro in place of the soaked bulgur. Add the full 3⁄4 tsp (3 mL) salt in step 2.

1 cup	fine or medium bulgur	250 mL
3⁄4 tsp	fine sea salt, divided	3 mL
1 cup	boiling water	250 mL
1	large cucumber, peeled, seeded and diced	1
2 cups	chopped tomatoes	500 mL
1 cup	packed fresh flat-leaf (Italian) parsley leaves, chopped	250 mL
3⁄4 cup	packed fresh mint leaves, chopped	175 mL
3⁄4 cup	chopped green onions	175 mL
2 tsp	ground cumin	10 mL
1⁄2 tsp	freshly cracked black pepper	2 mL
1⁄4 cup	freshly squeezed lemon juice	60 mL
3 tbsp	extra virgin olive oil	45 mL

1. In a large bowl, combine bulgur, 1⁄2 tsp (2 mL) of the salt and boiling water. Let stand for about 30 minutes or until water is absorbed. Fluff bulgur with a fork.
2. To the bulgur, add cucumber, tomatoes, parsley, mint, green onions, cumin, pepper, the remaining salt, lemon juice and oil, gently tossing to combine.

▸ Health Note

Super nourishment for body and mind, bulgur is rich in B vitamins for a healthy nervous system, as well as vitamin E and selenium — a dynamic duo of cancer-fighting antioxidants.

Nutrients per serving	
Calories	128
Total fat	6 g
Saturated fat	1 g
Cholesterol	0 mg
Sodium	275 mg
Carbohydrate	18 g
Fiber	3 g
Protein	3 g
Calcium	37 mg
Iron	1.7 mg

Bulgur Salad with Oranges, Cashews and Fresh Mint

Makes 12 side-dish servings

✪ Great for Steps 1, 2, 3, 4 and 5

This salad — a case of assertive opposites finding delicious balance — has been a favorite in my family for more than 20 years.

Tip

Look for roasted cashews lightly seasoned with sea salt.

Nutrients per serving	
Calories	156
Total fat	4 g
Saturated fat	1 g
Cholesterol	0 mg
Sodium	272 mg
Carbohydrate	28 g
Fiber	3 g
Protein	3 g
Calcium	30 mg
Iron	1.6 mg

1½ cups	medium or coarse bulgur	375 mL
1½ cups	boiling water	375 mL
1 tbsp	ground cumin	15 mL
1½ tsp	ground cinnamon	7 mL
1 tsp	fine sea salt	5 mL
½ tsp	freshly ground black pepper	2 mL
1 tbsp	finely grated orange zest	15 mL
⅓ cup	freshly squeezed orange juice	75 mL
2 tbsp	freshly squeezed lemon juice	30 mL
2 tbsp	extra virgin olive oil	30 mL
2 tbsp	liquid honey or agave nectar	30 mL
1 tbsp	Dijon mustard	15 mL
1	can (15 oz/425 mL) mandarin oranges packed in juice, drained (or 1½ cans, each 10 oz/287 mL)	1
1 cup	chopped green onions	250 mL
1 cup	packed fresh mint leaves, chopped	250 mL
½ cup	raisins	125 mL
⅓ cup	lightly salted roasted cashew pieces	75 mL

1. In a large bowl, combine bulgur and boiling water. Let stand for about 30 minutes or until water is absorbed. Fluff bulgur with a fork.
2. In a small bowl, whisk together cumin, cinnamon, salt, pepper, orange zest, orange juice, lemon juice, oil, honey and mustard.
3. To the bulgur, add oranges, green onions, mint and raisins. Add dressing and gently toss to coat. Cover and refrigerate for at least 1 hour, until chilled, or for up to 4 hours. Just before serving, add cashews and gently toss to combine.

Lentil and Bulgur Salad with Grapes and Mint

Makes 8 side-dish servings

✪ Great for Steps 1, 2, 3, 4 and 5

Not your typical side dish by any stretch, this whimsical take on tabbouleh breathes fresh air and plenty of style into a classic preparation.

1 cup	dried red lentils, rinsed	250 mL
5 cups	water	1.25 L
½ cup	fine bulgur	125 mL
1 tsp	ground coriander	5 mL
½ tsp	fine sea salt	2 mL
2 tbsp	extra virgin olive oil	30 mL
2 tbsp	freshly squeezed lime juice	30 mL
2 tsp	liquid honey or agave nectar	10 mL
2 cups	red seedless grapes, halved	500 mL
1 cup	packed fresh mint leaves, chopped	250 mL

1. In a medium saucepan, combine lentils and water. Bring to a boil over medium-high heat. Reduce heat and simmer for 15 to 18 minutes or until tender. Stir in bulgur. Cover, remove from heat and let stand for 15 minutes. Transfer to a large bowl and let cool completely. Gently fluff with a fork.
2. In a small bowl, whisk together coriander, salt, oil, lime juice and honey.
3. To the lentil mixture, add grapes and dressing, gently tossing to combine. Cover and refrigerate for at least 30 minutes, until chilled, or for up to 4 hours. Just before serving, add mint and gently toss to combine.

Superfood Spotlight

Grapes • Grapes may be small, but they're mighty. All grape varieties contain beneficial compounds, mainly polyphenols, most of which are found in the skin. Black, purple and red varieties also have particularly high levels of the flavonoids quercetin and anthocyanins (the dark pigments), which may help prevent cancer, heart disease and cardiovascular disease. The antioxidant benefits of paler grapes are mainly from catechin. Resveratrol, another antioxidant present in all grapes, has been linked to the prevention or inhibition of cancer and heart disease, degenerative nerve disease and viral infections, and may also protect against Alzheimer's disease.

Nutrients per serving

Calories	179
Total fat	4 g
Saturated fat	1 g
Cholesterol	0 mg
Sodium	181 mg
Carbohydrate	27 g
Fiber	5 g
Protein	8 g
Calcium	25 mg
Iron	1.9 mg

Pistachio and Citrus Couscous Salad

Makes 8 side-dish servings

✪ Great for Steps 1, 2, 3, 4 and 5

Pistachios have an exquisite, exotic taste all their own, but when joined by citrus, mint and whole wheat couscous, they hit even higher notes.

1 cup	freshly squeezed orange juice	250 mL
1 cup	water	250 mL
1/2 tsp	fine sea salt	2 mL
1 1/2 cups	whole wheat couscous	375 mL
1 tbsp	finely grated lemon zest	15 mL
2 tbsp	freshly squeezed lemon juice	30 mL
2 tbsp	extra virgin olive oil	30 mL
1 1/2 cups	diced seeded peeled cucumber	375 mL
1/2 cup	chopped dried apricots	125 mL
1/2 cup	chopped green onions	125 mL
1/2 cup	packed fresh mint leaves, chopped	125 mL
1/3 cup	coarsely chopped pistachios	75 mL

1. In a medium saucepan, combine orange juice, water and salt. Bring to a boil over high heat. Remove from heat and whisk in couscous. Cover and let stand for 5 minutes. Fluff with a fork. Transfer to a large bowl and let cool completely.
2. In a small bowl, whisk together lemon zest, lemon juice and oil.
3. To the couscous, add cucumber, apricots, green onions and mint. Add dressing and gently toss to coat. Sprinkle with pistachios.

Nutrients per serving	
Calories	402
Total fat	7 g
Saturated fat	1 g
Cholesterol	0 mg
Sodium	185 mg
Carbohydrate	85 g
Fiber	11 g
Protein	10 g
Calcium	77 mg
Iron	3.8 mg

Middle Eastern Couscous, Date and Chickpea Salad

Makes 6 main-dish servings

✪ Great for Steps 1, 3, 4 and 5

Whole wheat couscous combines with a symphony of Middle Eastern flavors — lemon, cardamom, cumin and olive oil — in this noteworthy salad. Protein-rich chickpeas and toasted almonds shift it from side dish to main dish.

Tip

To toast slivered almonds, place up to ½ cup (125 mL) almonds in a medium skillet set over medium heat. Cook, shaking the skillet, for 5 to 8 minutes or until almonds are golden brown and fragrant. Let cool completely before use.

Nutrients per serving	
Calories	380
Total fat	12 g
Saturated fat	1 g
Cholesterol	0 mg
Sodium	393 mg
Carbohydrate	61 g
Fiber	10 g
Protein	13 g
Calcium	77 mg
Iron	3.3 mg

2 cups	water	500 mL
½ tsp	fine sea salt	2 mL
1½ cups	whole wheat couscous	375 mL
1 tsp	ground cardamom	5 mL
1 tsp	ground cumin	5 mL
1 tbsp	finely grated lemon zest	15 mL
3 tbsp	freshly squeezed lemon juice	45 mL
2 tbsp	extra virgin olive oil	30 mL
1	can (14 to 19 oz/398 to 540 mL) chickpeas, drained and rinsed	1
¾ cup	packed fresh cilantro leaves, chopped	175 mL
½ cup	chopped pitted dates	125 mL
½ cup	thinly sliced green onions	125 mL
½ cup	slivered almonds, toasted (see tip, at left)	125 mL

1. In a medium saucepan, combine water and salt. Bring to a boil over high heat. Remove from heat and whisk in couscous. Cover and let stand for 5 minutes. Fluff with a fork. Transfer to a large bowl and let cool completely.
2. In a small bowl, whisk together cardamom, cumin, lemon zest, lemon juice and oil.
3. To the couscous, add chickpeas, cilantro and dates. Add dressing and gently toss to coat. Sprinkle with green onions and almonds.

Superfood Spotlight

Chickpeas • Chickpeas are a delicious protein food and a very good source of fiber. Their insoluble fiber, which binds to cholesterol and removes it from the body, also helps prevent digestive disorders such as diverticulitis. Their soluble fiber controls and lowers blood cholesterol and helps prevent strokes and heart disease. Chickpeas are extremely high in folate, which helps lower levels of blood homocysteine (a risk factor for cardiovascular disease). They are also rich in magnesium, which helps relax the arteries and protect against heart attacks.

Farro Salad with Arugula and Tomatoes

Makes 8 side-dish servings

✪ Great for Steps 1, 2, 4 and 5

Balsamic vinegar makes this otherwise understated salad pop, especially when combined with peppery arugula and sweet tomatoes — each flavor amps up the other.

Tip

The farro can be cooked a day in advance and refrigerated in an airtight container until ready to use.

$1\frac{1}{4}$ cups	semi-pearled farro	300 mL
3 tbsp	extra virgin olive oil	45 mL
$2\frac{1}{2}$ tbsp	balsamic vinegar	37 mL
$\frac{3}{4}$ tsp	fine sea salt	3 mL
$\frac{1}{4}$ tsp	freshly cracked black pepper	1 mL
2 cups	halved cherry or grape tomatoes	500 mL
1 cup	chopped drained roasted red bell peppers	250 mL
6 cups	packed arugula, roughly chopped	1.5 L

1. In a large saucepan of boiling water, cook farro for 25 to 30 minutes or until al dente. Drain well. Transfer to a large bowl and let cool completely.
2. In a small bowl, whisk together oil, vinegar, salt and pepper.
3. To the farro, add tomatoes and roasted peppers. Add dressing and gently toss to coat. Cover and refrigerate for at least 30 minutes, until chilled, or for up to 4 hours. Just before serving, add arugula and gently toss to combine.

Nutrients per serving	
Calories	178
Total fat	6 g
Saturated fat	1 g
Cholesterol	0 mg
Sodium	263 mg
Carbohydrate	28 g
Fiber	6 g
Protein	4 g
Calcium	41 mg
Iron	1.1 mg

Quinoa and Black Bean Salad

Makes 4 main-dish servings

✪ Great for Steps 1, 2, 3, 4 and 5

With black beans, tomatoes, cumin and cilantro, this quick quinoa salad takes a delectable Tex-Mex detour.

1 cup	quinoa, rinsed	250 mL
2 cups	water	500 mL
1½ tsp	ground cumin	7 mL
½ tsp	fine sea salt	2 mL
3 tbsp	extra virgin olive oil	45 mL
2 tsp	finely grated lime zest	10 mL
2 tbsp	freshly squeezed lime juice	30 mL
1 tsp	agave nectar or liquid honey	5 mL
1	can (14 to 19 oz/398 to 540 mL) black beans, drained and rinsed	1
2 cups	chopped tomatoes	500 mL
½ cup	thinly sliced green onions	125 mL
½ cup	packed fresh cilantro leaves, chopped	125 mL

1. In a medium saucepan, combine quinoa and water. Bring to a boil over medium-high heat. Reduce heat to low, cover and simmer for 15 to 18 minutes or until water is absorbed. Remove from heat and let cool completely.
2. In a small bowl, whisk together cumin, salt, oil, lime zest, lime juice and agave nectar.
3. In a large bowl, combine cooled quinoa, beans, tomatoes, green onions and cilantro. Add dressing and gently toss to coat. Cover and refrigerate for at least 30 minutes, until chilled, or for up to 4 hours.

Nutrients per serving	
Calories	357
Total fat	14 g
Saturated fat	2 g
Cholesterol	0 mg
Sodium	694 mg
Carbohydrate	47 g
Fiber	9 g
Protein	12 g
Calcium	69 mg
Iron	4.0 mg

Lemony Lentil and Quinoa Salad

Makes 6 main-dish servings

✪ Great for Steps 1, 3, 4 and 5

Among the many wonderful things about quinoa is that it cooks quickly and is substantial without being heavy, making it the perfect transition dinner from summer to fall.

6 cups	water, divided	1.5 L
1 cup	dried green lentils, rinsed	250 mL
1 cup	quinoa, rinsed	250 mL
1 tsp	dried tarragon	5 mL
1/2 tsp	fine sea salt	2 mL
1/4 tsp	freshly cracked black pepper	1 mL
2 tsp	finely grated lemon zest	10 mL
3 tbsp	freshly squeezed lemon juice	45 mL
2 tbsp	extra virgin olive oil	30 mL
1 tsp	Dijon mustard	5 mL
3/4 cup	thinly sliced green onions	175 mL
1 cup	packed fresh flat-leaf (Italian) parsley leaves, chopped	250 mL

1. In a medium saucepan, bring 4 cups (1 L) of the water to a boil over high heat. Add lentils, reduce heat and simmer for about 30 minutes or until tender but not mushy. Drain and let cool completely.
2. Meanwhile, in another medium saucepan, combine quinoa and the remaining water. Bring to a boil over medium-high heat. Reduce heat to low, cover and simmer for 15 to 18 minutes or until water is absorbed. Remove from heat and let cool completely.
3. In a small bowl, whisk together tarragon, salt, pepper, lemon zest, lemon juice, oil and mustard.
4. In a large bowl, combine cooled lentils, cooled quinoa and green onions. Add dressing and gently toss to coat. Cover and refrigerate for at least 1 hour, until chilled, or for up to 4 hours. Just before serving, add parsley and gently toss to combine.

Nutrients per serving	
Calories	254
Total fat	7 g
Saturated fat	1 g
Cholesterol	0 mg
Sodium	264 mg
Carbohydrate	38 g
Fiber	7 g
Protein	11 g
Calcium	44 mg
Iron	4.2 mg

Pomegranate and Quinoa Salad with Sunflower Seeds

Makes 6 side-dish servings

✪ Great for Steps 1, 3, 4 and 5

Enhanced with lemon, handfuls of herbs and a touch of agave nectar, this sensational combination of pomegranates, quinoa and sunflower seeds is worth making again and again.

Tip

To remove pomegranate seeds, score the fruit around the circumference and place it in a large bowl of water. Break the pomegranate open underwater to free the white seed sacs. The seeds will sink to the bottom of the bowl, and the membrane will float to the top. Strain out the seeds and put them in a separate bowl. Refrigerate or freeze any remaining seeds for another use.

Nutrients per serving	
Calories	227
Total fat	11 g
Saturated fat	2 g
Cholesterol	0 mg
Sodium	273 mg
Carbohydrate	27 g
Fiber	4 g
Protein	6 g
Calcium	25 mg
Iron	2.8 mg

1 cup	quinoa, rinsed	250 mL
2 cups	water	500 mL
2 tsp	finely grated lemon zest	10 mL
2 tbsp	freshly squeezed lemon juice	30 mL
2 tbsp	extra virgin olive oil	30 mL
1 tbsp	agave nectar or liquid honey	15 mL
1/2 tsp	fine sea salt	2 mL
3/4 cup	pomegranate seeds	175 mL
1/3 cup	lightly salted roasted sunflower seeds	75 mL
1/4 cup	packed fresh mint leaves, chopped	60 mL
1/4 cup	packed fresh cilantro leaves, chopped	60 mL

1. In a medium saucepan, combine quinoa and water. Bring to a boil over medium-high heat. Reduce heat to low, cover and simmer for 15 to 18 minutes or until water is absorbed. Transfer to a large bowl and let cool completely.
2. In a small bowl, whisk together lemon zest, lemon juice, oil, agave nectar and salt.
3. To the quinoa, add pomegranate seeds, sunflower seeds, mint and cilantro. Add dressing and gently toss to coat.

Variation

An equal amount of dried cranberries or chopped dried cherries may be used in place of the pomegranate seeds.

Indian-Spiced Quinoa, Watercress and Chickpea Salad

Makes 6 side-dish servings

✪ Great for Steps 1, 2, 3, 4 and 5

Here, strong flavors balance out mellow ones — chickpeas are roasted with garam masala and sweet raisins dance with tart lime and peppery watercress.

- **Preheat oven to 450°F (230°C)**
- **Large rimmed baking sheet, sprayed with nonstick cooking spray**

1 cup	quinoa, rinsed	250 mL
2 cups	water	500 mL
1	can (14 to 19 oz/398 to 540 mL) chickpeas, drained, rinsed and patted dry	1
1½ tsp	garam masala	7 mL
2 tbsp	extra virgin olive oil, divided	30 mL
1 tbsp	finely grated lime zest	15 mL
3 tbsp	freshly squeezed lime juice	45 mL
¼ tsp	fine sea salt	1 mL
6 cups	packed tender watercress sprigs	1.5 L
⅔ cup	golden raisins, roughly chopped	150 mL

1. In a medium saucepan, combine quinoa and water. Bring to a boil over medium-high heat. Reduce heat to low, cover and simmer for 15 to 18 minutes or until water is absorbed. Transfer to a large bowl and let cool completely.
2. Meanwhile, in a medium bowl, combine chickpeas, garam masala and half the oil. Spread in a single layer on prepared baking sheet. Roast in preheated oven for 10 to 15 minutes or until chickpeas are golden brown and crisp. Let cool completely in pan.
3. In a small bowl, whisk together lime zest, lime juice, the remaining oil and salt.
4. To the quinoa, add roasted chickpeas, watercress and raisins. Add dressing and gently toss to coat.

Nutrients per serving	
Calories	259
Total fat	7 g
Saturated fat	1 g
Cholesterol	0 mg
Sodium	285 mg
Carbohydrate	42 g
Fiber	5 g
Protein	8 g
Calcium	50 mg
Iron	2.4 mg

Wheat Berry, Pecan and Cherry Salad

Makes 8 side-dish servings

✪ Great for Steps 1, 3, 4 and 5

This salad stands a strong chance of becoming your go-to side dish for holiday meals. Then again, why wait?

Tip

See page 29 for instructions on toasting nuts.

6 cups	water	1.5 L
1½ cups	wheat berries	375 mL
2 tbsp	extra virgin olive oil	30 mL
2 tbsp	red wine vinegar	30 mL
1 tbsp	pure maple syrup or brown rice syrup	15 mL
½ tsp	fine sea salt	2 mL
½ tsp	freshly ground black pepper	2 mL
½ cup	dried cherries, chopped	125 mL
1 cup	packed fresh flat-leaf (Italian) parsley leaves, chopped	250 mL
½ cup	thinly sliced green onions	125 mL
⅓ cup	chopped toasted pecans	75 mL

1. In a medium saucepan, bring water to a boil over high heat. Add wheat berries, reduce heat and simmer for 60 to 75 minutes or until tender. Drain and rinse under cold water until cool. Transfer to a large bowl.
2. In a small bowl, whisk together oil, vinegar, maple syrup, salt and pepper.
3. To the wheat berries, add cherries and dressing, gently tossing to combine. Cover and refrigerate for at least 1 hour, until chilled, or for up to 24 hours. Just before serving, add parsley, green onions and pecans, gently tossing to combine.

Nutrients per serving	
Calories	220
Total fat	7 g
Saturated fat	1 g
Cholesterol	0 mg
Sodium	184 mg
Carbohydrate	35 g
Fiber	8 g
Protein	5 g
Calcium	34 mg
Iron	2.1 mg

Soba and Tofu Salad with Carrot Miso Dressing

Makes 6 main-dish servings

✪ Great for Steps 1, 2, 3, 4 and 5

Serenity by the forkful, this salad is so good, and so good for you. Gluten-free, high in protein and low on the glycemic index, buckwheat is one of the most nutritious grains around. But all you really need to know is that this salad is satisfying, energizing and undeniably delicious.

Tip

If the package of tofu you buy is slightly larger or smaller than 14 oz (400 g), just use the entire package (there is no need to add or subtract tofu to equal 14 oz/400 g).

Nutrients per serving	
Calories	302
Total fat	9 g
Saturated fat	0 g
Cholesterol	0 mg
Sodium	293 mg
Carbohydrate	44 g
Fiber	6 g
Protein	15 g
Calcium	193 mg
Iron	4.1 mg

- **Blender**

8 oz	soba (buckwheat) noodles	250 g
3 tsp	vegetable oil, divided	15 mL
14 oz	extra-firm tofu, drained, patted dry and cut into ½-inch (1 cm) cubes	400 g
4	green onions, trimmed and cut into 2-inch (5 cm) pieces	4
2 cups	broccoli florets	500 mL
2 cups	cremini or button mushrooms, trimmed and sliced	500 mL
2 cups	reduced-sodium ready-to-use chicken or vegetable broth	500 mL
12 oz	sugar snap peas, trimmed	375 g
1	clove garlic	1
½ cup	finely shredded carrot	125 mL
¼ cup	water	60 mL
2 tbsp	white or yellow miso	30 mL
1 tbsp	unseasoned rice vinegar	15 mL
2 tsp	toasted sesame oil	10 mL

1. In a large pot of boiling salted water, cook soba noodles according to package directions until just tender. Immediately drain and rinse under cold water until cool. Transfer to a large bowl.
2. In a large skillet, heat 2 tsp (10 mL) of the vegetable oil over medium-high heat. Add tofu and green onions; cook, stirring, for 3 to 4 minutes or until tofu is golden. Add to noodles.
3. Add the remaining vegetable oil to the skillet. Add broccoli and mushrooms, reduce heat to medium and cook, stirring, for 3 to 4 minutes or until mushrooms are softened. Add broth and peas; cook, stirring occasionally, for 2 to 4 minutes or until broccoli and peas are tender-crisp. Add to noodle mixture.
4. In blender, combine garlic, carrot, water, miso, vinegar and sesame oil; purée until smooth.
5. Pour dressing over noodle mixture, gently tossing to coat. Let cool to room temperature, then cover and refrigerate for at least 1 hour, until chilled, or for up to 2 hours.

Sesame Peanut Vegetable Noodle Salad

Makes 8 side-dish servings

✪ Great for Steps 3, 4 and 5

This rendition of an ever-popular takeout dish hits you over the head with its clear, true flavors. The key ingredient is natural peanut butter, which is loaded with flavor, protein and a range of antioxidants that rivals those found in berries.

Tip

Look for roasted peanuts lightly seasoned with sea salt.

8 oz	whole wheat or multigrain spaghetti	250 g
1⁄3 cup	unsweetened natural peanut butter	75 mL
1⁄4 cup	reduced-sodium ready-to-use vegetable or chicken broth	60 mL
3 tbsp	unseasoned rice vinegar	45 mL
3 tbsp	reduced-sodium tamari or soy sauce	45 mL
1 1⁄2 tbsp	agave nectar, brown rice syrup or liquid honey	22 mL
1 tbsp	toasted sesame oil	15 mL
2 tsp	ground ginger	10 mL
1⁄8 tsp	cayenne pepper	0.5 mL
1	large red bell pepper, cut into very thin strips	1
1⁄2 cup	thinly sliced green onions	125 mL
3⁄4 cup	packed fresh cilantro leaves, chopped	175 mL
1⁄4 cup	chopped lightly salted roasted peanuts	60 mL

1. In a large pot of boiling salted water, cook spaghetti according to package directions until al dente. Drain and rinse under cold water until cool.
2. In a small bowl, whisk together peanut butter, broth, vinegar, tamari, agave nectar, oil, ginger and cayenne.
3. In a large bowl, combine cold pasta, red pepper and green onions. Add dressing and gently toss to coat. Sprinkle with cilantro and peanuts.

Nutrients per serving	
Calories	240
Total fat	10 g
Saturated fat	1 g
Cholesterol	0 mg
Sodium	244 mg
Carbohydrate	32 g
Fiber	5 g
Protein	9 g
Calcium	18 mg
Iron	1.8 mg

Garden Pasta Salad

Makes 8 side-dish servings

✪ Great for Steps 1, 2, 3, 4 and 5

When you want to go all out without fuss, try this multi-hued salad. Crisp, purple cabbage is the surprise ingredient here, contributing subtle sweetness, nutrition and a distinctive crunch.

Tip

Make sure to use fine sea salt in the water you use to cook the pasta. Conventional table salt contains chemicals and additives, whereas sea salt contains an abundance of naturally occurring trace minerals.

8 oz	whole wheat rotini or other spiral pasta	250 g
3 cups	small broccoli florets (about 1 small head)	750 mL
2	cloves garlic, minced	2
½ tsp	fine sea salt	2 mL
¼ tsp	freshly cracked black pepper	1 mL
½ cup	nonfat plain yogurt	125 mL
3 tbsp	freshly squeezed lemon juice	45 mL
2 tbsp	extra virgin olive oil	30 mL
2 tsp	Dijon mustard	10 mL
3 cups	shredded purple cabbage	750 mL
2 cups	halved grape or cherry tomatoes	500 mL
½ cup	packed fresh basil leaves, chopped	125 mL
⅓ cup	pitted brine-cured black olives (such as kalamata), chopped	75 mL

1. In a large pot of boiling salted water, cook rotini according to package directions until al dente. Add broccoli during last 30 seconds of cooking. Drain and rinse under cold water until cool. Place in a large bowl.
2. In a small bowl, whisk together garlic, salt, pepper, yogurt, lemon juice, oil and mustard.
3. Add dressing to pasta mixture and gently toss to coat. Add cabbage, tomatoes, basil and olives, gently tossing to combine.

Superfood Spotlight

Cabbage • Cabbage is rich in phytonutrients, which may inhibit the growth of cancerous tumors and seem to have particular benefit in offering protection from colon, lung and hormone-based cancers such as breast cancer, probably by increasing the metabolism of estrogen. Cabbage is also rich in vitamins C and E, folate, fiber and minerals, and is a source of B vitamins, vitamin K, iron and beta-carotene. Its juice is a traditional remedy for peptic ulcers, and its indoles can help lower LDL ("bad") cholesterol.

Nutrients per serving

Calories	180
Total fat	5 g
Saturated fat	1 g
Cholesterol	0 mg
Sodium	205 mg
Carbohydrate	31 g
Fiber	5 g
Protein	7 g
Calcium	74 mg
Iron	2.0 mg

Orzo Salad with Fennel, Radishes and Goat Cheese

Makes 8 side-dish servings

✪ Great for Steps 1, 2, 4 and 5

Can a salad be sassy? Sure it can, when it's packed with crisp, boldly flavored vegetables and tangy goat cheese, then drizzled with a white balsamic dressing.

8 oz	whole wheat orzo or other small whole wheat pasta	250 g
1	medium-large bulb fennel	1
2 cups	halved grape or cherry tomatoes	500 mL
1½ cups	thinly sliced radishes (about 1 small bunch)	375 mL
3 tbsp	extra virgin olive oil	45 mL
2 tbsp	white balsamic or white wine vinegar	30 mL
½ tsp	fine sea salt	2 mL
2 oz	goat cheese, crumbled	60 g

1. In a large pot of boiling water, cook orzo according to package directions until al dente. Drain and rinse under cold water until cool. Transfer to a large bowl.
2. Cut stalks from fennel. Remove fronds, chopping enough to measure about ½ cup (125 mL). Discard any remaining fronds. Halve the fennel bulb lengthwise, cut off root end and chop fennel. Add chopped fennel and chopped fronds to orzo, along with tomatoes and radishes.
3. In a small bowl, whisk together oil, vinegar and salt. Add to orzo mixture and gently toss to coat. Fold in half the goat cheese. Sprinkle the remaining goat cheese over top.

Nutrients per serving

Calories	193
Total fat	7 g
Saturated fat	2 g
Cholesterol	4 mg
Sodium	231 mg
Carbohydrate	28 g
Fiber	4 g
Protein	7 g
Calcium	47 mg
Iron	1.7 mg

Healthy Know-How

Organic Vs. Natural

"Organic" and "natural" are common buzzwords in the world of food these days, but what exactly do the terms mean?

USDA Organic

To use the term "organic" on a food package, farmers and manufacturers must verify through an independent auditing agency that production processes have met all the organic guidelines set by the U.S. Department of Agriculture.

USDA-certified meat, dairy and egg products must come from animals that were given access to exercise, sunlight and, in the case of beef, a grazing pasture. Further, the animals cannot be treated with antibiotics or hormones, and their feed must be certified organic and free from animal by-products and genetic modifications.

USDA-certified organic produce comes from farms that have not used synthetic herbicides, pesticides, fertilizers or genetically modified seeds for at least three years.

Processed foods bearing the USDA emblem must contain at least 95% certified organic ingredients.

Natural

The term "natural" has far more nebulous criteria. For meat and poultry, the USDA requires the products to contain no added colors or artificial ingredients, and forbids processing that "fundamentally alter(s) the raw product." However, farmers and manufacturers are free to hire their own inspectors to meet these criteria. In addition, there are no requirements as to how the animal was raised.

Neither the USDA nor the FDA regulates or defines the term "natural" for any other food product, leaving the decision to use the term solely to the manufacturer.

A recent survey by the Shelton Group, an advertising agency, found that consumers trust the term "natural," which they believe to be federally regulated, more than the term "organic," which they believe to be "a fancy way of saying expensive." But in reality, "organic" is the only term with any federally regulated criteria.

Provençal Chicken and Orzo Salad

Makes 4 main-dish servings

✪ Great for Steps 1, 2, 3, 4 and 5

Boldly seasoned olives and marinated artichokes find perfect balance with chicken and whole wheat orzo in this pretty, crowd-pleasing salad.

Tip

The remaining artichoke marinade may be stored in the refrigerator (in the original jar) and used in salad dressings.

1 cup	whole wheat orzo	250 mL
1	jar (6 oz/170 mL) marinated artichoke hearts, with oil	1
3 cups	diced roasted or poached skinless chicken breast	750 mL
1 cup	halved cherry tomatoes	250 mL
½ cup	pitted brine-cured black olives (such as kalamata), coarsely chopped	125 mL
¼ cup	dried currants or chopped raisins	60 mL
1 tbsp	chopped fresh tarragon	15 mL
2 tbsp	white wine vinegar	30 mL
2 tsp	Dijon mustard	10 mL

1. In a large pot of boiling water, cook orzo according to package directions until al dente. Drain and rinse under cold water until cool. Transfer to a large bowl.
2. Drain artichoke hearts, reserving 2 tbsp (30 mL) marinade. Roughly chop artichoke hearts and add to orzo, along with chicken, tomatoes, olives and currants.
3. In a small bowl, whisk together tarragon, the reserved marinade, vinegar and mustard. Add to orzo mixture and gently toss to coat.

Nutrients per serving	
Calories	236
Total fat	4 g
Saturated fat	0 g
Cholesterol	53 mg
Sodium	649 mg
Carbohydrate	24 g
Fiber	3 g
Protein	26 g
Calcium	31 mg
Iron	3.1 mg

Thai Chicken Salad

Makes 6 main-dish servings

✪ Great for Steps 1, 2, 3 and 4

Herbs. Vegetables. Chicken. Lime. Mmm ... keep this recipe handy for your next potluck gathering.

Variations

Any variety of unsweetened natural nut or seed butter (e.g., cashew, almond, sunflower) may be used in place of the peanut butter.

Any other roasted or toasted chopped nut or seed (e.g., cashews, almonds, sunflower seeds or pepitas) may be used in place of the peanuts.

Substitute 12 oz (375 g) tempeh, diced, for the chicken.

Nutrients per serving	
Calories	285
Total fat	13 g
Saturated fat	2 g
Cholesterol	26 mg
Sodium	700 mg
Carbohydrate	22 g
Fiber	4 g
Protein	15 g
Calcium	54 mg
Iron	1.4 mg

- **Blender**

4	cloves garlic	4
1	1-inch (2.5 cm) piece gingerroot	1
1/4 tsp	cayenne pepper	1 mL
1/3 cup	freshly squeezed lime juice	75 mL
1/4 cup	reduced-sodium tamari or soy sauce	60 mL
2 tbsp	vegetable oil	30 mL
2 tbsp	agave nectar, brown rice syrup or liquid honey	30 mL
2 tbsp	unsweetened natural peanut butter	30 mL
3 cups	diced roasted or poached skinless chicken breast	750 mL
2	cucumbers, halved lengthwise, then thinly sliced crosswise	2
1	red bell pepper, cut into thin strips	1
3 cups	shredded napa cabbage	750 mL
1 cup	coarsely shredded carrots	250 mL
1/2 cup	thinly sliced red onion	125 mL
1/2 cup	packed fresh cilantro or mint leaves, chopped	125 mL
1/3 cup	coarsely chopped lightly salted roasted peanuts	75 mL

1. In blender, combine garlic, ginger, cayenne, lime juice, tamari, oil, agave nectar and peanut butter; purée until smooth.
2. In a large bowl, combine chicken, cucumbers, red pepper, cabbage, carrots, red onion and cilantro. Add dressing and gently toss to coat. Sprinkle with peanuts.

Summer Salmon Panzanella

Makes 4 main-dish servings

✪ Great for Steps 1, 2, 3, 4 and 5

Echo the breezy spirit of summer with a main dish that takes it in stride: an easy salmon salad with green beans, cherry tomatoes and crusty whole wheat baguette.

- **Steamer basket**

8 oz	green beans, trimmed and cut into 1-inch (2.5 cm) pieces	250 g
	Ice water	
1/2 tsp	fine sea salt	2 mL
1/4 tsp	freshly ground black pepper	1 mL
3 tbsp	extra virgin olive oil	45 mL
2 tbsp	red wine vinegar	30 mL
1/2 tsp	Dijon mustard	2 mL
4 cups	day-old whole-wheat baguette cubes	1 L
2 cups	halved cherry tomatoes	500 mL
1 cup	thinly sliced red onion	250 mL
1/2 cup	packed fresh basil leaves, thinly sliced	125 mL
1	can (15 oz/425 g) wild Alaskan salmon, drained (skin removed, if necessary)	1

1. Place green beans in a steamer basket set over a large pot of boiling water. Cover and steam for 4 to 6 minutes or until tender. Transfer to a large bowl of ice water to stop the cooking. Drain and pat dry with paper towels.
2. In a small bowl, whisk together salt, pepper, oil, vinegar and mustard.
3. In a large bowl, combine green beans, baguette cubes, tomatoes, red onion and basil. Add dressing and gently toss to coat. Let stand for 15 minutes to blend the flavors.
4. Flake salmon with a fork. Add to salad and gently toss to combine.

Nutrients per serving	
Calories	359
Total fat	14 g
Saturated fat	3 g
Cholesterol	41 mg
Sodium	500 mg
Carbohydrate	27 g
Fiber	8 g
Protein	29 g
Calcium	320 mg
Iron	2.0 mg

Balsamic Tuna Salad in Avocado Halves

Makes 2 main-dish servings

✪ Great for Steps 1, 2, 3 and 4

Nutrients per serving	
Calories	332
Total fat	16 g
Saturated fat	3 g
Cholesterol	15 mg
Sodium	321 mg
Carbohydrate	9 g
Fiber	7 g
Protein	27 g
Calcium	24 mg
Iron	1.8 mg

1	can (6 oz/170 g) tuna packed in olive oil, with oil	1
1 tsp	balsamic vinegar	5 mL
¼ tsp	Dijon mustard	1 mL
1	firm-ripe Hass avocado, peeled, halved and pitted	1

1. Drain tuna, reserving 2 tsp (10 mL) oil. In a small bowl, whisk together the reserved oil, vinegar and mustard. Set aside 1 tsp (5 mL) of the dressing. Add tuna to the remaining dressing, tossing gently to combine.
2. Fill avocado halves with tuna mixture. Drizzle with the reserved dressing.

Tuna and White Bean Salad

Makes 2 main-dish servings

✪ Great for Steps 1, 3 and 4

Nutrients per serving	
Calories	370
Total fat	7 g
Saturated fat	1 g
Cholesterol	15 mg
Sodium	629 mg
Carbohydrate	37 g
Fiber	11 g
Protein	39 g
Calcium	140 mg
Iron	4.9 mg

1	can (6 oz/170 g) tuna packed in olive oil, with oil	1
1 tbsp	red wine vinegar	15 mL
½ tsp	Dijon mustard	2 mL
1	can (14 to 19 oz/398 to 540 mL) white beans (see tip, page 135), drained and rinsed	1
½ cup	finely chopped celery	125 mL
¼ cup	finely chopped red onion	60 mL
⅓ cup	packed fresh flat-leaf (Italian) parsley leaves, chopped	75 mL
1 tsp	dried rosemary (optional)	5 mL

1. Drain tuna, reserving 1 tbsp (15 mL) oil. In a small bowl, whisk together the reserved oil, vinegar and mustard.
2. In a medium bowl, combine tuna, beans, celery, red onion, parsley and rosemary (if using). Add dressing and gently toss to coat.

Sicilian Tuna and Rice Salad

Makes 6 main-dish servings

✪ Great for Steps 1, 3, 4 and 5

This familiar, homey rice and tuna salad — versions of which can be found throughout Sicily — is hearty enough for the dinner table.

Tip

To hard-cook eggs, place eggs in a saucepan large enough to hold them in a single layer. Add enough cold water to cover eggs by 1 inch (2.5 cm). Heat over high heat until water is just boiling. Remove from heat and cover pan. Let stand for about 12 minutes for large eggs (9 minutes for medium eggs; 15 minutes for extra-large eggs). Drain eggs and cool completely under cold running water or in a bowl of ice water. Refrigerate until ready to eat.

Nutrients per serving	
Calories	275
Total fat	8 g
Saturated fat	2 g
Cholesterol	70 mg
Sodium	461 mg
Carbohydrate	20 g
Fiber	4 g
Protein	23 g
Calcium	65 mg
Iron	3.4 mg

2	cans (each 6 oz/170 g) tuna packed in olive oil, with oil	2
2 tsp	finely grated lemon zest	10 mL
1/4 cup	freshly squeezed lemon juice	60 mL
3 cups	cooked brown basmati or other long-grain brown rice (see page 438), cooled slightly	750 mL
1	large red bell pepper, chopped	1
1 1/4 cups	thinly sliced green onions	300 mL
1 cup	chopped celery	250 mL
1/2 cup	pitted kalamata or other brine-cured black olives, chopped	125 mL
3 tbsp	drained capers	45 mL
2	hard-cooked large eggs (see tip at left), peeled and chopped	2
1 cup	packed fresh flat-leaf (Italian) parsley leaves, chopped	250 mL

1. Drain tuna, reserving 2 tbsp (30 mL) oil. In a small bowl, whisk together the reserved oil, lemon zest and lemon juice.
2. In a large bowl, combine tuna, rice, red pepper, green onions, celery, olives and capers. Add dressing and gently toss to coat. Cover and refrigerate for at least 1 hour, until chilled, or for up to 6 hours. Just before serving, add eggs and parsley, gently tossing to combine.

Crab and Papaya Salad with Mint Dressing

Makes 2 main-dish servings

✪ Great for Steps 1, 2, 3 and 4

No ordinary crab dish could cut it on a wiltingly hot day. But this no-cook crab salad, with luscious tropical papaya, crisp red pepper and the clean flavors of lime and mint, exudes cool pleasure and satisfaction.

Tips

Jumbo lump crabmeat is typically larger chunks of crabmeat from larger crabs. It works well in salads and crab cakes.

Two 6-oz (175 g) cans of lump crabmeat, drained, may be used in place of the fresh crabmeat.

1 tsp	finely grated lime zest	5 mL
1 tbsp	freshly squeezed lime juice	15 mL
1 tbsp	vegetable oil	15 mL
1½ tsp	agave nectar or liquid honey	7 mL
1 tsp	fish sauce (nam pla)	5 mL
6 oz	cooked jumbo lump crabmeat, picked over	175 g
1	large red bell pepper, finely chopped	1
1½ cups	diced papaya (about 1 medium)	375 mL
¼ cup	packed fresh mint leaves, chopped	60 mL

1. In a small bowl, whisk together lime zest, lime juice, oil, agave nectar and fish sauce.
2. In a large bowl, combine crabmeat, red pepper, papaya and mint. Add dressing and gently toss to coat.

Superfood Spotlight

Crabmeat • Crabmeat is low in total fat and saturates and rich in minerals. It is a good source of l-tyrosine, an amino acid that has been shown to improve brain power. It contains as much protein as a similar weight of lean beef and is therefore ideal for vegetarians who eat fish and seafood. A 3½ oz (100 g) portion of crab provides over half a day's recommended intake of selenium — a powerful mineral with anticancer action — as well as a quarter of a day's folate, which protects against birth defects and is linked to a reduction in blood homocysteine (a contributing factor in heart disease).

Nutrients per serving	
Calories	237
Total fat	8 g
Saturated fat	1 g
Cholesterol	62 mg
Sodium	564 mg
Carbohydrate	22 g
Fiber	4 g
Protein	20 g
Calcium	101 mg
Iron	1.2 mg

Shrimp, Grapefruit and Watercress Salad

Makes 4 main-dish servings

✪ Great for Steps 1, 2, 3 and 4

A study in pink and green, this recipe is one for the "secret weapon" file. Watercress and fresh mint dress up ready-cooked shrimp from the supermarket, while bittersweet grapefruit brightens all.

Tip

Avocados come in several varieties, but Hass are the most widely available. A Hass avocado — notable for its dark, bumpy skin and rich, buttery flesh — is ideal in this simple salad, but any other variety may be used in its place.

2	red grapefruit	2
2 tsp	extra virgin olive oil	10 mL
1 tsp	liquid honey or agave nectar	5 mL
1/2 tsp	fine sea salt	2 mL
1/8 tsp	freshly ground black pepper	0.5 mL
12 oz	cooked peeled deveined medium shrimp	375 g
4 cups	packed tender watercress	1 L
1	small firm-ripe Hass avocado, diced	1
1 tbsp	minced fresh mint	15 mL

1. Using a sharp knife, cut peel and pith from grapefruit. Working over a large bowl, cut between membranes to release segments.
2. Squeeze any remaining juice from grapefruit membranes into a small bowl. Whisk in oil, honey, salt and pepper.
3. To the grapefruit segments, add shrimp and dressing, gently tossing to coat.
4. Divide watercress among four plates. Arrange shrimp mixture, avocado and mint on top.

Superfood Spotlight

Grapefruit • Grapefruits are high in antioxidants, which can boost the immune system, protect the heart and help prevent prostate and other cancers. Pink-fleshed grapefruit has more health benefits than white — the pink pigment indicates the presence of the antioxidant lycopene. Like other citrus fruits, grapefruits contain flavonoids, compounds that appear to increase the benefits of vitamin C. Grapefruits are low on the glycemic index and very low in calories, making them a good option for dieters and those watching their blood sugar levels. Because grapefruit juice can alter the effect of certain drugs (e.g., drugs that lower blood pressure), people on medication should check with their doctors before they consume the fruit.

Nutrients per serving	
Calories	270
Total fat	11 g
Saturated fat	2 g
Cholesterol	143 mg
Sodium	440 mg
Carbohydrate	22 g
Fiber	6 g
Protein	22 g
Calcium	137 mg
Iron	2.6 mg

Soups, Stews and Chilis

Beet Soup with Fresh Ginger . . . 166
Bok Choy and Mushroom Soup . . . 167
Creamy Broccoli Soup . . . 168
Velvety Carrot Soup . . . 169
Roasted Cauliflower Soup . . . 170
Thai Curry Pumpkin Soup . . . 171
Butternut Squash Soup with Sage and Thyme . . . 172
Sweet Potato Bisque with West Indian Spices . . . 173
Classic Tomato Soup . . . 174
Farmers' Market Gazpacho . . . 175
Vegetable Minestrone . . . 176
Quick Kale and Quinoa Minestrone . . . 177
Healthy Know-How: Frozen Vegetables and Fruit — A Great Addition to Your Diet . . . 178
So-Easy Spring Pea Soup . . . 178
Swedish Yellow Split Pea Soup with Fresh Dill . . . 179
Black-Eyed Pea Soup with Indian Spices . . . 180
Lemony Chickpea and Quinoa Soup with Parmesan . . . 181
Tunisian Chickpea, Quinoa and Lentil Soup . . . 182
French Lentil Soup . . . 183
Red Lentil Mulligatawny . . . 184
Tabbouleh Soup with Lentils and Bulgur . . . 185
Black Bean Pumpkin Soup . . . 186
Tuscan Farro and White Bean Soup . . . 187
Mushroom and Barley Soup . . . 188
Summer Vegetable Orzo Soup . . . 189

Curried Orzo Soup . . . 190
Brown Rice, Greens and Miso Soup . . . 191
Miso Soup with Soba and Vegetables. . . 192
Spinach Egg Drop Soup . . . 193
Asian Chicken Noodle Soup . . . 194
Spiced Chicken and Couscous Soup. . . 195
Turkey Soup with Sweet Potatoes and Mustard Greens . . . 196
Vietnamese Pho. . . 197
Beef and Snow Pea Soup . . . 198
Middle Eastern Beef, Bulgur and Chickpea Soup . . . 199
Salmon Chowder. . . 200
Pasta e Fagioli . . . 201
Butternut Squash, White Bean and Kale Stew . . . 202
Red Lentil and Kale Stew. . . 203
Barley, Mushroom and Kale Stew . . . 204
Farro Stew with Spring Peas and Mint. . . 205
Healthy Know-How: Understanding Sodium Labels on Food Packages . . . 206
Red Fish Stew . . . 206
Black Bean Chipotle Chili . . . 207
Sweet Potato, Swiss Chard and Black Bean Chili . . . 208
Indian-Spiced Chickpea Chili . . . 209
White Turkey Chili . . . 210
Green Chile and Pork Pozole . . . 211
Lean Beef and Bean Cowboy Chili . . . 212
Quick Moroccan Beef and Chickpea Chili. . . 213

Beet Soup with Fresh Ginger

Makes 6 servings

✪ Great for Steps 1, 2, 3 and 4

What you find here — aside from a striking ruby and white presentation — is an equally beautiful expression of flavors.

Tip

When puréeing the soup in a food processor or blender, fill the bowl or jug no more than halfway full at a time.

Storage Tip

Store the cooled soup in an airtight container in the refrigerator for up to 2 days or in the freezer for up to 6 months. Thaw overnight in the refrigerator or in the microwave using the Defrost function. Warm soup in a medium saucepan over medium-low heat.

Nutrients per serving	
Calories	102
Total fat	3 g
Saturated fat	0 g
Cholesterol	0 mg
Sodium	174 mg
Carbohydrate	17 g
Fiber	4 g
Protein	4 g
Calcium	53 mg
Iron	1.1 mg

- **Food processor, blender or immersion blender**

4 cups	diced peeled beets	1 L
4 cups	reduced-sodium ready-to-use vegetable broth, divided	1 L
1 tbsp	extra virgin olive oil	15 mL
2 cups	chopped onions	500 mL
2 tbsp	grated gingerroot	30 mL
1 tsp	garam masala	5 mL
1/2 cup	nonfat plain Greek yogurt	125 mL

1. In a medium microwave-safe bowl, combine beets and 2 cups (500 mL) of the broth. Loosely cover and microwave on High for 15 to 20 minutes or until beets are very tender.
2. In a medium saucepan, heat oil over medium-high heat. Add onions and cook, stirring, for 6 to 8 minutes or until softened. Add beet mixture, ginger, garam masala and 1 cup (250 mL) of the broth. Reduce heat to low, cover and simmer for 5 minutes.
3. Working in batches, transfer soup to food processor (or use immersion blender in pot) and purée until smooth. Return soup to pan (if necessary) and whisk in the remaining broth. Warm over medium heat, stirring, for 1 minute. Serve dolloped with yogurt.

Bok Choy and Mushroom Soup

Makes 4 servings

✪ Great for Steps 1, 2, 3 and 4

Bok choy may sound exotic, but this mild, versatile vegetable with crunchy white stalks and tender dark green leaves is commonly available and well priced at most supermarkets. It has a light, sweet flavor and crisp texture that comes from its high water content, which makes it perfect for fast, flavorful soups, because it takes just minutes to wilt. As for nutrition, bok choy is very high in vitamin A, vitamin C, calcium and fiber, and very low in calories.

Storage Tip

Store the cooled soup in an airtight container in the refrigerator for up to 2 days. Warm soup in a medium saucepan over medium-low heat.

Nutrients per serving	
Calories	141
Total fat	5 g
Saturated fat	0 g
Cholesterol	0 mg
Sodium	557 mg
Carbohydrate	16 g
Fiber	4 g
Protein	11 g
Calcium	292 mg
Iron	3.8 mg

3	cloves garlic, minced	3
1 tbsp	minced gingerroot	15 mL
6 cups	reduced-sodium ready-to-use chicken or vegetable broth	1.5 L
2 tbsp	reduced-sodium tamari or soy sauce	30 mL
2 tbsp	unseasoned rice vinegar	30 mL
1 tbsp	toasted sesame oil	15 mL
1 lb	cremini or button mushrooms, trimmed and sliced	500 g
8 oz	firm tofu, drained and cut into 1/2-inch (1 cm) cubes	250 g
6 cups	sliced bok choy	1.5 L
2/3 cup	thinly sliced green onions	150 mL

1. In a large saucepan, combine garlic, ginger, broth, tamari, vinegar and oil. Bring to a boil over medium-high heat. Stir in mushrooms, reduce heat and simmer, stirring occasionally, for 5 minutes or until mushrooms are tender. Stir in tofu, bok choy and green onions; simmer for 3 to 4 minutes or until bok choy is wilted and tofu is heated through.

Superfood Spotlight

Mushrooms • Mushrooms are low in carbohydrates, calories and sodium and are cholesterol- and fat-free. They are also rich in B vitamins, which can help maintain a healthy metabolism. Mushrooms are an excellent source of potassium, a mineral that helps lower elevated blood pressure and reduces the risk of stroke. One medium portobello mushroom, for example, has even more potassium than a banana or a glass of orange juice. Further, mushrooms are a rich source of riboflavin, niacin and selenium (an antioxidant that works with vitamin E to protect cells from the damaging effects of free radicals). Research indicates that regular ingestion of mushrooms over a long period of time may decrease the amount of cancerous cells in the body, as well as help prevent more of such cells from forming.

Creamy Broccoli Soup

Makes 4 servings

✪ Great for Steps 1, 2, 3, 4 and 5

Rich in nutrients, but low in fat and calories, this creamy broccoli soup is elegant enough for company, but also just right for an easy weeknight supper. The oats may seem like an unusual addition, but they melt away as the soup simmers, making it all the more velvety.

Storage Tip

Store the cooled soup in an airtight container in the refrigerator for up to 2 days or in the freezer for up to 6 months. Thaw overnight in the refrigerator or in the microwave using the Defrost function. Warm soup in a medium saucepan over medium-low heat.

Nutrients per serving	
Calories	173
Total fat	8 g
Saturated fat	1 g
Cholesterol	0 mg
Sodium	189 mg
Carbohydrate	22 g
Fiber	8 g
Protein	7 g
Calcium	119 mg
Iron	2.4 mg

- **Food processor, blender or immersion blender**

1 tbsp	extra virgin olive oil	15 mL
1½ cups	chopped onions	375 mL
2	cloves garlic, minced	2
2 tsp	dried basil	10 mL
¼ tsp	freshly ground black pepper	1 mL
1½ lbs	broccoli, coarsely chopped (both florets and peeled stems)	750 g
⅓ cup	large-flake (old-fashioned) rolled oats	75 mL
4 cups	reduced-sodium ready-to-use vegetable broth	1 L
1½ cups	water	375 mL

1. In a large saucepan, heat oil over medium-high heat. Add onions and cook, stirring, for 5 to 6 minutes or until softened. Add garlic, basil and pepper; cook, stirring, for 30 seconds.
2. Stir in broccoli, oats, broth and water. Bring to a boil. Reduce heat and simmer, stirring occasionally, for 15 to 18 minutes or until broccoli is tender.
3. Working in batches, transfer soup to food processor (or use immersion blender in pot) and purée until smooth. Return soup to pan (if necessary). Warm over medium heat, stirring, for 1 minute.

Superfood Spotlight

Broccoli • Broccoli is a rich source of vitamin A, which is good for growth and the repair of body tissues. It is also brimming with calcium, selenium, vitamin C and vitamin K, which is important for normal blood clotting and healthy bones. But it is broccoli's cancer-combating powers that make it something of a nutritional show-stopper. Part of the Brassica family, broccoli contains isothiocyanates — chemicals that stimulate the body's production of its own cancer-fighting substances. It is also rich in indole-3-carbinol, a compound that may reduce the danger of hormone-dependent cancers, and sulforaphane, a phytochemical that helps destroy carcinogens. Early research indicates that broccoli, along with four other fruits and vegetables (potatoes, oranges, apples and radishes), contains substances that act in the same way as the drugs used to treat Alzheimer's disease. Of the five, broccoli is the most potent.

Velvety Carrot Soup

Makes 6 servings

✪ Great for Steps 1, 2, 3 and 4

This soup is perfectly outfitted for any season, with a readily available blend of carrots and onions and a tart finish of lemon juice and yogurt for zing. Every spoonful is packed with nutrition, too.

Tip

When puréeing the soup in a food processor or blender, fill the bowl no more than halfway full at a time.

Storage Tip

Store the cooled soup in an airtight container in the refrigerator for up to 2 days or in the freezer for up to 6 months. Thaw overnight in the refrigerator or in the microwave using the Defrost function. Warm soup in a medium saucepan over medium-low heat.

Nutrients per serving	
Calories	98
Total fat	3 g
Saturated fat	0 g
Cholesterol	0 mg
Sodium	165 mg
Carbohydrate	17 g
Fiber	4 g
Protein	2 g
Calcium	78 mg
Iron	0.8 mg

- **Food processor, blender or immersion blender**

1 tbsp	extra virgin olive oil	15 mL
1 cup	chopped onion	250 mL
1 lb	carrots, chopped	500 g
2 tsp	ground cumin	10 mL
4 cups	reduced-sodium ready-to-use chicken or vegetable broth	1 L
1 tbsp	liquid honey	15 mL
1 tbsp	freshly squeezed lemon juice	15 mL
½ cup	nonfat plain yogurt	125 mL
¼ cup	minced fresh chives (optional)	60 mL

1. In a large saucepan, heat oil over medium-high heat. Add onions and cook, stirring, for 5 to 6 minutes or until softened.
2. Stir in carrots, cumin and broth. Bring to a boil. Reduce heat and simmer, stirring occasionally, for 25 to 30 minutes or until carrots are very soft.
3. Working in batches, transfer soup to food processor (or use immersion blender in pot) and purée until smooth. Return soup to pan (if necessary) and whisk in honey and lemon juice. Warm over medium heat, stirring, for 1 minute. Serve dolloped with yogurt and sprinkled with chives (if using).

▶ Health Note

In a study published in 2011, researchers from the Centers for Disease Control and Prevention (CDC) reported that the antioxidant known as alpha carotene — which is present in exceedingly high amounts in carrots — appears to be associated with longevity. Perhaps a double batch of this soup is in order.

Roasted Cauliflower Soup

Makes 8 servings

✪ Great for Steps 1, 2 and 4

Get ready: with its sublime balance of spices, subtle sweetness and buttery, velvety texture, this seemingly simple soup has a serious wow factor.

Tip

When puréeing the soup in a food processor or blender, fill the bowl no more than halfway full at a time.

Storage Tip

Store the cooled soup in an airtight container in the refrigerator for up to 2 days or in the freezer for up to 6 months. Thaw overnight in the refrigerator or in the microwave using the Defrost function. Warm soup in a medium saucepan over medium-low heat.

Nutrients per serving	
Calories	63
Total fat	3 g
Saturated fat	0 g
Cholesterol	0 mg
Sodium	238 mg
Carbohydrate	9 g
Fiber	3 g
Protein	2 g
Calcium	39 mg
Iron	0.8 mg

- **Preheat oven to 450°F (230°C)**
- **Large rimmed baking sheet, lined with foil and sprayed with nonstick cooking spray (preferably olive oil)**
- **Food processor, blender or immersion blender**

6 cups	cauliflower florets (about 1 large head)	1.5 L
4 tsp	extra virgin olive oil, divided	20 mL
1/2 tsp	fine sea salt, divided	2 mL
2 cups	chopped onions	500 mL
2 tsp	ground cumin	10 mL
2 cups	reduced-sodium ready-to-use chicken or vegetable broth	500 mL
4 cups	water	1 L
1 tbsp	freshly squeezed lemon juice	15 mL
1/4 cup	packed fresh parsley leaves, roughly chopped	60 mL

1. On prepared baking sheet, toss cauliflower with half the oil and half the salt. Spread in a single layer. Roast in preheated oven for 35 to 40 minutes, stirring occasionally, until golden-brown and tender.
2. Meanwhile, in a large saucepan, heat the remaining oil over medium-high heat. Add onions and cook, stirring, for 6 to 8 minutes or until softened.
3. Stir in roasted cauliflower, cumin, the remaining salt, broth and water. Bring to a boil. Reduce heat and simmer, stirring occasionally, for 20 minutes or until cauliflower is very soft.
4. Working in batches, transfer soup to food processor (or use immersion blender in pot) and purée until smooth. Return soup to pan (if necessary) and whisk in lemon juice. Warm over medium heat, stirring, for 1 minute. Serve sprinkled with parsley.

▶ Health Note

Cauliflower offers high fiber and exceptionally high levels of vitamin C, while the onions deliver a trifecta of disease-fighting compounds: fructans, flavonoids and organosulfur. Fructans thwart infections by encouraging the growth of beneficial bacteria in the gut, flavonoids prevent DNA damage that might lead to cancer, and organosulfur may reduce the risk of blood clots.

Thai Curry Pumpkin Soup

Makes 8 servings

✪ Great for Steps 1, 2 and 4

You'll love the layers of flavor that come through in this super-fast and easy Thai soup.

Tip

If 15-oz (425 mL) cans of pumpkin aren't available, purchase two 28-oz (796 mL) cans and measure out 3¾ cups (925 mL). Refrigerate extra pumpkin in an airtight container for up to 1 week.

Storage Tip

Store the cooled soup in an airtight container in the refrigerator for up to 2 days or in the freezer for up to 6 months. Thaw overnight in the refrigerator or in the microwave using the Defrost function. Warm soup in a medium saucepan over medium-low heat.

Nutrients per serving	
Calories	131
Total fat	7 g
Saturated fat	5 g
Cholesterol	0 mg
Sodium	63 mg
Carbohydrate	17 g
Fiber	5 g
Protein	4 g
Calcium	29 mg
Iron	2.1 mg

4	cloves garlic, minced	4
2	cans (each 15 oz/425 mL) pumpkin purée (not pie filling)	2
4 cups	reduced-sodium ready-to-use chicken broth	1 L
3 tbsp	brown rice syrup, liquid honey or agave nectar	45 mL
1 tbsp	Thai red curry paste	15 mL
½ cup	packed fresh cilantro leaves, chopped, divided	125 mL
1 cup	light coconut milk	250 mL
1 tbsp	freshly squeezed lime juice	15 mL

1. In a large saucepan, whisk together garlic, pumpkin, broth, brown rice syrup and curry paste. Bring to a simmer over medium-low heat. Reduce heat and simmer, stirring occasionally, for 5 minutes to blend the flavors. Whisk in half the cilantro, coconut milk and lime juice; simmer, stirring, for 1 to 2 minutes or until heated through. Serve sprinkled with the remaining cilantro.

▸ Health Note

If you think canned pumpkin isn't as healthy as fresh, think again: it has slightly less fiber, but otherwise has a similar nutrition profile and provides more bio-available beta carotene due to heat used in the canning process.

Butternut Squash Soup with Sage and Thyme

Makes 8 servings

✪ Great for Steps 1, 2 and 4

This soup is so velvety it's hard to believe there's no cream and only a small amount of butter. The buttermilk adds richness and complexity without the high fat and calorie content of heavy cream, and also brightens the sweetness of the squash.

Storage Tip

Store the cooled soup in an airtight container in the refrigerator for up to 2 days or in the freezer for up to 6 months. Thaw overnight in the refrigerator or in the microwave using the Defrost function. Warm soup in a medium saucepan over medium-low heat.

Nutrients per serving	
Calories	100
Total fat	1 g
Saturated fat	0 g
Cholesterol	0 mg
Sodium	450 mg
Carbohydrate	22 g
Fiber	6 g
Protein	2 g
Calcium	90 mg
Iron	1.2 mg

- **Food processor, blender or immersion blender**

2 tsp	extra virgin olive oil	10 mL
1¼ cups	chopped onions	300 mL
1	butternut squash (about 3 lbs/1.5 kg), peeled and diced	1
2 tsp	dried rubbed sage	10 mL
1 tsp	dried thyme	5 mL
¼ tsp	freshly ground black pepper	1 mL
5 cups	reduced-sodium ready-to-use chicken or vegetable broth	1.25 L
⅓ cup	buttermilk	75 mL
1 tbsp	liquid honey or brown rice syrup	15 mL
3 tbsp	minced fresh chives (optional)	45 mL

1. In a large saucepan, heat oil over medium-high heat. Add onions and cook, stirring, for 5 to 6 minutes or until softened.
2. Stir in squash, sage, thyme, pepper and broth. Bring to a boil. Reduce heat and simmer, stirring occasionally, for 30 to 35 minutes or until squash is very tender.
3. Working in batches, transfer soup to food processor (or use immersion blender in pot) and purée until smooth. Return soup to pan (if necessary). Warm over medium heat, stirring, for 1 minute. Whisk in buttermilk and honey; heat for 30 seconds. Serve sprinkled with chives, if desired.

Superfood Spotlight

Butternut Squash • Squashes are related to pumpkin, cucumber and melon, and have a lightly nutty flavor that is ideal in both sweet and savory cooking. The orange-fleshed varieties, notably butternut, tend to contain the highest levels of beneficial nutrients. Butternut squash is one of the richest sources of beta-cryptoxanthin, a carotene linked with protection from lung cancer. The other carotenes it contains reduce the risk of colon cancer and prostate problems in men, and may help reduce inflammation associated with conditions such as asthma and arthritis. The vegetable is also a very good source of several vitamins and minerals, including the antioxidant vitamins C and E, calcium, iron and magnesium.

Sweet Potato Bisque with West Indian Spices

Makes 6 servings

✪ Great for Steps 1, 2, 3 and 4

As an avowed lover of all things sweet potato, I am unabashedly beholden to this soup. It has just the right balance of sweet, savory and spicy.

Tip

When puréeing the soup in a food processor or blender, fill the bowl no more than halfway full at a time.

Storage Tip

Store the cooled soup in an airtight container in the refrigerator for up to 2 days or in the freezer for up to 6 months. Thaw overnight in the refrigerator or in the microwave using the Defrost function. Warm soup in a medium saucepan over medium-low heat.

Nutrients per serving	
Calories	151
Total fat	3 g
Saturated fat	2 g
Cholesterol	0 mg
Sodium	150 mg
Carbohydrate	29 g
Fiber	5 g
Protein	3 g
Calcium	78 mg
Iron	1.2 mg

- **Food processor, blender or immersion blender**

2 lbs	sweet potatoes, peeled and shredded	1 kg
1½ tsp	mild curry powder	7 mL
1 tsp	finely grated lime zest	5 mL
½ tsp	ground allspice	2 mL
4 cups	reduced-sodium ready-to-use chicken or vegetable broth	1 L
½ cup	packed fresh cilantro leaves, chopped, divided	125 mL
1 cup	light coconut milk	250 mL
⅓ cup	plain nonfat yogurt	75 mL
1 tbsp	freshly squeezed lime juice	15 mL

1. In a large saucepan, combine sweet potatoes, curry powder, lime zest, allspice and broth. Bring to a boil over medium-high heat. Reduce heat and simmer, stirring occasionally, for 25 to 30 minutes or until sweet potatoes are very soft.
2. Working in batches, transfer soup to food processor (or use immersion blender in pot) and purée until smooth. Return soup to pan (if necessary) and whisk in half the cilantro and coconut milk. Warm over medium heat, stirring, for 1 minute.
3. In a small bowl, whisk together yogurt and lime juice until smooth. Serve soup drizzled with yogurt mixture and sprinkled with the remaining cilantro.

Classic Tomato Soup

Makes 4 servings

✪ Great for Steps 1, 2 and 4

Canned tomatoes vary in their sweetness, so taste for sweetness in the finished soup — you may want to add a bit of agave nectar to balance the acidity of the tomatoes.

Tip

When puréeing the soup in a food processor or blender, fill the bowl no more than halfway full at a time.

Storage Tip

Store the cooled soup in an airtight container in the refrigerator for up to 2 days or in the freezer for up to 6 months. Thaw overnight in the refrigerator or in the microwave using the Defrost function. Warm soup in a medium saucepan over medium-low heat.

Nutrients per serving	
Calories	109
Total fat	4 g
Saturated fat	1 g
Cholesterol	0 mg
Sodium	744 mg
Carbohydrate	17 g
Fiber	3 g
Protein	3 g
Calcium	46 mg
Iron	1.6 mg

- **Food processor, blender or immersion blender**

1 tbsp	extra virgin olive oil	15 mL
1¼ cups	chopped onions	300 mL
2 tsp	dried basil	10 mL
¾ tsp	fine sea salt	3 mL
⅛ tsp	cayenne pepper	0.5 mL
2	cans (each 14 to 15 oz/398 to 425 mL) diced tomatoes, with juice	2
2 tbsp	tomato paste	30 mL
2 cups	water	500 mL

1. In a large saucepan, heat oil over medium-high heat. Add onions and cook, stirring, for 5 to 6 minutes or until softened. Add basil, salt and cayenne; cook, stirring, for 30 seconds.
2. Stir in tomatoes with juice, tomato paste and water. Bring to a boil. Reduce heat and simmer, stirring occasionally, for about 20 minutes to blend the flavors.
3. Working in batches, transfer soup to food processor (or use immersion blender in pot) and purée until smooth. Return soup to pan (if necessary). Warm over medium heat, stirring, for 1 minute.

Superfood Spotlight

Tomatoes • Tomatoes are our major source of dietary lycopene, a carotene antioxidant that fights heart disease and may help to prevent prostate cancer. Tomatoes also have an anticoagulant effect because of their salicylates, and they contain several other antioxidants, including quercetin and lutein, which help to prevent cataracts and keep heart and eyes healthy. Tomatoes are an excellent source of vitamin C — one medium tomato contains nearly a quarter of the day's recommended intake for an adult — and are rich in potassium to help regulate body fluids. Tomatoes are low in calories and contain significant amounts of fiber.

Farmers' Market Gazpacho

Makes 4 servings

✪ Great for Steps 1, 2 and 4

Gazpacho is a cold summertime soup typically made from a puréed mixture of fresh tomatoes, bell peppers, onions, celery, cucumber, bread crumbs, garlic, olive oil, vinegar and sometimes lemon juice — though variations are too numerous to count.

Tip

For a smoother texture, process the soup until very smooth, then press it through a sieve set over a bowl, discarding the solids.

Storage Tip

Store the cooled soup in an airtight container in the refrigerator for up to 1 day.

Nutrients per serving	
Calories	91
Total fat	4 g
Saturated fat	1 g
Cholesterol	0 mg
Sodium	362 mg
Carbohydrate	13 g
Fiber	4 g
Protein	3 g
Calcium	38 mg
Iron	0.9 mg

- **Food processor**

5	cloves garlic, coarsely chopped	5
1½ lbs	tomatoes, cut into quarters (about 4)	750 g
1 cup	coarsely chopped seeded peeled cucumber	250 mL
½ cup	chopped sweet onion	125 mL
½ cup	chopped red bell pepper	125 mL
½ cup	chopped green bell pepper	125 mL
½ tsp	fine sea salt	2 mL
½ tsp	ground cumin	2 mL
3 tbsp	sherry vinegar or red wine vinegar	45 mL
1 tbsp	extra virgin olive oil	15 mL
½ tsp	agave nectar	2 mL

1. In food processor, combine garlic, tomatoes, cucumber, onion, red pepper, green pepper, salt, cumin, vinegar, oil and agave nectar; pulse until mostly but not entirely smooth. Cover and refrigerate for at least 30 minutes, to blend the flavors, or for up to 24 hours.

Vegetable Minestrone

Makes 8 servings

✪ Great for Steps 1, 2, 3, 4 and 5

The depth of flavor from the sautéed onions, carrots, celery and garlic in this minestrone is so savory that there's no need for broth; water, canned tomatoes and Italian seasoning work beautifully.

Tip

An equal amount of frozen cut green beans (no need to thaw) may be used in place of the fresh green beans.

Storage Tip

Store the cooled soup in an airtight container in the refrigerator for up to 2 days or in the freezer for up to 6 months. Thaw overnight in the refrigerator or in the microwave using the Defrost function. Warm soup in a medium saucepan over medium-low heat.

Nutrients per serving	
Calories	132
Total fat	2 g
Saturated fat	0 g
Cholesterol	0 mg
Sodium	728 mg
Carbohydrate	25 g
Fiber	6 g
Protein	7 g
Calcium	135 mg
Iron	2.6 mg

2 tsp	extra virgin olive oil	10 mL
3	cloves garlic, minced	3
1½ cups	chopped onions	375 mL
1 cup	chopped carrots	250 mL
1 cup	chopped celery	250 mL
1 tbsp	dried Italian seasoning	15 mL
1 tsp	fine sea salt	5 mL
2	cans (each 14 to 15 oz/398 to 425 mL) diced tomatoes, with juice	2
1	can (14 to 19 oz/398 to 540 mL) white beans, drained and rinsed	1
4 cups	chopped kale (tough stems and center ribs removed)	1 L
⅓ cup	whole wheat or multigrain tiny pasta (such as ditalini or orzo)	75 mL
8 cups	water	2 L
8 oz	green beans, trimmed and cut into 1-inch (2.5 cm) pieces	250 g

1. In a large saucepan, heat oil over medium-high heat. Add garlic, onions, carrots, celery, Italian seasoning and salt; cook, stirring, for 6 to 8 minutes or until vegetables are softened. Stir in tomatoes and cook for 2 minutes or until some of the liquid is evaporated.
2. Stir in beans, kale, pasta and water. Bring to a boil. Reduce heat and simmer, stirring occasionally, for 15 minutes. Stir in green beans and simmer, stirring occasionally, for 10 to 15 minutes or until vegetables are soft and soup has thickened.

Quick Kale and Quinoa Minestrone

Makes 8 servings

✪ Great for Steps 1, 2, 3, 4 and 5

Hearty fare without being heavy, this lovely green, red and white soup looks and tastes like a bowlful of Italy. The addition of quinoa, however, is decidedly New World. And while any dark, leafy green will work here, consider sticking with kale, as it contains the highest levels of antioxidants of all vegetables and is a very good source of vitamin C.

Storage Tip

Store the cooled soup in an airtight container in the refrigerator for up to 2 days or in the freezer for up to 6 months. Thaw overnight in the refrigerator or in the microwave using the Defrost function. Warm soup in a medium saucepan over medium-low heat.

Nutrients per serving	
Calories	205
Total fat	3 g
Saturated fat	0 g
Cholesterol	0 mg
Sodium	434 mg
Carbohydrate	37 g
Fiber	8 g
Protein	9 g
Calcium	226 mg
Iron	5.0 mg

2 tsp	extra virgin olive oil	10 mL
1½ cups	chopped onions	375 mL
1¼ cups	chopped carrots	300 mL
1 cup	chopped celery	250 mL
4	cloves garlic, minced	4
8 cups	chopped kale (tough stems and center ribs removed)	2 L
1½ tbsp	dried Italian seasoning	22 mL
⅔ cup	quinoa, rinsed	150 mL
1	jar (26 oz/700 mL) reduced-sodium marinara sauce	1
8 cups	reduced-sodium ready-to-use vegetable or chicken broth	2 L
1	can (14 to 19 oz/398 to 540 mL) white beans, drained and rinsed	1

1. In a large saucepan, heat oil over medium-high heat. Add onions, carrots and celery; cook, stirring, for 6 to 8 minutes or until softened. Add garlic, kale and Italian seasoning; cook, stirring, for 1 minute.
2. Stir in quinoa, marinara sauce and broth. Bring to a boil. Reduce heat, cover, leaving lid ajar, and simmer, stirring occasionally, for 20 minutes or until quinoa is tender.
3. In a small bowl, mash half the beans with a fork. Stir mashed and whole beans into soup and simmer, stirring occasionally, for 5 to 10 minutes or until soup is slightly thickened.

Healthy Know-How

Frozen Vegetables and Fruit — A Great Addition to Your Diet

For a significant part of the year, fresh produce is both limited and expensive. So what's a health-minded, produce-loving home cook to do? Head to the frozen foods section of the supermarket, that's what. Counter to popular belief that frozen fruits and vegetables are lacking in nutrients, they may be even more healthful than some of the fresh produce sold in supermarkets. The explanation is twofold. First, fruits and vegetables destined for freezing tend to be processed at the peak of ripeness, a time when they are most nutrient-packed. They are then flash-frozen (vegetables get a quick steam-blanching), which preserves them in a relatively nutrient-rich state. On the other hand, fruits and vegetables destined to be shipped to fresh produce aisles around the country are typically picked before they are ripe, which gives them less time to develop a full spectrum of vitamins and minerals. Additionally, exposure to light and heat during shipping degrades delicate nutrients such vitamins C and B.

In sum, buy fresh, ripe produce when it's in season, but when it's not, frozen is a great option. If you live in the United States, choose packages marked with the USDA's "U.S. Fancy" shield, which designates produce of the best size, shape and color. Steam or microwave your produce rather than boiling it to minimize the loss of water-soluble vitamins.

So-Easy Spring Pea Soup

Makes 4 servings

✪ Great for Steps 2, 3 and 4

- **Blender**

3 cups	frozen petite peas, thawed	750 mL
2 tbsp	chopped fresh mint or basil	30 mL
2 cups	reduced-sodium ready-to-use vegetable broth	500 mL

1. In blender, combine peas, mint and broth; purée until smooth.
2. Transfer purée to a medium saucepan. Warm over medium heat, stirring often, for 4 to 5 minutes or until hot but not boiling.

Nutrients per serving	
Calories	102
Total fat	0 g
Saturated fat	0 g
Cholesterol	0 mg
Sodium	157 mg
Carbohydrate	19 g
Fiber	7 g
Protein	6 g
Calcium	41 mg
Iron	2.0 mg

Swedish Yellow Split Pea Soup with Fresh Dill

Makes 6 servings

✪ Great for Steps 1, 2, 3 and 4

Yellow pea soup with ham is traditionally served every Thursday night in Sweden. If you've ever wondered why bags of yellow split peas are sold at IKEA, that's why.

Tip

An equal amount of dried yellow lentils or green split peas may be used in place of the yellow split peas.

Storage Tip

Store the cooled soup in an airtight container in the refrigerator for up to 2 days or in the freezer for up to 6 months. Thaw overnight in the refrigerator or in the microwave using the Defrost function. Warm soup in a medium saucepan over medium-low heat.

Nutrients per serving	
Calories	229
Total fat	3 g
Saturated fat	1 g
Cholesterol	0 mg
Sodium	292 mg
Carbohydrate	40 g
Fiber	6 g
Protein	12 g
Calcium	104 mg
Iron	3.6 mg

- **Food processor or blender**

1 tbsp	extra virgin olive oil	15 mL
2 cups	chopped onions	500 mL
1½ cups	chopped carrots	375 mL
¼ tsp	fine sea salt	1 mL
¼ tsp	freshly cracked black pepper	1 mL
1⅓ cups	dried yellow split peas, rinsed	325 mL
6 cups	reduced-sodium ready-to-use chicken or vegetable broth	1.5 L
¾ cup	water	175 mL
¼ cup	chopped fresh dill, divided	60 mL

1. In a large saucepan, heat oil over medium-high heat. Add onions, carrots, salt and pepper; cook, stirring, for 6 to 8 minutes or until vegetables are softened.
2. Stir in peas and broth. Bring to a boil. Reduce heat to medium-low, cover and simmer, stirring occasionally, for 35 to 40 minutes or until peas are very tender.
3. Transfer 1 cup (250 mL) of the soup solids to food processor. Add water and purée until smooth. Return purée to pan and stir in half the dill. Simmer, stirring often, for 5 minutes to blend the flavors, thinning soup with water if too thick. Serve sprinkled with the remaining dill.

Superfood Spotlight

Split Peas • Dried split peas, like other legumes, are rich in soluble fiber. This forms a gel-like substance in the digestive tract that binds cholesterol-containing bile and carries it out of the body. Split peas also contain an isoflavone called daidzein, which acts like weak estrogen in the body. The consumption of daidzein has been linked to a reduced risk of certain health conditions, including breast and prostate cancer. Split peas are particularly rich in potassium, a mineral that can help lower blood pressure and control fluid retention, and may help limit the growth of potentially damaging plaques in the blood vessels.

Black-Eyed Pea Soup with Indian Spices

Makes 6 servings

✪ Great for Steps 1, 2, 3 and 4

Black-eyed peas pack a spicy soup with plenty of folate, while onions infuse it with vitamin C.

Tip

Two 14- to 19-oz (398 to 540 mL) cans of black-eyed peas, drained and rinsed, may be used in place of the frozen peas. Reduce the simmering time in step 2 to 20 minutes.

Storage Tip

Store the cooled soup in an airtight container in the refrigerator for up to 2 days or in the freezer for up to 6 months. Thaw overnight in the refrigerator or in the microwave using the Defrost function. Warm soup in a medium saucepan over medium-low heat.

Nutrients per serving	
Calories	175
Total fat	3 g
Saturated fat	0 g
Cholesterol	0 mg
Sodium	252 mg
Carbohydrate	30 g
Fiber	6 g
Protein	10 g
Calcium	47 mg
Iron	2.9 mg

- **Food processor, blender or immersion blender**

2 tsp	vegetable oil	10 mL
1½ cups	chopped onions	375 mL
¾ cup	chopped celery	175 mL
1 tbsp	mild or hot curry powder	15 mL
1 tsp	garam masala	5 mL
¾ tsp	ground cumin	3 mL
½ tsp	fine sea salt	2 mL
¼ tsp	cayenne pepper	1 mL
2	packages (each 10 oz/300 g) frozen black-eyed peas	2
6 cups	water	1.5 L
1 cup	packed fresh cilantro leaves, chopped, divided	250 mL

1. In a large saucepan, heat oil over medium-high heat. Add onions and celery; cook, stirring, for 6 to 8 minutes or until softened. Add curry powder, garam masala, cumin, salt and cayenne; cook, stirring, for 30 seconds.
2. Stir in peas and water. Bring to a boil. Reduce heat to low, cover and simmer, stirring occasionally, for 35 to 40 minutes or until peas are very tender.
3. Transfer 2 cups (500 mL) of the soup solids and ½ cup (125 mL) of the soup liquid to food processor and purée until smooth (or, using an immersion blender in the pan, pulse the soup in three or four quick spurts to partially blend it, leaving it chunky). Return purée to pan (if necessary) and stir in half the cilantro. Simmer, stirring, for 2 to 3 minutes to blend the flavors. Serve sprinkled with the remaining cilantro.

Lemony Chickpea and Quinoa Soup with Parmesan

Makes 6 servings

✪ Great for Steps 1, 2, 3, 4 and 5

Lemon zest and lemon juice bring a touch of sunshine to this delicious soup, which can be made as spicy or as mellow as you like.

Storage Tip

Store the cooled soup in an airtight container in the refrigerator for up to 2 days or in the freezer for up to 6 months. Thaw overnight in the refrigerator or in the microwave using the Defrost function. Warm soup in a medium saucepan over medium-low heat.

Nutrients per serving	
Calories	257
Total fat	6 g
Saturated fat	2 g
Cholesterol	9 mg
Sodium	600 mg
Carbohydrate	39 g
Fiber	8 g
Protein	10 g
Calcium	170 mg
Iron	3.1 mg

2 tsp	extra virgin olive oil	10 mL
2 cups	chopped onions	500 mL
3	cloves garlic, minced	3
1 tbsp	dried Italian seasoning	15 mL
1/8 tsp	cayenne pepper	0.5 mL
2	cans (each 14 to 19 oz/398 to 540 mL) chickpeas, drained and rinsed	2
1/2 cup	quinoa, rinsed	125 mL
8 cups	reduced-sodium ready-to-use chicken or vegetable broth	2 L
1 cup	packed fresh parsley leaves, chopped	250 mL
1 tsp	finely grated lemon zest	5 mL
3 tbsp	freshly squeezed lemon juice	45 mL
1/3 cup	freshly grated Parmesan cheese	75 mL

1. In a large saucepan, heat oil over medium-high heat. Add onions and cook, stirring, for 6 to 8 minutes or until softened. Add garlic, Italian seasoning and cayenne; cook, stirring, for 1 minute.
2. Stir in chickpeas, quinoa and broth. Bring to a boil. Reduce heat to medium-low, cover, leaving lid ajar, and simmer, stirring occasionally, for 20 minutes or until quinoa is tender. Stir in parsley, lemon zest and lemon juice. Serve sprinkled with cheese.

Tunisian Chickpea, Quinoa and Lentil Soup

Makes 8 servings

✪ Great for Steps 1, 2, 3, 4 and 5

Hearty enough to satisfy the biggest appetites, this exotically spiced dish is based on a North African soup called harira. It's typical for harira to have chickpeas, lentils and rice, but I've swapped the rice for quinoa. It's just as spectacularly delicious, especially on day two, when the flavors have had further chance to mingle.

Storage Tip

Store the cooled soup in an airtight container in the refrigerator for up to 2 days or in the freezer for up to 6 months. Thaw overnight in the refrigerator or in the microwave using the Defrost function. Warm soup in a medium saucepan over medium-low heat.

Nutrients per serving	
Calories	262
Total fat	5 g
Saturated fat	0 g
Cholesterol	3 mg
Sodium	389 mg
Carbohydrate	43 g
Fiber	10 g
Protein	12 g
Calcium	94 mg
Iron	4.1 mg

1 tbsp	extra virgin olive oil	15 mL
2 cups	chopped onions	500 mL
1 tbsp	ground cumin	15 mL
2 tsp	ground ginger	10 mL
1	can (28 oz/796 mL) crushed tomatoes, with juice	1
2⁄3 cup	dried brown lentils, rinsed	150 mL
8 cups	reduced-sodium ready-to-use chicken or vegetable broth	2 L
1	can (14 to 19 oz/398 to 540 mL) chickpeas, drained and rinsed	1
2⁄3 cup	quinoa, rinsed	150 mL
1 cup	packed fresh cilantro leaves, chopped	250 mL
1 cup	packed fresh flat-leaf (Italian) parsley leaves, chopped	250 mL
1 tbsp	freshly squeezed lemon juice	15 mL

1. In a large saucepan, heat oil over medium-high heat. Add onions and cook, stirring, for 6 to 8 minutes or until softened. Add cumin and ginger; cook, stirring, for 30 seconds.
2. Stir in tomatoes with juice, lentils and broth. Bring to a boil. Reduce heat to low, cover, leaving lid ajar, and simmer for 30 minutes. Stir in chickpeas and quinoa; cover, leaving lid ajar, and simmer, stirring occasionally, for 20 minutes or until lentils are very tender. Stir in cilantro, parsley and lemon juice.

French Lentil Soup

Makes 6 servings

✪ Great for Steps 1, 2, 3 and 4

It won't take more than a spoonful or two for you to understand why this soup is a classic. Soaking the lentils in hot water helps them cook a bit more quickly when they're added to the soup. Leftovers are great, as most legume soups benefit from being made a day ahead so their flavors can meld. Stir in a little water when you reheat the soup if it's too thick.

Storage Tip

Store the cooled soup in an airtight container in the refrigerator for up to 2 days or in the freezer for up to 6 months. Thaw overnight in the refrigerator or in the microwave using the Defrost function. Warm soup in a medium saucepan over medium-low heat.

Nutrients per serving	
Calories	219
Total fat	4 g
Saturated fat	0 g
Cholesterol	0 mg
Sodium	171 mg
Carbohydrate	36 g
Fiber	9 g
Protein	13 g
Calcium	69 mg
Iron	3.4 mg

- **Food processor, blender or immersion blender**

1¼ cups	dried green lentils, rinsed	300 mL
2 cups	boiling water	500 mL
1 tbsp	extra virgin olive oil	15 mL
2 cups	chopped onions	500 mL
1 cup	chopped celery	250 mL
1 cup	chopped carrots	250 mL
	Fine sea salt and cracked black pepper	
3	cloves garlic, minced	3
2 tsp	chopped fresh rosemary	10 mL
1	can (14 to 15 oz/398 to 425 mL) crushed tomatoes, with juice	1
6 cups	water	1.5 L
2 tsp	red wine vinegar	10 mL
½ cup	chopped celery leaves (optional)	125 mL

1. In a medium bowl, combine lentils and boiling water. Let stand for 10 minutes.
2. Meanwhile, in a large saucepan, heat oil over medium-high heat. Add onions, celery, carrots, ¾ tsp (3 mL) salt and ¼ tsp (1 mL) pepper; cook, stirring, for 6 to 8 minutes or until vegetables are softened. Add garlic and rosemary; cook, stirring, for 1 minute.
3. Drain lentils and add to the pan, along with tomatoes with juice and 6 cups (1.5 L) water. Bring to a boil. Reduce heat to medium-low, cover and simmer, stirring occasionally, for 35 to 40 minutes or until lentils are tender.
4. Transfer 2 cups (500 mL) of the soup (mostly solids) to food processor and purée until smooth (or, using an immersion blender in the pan, pulse the soup in three or four quick spurts to partially blend it, leaving it chunky). Return purée to pan (if necessary) and stir in vinegar. Season to taste with salt and pepper. Simmer, stirring often, for 5 minutes. Serve garnished with celery leaves, if desired.

Red Lentil Mulligatawny

Makes 8 servings

✪ Great for Steps 1, 2, 3, 4 and 5

The name of this highly seasoned Indian soup means "pepper water." Although most often made with chicken, this version gets its body from red lentils. The soup gets quite a kick from the combination of curry powder, ginger, cumin and cayenne.

Storage Tip

Store the cooled soup in an airtight container in the refrigerator for up to 2 days or in the freezer for up to 6 months. Thaw overnight in the refrigerator or in the microwave using the Defrost function. Warm soup in a medium saucepan over medium-low heat.

Nutrients per serving	
Calories	353
Total fat	5 g
Saturated fat	2 g
Cholesterol	0 mg
Sodium	157 mg
Carbohydrate	61 g
Fiber	11 g
Protein	16 g
Calcium	68 mg
Iron	3.8 mg

2 tsp	vegetable oil	10 mL
2 cups	chopped onions	500 mL
5	cloves garlic, minced	5
1	large Granny Smith or other tart apple, peeled and chopped	1
1½ tbsp	garam masala	22 mL
1 tbsp	mild curry powder	15 mL
½ tsp	cayenne pepper	2 mL
2 cups	dried red lentils, rinsed	500 mL
8 cups	reduced-sodium ready-to-use vegetable or chicken broth	2 L
1 cup	light coconut milk	250 mL
3 tbsp	freshly squeezed lime juice	45 mL
½ cup	packed fresh cilantro leaves, roughly chopped	125 mL
3¾ cups	hot cooked brown basmati or other long-grain brown rice (see page 438)	925 mL

1. In a large saucepan, heat oil over medium-high heat. Add onions and cook, stirring, for 6 to 8 minutes or until softened. Add garlic, apple, garam masala, curry powder and cayenne; cook, stirring, for 1 minute.
2. Stir in lentils and broth. Bring to a boil. Reduce heat to medium-low, cover, leaving lid ajar, and simmer, stirring occasionally, for 25 to 30 minutes or until lentils are falling apart. Stir in coconut milk and lime juice; simmer, stirring occasionally, for 5 minutes to blend the flavors. Stir in cilantro.
3. Divide rice among eight soup bowls and ladle soup over top.

Tabbouleh Soup with Lentils and Bulgur

Makes 8 servings

✪ Great for Steps 1, 2, 3, 4 and 5

A reminder of summer in a winter bowl, this soup includes all the ingredients contained in a great tabbouleh: bulgur wheat, tomatoes, lemon juice and plenty of parsley and mint. Lentils join the cast for added heartiness, as well as nutrition.

Storage Tip

Store the cooled soup in an airtight container in the refrigerator for up to 2 days or in the freezer for up to 6 months. Thaw overnight in the refrigerator or in the microwave using the Defrost function. Warm soup in a medium saucepan over medium-low heat.

Nutrients per serving	
Calories	212
Total fat	3 g
Saturated fat	0 g
Cholesterol	0 mg
Sodium	521 mg
Carbohydrate	38 g
Fiber	8 g
Protein	11 g
Calcium	66 mg
Iron	3.3 mg

1 tbsp	extra virgin olive oil	15 mL
2 cups	chopped onions	500 mL
3	cloves garlic, minced	3
1 tbsp	ground cumin	15 mL
3/4 tsp	fine sea salt	3 mL
1/4 tsp	cracked black pepper	1 mL
1 cup	dried brown lentils, rinsed	250 mL
1 cup	fine or medium bulgur	250 mL
6 cups	water	1.5 L
2	cans (each 14 to 15 oz/398 to 425 mL) diced tomatoes, with juice	2
1 cup	packed fresh flat-leaf (Italian) parsley leaves, chopped, divided	250 mL
1/2 cup	packed fresh mint leaves, chopped, divided	125 mL
3 tbsp	freshly squeezed lemon juice	45 mL

1. In a large saucepan, heat oil over medium-high heat. Add onions and cook, stirring, for 6 to 8 minutes or until softened. Add garlic, cumin, salt and pepper; cook, stirring, for 1 minute.
2. Stir in lentils, bulgur and water. Bring to a boil. Reduce heat to medium-low, cover, leaving lid ajar, and simmer, stirring occasionally, for 40 to 45 minutes or until lentils are tender. Stir in tomatoes with juice, half the parsley and half the mint; simmer, stirring occasionally, for 5 minutes. Stir in the remaining parsley, the remaining mint and lemon juice.

Black Bean Pumpkin Soup

Makes 10 servings

✪ Great for Steps 1, 2, 3 and 4

Your search for the best black bean soup has ended. You won't taste the pumpkin — it just adds a voluptuous richness.

Tips

If you can only find 19-oz (540 mL) cans of black beans, buy three, but only use half of the third can.

If you only have sweet smoked paprika, add 1⁄8 tsp (0.5 mL) cayenne pepper.

If you can't find a 15-oz (425 mL) can of pumpkin, buy a larger can and measure out 1 3⁄4 cups (425 mL). Refrigerate extra pumpkin in an airtight container for up to 1 week.

Storage Tip

See page 187.

Nutrients per serving	
Calories	168
Total fat	2 g
Saturated fat	0 g
Cholesterol	0 mg
Sodium	698 mg
Carbohydrate	29 g
Fiber	9 g
Protein	9 g
Calcium	110 mg
Iron	2.8 mg

- **Food processor**

3	cans (each 14 to 15 oz/398 to 425 mL) black beans, drained and rinsed	3
2	cans (each 10 oz/284 mL) diced tomatoes with chiles, with juice	2
2 tsp	extra virgin olive oil	10 mL
2 cups	chopped onions	500 mL
4	cloves garlic, minced	4
2 tbsp	ground cumin	30 mL
2 tsp	dried oregano	10 mL
1 tsp	chipotle chile powder or hot smoked paprika	5 mL
1⁄2 tsp	fine sea salt	2 mL
1	can (15 oz/425 mL) pumpkin purée (not pie filling)	1
6 cups	water	1.5 L
3 tbsp	freshly squeezed lime juice	45 mL
3⁄4 cup	nonfat plain yogurt	175 mL
1⁄2 cup	packed fresh cilantro leaves, chopped	125 mL

1. In food processor, pulse beans and tomatoes with juice until blended but not completely smooth.
2. In a large saucepan, heat oil over medium-high heat. Add onions and cook, stirring, for 6 to 8 minutes or until softened. Add garlic, cumin, oregano, chile powder and salt; cook, stirring, for 1 minute.
3. Stir in bean mixture, pumpkin and water. Bring to a boil. Reduce heat and simmer, stirring occasionally, for 25 to 30 minutes or until thickened. Stir in lime juice. Serve dolloped with yogurt and sprinkled with cilantro.

Tuscan Farro and White Bean Soup

Makes 8 servings

✪ Great for Steps 1, 2, 3, 4 and 5

Farro is an ancient variety of wheat cultivated in Italy that has recently caught the attention of cooks in North America. It has a nutty flavor and a firm, chewy texture that resembles barley more than wheat. Italians put farro in salads, stuffings and especially soups.

Storage Tip

Store the cooled soup in an airtight container in the refrigerator for up to 2 days or in the freezer for up to 6 months. Thaw overnight in the refrigerator or in the microwave using the Defrost function. Warm soup in a medium saucepan over medium-low heat.

Variation

Substitute pearl barley for the farro.

Nutrients per serving	
Calories	211
Total fat	2 g
Saturated fat	0 g
Cholesterol	0 mg
Sodium	398 mg
Carbohydrate	41 g
Fiber	9 g
Protein	7 g
Calcium	76 mg
Iron	2.2 mg

1 tbsp	extra virgin olive oil	15 mL
1½ cups	chopped onions	375 mL
1 cup	chopped carrots	250 mL
1 cup	chopped celery	250 mL
3	cloves garlic, minced	3
1 cup	diced peeled waxy potatoes (such as red-skinned potatoes)	250 mL
2 tsp	dried rubbed sage	10 mL
2 tsp	dried rosemary	10 mL
½ tsp	freshly cracked black pepper	2 mL
1	can (14 to 15 oz/398 to 425 mL) diced tomatoes, with juice	1
6 cups	reduced-sodium ready-to-use chicken or vegetable broth	1.5 L
2½ cups	water	625 mL
1	can (14 to 19 oz/398 to 540 mL) white beans, drained and rinsed	1
1 cup	semi-pearled farro	250 mL

1. In a large pot, heat oil over medium-high heat. Add onions, carrots and celery; cook, stirring, for 6 to 8 minutes or until softened. Add garlic, potatoes, sage, rosemary and pepper; cook, stirring, for 1 minute.
2. Stir in tomatoes with juice, broth and water. Bring to a boil. Stir in beans and farro. Reduce heat to low, cover and simmer, stirring occasionally, for 25 to 30 minutes or until farro is tender.

Superfood Spotlight

Sage • Native to the Mediterranean, sage has one of the longest histories of use of any medicinal herb. It contains a variety of volatile oils, flavonoids and phenolic acids. Sage is in the top ten of herbs that have the most powerful antioxidant effect, neutralizing the cell-damaging free radicals that are thought to be linked with the aging process. Herbalists have long believed that sage is an outstanding memory enhancer; in trials, even small amounts significantly improved short-term recall. Because sage is antibacterial, it can help reduce the number of hot flashes in menopausal women and is recommended for people with inflammatory conditions such as rheumatoid arthritis and asthma.

Mushroom and Barley Soup

Makes 8 servings

✪ Great for Steps 1, 2, 4 and 5

It may not be a new flavor combination, but mushroom and barley soup is so satisfying that you'll wonder anew at how such modest ingredients can conspire to create something so delightful.

1 tbsp	extra virgin olive oil	15 mL
1 lb	cremini or button mushrooms, chopped	500 g
2 cups	chopped onions	500 mL
1½ cups	chopped carrots	375 mL
1½ cups	chopped celery	375 mL
¼ tsp	fine sea salt	1 mL
¼ tsp	freshly ground black pepper	1 mL
1 cup	pearl barley	250 mL
8 cups	reduced-sodium ready-to-use beef or vegetable broth	2 L
2 cups	water	500 mL
2 tbsp	chopped fresh dill	30 mL

1. In a large pot, heat oil over medium-high heat. Add mushrooms, onions, carrots, celery, salt and pepper; cook, stirring, for 6 to 8 minutes or until slightly softened. Reduce heat to medium-low and cook, stirring occasionally, for 15 to 20 minutes or until vegetables are browned.
2. Stir in barley, broth and water. Increase heat to medium-high and bring to a boil, stirring often. Reduce heat to medium, cover, leaving lid ajar, and simmer, stirring occasionally, for 1 hour or until barley is tender and soup is starting to thicken. Stir in dill.

Storage Tip

Store the cooled soup in an airtight container in the refrigerator for up to 2 days or in the freezer for up to 6 months. Thaw overnight in the refrigerator or in the microwave using the Defrost function. Warm soup in a medium saucepan over medium-low heat.

Superfood Spotlight

Carrots • Carrots are an excellent source of antioxidant compounds and the richest vegetable source of carotenes, which give them their bright orange color and may reduce the incidence of heart disease by about 45%. A high intake of carotenes has been linked with a 20% decrease in postmenopausal breast cancer and up to a 50% decrease in cancers of the cervix, bladder, colon, prostate, larynx and esophagus. Extensive studies have shown that a diet that includes at least one carrot per day could cut the rate of lung cancer in half.

Carrots also offer an excellent source of fiber, vitamin K and biotin, the latter of which is beneficial for strong nails and hair. They are a good source of vitamins B6, C and E, potassium, calcium and thiamine. A chemical in carrots, falcarinol, has been shown to suppress tumors in animals by a third.

Nutrients per serving

Calories	165
Total fat	3 g
Saturated fat	0 g
Cholesterol	0 mg
Sodium	268 mg
Carbohydrate	32 g
Fiber	7 g
Protein	5 g
Calcium	75 mg
Iron	1.7 mg

Summer Vegetable Orzo Soup

Makes 6 servings

✪ Great for Steps 1, 2, 4 and 5

This satisfying soup gets a hint of sweetness from fresh summer corn, and is made dinner-worthy by the addition of high-fiber whole wheat orzo.

Storage Tip

Store the cooled soup in an airtight container in the refrigerator for up to 2 days or in the freezer for up to 6 months. Thaw overnight in the refrigerator or in the microwave using the Defrost function. Warm soup in a medium saucepan over medium-low heat.

2 tsp	extra virgin olive oil	10 mL
1½ cups	chopped onions	375 mL
2	cloves garlic, minced	2
½ tsp	fine sea salt	2 mL
¼ tsp	cracked black pepper	1 mL
4	small zucchini, halved lengthwise and thinly sliced	4
2	cans (each 14 to 15 oz/398 to 425 mL) diced tomatoes, with juice	2
1½ cups	fresh corn kernels	375 mL
6 cups	water	1.5 L
8 oz	green beans, trimmed and cut into thirds	250 g
½ cup	whole wheat orzo	125 mL
1 cup	packed fresh basil leaves, chopped, divided	250 mL

1. In a large saucepan, heat oil over medium-high heat. Add onions and cook, stirring, for 5 to 6 minutes or until softened. Add garlic, salt and pepper; cook, stirring, for 1 minute.
2. Stir in zucchini, tomatoes with juice, corn and water. Bring to a boil. Reduce heat and simmer, stirring occasionally, for 15 minutes. Stir in beans, orzo and half the basil; simmer, stirring occasionally, for 15 to 20 minutes or until orzo is al dente. Stir in the remaining basil.

Nutrients per serving	
Calories	166
Total fat	2 g
Saturated fat	0 g
Cholesterol	0 mg
Sodium	570 mg
Carbohydrate	32 g
Fiber	6 g
Protein	5 g
Calcium	50 mg
Iron	1.6 mg

Curried Orzo Soup

Makes 4 servings

✪ Great for Steps 1, 2, 4 and 5

How could something so easy to make taste so complex and exotic? This little soup pulls it off, while packing in a slew of good-for-you things, too.

Tip

If you can't find fire-roasted tomatoes, you can used regular diced tomatoes.

Storage Tip

Store the cooled soup in an airtight container in the refrigerator for up to 2 days or in the freezer for up to 6 months. Thaw overnight in the refrigerator or in the microwave using the Defrost function. Warm soup in a medium saucepan over medium-low heat.

Nutrients per serving	
Calories	182
Total fat	3 g
Saturated fat	0 g
Cholesterol	0 mg
Sodium	427 mg
Carbohydrate	35 g
Fiber	8 g
Protein	5 g
Calcium	76 mg
Iron	2.7 mg

2 tsp	extra virgin olive oil	10 mL
1 cup	chopped onion	250 mL
2	cloves garlic, minced	2
1/2 cup	whole wheat orzo	125 mL
2 tsp	mild curry powder	10 mL
1	can (14 to 15 oz/398 to 425 mL) fire-roasted tomatoes, with juice	1
4 cups	reduced-sodium ready-to-use chicken or vegetable broth	1 L
4 cups	packed baby spinach, roughly chopped	1 L
2 tsp	freshly squeezed lime juice	10 mL

1. In a large saucepan, heat oil over medium-high heat. Add onion and cook, stirring, for 5 to 6 minutes or until softened. Add garlic, orzo and curry powder; cook, stirring, for 30 seconds.
2. Stir in tomatoes with juice and broth. Bring to a boil. Reduce heat and simmer, stirring occasionally, for 6 minutes or until the orzo is almost tender. Stir in spinach and simmer, stirring, for 1 to 2 minutes or until wilted. Stir in lime juice.

Brown Rice, Greens and Miso Soup

Makes 6 servings

✪ Great for Steps 1, 2, 3, 4 and 5

Some soups genuinely do inspire fidelity akin to love, and this is one of them. In the cold of winter, when I mull over the matter of what soup to cook up to provide comfort all weekend long, I decide with remarkable frequency to make this one. Make the rice ahead of time, or use frozen brown rice to further speed along the prep time.

Storage Tip

Store the cooled soup in an airtight container in the refrigerator for up to 2 days or in the freezer for up to 6 months. Thaw overnight in the refrigerator or in the microwave using the Defrost function. Warm soup in a medium saucepan over medium-low heat.

Nutrients per serving	
Calories	242
Total fat	4 g
Saturated fat	0 g
Cholesterol	0 mg
Sodium	413 mg
Carbohydrate	45 g
Fiber	6 g
Protein	10 g
Calcium	182 mg
Iron	3.4 mg

2 tsp	vegetable oil	10 mL
1½ cups	chopped onions	375 mL
3	cloves garlic, minced	3
12 oz	cremini or button mushrooms, trimmed and sliced	375 g
¼ tsp	fine sea salt	1 mL
1½ tsp	ground ginger	7 mL
6 cups	water	1.5 L
2 tbsp	yellow miso	30 mL
1	can (14 to 19 oz/398 to 540 mL) chickpeas, drained and rinsed	1
6 cups	chopped kale or mustard greens (tough stems and center ribs removed)	1.5 L
3 cups	cooked long-grain brown rice (see page 438)	750 mL

1. In a large saucepan, heat oil over medium-high heat. Add onions and cook, stirring, for 6 to 8 minutes or until softened. Add garlic, mushrooms and salt; cook, stirring, for 5 minutes or until mushrooms are softened.
2. Stir in ginger, water and miso. Bring to a boil. Add chickpeas, kale and rice; reduce heat and simmer, stirring occasionally, for 5 minutes or until kale is wilted.

Superfood Spotlight

Onions • Although often considered a supporting flavor rather than a star food, onions have potent health-enhancing qualities that make them worthy of superfood status. They increase the production of glutathione, a tripeptide that serves as an antioxidant for the liver, aiding the elimination of toxins and carcinogens from the body. It is believed that anticancer benefits come from the sulfur compounds known as allyl sulfides, which give onions their strong smell and help prevent cancer by blocking the effects of carcinogens in the body. Onions also contain numerous flavonoids, such as quercetin, that help prevent blood clots and protect against heart disease and cancer. Onions have anti-inflammatory and antibacterial effects and can help minimize the nasal congestion of a cold. Finally, onions are very rich in chromium, a trace mineral that helps cells respond to insulin, and are a good source of vitamin C and other trace elements.

Miso Soup with Soba and Vegetables

Makes 6 servings

✪ Great for Steps 1, 2, 3, 4 and 5

Tips

Soba noodles (brown Japanese noodles made from buckwheat), instant dashi (a powdered form of Japanese soup broth made from dried bonito tuna flakes and kombu) and miso (fermented soybean paste) can be found at Asian markets and in the Asian foods section of well-stocked supermarkets.

For the best flavor and texture, use fresh (refrigerated) tofu, not shelf-stable tofu in Tetra Paks.

Two tsp (10 mL) Thai fish sauce may be used in place of the instant dashi.

8 oz	soba (buckwheat) noodles	250 g
8 cups	water	2 L
4 tsp	instant dashi	20 mL
½ cup	reduced-sodium tamari or soy sauce	125 mL
1 tbsp	brown rice syrup or agave nectar	15 mL
3	carrots, cut crosswise into thin slices	3
1	package (12 to 16 oz/340 to 454 g) fresh soft silken tofu, drained and cut into ½-inch (1 cm) cubes	1
6 cups	packed spinach, trimmed and coarsely chopped	1.5 L
¼ cup	yellow miso	60 mL
¾ cup	thinly sliced green onions	175 mL

1. In a large pot of boiling water, cook soba noodles according to package directions until al dente (be careful not to overcook). Drain and rinse briefly under cold water to stop the cooking.
2. In the same pot, bring 8 cups (2 L) water to a boil over high heat. Stir in dashi, reduce heat and simmer, stirring occasionally, for 3 minutes. Stir in tamari and brown rice syrup; simmer for 5 minutes. Stir in carrots and simmer, stirring occasionally, for 5 minutes. Stir in tofu and spinach; simmer for 1 minute.
3. In a small bowl, combine miso and ½ cup (125 mL) of the hot soup broth. Stir into soup.
4. Divide noodles among six soup bowls. Ladle hot soup over top and sprinkle with green onions.

Nutrients per serving	
Calories	355
Total fat	6 g
Saturated fat	0 g
Cholesterol	0 mg
Sodium	736 mg
Carbohydrate	64 g
Fiber	4 g
Protein	16 g
Calcium	91 mg
Iron	3.6 mg

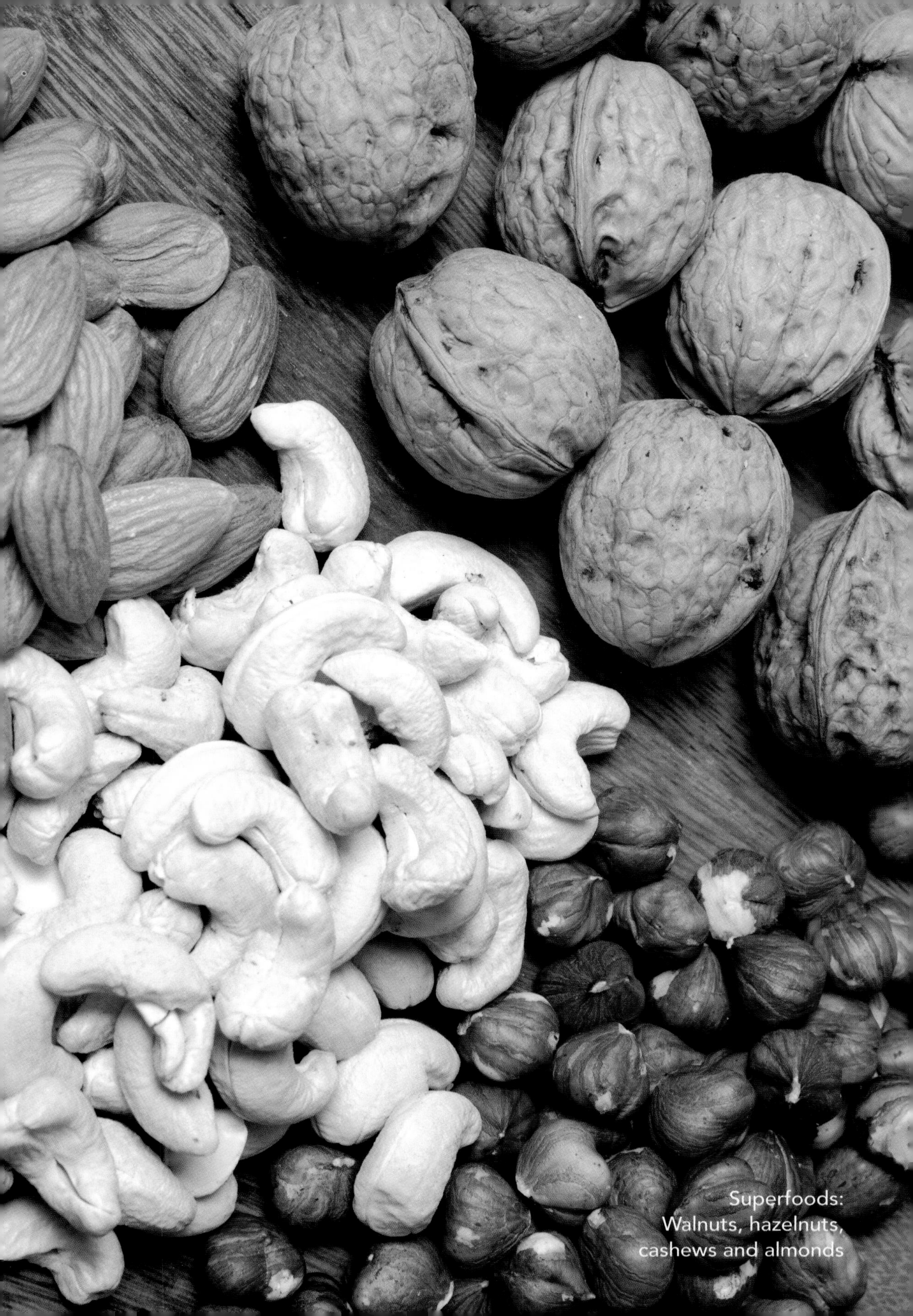

Superfoods:
Walnuts, hazelnuts,
cashews and almonds

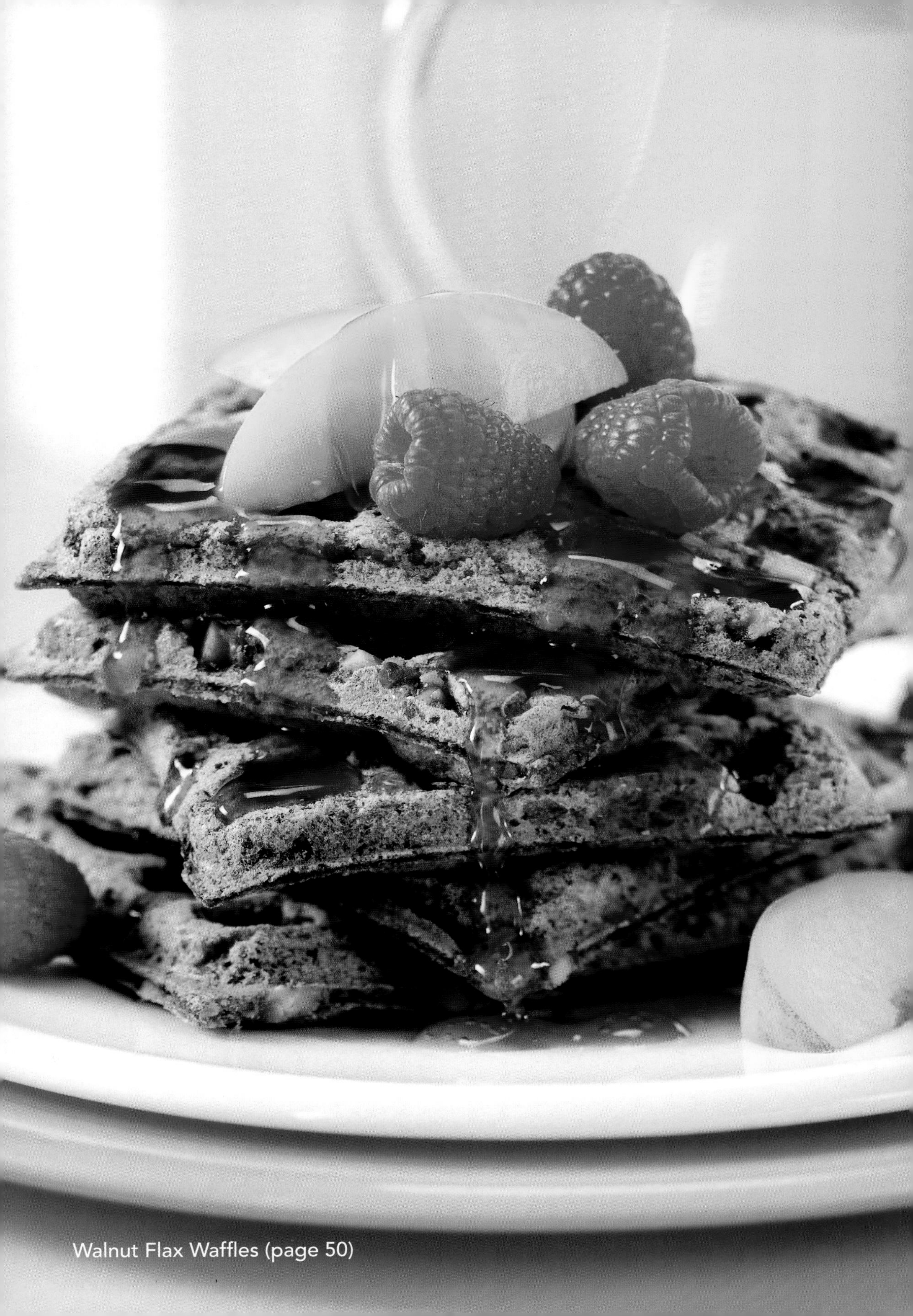

Walnut Flax Waffles (page 50)

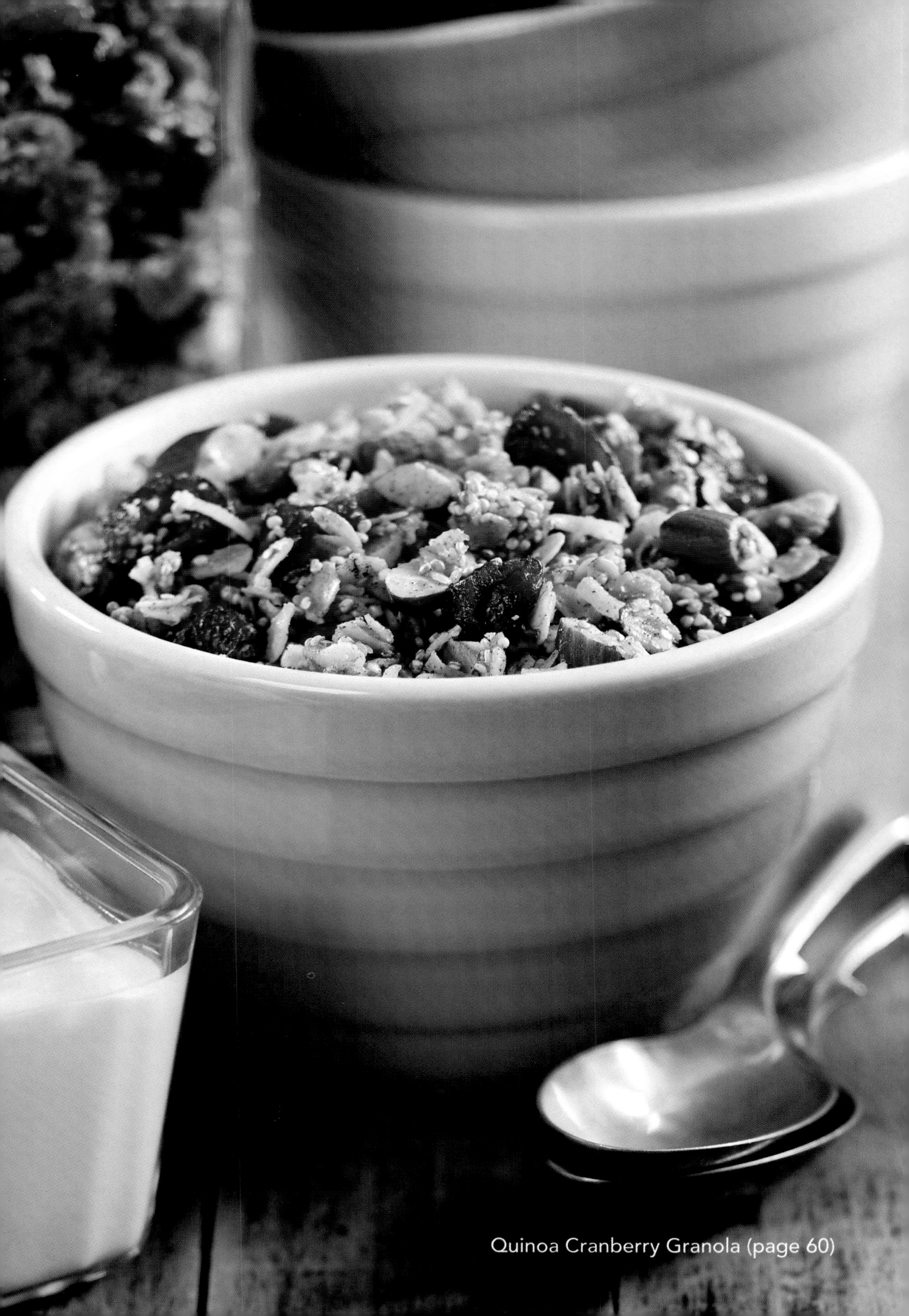
Quinoa Cranberry Granola (page 60)

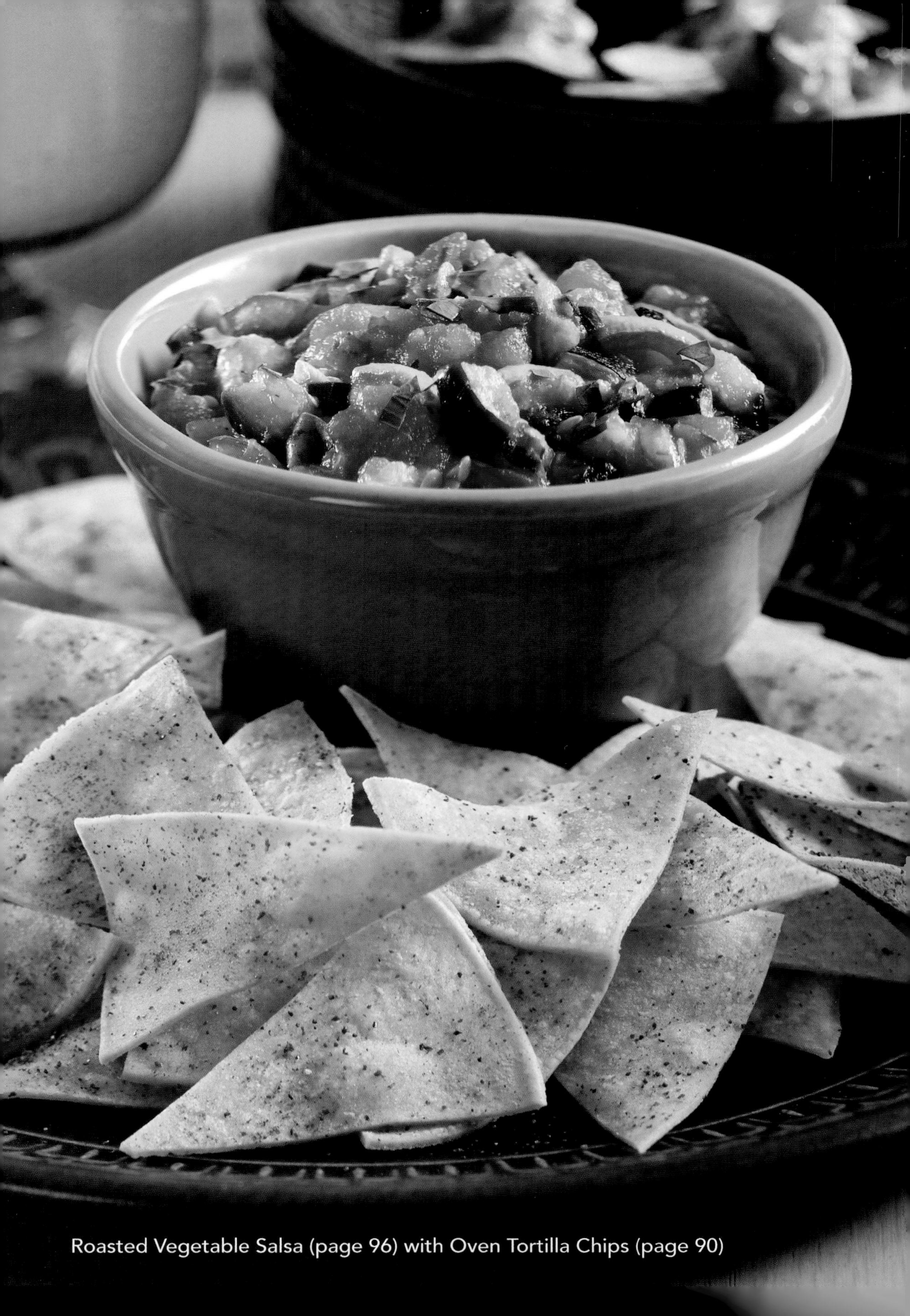

Roasted Vegetable Salsa (page 96) with Oven Tortilla Chips (page 90)

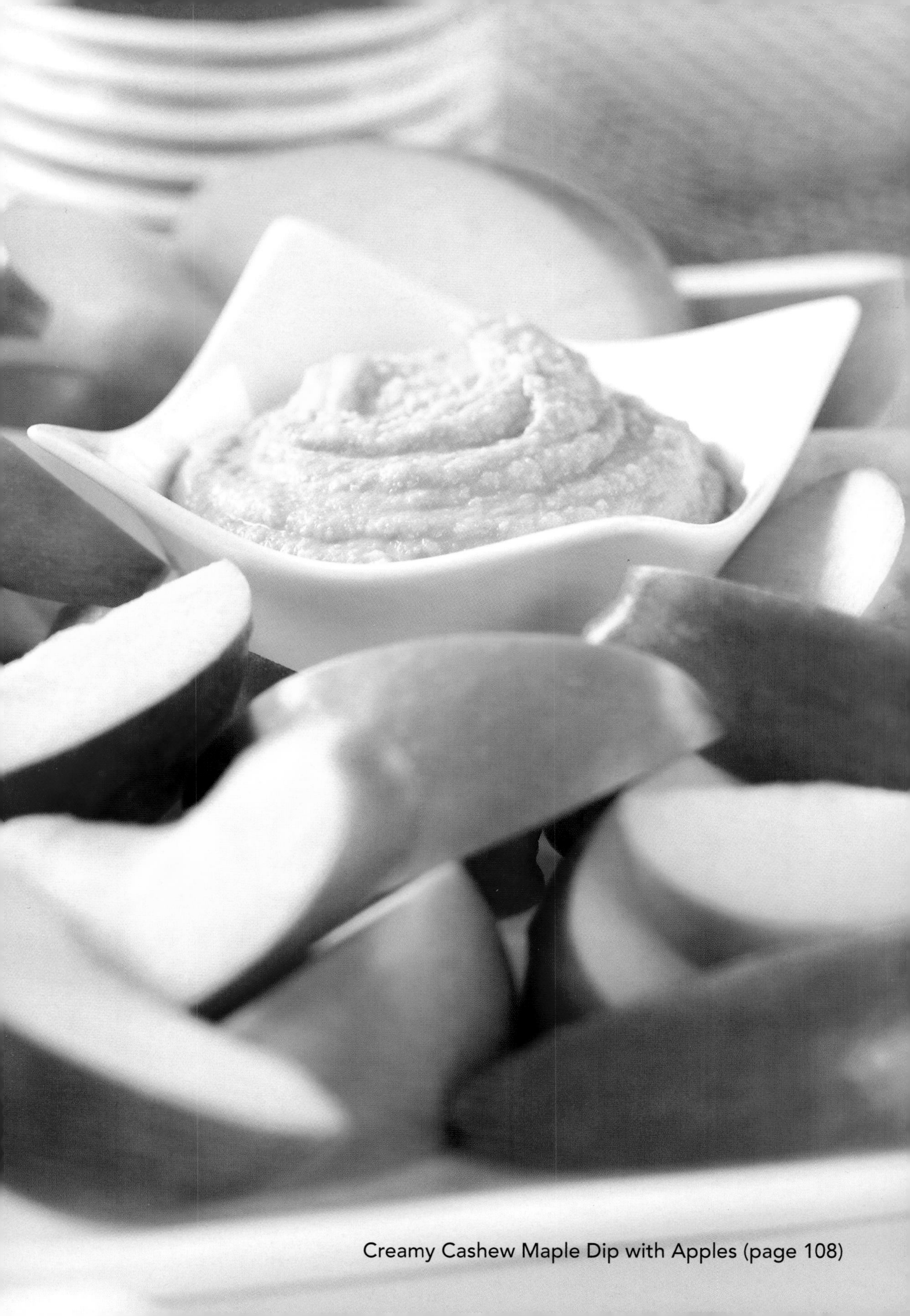

Creamy Cashew Maple Dip with Apples (page 108)

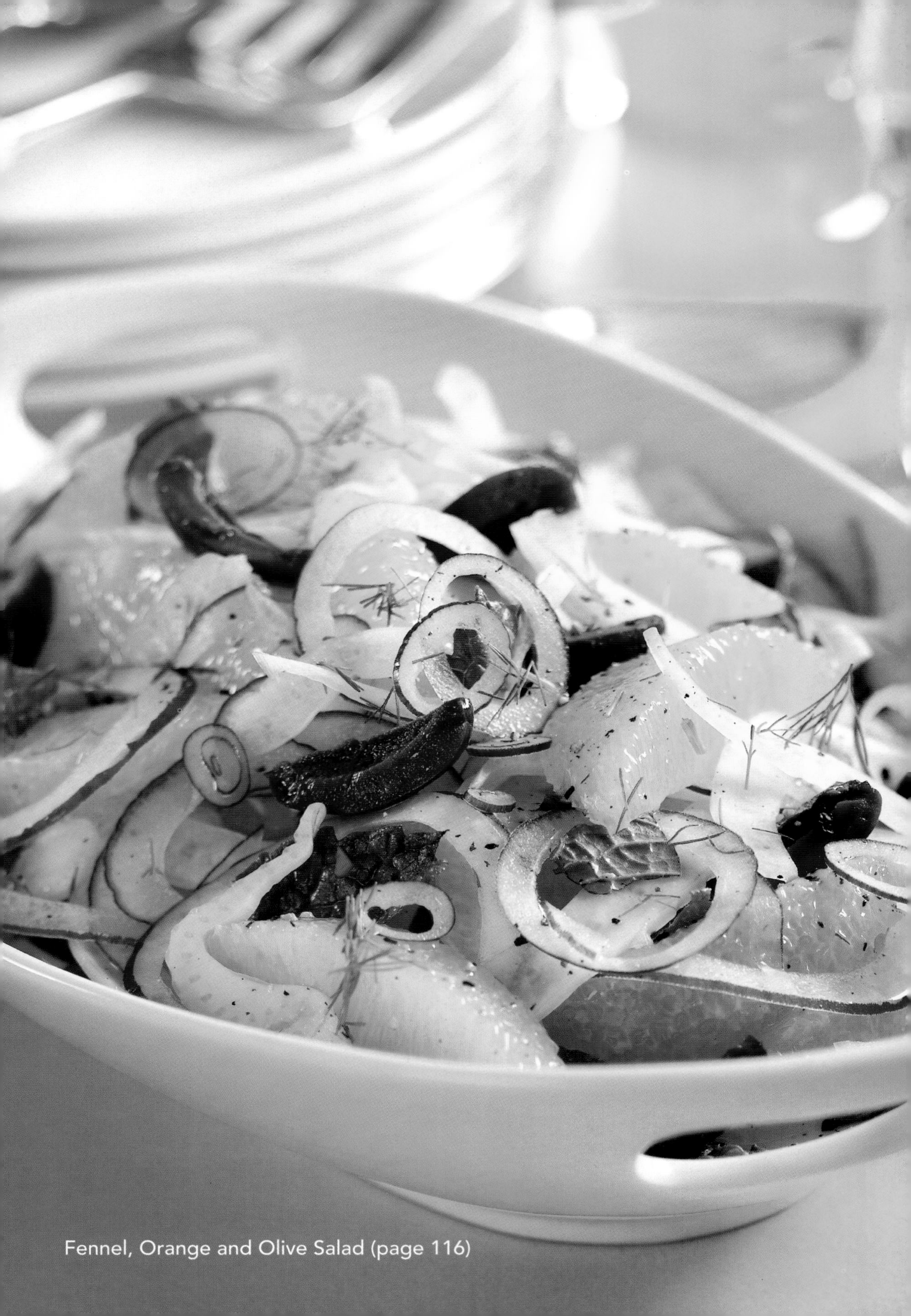

Fennel, Orange and Olive Salad (page 116)

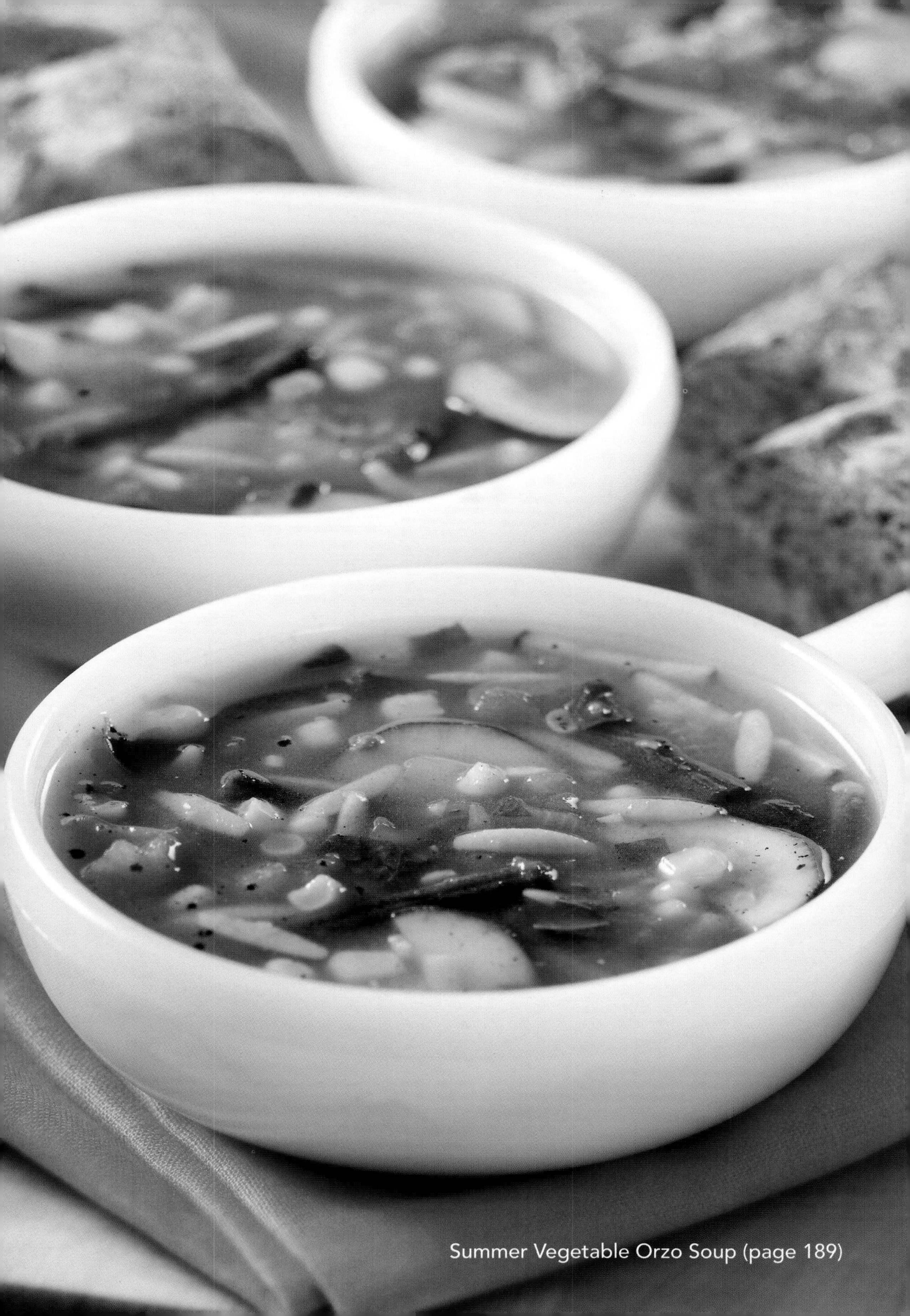
Summer Vegetable Orzo Soup (page 189)

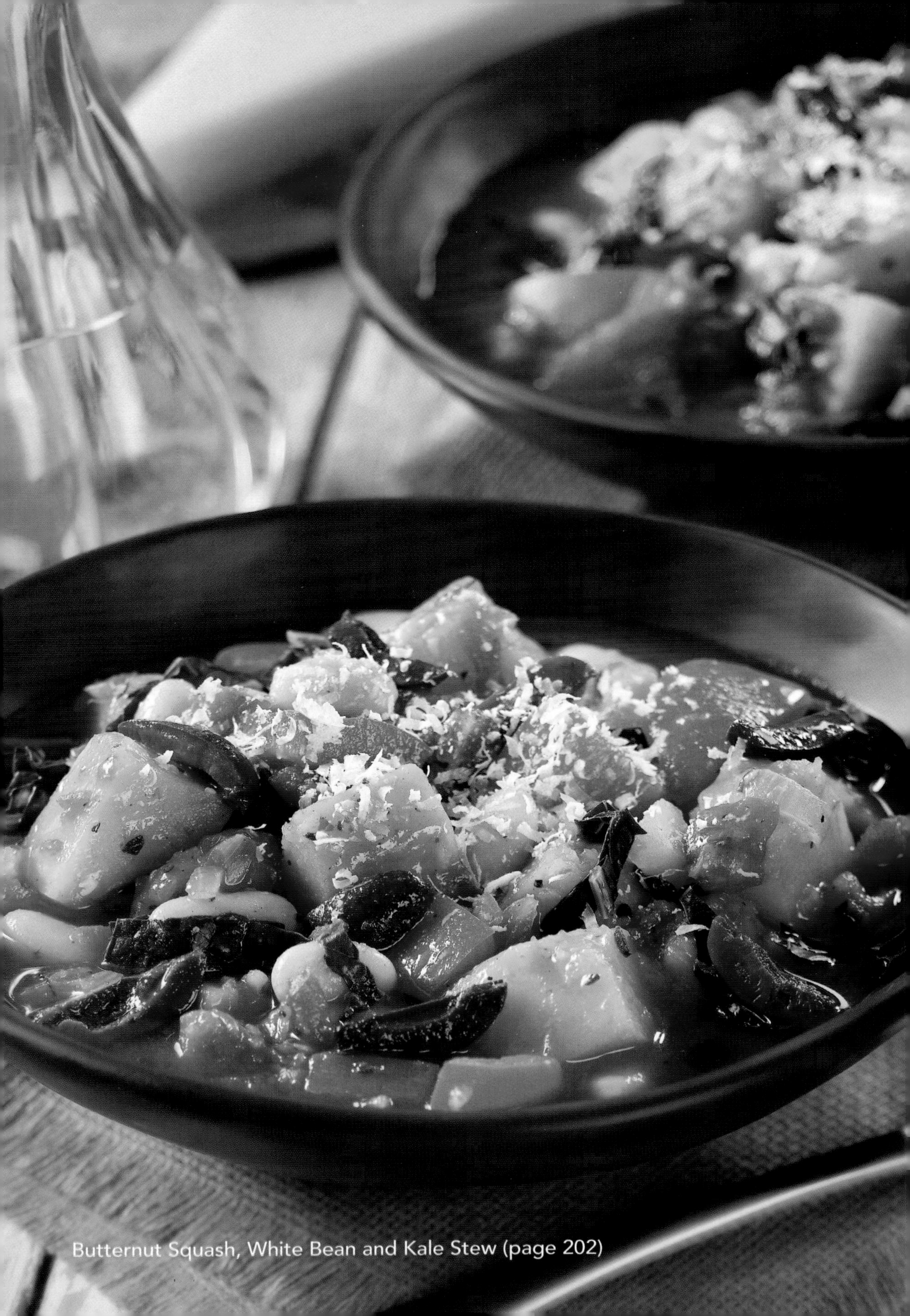

Butternut Squash, White Bean and Kale Stew (page 202)

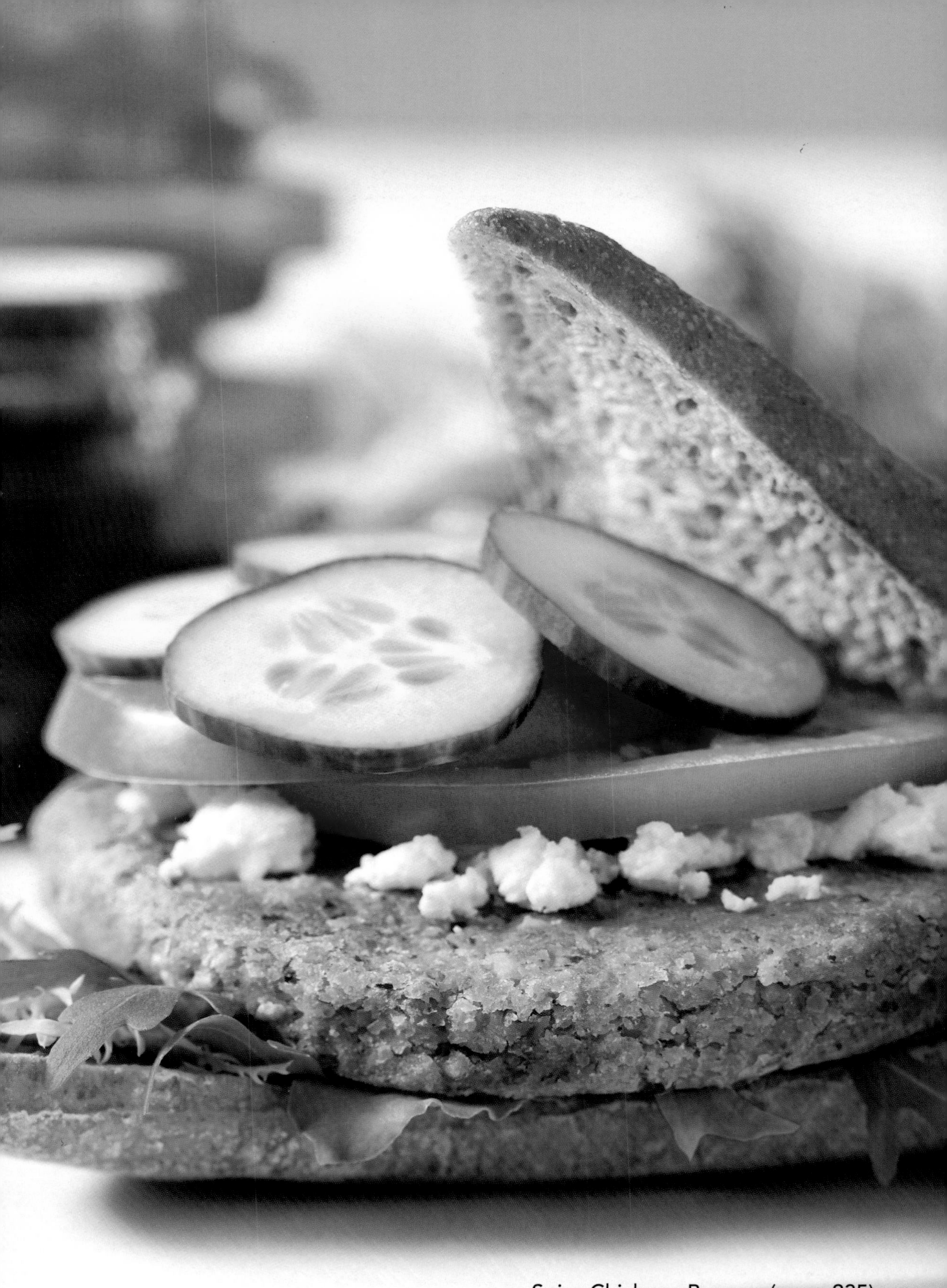

Spicy Chickpea Burgers (page 235)

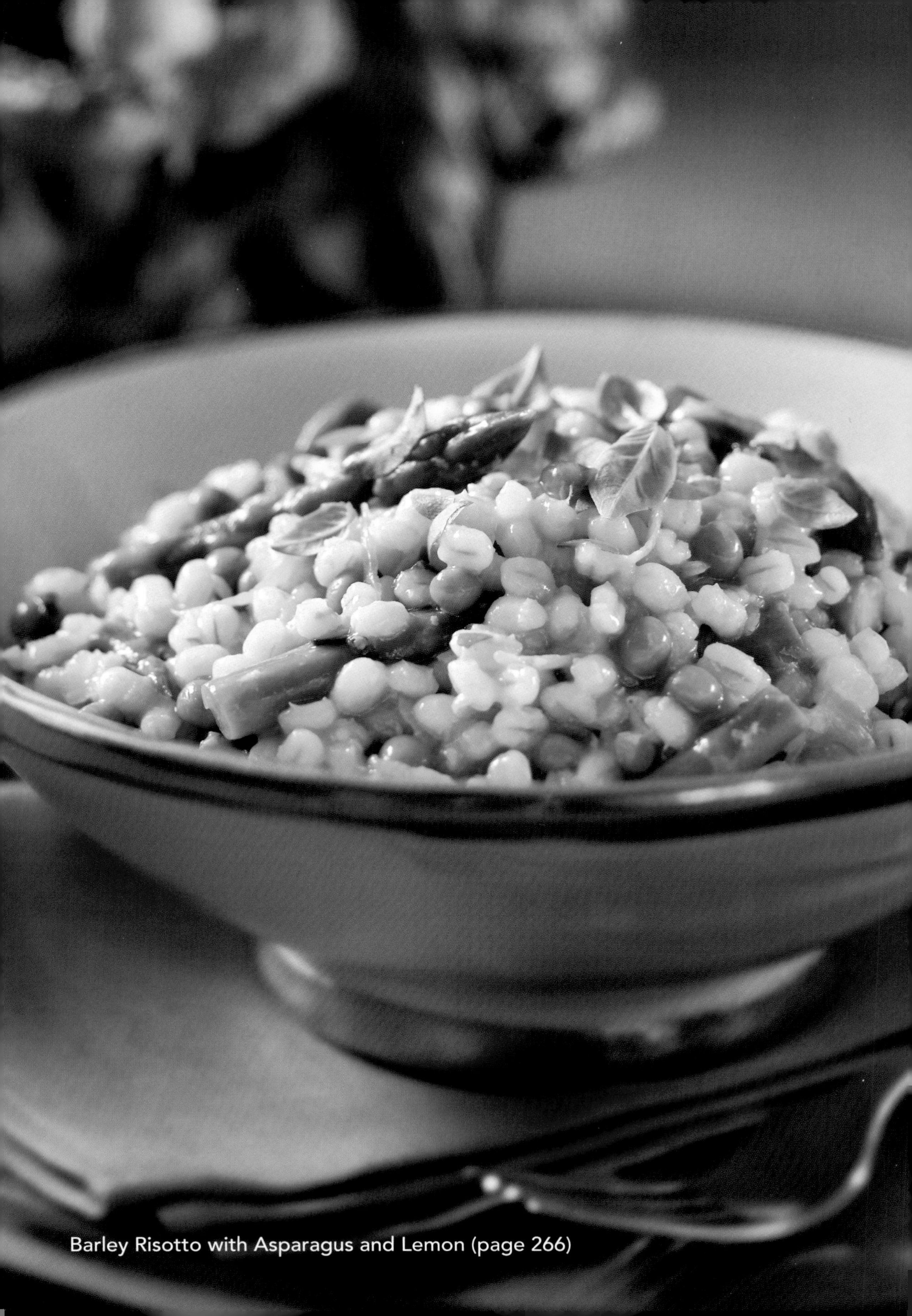

Barley Risotto with Asparagus and Lemon (page 266)

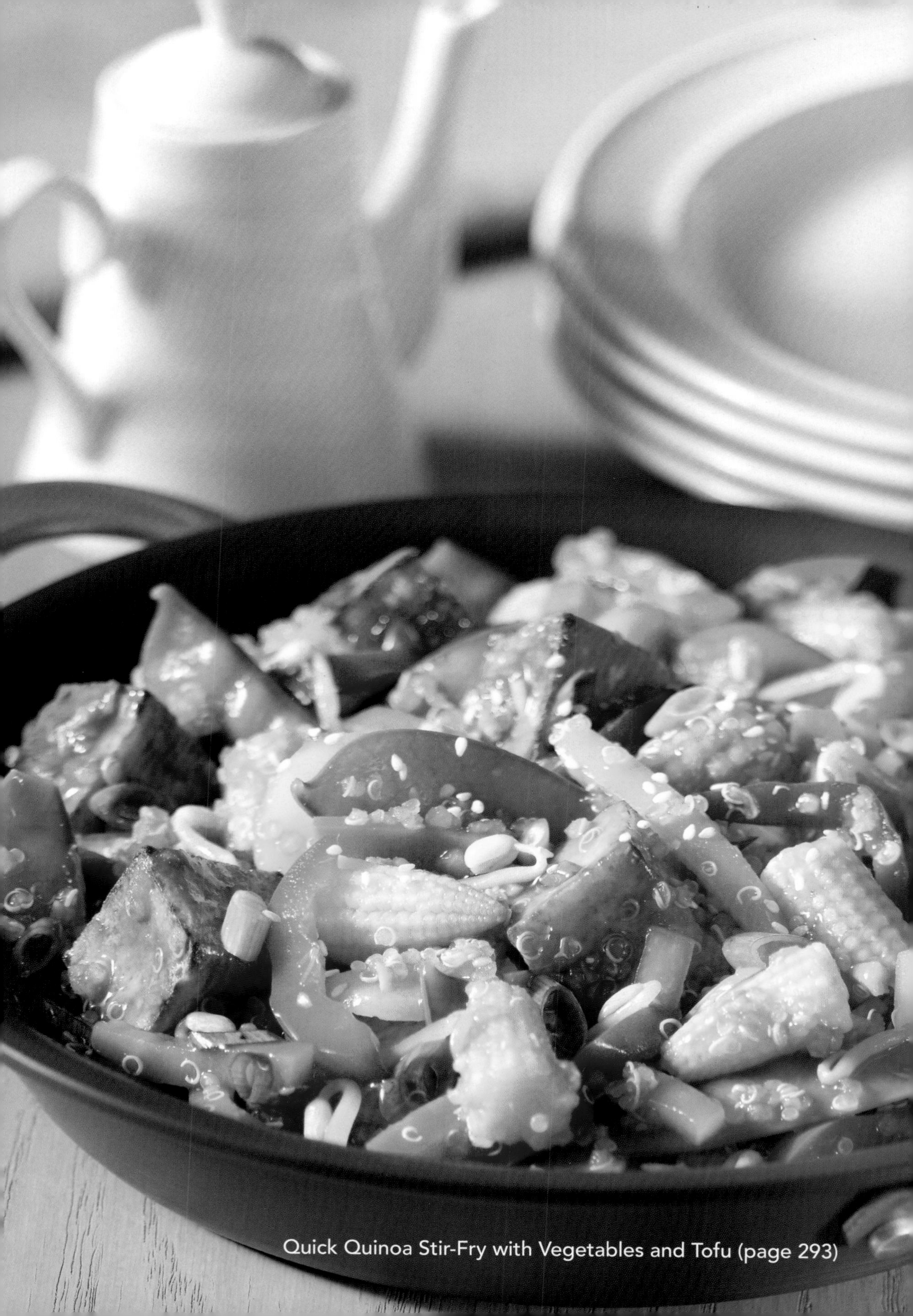
Quick Quinoa Stir-Fry with Vegetables and Tofu (page 293)

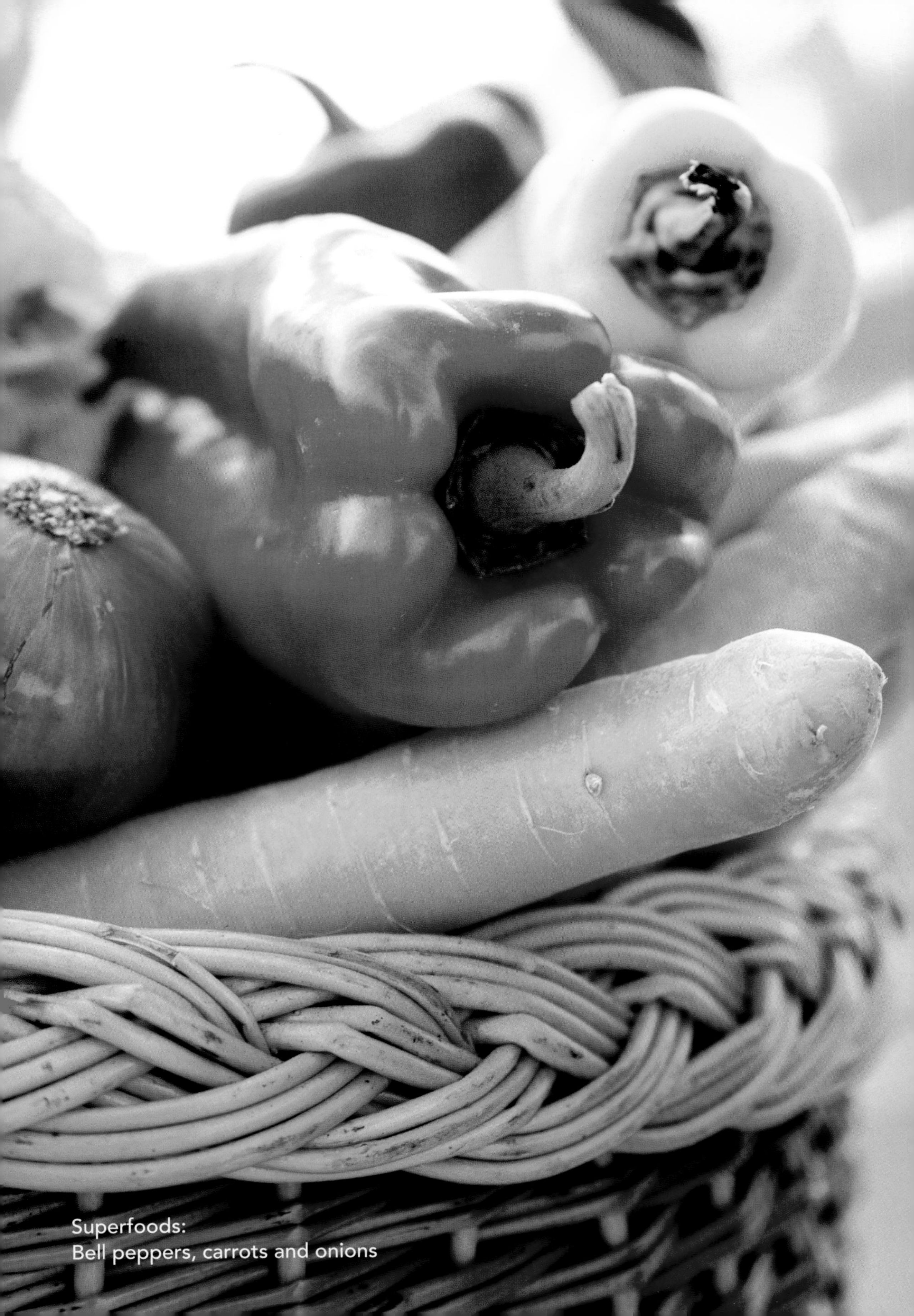

Superfoods:
Bell peppers, carrots and onions

Spinach Egg Drop Soup

Makes 4 servings

✪ Great for Steps 1, 2 and 4

Egg drop soup, also known as egg flower soup, is one of the easiest (and most frugal) soups to prepare. The trick is how the eggs are handled. For ribbons of egg throughout the soup, lightly beat the eggs so that no bubbles form and turn off the heat before pouring them in (this produces silkier threads). Pour the eggs in a very slow stream, stirring — in one direction only — as soon as you start pouring.

Storage Tip

Store the cooled soup in an airtight container in the refrigerator for up to 2 days. Warm soup in a medium saucepan over medium-low heat.

Nutrients per serving	
Calories	63
Total fat	2 g
Saturated fat	1 g
Cholesterol	90 mg
Sodium	250 mg
Carbohydrate	6 g
Fiber	2 g
Protein	4 g
Calcium	47 mg
Iron	1.3 mg

1	3-inch (7.5 cm) piece gingerroot	1
5 cups	reduced-sodium ready-to-use chicken or vegetable broth	1.25 L
1/2 tsp	Asian chili-garlic sauce	2 mL
2	large eggs, lightly beaten	2
2 cups	packed baby spinach	500 mL

1. Cut ginger crosswise into thin slices. Cut half the slices into julienne.
2. In a medium saucepan, combine whole ginger slices, broth and chili-garlic sauce. Bring to a boil over medium-high heat. Reduce heat to low, cover and simmer for 5 minutes. Using a slotted spoon, remove and discard ginger.
3. Add julienned ginger to the pan and return to a simmer. Remove from heat and gradually pour in eggs, swirling in one direction with a chopstick or fork to create long strands. Stir in spinach, cover and let stand for 1 minute or until spinach is wilted. Serve immediately.

Asian Chicken Noodle Soup

Makes 6 servings

✪ Great for Steps 1, 3, 4 and 5

Wonderfully fragrant and so satisfying when the chill of autumn returns, this Asian-inspired take on chicken noodle soup will ward off the slightest sign of a cold. Place a bottle of Asian chili sauce (such as Sriracha) on the table so daring diners (or the especially congested) can add a few drops.

Storage Tip

Store the cooled soup in an airtight container in the refrigerator for up to 2 days or in the freezer for up to 6 months. Thaw overnight in the refrigerator or in the microwave using the Defrost function. Warm soup in a medium saucepan over medium-low heat.

Nutrients per serving	
Calories	245
Total fat	5 g
Saturated fat	0 g
Cholesterol	33 mg
Sodium	663 mg
Carbohydrate	31 g
Fiber	4 g
Protein	19 g
Calcium	108 mg
Iron	2.9 mg

1 tbsp	vegetable oil	15 mL
3	cloves garlic, minced	3
2 tbsp	minced gingerroot	30 mL
6 cups	reduced-sodium ready-to-use chicken or vegetable broth, divided	1.5 L
12 oz	boneless skinless chicken breasts, trimmed (about 2 medium)	375 g
2 tbsp	reduced-sodium tamari or soy sauce	30 mL
2 tsp	toasted sesame oil	10 mL
1 tbsp	brown rice syrup or agave nectar	15 mL
6 oz	multigrain or whole wheat angel hair pasta, broken in half	175 g
6 cups	chopped bok choy	1.5 L
1/2 cup	thinly sliced green onions	125 mL

1. In a large saucepan, heat oil over medium-high heat. Add garlic and ginger; cook, stirring, for 30 seconds.
2. Stir in 2 cups (500 mL) of the broth. Bring to a boil. Add chicken, reduce heat to medium-low, cover and simmer for 5 minutes or until chicken is no longer pink inside. Using tongs, transfer chicken to a cutting board and slice crosswise into strips.
3. Add the remaining broth, tamari, sesame oil and brown rice syrup to the pan. Increase heat to medium-high and bring to a boil. Add pasta and boil, uncovered, for 3 minutes. Add bok choy and boil, stirring occasionally, for 3 to 4 minutes or until pasta is al dente and bok choy is wilted.
4. Ladle soup into bowls and top with chicken strips and green onions.

Spiced Chicken and Couscous Soup

Makes 6 servings

✪ Great for Steps 1, 3, 4 and 5

If ever there was an easy, exotic dinner to brighten winter's gloom, this is it. The fresh cilantro is a must, providing bright contrast to the earthy whole wheat couscous and spicy broth.

Storage Tip

Store the cooled soup in an airtight container in the refrigerator for up to 2 days or in the freezer for up to 6 months. Thaw overnight in the refrigerator or in the microwave using the Defrost function. Warm soup in a medium saucepan over medium-low heat.

2 tsp	extra virgin olive oil	10 mL
$1\frac{1}{2}$ cups	chopped onions	375 mL
1 tbsp	pumpkin pie spice	15 mL
1 tsp	sweet or hot smoked paprika	5 mL
1 tsp	ground cumin	5 mL
1	can (28 oz/796 mL) diced tomatoes, with juice	1
6 cups	reduced-sodium ready-to-use chicken or vegetable broth	1.5 L
3 cups	diced or shredded cooked chicken breast	750 mL
$\frac{2}{3}$ cup	whole wheat couscous	150 mL
1 cup	packed fresh cilantro leaves, chopped	250 mL
2 tbsp	freshly squeezed lemon juice	30 mL

1. In a large saucepan, heat oil over medium-high heat. Add onions and cook, stirring, for 5 to 6 minutes or until softened. Add pumpkin pie spice, paprika and cumin; cook, stirring, for 30 seconds.
2. Stir in tomatoes with juice and broth. Bring to a gentle boil. Stir in chicken and couscous; reduce heat to low, cover, leaving lid ajar, and simmer, stirring occasionally, for 5 to 6 minutes. Stir in cilantro and lemon juice.

Nutrients per serving	
Calories	325
Total fat	9 g
Saturated fat	2 g
Cholesterol	52 mg
Sodium	738 mg
Carbohydrate	33 g
Fiber	6 g
Protein	30 g
Calcium	74 mg
Iron	3.3 mg

Turkey Soup with Sweet Potatoes and Mustard Greens

Makes 6 servings

✪ Great for Steps 1, 3 and 4

A few fresh vegetables and some leftover turkey is all you'll need to create this soul-satisfying soup.

2 tsp	extra virgin olive oil	10 mL
1¼ cups	chopped onions	300 mL
2	cloves garlic, minced	2
¼ tsp	freshly cracked black pepper	1 mL
1	large sweet potato (about 1 lb/500 g), peeled and cut into ½-inch (1 cm) cubes	1
1	can (14 to 15 oz/398 to 425 mL) diced tomatoes, with juice	1
1 tbsp	chopped fresh rosemary	15 mL
4 cups	reduced-sodium ready-to-use chicken or vegetable broth	1 L
3 tbsp	tomato paste	45 mL
6 cups	packed sliced mustard greens, tough stems removed	1.5 L
2 cups	diced cooked turkey breast	500 mL
1 tsp	Dijon mustard	5 mL

1. In a large saucepan, heat oil over medium-high heat. Add onions and cook, stirring, for 5 to 6 minutes or until softened. Add garlic and pepper; cook, stirring, for 30 seconds.
2. Stir in sweet potato, tomatoes with juice, rosemary, broth and tomato paste. Bring to a boil. Reduce heat to low, cover, leaving lid ajar, and simmer, stirring occasionally, for 25 to 30 minutes or until sweet potatoes are very tender but not falling apart. Stir in mustard greens, turkey and mustard. Cover and simmer for 5 minutes or until greens are wilted.

Tip

To save time, look for bags of ready-cut mustard greens. Alternatively, use a 12-oz (375 g) bag of frozen chopped mustard greens.

Storage Tip

Store the cooled soup in an airtight container in the refrigerator for up to 2 days or in the freezer for up to 6 months. Thaw overnight in the refrigerator or in the microwave using the Defrost function. Warm soup in a medium saucepan over medium-low heat.

Superfood Spotlight

Rosemary • Traditionally, rosemary has been used as a mental stimulant, memory booster, general tonic and circulation aid. Herbalists have long recommended rosemary tea to treat colds, flu and rheumatism. Like several other herbs, rosemary has been shown to fight bacteria that can cause throat infections, such as *E. coli* and staphylococcus, so an infusion of rosemary makes a good gargle. In addition, recent research has found that rosemary is one of the leading herbs for antioxidant activity, helping to reduce the risk of diseases and the effects of aging.

Nutrients per serving	
Calories	153
Total fat	2 g
Saturated fat	0 g
Cholesterol	8 mg
Sodium	635 mg
Carbohydrate	27 g
Fiber	6 g
Protein	8 g
Calcium	118 mg
Iron	2.5 mg

Vietnamese Pho

Makes 4 servings

✪ Great for Steps 1, 3, 4 and 5

In Vietnam, people are fiercely loyal to their favorite version of pho. After a taste of this quick, light version, you'll start to feel the same sense of loyalty. Serve it with Asian chili sauce (such as Sriracha) for diners who want to add some heat.

Tip

For best results, select a deli roast beef that does not have additional flavorings (such as Italian herbs or barbecue seasoning).

Storage Tip

See page 196.

2 tbsp	finely grated gingerroot	30 mL
3 cups	reduced-sodium ready-to-use chicken broth	750 mL
3 cups	water	750 mL
2 tbsp	reduced-sodium tamari or soy sauce	30 mL
1 tbsp	brown rice syrup or agave nectar	15 mL
8 oz	whole wheat or multigrain spaghetti, broken	250 g
2 tbsp	freshly squeezed lime juice	30 mL
8 oz	sliced deli roast beef, halved crosswise and cut lengthwise into 1-inch (2.5 cm) strips	250 g
1 cup	mung bean sprouts	250 mL
1 cup	packed fresh basil leaves, sliced	250 mL
1/2 cup	packed fresh cilantro leaves	125 mL
1/2 cup	chopped green onions	125 mL

1. In a large saucepan, combine ginger, broth, water, tamari and brown rice syrup. Bring to a boil over medium-high heat. Add spaghetti and boil, stirring once or twice, for 6 to 8 minutes or until al dente. Stir in lime juice.
2. Using tongs, divide pasta among four soup bowls. Top with roast beef. Ladle hot soup broth over top. Top with bean sprouts, basil, cilantro and green onions.

Variation

This soup is easily converted to a vegetarian dish; simply use vegetable broth in place of the chicken broth, and diced firm tofu in place of the roast beef.

Nutrients per serving	
Calories	327
Total fat	4 g
Saturated fat	1 g
Cholesterol	31 mg
Sodium	644 mg
Carbohydrate	57 g
Fiber	9 g
Protein	26 g
Calcium	478 mg
Iron	5.2 mg

Beef and Snow Pea Soup

Makes 6 servings

✪ Great for Steps 1, 3, 4 and 5

Who needs takeout? You can make beef and snow pea soup just as fast yourself.

Tips

For best results, select a deli roast beef that does not have additional flavorings (such as Italian herbs or barbecue seasoning).

To add more protein to this soup, replace the rice with hot cooked quinoa.

Storage Tip

Store the cooled soup in an airtight container in the refrigerator for up to 2 days or in the freezer for up to 6 months. Thaw overnight in the refrigerator or in the microwave using the Defrost function. Warm soup in a medium saucepan over medium-low heat.

Nutrients per serving	
Calories	238
Total fat	5 g
Saturated fat	1 g
Cholesterol	25 mg
Sodium	709 mg
Carbohydrate	34 g
Fiber	5 g
Protein	13 g
Calcium	62 mg
Iron	3.2 mg

3 tbsp	minced gingerroot	45 mL
6 cups	reduced-sodium ready-to-use beef or vegetable broth	1.5 L
1	large red bell pepper, cut into very thin strips	1
12 oz	snow peas, threads removed, cut in half on the diagonal	375 g
8 oz	thinly sliced deli roast beef, cut into ½-inch (1 cm) wide strips	250 g
1 cup	thinly sliced green onions	250 mL
2 tbsp	reduced-sodium tamari or soy sauce	30 mL
2 tbsp	unseasoned rice vinegar	30 mL
1 tbsp	toasted sesame oil	15 mL
3 cups	hot cooked short- or medium-grain brown rice (see page 438)	750 mL

1. In a large saucepan, combine ginger and broth. Bring to a gentle boil over medium-high heat. Add red pepper and peas; boil for 1 minute. Add beef and green onions; reduce heat and simmer for 1 minute. Remove from heat and stir in tamari, vinegar and oil.
2. Divide rice among six soup bowls and ladle soup over top.

Middle Eastern Beef, Bulgur and Chickpea Soup

Makes 6 servings

✪ Great for Steps 1, 3, 4 and 5

With its notes of cumin, cinnamon and coriander playing off the gentle heat of black pepper, this Middle Eastern soup combines the best parts of meaty kefta and vegetarian beans and grains. Its rich body makes it a seriously satisfying dinner any night of the week.

Storage Tip

Store the cooled soup in an airtight container in the refrigerator for up to 2 days or in the freezer for up to 6 months. Thaw overnight in the refrigerator or in the microwave using the Defrost function. Warm soup in a medium saucepan over medium-low heat.

Nutrients per serving	
Calories	202
Total fat	4 g
Saturated fat	1 g
Cholesterol	23 mg
Sodium	446 mg
Carbohydrate	27 g
Fiber	6 g
Protein	14 g
Calcium	66 mg
Iron	2.7 mg

8 oz	extra-lean ground beef	250 g
1½ cups	chopped onions	375 mL
3	cloves garlic, minced	3
2 tsp	ground cumin	10 mL
1 tsp	ground cinnamon	5 mL
¾ tsp	ground coriander	3 mL
¼ tsp	fine sea salt	1 mL
¼ tsp	freshly ground black pepper	1 mL
1	can (14 to 19 oz/398 to 540 mL) chickpeas, drained and rinsed	1
½ cup	fine or medium bulgur	125 mL
6 cups	reduced-sodium ready-to-use beef or vegetable broth	1.5 L
2 cups	water	500 mL
½ cup	packed fresh cilantro or mint leaves, chopped	125 mL
1 tsp	finely grated lemon zest	5 mL
1 tbsp	freshly squeezed lemon juice	15 mL

1. In a large saucepan, cook beef over medium-high heat, breaking it up with a spoon, for 3 to 5 minutes or until no longer pink. Drain off any excess fat. Add onions and cook, stirring, for 6 to 8 minutes or until softened. Add garlic, cumin, cinnamon, coriander, salt and pepper; cook, stirring, for 1 minute.
2. Stir in chickpeas, bulgur, broth and water. Bring to a boil. Reduce heat to medium-low, cover, leaving lid ajar, and simmer, stirring occasionally, for 15 to 20 minutes or until bulgur is tender. Stir in cilantro, lemon zest and lemon juice.

Salmon Chowder

Makes 4 servings

✪ Great for Steps 1, 3 and 4

Making salmon chowder is usually impractical for the home cook, especially on a weeknight. But this simple version offers a shortcut that works with great success: canned Alaskan salmon, including the canning liquid (the latter enriches the broth).

Tip

Sweet smoked paprika is used here to add a nuanced, smoky flavor without heat. Avoid using hot smoked paprika unless you want to add heat to the chowder.

Storage Tip

Store the cooled chowder in an airtight container in the refrigerator for up to 1 day. Warm chowder in a medium saucepan over medium-low heat.

Nutrients per serving	
Calories	419
Total fat	9 g
Saturated fat	1 g
Cholesterol	7 mg
Sodium	303 mg
Carbohydrate	47 g
Fiber	4 g
Protein	38 g
Calcium	500 mg
Iron	3.9 mg

2 tsp	extra virgin olive oil	10 mL
1 lb	small waxy potatoes (such as red-skinned), peeled and diced	500 g
1½ cups	chopped onions	375 mL
1 cup	chopped celery	250 mL
1 tsp	sweet smoked paprika (not hot)	5 mL
1	bottle (8 oz/227 mL) clam juice	1
¾ cup	water	175 mL
2 cups	evaporated skim milk	500 mL
1	can (15 oz/425 g) wild Alaskan salmon, with liquid (skin removed, if necessary)	1
2 tbsp	chopped fresh dill	30 mL

1. In a large saucepan, heat oil over medium-high heat. Add potatoes, onions and celery; cook, stirring, for 6 to 8 minutes or until potatoes are golden and onions and celery are softened. Add paprika and cook, stirring, for 1 minute.
2. Stir in clam juice and water. Bring to a boil. Reduce heat to medium-low, cover, leaving lid ajar, and simmer, stirring once or twice, for 12 minutes or until potatoes are barely tender. Stir in milk. Reduce heat and simmer, uncovered, stirring once or twice, for 5 to 6 minutes or until potatoes are tender. Stir in salmon with liquid and dill, gently breaking salmon into chunks with a spoon. Simmer, stirring gently, for 3 to 4 minutes to warm through and blend the flavors.

Pasta e Fagioli

Makes 8 servings

✪ Great for Steps 1, 2, 3, 4 and 5

This cannellini-rich dish — part soup and part stew — is saucy and comforting. Once you try it, you'll understand why Tuscans proudly call themselves mangiafagioli, *or bean eaters.*

Tip

If using the larger 19-oz (540 mL) cans of beans, you may want to add up to ½ cup (125 mL) extra broth to thin the soup.

Storage Tip

Store the cooled soup in an airtight container in the refrigerator for up to 2 days or in the freezer for up to 6 months. Thaw overnight in the refrigerator or in the microwave using the Defrost function. Warm soup in a medium saucepan over medium-low heat.

Nutrients per serving	
Calories	200
Total fat	3 g
Saturated fat	1 g
Cholesterol	5 mg
Sodium	718 mg
Carbohydrate	34 g
Fiber	9 g
Protein	10 g
Calcium	161 mg
Iron	2.8 mg

2 tsp	extra virgin olive oil	10 mL
2 cups	chopped onions	500 mL
1¼ cups	chopped celery	300 mL
1¼ cups	chopped carrots	300 mL
3	cloves garlic, minced	3
1 tbsp	dried Italian seasoning	15 mL
¼ tsp	freshly cracked black pepper	1 mL
2	cans (each 14 to 19 oz/398 to 540 mL) cannellini (white kidney) beans, drained and rinsed	2
1	can (28 oz/796 mL) diced tomatoes, with juice	1
⅔ cup	whole wheat elbow macaroni or other small tubular pasta	150 mL
6 cups	reduced-sodium ready-to-use chicken or vegetable broth	1.5 L
½ cup	packed fresh flat-leaf (Italian) parsley leaves, chopped	125 mL
¼ cup	freshly grated Parmesan cheese	60 mL

1. In a large saucepan, heat oil over medium-high heat. Add onions, celery and carrots; cook, stirring, for 6 to 8 minutes or until softened. Add garlic, Italian seasoning and pepper; cook, stirring, for 30 seconds.
2. In a small bowl, mash ½ cup (125 mL) of the beans with a fork. Stir mashed beans, whole beans, tomatoes with juice, pasta and broth into the pan. Bring to a boil. Reduce heat to medium-low, cover and simmer, stirring occasionally, for 10 minutes or until pasta is al dente. Remove from heat and let stand for 5 minutes. Stir in parsley. Serve sprinkled with cheese.

Butternut Squash, White Bean and Kale Stew

Makes 8 servings

✪ Great for Steps 1, 2, 3 and 4

Call it a stew or call it chili, you'll definitely call it delectable. Far from being a retiring meatless dish on the sidelines, this is a take-center-stage attention-grabber.

Storage Tip

Store the cooled stew in an airtight container in the refrigerator for up to 2 days or in the freezer for up to 6 months. Thaw overnight in the refrigerator or in the microwave using the Defrost function. Warm stew in a medium saucepan over medium-low heat.

2 tsp	extra virgin olive oil	10 mL
2	red bell peppers, cut into 1-inch (2.5 cm) pieces	2
1	butternut squash (about 2 lbs/1 kg), peeled and cut into 1-inch (2.5 cm) cubes	1
1½ cups	chopped onions	375 mL
2½ tsp	dried rubbed sage	12 mL
½ tsp	fine sea salt	2 mL
¼ tsp	freshly cracked black pepper	1 mL
1	can (14 to 15 oz/398 to 425 mL) diced tomatoes, with juice	1
1½ cups	reduced-sodium ready-to-use vegetable or chicken broth	375 mL
2	cans (each 14 to 19 oz/398 to 540 mL) cannellini (white kidney) beans, drained and rinsed	2
1	large bunch kale, stems and ribs removed, very thinly sliced crosswise (about 5 cups/1.25 L)	1
¼ cup	pitted brine-cured black olives (such as kalamata), quartered	60 mL
¼ cup	freshly grated Romano cheese	60 mL

1. In a large saucepan, heat oil over medium-high heat. Add red peppers, squash and onions; cook, stirring, for 12 to 15 minutes or until squash is slightly softened. Add sage, salt and pepper; cook, stirring, for 1 minute.
2. Stir in tomatoes with juice and broth. Bring to a boil. Reduce heat to medium-low, cover and simmer, stirring occasionally, for 15 to 20 minutes or until squash is tender. Stir in beans and kale. Cover and simmer, stirring occasionally, for 5 to 6 minutes or until kale is wilted. Serve sprinkled with olives and cheese.

▸ Health Note

Herbalists have recognized sage's health-promoting qualities for thousands of years. The ancient Greeks used it to help preserve meat, and 10th-century physicians in Arabia believed it helped promote immortality.

Nutrients per serving	
Calories	214
Total fat	3 g
Saturated fat	1 g
Cholesterol	3 mg
Sodium	738 mg
Carbohydrate	39 g
Fiber	11 g
Protein	11 g
Calcium	233 mg
Iron	4.0 mg

Red Lentil and Kale Stew

Makes 8 servings

✪ Great for Steps 1, 2, 3 and 4

Red lentils, which cook more quickly than other lentil varieties, are the foundation of this earthy, rustic stew.

Storage Tip

Store the cooled stew in an airtight container in the refrigerator for up to 2 days or in the freezer for up to 6 months. Thaw overnight in the refrigerator or in the microwave using the Defrost function. Warm stew in a medium saucepan over medium-low heat.

Nutrients per serving	
Calories	289
Total fat	4 g
Saturated fat	0 g
Cholesterol	0 mg
Sodium	286 mg
Carbohydrate	48 g
Fiber	11 g
Protein	18 g
Calcium	213 mg
Iron	5.8 mg

1 tbsp	extra virgin olive oil	15 mL
1½ cups	chopped onions	375 mL
1 tbsp	ground cumin	15 mL
1 tsp	ground coriander	5 mL
¼ tsp	cayenne pepper	1 mL
8 cups	packed coarsely chopped kale (tough stems and center ribs removed)	2 L
6 cups	reduced-sodium ready-to-use vegetable or chicken broth	1.5 L
1	can (14 to 19 oz/398 to 540 mL) chickpeas, drained and rinsed	1
2 cups	dried red lentils, rinsed	500 mL
2 tsp	red wine vinegar	10 mL
½ cup	nonfat plain yogurt	125 mL
1 tbsp	freshly squeezed lime juice	15 mL

1. In a large saucepan, heat oil over medium-high heat. Add onions and cook, stirring, for 5 to 6 minutes or until softened. Add cumin, coriander and cayenne; cook, stirring, for 30 seconds.
2. Stir in kale and broth. Bring to a boil. Stir in chickpeas and lentils. Reduce heat to medium, cover, leaving lid ajar, and simmer, stirring occasionally, for 15 to 20 minutes or until lentils are very tender. Stir in vinegar.
3. In a small bowl, whisk together yogurt and lime juice. Serve stew drizzled with yogurt mixture.

▸ Health Note

Red lentils are one fast food worth craving: a mere ½-cup (125 mL) serving provides 75 µg of riboflavin, 179 µg of folate, 19 mg of calcium, 1.25 mg of zinc and 3.30 mg of iron.

Barley, Mushroom and Kale Stew

Makes 8 servings

✪ Great for Steps 1, 2, 4 and 5

You'll reach for this recipe again and again for its incredible simplicity and ability to satisfy.

Storage Tip

Store the cooled stew in an airtight container in the refrigerator for up to 2 days or in the freezer for up to 6 months. Thaw overnight in the refrigerator or in the microwave using the Defrost function. Warm stew in a medium saucepan over medium-low heat.

1 tbsp	extra virgin olive oil	15 mL
2 cups	chopped onions	500 mL
3	cloves garlic, minced	3
12 oz	cremini or button mushrooms, trimmed and sliced	375 g
1 tbsp	minced fresh rosemary	15 mL
1	can (28 oz/796 mL) diced tomatoes, with juice	1
1 cup	pearl barley	250 mL
5 cups	reduced-sodium ready-to-use vegetable or chicken broth	1.25 L
8 cups	packed chopped kale (tough stems and center ribs removed)	2 L
1/3 cup	freshly grated Parmesan cheese	75 mL

1. In a large saucepan, heat oil over medium-high heat. Add onions and cook, stirring, for 6 to 8 minutes or until softened. Add garlic, mushrooms and rosemary; cook, stirring, for 6 to 7 minutes or until mushrooms are browned. Add tomatoes with juice and cook, stirring, for 1 minute.
2. Stir in barley and broth. Bring to a boil. Reduce heat to low, cover and simmer, stirring occasionally, for 40 to 45 minutes or until barley is tender. Stir in kale and cook, stirring, for 5 to 6 minutes or until wilted. Serve sprinkled with cheese.

Nutrients per serving	
Calories	218
Total fat	4 g
Saturated fat	1 g
Cholesterol	6 mg
Sodium	452 mg
Carbohydrate	38 g
Fiber	8 g
Protein	8 g
Calcium	256 mg
Iron	3.7 mg

Farro Stew with Spring Peas and Mint

Makes 6 servings

✪ Great for Steps 1, 2, 3, 4 and 5

The chewy grains of farro work as an earthy foil to the decidedly spring flavors of green peas, mint and radishes.

Storage Tip

Store the cooled stew in an airtight container in the refrigerator for up to 2 days or in the freezer for up to 6 months. Thaw overnight in the refrigerator or in the microwave using the Defrost function. Warm stew in a medium saucepan over medium-low heat.

- **Food processor**

4 tsp	extra virgin olive oil, divided	20 mL
1¼ cups	chopped onions	300 mL
4	cloves garlic, minced	4
½ tsp	fine sea salt	2 mL
¼ tsp	freshly cracked black pepper	1 mL
1½ cups	semi-pearled farro or pearl barley	375 mL
½ cup	dry white wine	125 mL
2 cups	reduced-sodium ready-to-use vegetable or chicken broth	500 mL
2 cups	water	500 mL
1 cup	frozen petite peas, thawed	250 mL
½ cup	coarsely chopped green onions	125 mL
½ cup	packed fresh mint leaves	125 mL
2 tbsp	freshly squeezed lemon juice	30 mL
1 cup	chopped radishes	250 mL
½ cup	crumbled soft goat cheese (optional)	125 mL

1. In a large saucepan, heat half the oil over medium-high heat. Add onions and cook, stirring, for 5 to 6 minutes or until softened. Add garlic, salt and pepper; cook, stirring, for 30 seconds. Add farro and cook, stirring, for 2 minutes. Add wine and boil until most of the liquid is absorbed.
2. Stir in broth and water. Bring to a boil. Reduce heat to medium-low, cover and simmer, stirring occasionally, for 25 to 30 minutes or until farro is tender.
3. Meanwhile, in food processor, combine peas, green onions, mint, lemon juice and the remaining oil; pulse until chopped. Stir into stew, cover and simmer for 5 minutes.
4. Serve stew topped with radishes and goat cheese (if using).

▶ Health Note

Peas are rich in immune-supportive vitamin C, bone-building vitamin K and manganese, heart-healthy dietary fiber and folate, and energy-producing thiamin (vitamin B_1).

Nutrients per serving

Calories	257
Total fat	4 g
Saturated fat	1 g
Cholesterol	0 mg
Sodium	313 mg
Carbohydrate	49 g
Fiber	11 g
Protein	7 g
Calcium	45 mg
Iron	2.2 mg

Healthy Know-How

Understanding Sodium Labels on Food Packages

Food manufacturers' sodium claims can be confusing at best, incomprehensible at worst. Here's how the US Food and Drug Administration defines those claims:

- **Sodium-Free:** Less than 5 mg sodium per serving.
- **Very Low Sodium:** 35 mg sodium or less per serving.
- **Low Sodium:** 140 mg sodium or less per serving.
- **Reduced Sodium:** 25% less sodium than the original item.
- **Light in Sodium:** 50% less sodium than the original item.

Red Fish Stew

Makes 6 servings

✪ Great for Steps 1, 2, 3 and 4

Onions, tomatoes and roasted peppers go velvety when simmered ensemble, and when halibut follows suit, it picks up hints of the vegetables' flavor and becomes delicately nuanced.

2 tsp	extra virgin olive oil	10 mL
1½ cups	chopped onions	375 mL
2	cloves garlic, minced	2
2	cans (each 14 to 15 oz/398 to 425 mL) diced tomatoes, with juice	2
1	jar (12 oz/340 mL) roasted red bell peppers, drained and chopped	1
1¼ lbs	skinless cod or halibut fillets, cut into 1-inch (2.5 mL) pieces	625 g
2 tsp	finely grated lemon zest	10 mL
½ cup	packed fresh flat-leaf (Italian) parsley leaves, chopped	125 mL
2 tbsp	freshly squeezed lemon juice	30 mL
	Fine sea salt and freshly ground black pepper	

1. In a large saucepan, heat oil over medium-high heat. Add onions and cook, stirring, for 5 to 6 minutes or until softened. Add garlic and cook, stirring, for 30 seconds.
2. Stir in tomatoes with juice and roasted peppers. Reduce heat and simmer, stirring occasionally, for 10 minutes. Stir in cod and lemon zest; reduce heat to low, cover and simmer for about 5 minutes or until cod is opaque and flakes easily when tested with a fork. Stir in parsley and lemon juice. Season to taste with salt and pepper.

Nutrients per serving	
Calories	190
Total fat	4 g
Saturated fat	1 g
Cholesterol	33 mg
Sodium	522 mg
Carbohydrate	13 g
Fiber	2 g
Protein	24 g
Calcium	93 mg
Iron	2.3 mg

Black Bean Chipotle Chili

Makes 8 servings

✪ Great for Steps 1, 2, 3 and 4

This homey vegetarian chili — a piquant main dish that's always in fashion — gets its fire from chipotle chile powder.

Tip

If using the larger 19-oz (540 mL) cans of beans, you may want to add up to ½ cup (125 mL) reduced-sodium vegetable broth or water to thin the chili.

Storage Tip

Store the cooled chili in an airtight container in the refrigerator for up to 2 days or in the freezer for up to 6 months. Thaw overnight in the refrigerator or in the microwave using the Defrost function. Warm chili in a medium saucepan over medium-low heat.

Nutrients per serving	
Calories	203
Total fat	2 g
Saturated fat	0 g
Cholesterol	0 mg
Sodium	685 mg
Carbohydrate	33 g
Fiber	8 g
Protein	12 g
Calcium	111 mg
Iron	3.0 mg

2 tsp	vegetable oil	10 mL
2 cups	chopped onions	500 mL
4	cloves garlic, minced	4
3 tbsp	chili powder	45 mL
1½ tbsp	ground cumin	22 mL
2 tsp	dried oregano	10 mL
1½ tsp	chipotle chile powder	7 mL
3	cans (each 14 to 19 oz/398 to 540 mL) black beans, drained and rinsed	3
1	can (28 oz/796 mL) crushed tomatoes, with juice	1
⅓ cup	water	75 mL
1 tbsp	finely grated lime zest	15 mL
¼ cup	freshly squeezed lime juice	60 mL
1 cup	nonfat plain Greek yogurt	250 mL

Suggested Accompaniments

Fresh cilantro leaves
Chopped green onions
Chopped radishes
Crumbled queso fresco

1. In a large saucepan, heat oil over medium-high heat. Add onions and cook, stirring, for 6 to 8 minutes or until softened. Add garlic, chili powder, cumin, oregano and chipotle chile powder; cook, stirring, for 1 minute.
2. In a small bowl, coarsely mash one-third of the beans with a potato masher or fork. Stir mashed beans, whole beans, tomatoes with juice and water into the pan. Bring to a boil. Reduce heat and simmer, stirring often, for about 15 minutes to blend the flavors. Stir in lime zest and lime juice. Serve topped with yogurt and any of the suggested accompaniments, as desired.

▸ Health Note

One cup (250 mL) of beans packs half a day's supply of folate, blood pressure–regulating magnesium and energizing iron.

Sweet Potato, Swiss Chard and Black Bean Chili

Makes 8 servings

✪ Great for Steps 1, 2, 3 and 4

The earthiness of the Swiss chard is a natural complement to the sweet potatoes and spices.

Tips

If using the larger 19-oz (540 mL) cans of beans, you may want to add up to ½ cup (125 mL) reduced-sodium vegetable broth or water to thin the chili.

Regular diced tomatoes may be used in place of the tomatoes with chiles. You'll need about 3¾ cups (925 mL) tomatoes with juice for this recipe.

Storage Tip

See page 207.

Nutrients per serving	
Calories	243
Total fat	3 g
Saturated fat	0 g
Cholesterol	0 mg
Sodium	691 mg
Carbohydrate	43 g
Fiber	10 g
Protein	11 g
Calcium	123 mg
Iron	3.8 mg

1 tbsp	extra virgin olive oil	15 mL
2 cups	chopped onions	500 mL
4	cloves garlic, minced	4
3 cups	cubed peeled sweet potatoes (½-inch/1 cm cubes)	750 mL
¼ cup	chili powder	60 mL
1 tbsp	ground cumin	15 mL
3	cans (each 14 to 19 oz/398 to 540 mL) black beans, drained and rinsed	3
3	cans (each 10 oz/284 mL) diced tomatoes with chiles, with juice	3
1 cup	chopped Swiss chard stems	250 mL
2 cups	reduced-sodium ready-to-use vegetable or chicken broth	500 mL
3 cups	packed coarsely chopped Swiss chard leaves	750 mL

1. In a large saucepan, heat oil over medium-high heat. Add onions and cook, stirring, for 6 to 8 minutes or until softened. Add garlic, sweet potatoes, chili powder and cumin; cook, stirring, for 2 minutes.
2. Stir in beans, tomatoes with juice, Swiss chard stems and broth. Bring to a boil. Reduce heat to medium-low, cover, leaving lid ajar, and simmer, stirring occasionally, for 20 to 25 minutes or until sweet potatoes are very tender. Stir in Swiss chard leaves and simmer, stirring occasionally, for 4 to 5 minutes or until leaves are tender but still bright green.

Indian-Spiced Chickpea Chili

Makes 6 servings

✪ Great for Steps 1, 2, 3 and 4

You can tell that the inspiration for this dish comes from hot, humid lands because of the way the first bite causes a light sweat at the temples. But the harmony of spices continues to evolve and mellow with each subsequent bite.

Tip

Regular diced tomatoes may be used in place of the tomatoes with chiles. You'll need about 2½ cups (625 mL) tomatoes with juice for this recipe.

Storage Tip

See page 207.

Nutrients per serving	
Calories	195
Total fat	4 g
Saturated fat	0 g
Cholesterol	0 mg
Sodium	699 mg
Carbohydrate	34 g
Fiber	8 g
Protein	8 g
Calcium	73 mg
Iron	2.7 mg

2 tsp	vegetable oil	10 mL
1½ cups	chopped onions	375 mL
1 cup	chopped celery	250 mL
1 cup	chopped carrots	250 mL
1 tbsp	mild curry powder	15 mL
2 tsp	garam masala	10 mL
1 tsp	ground ginger	5 mL
¼ tsp	fine sea salt	1 mL
¼ tsp	cayenne pepper	1 mL
2	cans (each 14 to 19 oz/398 to 540 mL) chickpeas, drained and rinsed	2
2	cans (each 10 oz/284 mL) diced tomatoes with chiles, with juice	2
1½ cups	water	375 mL
2 tbsp	tomato paste	30 mL
⅓ cup	packed fresh cilantro leaves, chopped	75 mL
1 tsp	finely grated lime zest	5 mL
1 tbsp	freshly squeezed lime juice	15 mL

1. In a large saucepan, heat oil over medium-high heat. Add onions, celery and carrots; cook, stirring, for 6 to 8 minutes or until softened. Add curry powder, garam masala, ginger, salt and cayenne; cook, stirring, for 1 minute.
2. Stir in chickpeas, tomatoes with juice, water and tomato paste. Bring to a boil. Reduce heat to medium-low, cover, leaving lid ajar, and simmer, stirring occasionally, for 20 minutes or until slightly thickened. Stir in cilantro, lime zest and lime juice; simmer for 1 minute.

Superfood Spotlight

Celery • Celery has long been regarded as an ideal food for dieters because of its high water content and therefore low calorie content. But it offers so much more. It is a good source of potassium and is surprisingly high in calcium, vital for healthy bones, healthy blood pressure levels and nerve function. The darker green stalks and the leaves contain carotenes and more of the minerals and vitamin C than the paler stalks, so don't discard them. Celery also contains polyacetylenes and phthalides, compounds that may protect against inflammation and high blood pressure.

White Turkey Chili

Makes 6 servings

✪ Great for Steps 3 and 4

White beans and ground turkey, a dynamic duo of lean protein, work in harmony with the round and lemony flavor of tomatillo salsa to give this easy chili its Southwestern flavor and flair. With the addition of some fresh and flavorful toppings — lime, cilantro and Greek yogurt — it's a surefire winner.

Tips

Any other variety of white beans may be used in place of the cannellini beans.

If reduced-sodium salsa verde in not available, use regular salsa verde and omit the salt.

Storage Tip

See page 211.

Nutrients per serving	
Calories	258
Total fat	5 g
Saturated fat	1 g
Cholesterol	43 mg
Sodium	719 mg
Carbohydrate	28 g
Fiber	7 g
Protein	26 g
Calcium	117 mg
Iron	4.0 mg

1 lb	lean ground turkey	500 g
1 tbsp	ground cumin	15 mL
2 tsp	dried oregano	10 mL
1⁄4 tsp	fine sea salt	1 mL
2	cans (each 14 to 19 oz/398 to 540 mL) cannellini (white kidney) beans, drained and rinsed	2
2	jars (each 12 oz/340 mL) reduced-sodium salsa verde	2
2⁄3 cup	water	150 mL
3⁄4 cup	packed fresh cilantro leaves, chopped, divided	175 mL
1 tsp	finely grated lime zest	5 mL
3 tbsp	freshly squeezed lime juice, divided	45 mL
2⁄3 cup	nonfat plain Greek yogurt	150 mL

1. In a large saucepan, cook turkey over medium-high heat, breaking it up with a spoon, for 7 to 10 minutes or until no longer pink. Add cumin, oregano and salt; cook, stirring, for 1 minute.
2. In a small bowl, coarsely mash half the beans with a potato masher or fork. Stir mashed beans, whole beans, salsa and water into the pan. Bring to a boil. Reduce heat to medium-low, cover, leaving lid ajar, and simmer, stirring occasionally, for 10 to 15 minutes or until slightly thickened. Stir in half the cilantro, lime zest and 2 tbsp (30 mL) lime juice. Simmer, uncovered, for 2 minutes.
3. In a small bowl, whisk together yogurt and the remaining lime juice. Serve chili topped with yogurt mixture and the remaining cilantro.

Variation

Substitute lean ground chicken or extra-lean ground pork for the turkey.

Green Chile and Pork Pozole

Makes 6 servings

✪ Great for Steps 1, 3 and 4

This revamped version of white chili showcases the citrusy flavor of tomatillos.

Storage Tip

Store the cooled chili in an airtight container in the refrigerator for up to 2 days or in the freezer for up to 6 months. Thaw overnight in the refrigerator or in the microwave using the Defrost function. Warm chili in a medium saucepan over medium-low heat.

Variation

Substitute lean ground chicken or turkey for the pork.

Nutrients per serving	
Calories	356
Total fat	11 g
Saturated fat	4 g
Cholesterol	49 mg
Sodium	697 mg
Carbohydrate	41 g
Fiber	6 g
Protein	20 g
Calcium	37 mg
Iron	5.6 mg

- **Food processor**

2	cans (each 12 oz/340 mL) whole tomatillos, with juice	2
2 tsp	vegetable oil	10 mL
2 cups	chopped onions	500 mL
1 lb	extra-lean ground pork	500 g
4	cloves garlic, minced	4
1 tbsp	minced seeded jalapeño pepper	15 mL
2½ tsp	ground cumin	12 mL
1 cup	packed fresh cilantro leaves, chopped, divided	250 mL
2	cans (each 15 oz/425 mL) yellow hominy, drained	2
2 cups	reduced-sodium ready-to-use vegetable or chicken broth	500 mL

1. In food processor, purée tomatillos and their juice. Set aside.
2. In a large saucepan, heat oil over medium-high heat. Add onions and cook, stirring, for 6 to 8 minutes or until softened. Add pork, garlic, jalapeño and cumin; cook, breaking pork up with spoon, for 7 to 10 minutes or until pork is no longer pink. Drain off any excess fat.
3. Stir in tomatillo purée, half the cilantro, hominy and broth. Bring to a boil. Reduce heat to medium-low, cover, leaving lid ajar, and simmer, stirring occasionally, for 10 minutes. Serve sprinkled with the remaining cilantro.

Lean Beef and Bean Cowboy Chili

Makes 8 servings

✪ Great for Steps 1, 3 and 4

Don't be fooled by the short ingredient list — this quick chili tastes surprisingly complex. A bit of cocoa powder sneaks in, instantly deepening the flavor.

Tip

Regular diced tomatoes may be used in place of the tomatoes with chiles. You'll need about 3¾ cups (925 mL) tomatoes with juice for this recipe.

Storage Tip

Store the cooled chili in an airtight container in the refrigerator for up to 2 days or in the freezer for up to 6 months. Thaw overnight in the refrigerator or in the microwave using the Defrost function. Warm chili in a medium saucepan over medium-low heat.

Nutrients per serving	
Calories	241
Total fat	6 g
Saturated fat	2 g
Cholesterol	31 mg
Sodium	678 mg
Carbohydrate	27 g
Fiber	9 g
Protein	19 g
Calcium	63 mg
Iron	3.7 mg

2 tsp	vegetable oil	10 mL
1½ cups	chopped onions	375 mL
4	cloves garlic, minced	4
3 tbsp	chili powder	45 mL
2 tsp	ground cumin	10 mL
2 tbsp	unsweetened cocoa powder (not Dutch process)	30 mL
1 lb	extra-lean ground beef	500 g
2 tbsp	tomato paste	30 mL
3	cans (each 10 oz/284 mL) diced tomatoes with chiles, with juice	3
2	cans (each 14 to 19 oz/398 to 540 mL) red kidney beans, drained and rinsed	2

Suggested Accompaniments

Fresh cilantro leaves
Chopped green onions
Nonfat plain Greek yogurt
Crumbled queso fresco
Chopped radishes

1. In a large saucepan, heat oil over medium-high heat. Add onions and cook, stirring, for 5 to 6 minutes or until softened. Add garlic, chili powder, cumin and cocoa powder; cook, stirring, for 1 minute. Add beef and tomato paste; cook, breaking beef up with a spoon, for 7 to 10 minutes or until beef is no longer pink.
2. Stir in tomatoes with juice and beans. Bring to a boil. Reduce heat to medium-low, cover, leaving lid ajar, and simmer, stirring occasionally, for 20 minutes or until slightly thickened. Serve with any of the suggested accompaniments, as desired.

Variation

Substitute lean ground turkey or extra-lean ground pork for the beef.

Quick Moroccan Beef and Chickpea Chili

Makes 8 servings

✪ Great for Steps 1, 3 and 4

Spicy, tangy and slightly sweet, this filling chili elevates ground beef in an enchanting new way. Serve with whole wheat couscous or quinoa.

Storage Tip

Store the cooled chili in an airtight container in the refrigerator for up to 2 days or in the freezer for up to 6 months. Thaw overnight in the refrigerator or in the microwave using the Defrost function. Warm chili in a medium saucepan over medium-low heat.

2 tsp	extra virgin olive oil	10 mL
1½ cups	chopped onions	375 mL
1 cup	chopped carrots	250 mL
1 lb	extra-lean ground beef	500 g
2	cloves garlic, minced	2
2 tsp	sweet smoked paprika	10 mL
1½ tsp	ground cumin	7 mL
1½ tsp	ground cinnamon	7 mL
2	cans (each 14 to 19 oz/398 to 540 mL) chickpeas, drained and rinsed	2
1	can (28 oz/796 mL) diced tomatoes, with juice	1
½ cup	golden raisins	125 mL
2 cups	reduced-sodium ready-to-use beef broth	500 mL
1 tsp	finely grated orange zest	5 mL
¼ cup	freshly squeezed orange juice	60 mL
¼ cup	pitted brine-cured black olives (such as kalamata), quartered	60 mL
¾ cup	packed fresh flat-leaf (Italian) parsley leaves, chopped	175 mL

1. In a large saucepan, heat oil over medium-high heat. Add onions and carrots; cook, stirring, for 6 to 8 minutes or until softened. Add beef, garlic, paprika, cumin and cinnamon; cook, breaking beef up with spoon, for 7 to 10 minutes or until beef is no longer pink.
2. Stir in chickpeas, tomatoes with juice, raisins, broth, orange zest and orange juice. Bring to a boil. Reduce heat to medium-low, cover, leaving lid ajar, and simmer, stirring occasionally, for 10 minutes. Stir in olives. Serve sprinkled with parsley.

Nutrients per serving	
Calories	272
Total fat	8 g
Saturated fat	2 g
Cholesterol	31 mg
Sodium	408 mg
Carbohydrate	34 g
Fiber	7 g
Protein	19 g
Calcium	79 mg
Iron	4.0 mg

Sandwiches, Wraps, Burgers and Pizzas

Green Club Sandwich 216
Roasted Beet and Hummus Heroes 216
Cannellini and Artichoke Sandwiches 217
Goat Cheese, Carrot and Golden Raisin Sandwich 217
Tofu Salad Sandwiches 218
Egg Salad Sandwiches on Dark Rye 218
Chicken Salad Sandwiches with Apricots and Almonds 219
Vietnamese-Style Chicken Sandwiches 220
Herbed Cheese, Turkey and Sprouts Sandwiches 221
Spicy Salsa Joes 221
Healthy Know-How: How Much Salt Do We Need? 222
Mediterranean Tuna Sandwich 222
Grilled Salmon Sandwiches with Creamy Lime Coleslaw 223
Cherry Tomato, Avocado and Cucumber Pitas 224
Greek Salad Pitas 224
Tunisian Tuna and Egg Salad Pitas 225
Black Bean and Spinach Burritos 226
Lentil, Mushroom and Kale Burritos 227
California Vegetable Wraps 228
Goat Cheese, Edamame and Roasted Pepper Wraps 228
Quinoa and Chickpea Wraps 229

Cashew Butter and Banana Wraps 229
Tempeh Fajita Wraps. 230
Turkey, Kale and Cranberry Wraps 230
Smoked Turkey, Avocado and Mango Wraps 231
Southeast Asian Roast Beef Wraps 232
Niçoise Salad Wraps 232
Portobello Pesto Burgers. 233
Best Black Bean Burgers 234
Spicy Chickpea Burgers. 235
Bulgur Burgers. 236
Texas BBQ Turkey Burgers 237
Beef and Quinoa Power Burgers. 238
Anytime Tuna Burgers 239
Thai Salmon Burgers 240
Skillet Pizza Marinara 241
Pizza Margherita 242
Artichoke and Ricotta Pizza 243
Greek Pizza 244
Asparagus and Goat Cheese Pizza 245
Mushroom, Pepper and Arugula Pizza 246
Pumpkin, Sausage and Smoked Gouda Pizza 247

Green Club Sandwich

Makes 2 servings

✪ Great for Steps 1, 2, 3, 4 and 5

Nutrients per serving	
Calories	317
Total fat	12 g
Saturated fat	2 g
Cholesterol	0 mg
Sodium	467 mg
Carbohydrate	54 g
Fiber	20 g
Protein	13 g
Calcium	117 mg
Iron	3.2 mg

1	small firm-ripe Hass avocado, sliced	1
1⁄8 tsp	fine sea salt	0.5 mL
2 tsp	freshly squeezed lemon juice	10 mL
3	slices seeded whole-grain sandwich bread	3
3 tbsp	hummus	45 mL
2	plum (Roma) tomatoes, sliced crosswise	2
1 cup	packed tender watercress sprigs or arugula	250 mL

1. Sprinkle avocado slices with salt and lemon juice.
2. Spread one side of each bread slice with hummus. Top one slice with half each of the avocado, tomato and watercress. Cover with another slice of bread, hummus side up. Top with the remaining avocado, tomato and watercress. Cover with the third bread slice, hummus side down, pressing down gently. Cut sandwich in half.

Roasted Beet and Hummus Heroes

Makes 2 servings

✪ Great for Steps 1, 2, 3, 4 and 5

Nutrients per serving	
Calories	255
Total fat	10 g
Saturated fat	3 g
Cholesterol	17 mg
Sodium	428 mg
Carbohydrate	26 g
Fiber	5 g
Protein	9 g
Calcium	183 mg
Iron	2.7 mg

- **Preheat oven to 425°F (220°C)**

2	beets, greens removed	2
1⁄8 tsp	fine sea salt	0.5 mL
1⁄8 tsp	freshly ground black pepper	0.5 mL
2 tsp	extra virgin olive oil	10 mL
1⁄4 cup	hummus	60 mL
2	whole-grain rolls, split	2
1 cup	packed arugula	250 mL
1⁄4 cup	crumbled feta cheese	60 mL

1. Tightly wrap beets in foil. Roast directly on oven rack in preheated oven for 45 to 60 minutes or until tender. Unwrap foil and let cool completely on a wire rack, then peel and slice beets. Sprinkle with salt and pepper, and drizzle with oil.
2. Spread hummus on split sides of rolls, then stuff with beets, arugula and feta, dividing evenly. Press to close.

Cannellini and Artichoke Sandwiches

Makes 2 servings

✪ Great for Steps 1, 2, 3, 4 and 5

Nutrients per serving	
Calories	306
Total fat	7 g
Saturated fat	1 g
Cholesterol	0 mg
Sodium	465 mg
Carbohydrate	64 g
Fiber	12 g
Protein	18 g
Calcium	128 mg
Iron	5.8 mg

2 tsp	extra virgin olive oil	10 mL
1	clove garlic, minced	1
3 cups	packed baby spinach	750 mL
1⁄8 tsp	fine sea salt	0.5 mL
1⁄8 tsp	freshly ground black pepper	0.5 mL
4	slices dark rye bread, toasted	4
1 cup	rinsed drained canned cannellini (white kidney) beans, mashed with a fork	250 mL
1⁄2 cup	drained canned or thawed frozen artichoke hearts	125 mL

1. In a large skillet, heat oil over medium-high heat. Add garlic and cook, stirring, for 30 seconds. Add spinach and cook, stirring, for about 2 minutes or until wilted. Sprinkle with salt and pepper.
2. Spread one side of 2 toast slices with mashed beans. Top with spinach mixture and artichoke hearts, dividing evenly. Cover with the remaining bread slices, pressing down gently. Cut sandwiches in half.

Goat Cheese, Carrot and Golden Raisin Sandwich

Makes 1 serving

✪ Great for Steps 1, 2, 4 and 5

Nutrients per serving	
Calories	291
Total fat	8 g
Saturated fat	4 g
Cholesterol	17 mg
Sodium	521 mg
Carbohydrate	38 g
Fiber	6 g
Protein	13 g
Calcium	155 mg
Iron	3.2 mg

1⁄2 cup	coarsely grated carrot	125 mL
1⁄8 tsp	fine sea salt	0.5 mL
2	slices seeded whole-grain sandwich bread	2
1⁄4 cup	packed mild soft goat cheese	60 mL
1 cup	packed arugula or baby spinach	250 mL
1 tbsp	golden raisins or other dried fruit	15 mL

1. In a small bowl, combine carrots and salt.
2. Spread one side of each bread slice with goat cheese. Top one slice with carrots, arugula and raisins. Cover with the remaining bread slice, goat cheese side down, pressing down gently. Cut sandwich in half.

Tofu Salad Sandwiches

Makes 4 servings

✪ Great for Steps 1, 3, 4 and 5

Here, tofu is a delicate canvas for an old-fashioned, egg salad–style sandwich filling.

Nutrients per serving	
Calories	263
Total fat	9 g
Saturated fat	1 g
Cholesterol	5 mg
Sodium	375 mg
Carbohydrate	35 g
Fiber	5 g
Protein	11 g
Calcium	287 mg
Iron	3.2 mg

8 oz	extra-firm tofu (see tip, page 192)	250 g
1/8 tsp	dried dillweed	0.5 mL
1/8 tsp	fine sea salt	0.5 mL
1/8 tsp	freshly ground black pepper	0.5 mL
2 tbsp	olive oil mayonnaise or vegan mayonnaise	30 mL
1 tbsp	sweet or dill pickle relish	15 mL
1 tsp	Dijon mustard	5 mL
4	multigrain English muffins, split and toasted	4
4	large tomato slices	4
2 cups	packed arugula or baby spinach	500 mL

1. Drain tofu and press dry between paper towels, then cut into 1/4-inch (0.5 cm) cubes.
2. In a medium bowl, whisk together dill, salt, pepper, mayonnaise, relish and mustard. Add half the tofu, mashing with the back of a spoon. Gently stir in the remaining tofu.
3. Top bottom halves of English muffins with tofu salad, tomato and arugula, dividing evenly. Cover with top halves, pressing down gently.

Egg Salad Sandwiches on Dark Rye

Makes 2 servings

✪ Great for Steps 1, 3, 4 and 5

Nutrients per serving	
Calories	302
Total fat	8 g
Saturated fat	2 g
Cholesterol	270 mg
Sodium	569 mg
Carbohydrate	43 g
Fiber	5 g
Protein	22 g
Calcium	146 mg
Iron	4.3 mg

1 tsp	ground cumin	5 mL
1/8 tsp	fine sea salt	0.5 mL
1/8 tsp	freshly ground black pepper	0.5 mL
1/3 cup	nonfat plain Greek yogurt	75 mL
1 tsp	Dijon mustard	5 mL
4	hard-cooked eggs (see tip, page 161), cooled, peeled and chopped	4
1	small red bell pepper, chopped	1
4	slices dark rye bread, toasted	4
2 cups	packed tender watercress sprigs or arugula	500 mL

1. In a medium bowl, whisk together cumin, salt, pepper, yogurt and mustard. Fold in eggs and red pepper.
2. Spread one side of 2 toast slices with egg salad. Top with watercress, dividing evenly. Cover with the remaining bread slices, pressing down gently. Cut sandwiches in half.

Chicken Salad Sandwiches with Apricots and Almonds

Makes 2 servings

✪ Great for Steps 1, 3, 4 and 5

Tangy Greek yogurt, sharp Dijon mustard, sweet dried apricots and crunchy almonds make this chicken sandwich a standout.

Tips

When buying dried apricots, choose an organic variety if you can, because these do not contain sulfur dioxide, which some people are allergic to.

Look for roasted almonds lightly seasoned with sea salt. If your almonds seem heavily salted, rub off some of the salt with a paper towel before chopping. If using unsalted roasted almonds (or toasted almonds), add another pinch of fine sea salt to the recipe.

Nutrients per serving	
Calories	329
Total fat	5 g
Saturated fat	0 g
Cholesterol	18 mg
Sodium	506 mg
Carbohydrate	64 g
Fiber	15 g
Protein	31 g
Calcium	155 mg
Iron	3.7 mg

1⁄8 tsp	fine sea salt	0.5 mL
1⁄8 tsp	freshly cracked black pepper	0.5 mL
1⁄3 cup	nonfat plain Greek yogurt	75 mL
1 tsp	Dijon mustard	5 mL
1 1⁄2 cups	chopped cooked chicken breast or turkey breast	375 mL
2 tbsp	chopped dried apricots	30 mL
2 tbsp	chopped lightly salted roasted almonds	30 mL
4	slices seeded multigrain sandwich bread, toasted	4
2 cups	mesclun (mixed baby lettuce)	500 mL

1. In a medium bowl, whisk together salt, pepper, yogurt and mustard. Stir in chicken, apricots and almonds.
2. Top 2 toast slices with chicken salad and mesclun, dividing evenly. Cover with the remaining toast slices, pressing down gently. Cut sandwiches in half.

Superfood Spotlight

Apricots • Both fresh and dried apricots are highly nutritious and have a low glycemic index, making them an excellent food for sweet-toothed dieters. Fresh apricots contain vitamin C, folate, potassium and vitamin E. They are rich in beta carotene, an important antioxidant that helps to prevent some cancers. They are also ideal for weight maintenance, as they are a good source of fiber and are fat-free. The semidried, plumped fruit is a very good source of potassium and iron, but the drying process diminishes the vitamin C and carotene content.

Vietnamese-Style Chicken Sandwiches

Makes 4 servings

✪ Great for Steps 1, 3, 4 and 5

Despite the exotic inspiration for this sandwich, you can get all the ingredients right at the supermarket.

Variation

Use 8 oz (250 g) plain or Asian-flavored tempeh, thinly sliced, in place of the chicken.

2	cloves garlic, minced	2
1 tsp	ground ginger	5 mL
1 tsp	finely grated lime zest	5 mL
1/8 tsp	cayenne pepper	0.5 mL
3 tbsp	unseasoned rice vinegar	45 mL
1 tsp	agave nectar or liquid honey	5 mL
1/2 tsp	Asian fish sauce (nam pla)	2 mL
3 cups	shredded coleslaw mix (shredded cabbage and carrots)	750 mL
1 cup	thinly sliced red onion	250 mL
1	multigrain baguette, cut crosswise into 4 sections	1
8 oz	thinly sliced deli roasted chicken breast	250 g
1/4 cup	packed fresh cilantro leaves	60 mL

1. In a large bowl, whisk together garlic, ginger, lime zest, cayenne, vinegar, agave nectar and fish sauce. Add coleslaw mix and red onion, tossing to combine. Let stand for 5 minutes.
2. Slice baguette sections horizontally almost all the way through, leaving the halves attached at one side. Mound coleslaw mixture, chicken and cilantro on the bottom halves, dividing evenly, and gently press sandwiches closed.

Nutrients per serving	
Calories	201
Total fat	5 g
Saturated fat	2 g
Cholesterol	24 mg
Sodium	603 mg
Carbohydrate	27 g
Fiber	3 g
Protein	19 g
Calcium	46 mg
Iron	0.8 mg

Herbed Cheese, Turkey and Sprouts Sandwiches

Makes 2 servings

✪ Great for Steps 1, 3, 4 and 5

Nutrients per serving	
Calories	305
Total fat	6 g
Saturated fat	2 g
Cholesterol	44 mg
Sodium	563 mg
Carbohydrate	40 g
Fiber	4 g
Protein	30 g
Calcium	140 mg
Iron	4.1 mg

- **Blender or small food processor**

1 tbsp	chopped fresh flat-leaf (Italian) parsley leaves	15 mL
½ tsp	dried thyme	2 mL
⅛ tsp	freshly cracked black pepper	0.5 mL
½ cup	nonfat cottage cheese	125 mL
4	slices whole-grain sandwich bread	4
1	tomato, sliced	1
5 oz	sliced roast deli turkey	150 g
½ cup	alfalfa, radish or pea sprouts	125 mL

1. In blender, combine parsley, thyme, pepper and cottage cheese; purée until smooth.
2. Spread one side of each bread slice with cheese spread. Top 2 slices with tomato, turkey and sprouts, dividing evenly. Cover with the remaining bread slices, cheese spread side down, pressing down gently. Cut sandwiches in half.

Spicy Salsa Joes

Makes 4 servings

✪ Great for Steps 1, 3, 4 and 5

These are the zesty cousins of the original sloppy joes.

Nutrients per serving	
Calories	328
Total fat	11 g
Saturated fat	2 g
Cholesterol	65 mg
Sodium	337 mg
Carbohydrate	38 g
Fiber	7 g
Protein	28 g
Calcium	166 mg
Iron	4.1 mg

1 tbsp	extra virgin olive oil	15 mL
1 lb	lean ground turkey	500 g
1 cup	chipotle salsa	250 mL
4	multigrain English muffins, split and toasted	4
1	small firm-ripe Hass avocado, diced	1
¼ cup	packed fresh cilantro leaves, chopped	60 mL

1. In a large skillet, heat oil over medium-high heat. Add turkey and cook, breaking it up with a spoon, for 3 to 5 minutes or until no longer pink. Stir in salsa, reduce heat and simmer, stirring once or twice, for 2 minutes.
2. Top bottom halves of English muffins with turkey mixture, avocado and cilantro, dividing evenly. Cover with top halves, pressing down gently.

Variation

Substitute extra-lean ground beef or pork for the turkey.

Healthy Know-How

How Much Salt Do We Need?

Scientists estimate that most people need only 250 to 500 mg of sodium per day for physiological functions such as muscle contractions and nerve transmissions, although it does vary by individual. Americans consume an average of 3,400 mg of sodium per day.

The U.S. government's 2011 update of the Dietary Guidelines continues to recommend a much lower amount: 2,300 mg per day for adults. (For African-Americans, people with hypertension and anyone over the age of 51, the recommendation drops to 1,500 mg.)

The good news is that cutting back on salt is much easier than most people realize. One of the simplest ways to reduce sodium is to eliminate most or all processed and restaurant foods, which account for 77% of the sodium in the average American diet. Only 10% to 11% is added at the table; the remainder is added by cooks or occurs naturally in foods.

Mediterranean Tuna Sandwich

Makes 4 servings

✪ Great for Steps 1, 3, 4 and 5

Variation

Substitute an equal amount of canned chicken breast or salmon (any skin and bones removed) in place of the tuna.

Nutrients per serving	
Calories	206
Total fat	5 g
Saturated fat	1 g
Cholesterol	26 mg
Sodium	249 mg
Carbohydrate	15 g
Fiber	1 g
Protein	31 g
Calcium	23 mg
Iron	1.8 mg

2 tbsp	red wine vinegar	30 mL
1 tbsp	extra virgin olive oil	15 mL
1 tbsp	Dijon mustard	15 mL
2	cans (each 6 oz/170 g) chunk light tuna in water, drained	2
1⁄4 cup	finely chopped red onion	60 mL
1⁄4 cup	pitted brine-cured black olives (such as kalamata), coarsely chopped	60 mL
2 tbsp	chopped fresh parsley leaves	30 mL
2 tsp	drained capers, chopped	10 mL
1	multigrain baguette, cut crosswise into 4 sections	1
4	large lettuce leaves	4
1	large firm-ripe tomato, sliced	1

1. In a medium bowl, whisk together vinegar, oil and mustard. Add tuna, red onion, olives, parsley and capers, gently tossing to flake tuna slightly and coat with dressing.
2. Split baguette sections horizontally almost all the way through, leaving the halves attached at one side. Mound tuna salad, lettuce and tomato on the bottom halves, dividing evenly, and gently press sandwiches closed.

Grilled Salmon Sandwiches with Creamy Lime Coleslaw

Makes 4 servings

✪ Great for Steps 1, 3, 4 and 5

This is a sandwich worth bragging about. The bold flavors begin with grilled salmon fillets glazed with barbecue sauce and nestled on tender whole wheat buns. Then comes the clincher: a creamy lime coleslaw with piquant green onions and citrusy cilantro.

Tip

For reasons of both convenience and frugality, consider using thawed frozen salmon fillets for this recipe.

- **Preheat barbecue grill to medium-high**

Pinch	fine sea salt	Pinch
3 tbsp	nonfat plain yogurt	45 mL
1 tsp	finely grated lime zest	5 mL
1 tbsp	freshly squeezed lime juice	15 mL
1½ cups	shredded coleslaw mix (shredded cabbage and carrots)	375 mL
¼ cup	packed fresh cilantro leaves, chopped	60 mL
¼ cup	chopped green onions	60 mL
4	skinless salmon fillets (each about 5 oz/150 g)	4
	Nonstick cooking spray	
¼ cup	barbecue sauce	60 mL
4	whole wheat hot dog buns, split	4

1. In a medium bowl, whisk together salt, yogurt, lime zest and lime juice. Add coleslaw mix, cilantro and green onions, tossing to coat.
2. Lightly spray salmon with cooking spray. Place salmon on preheated barbecue and grill for 3 minutes. Turn and brush generously with barbecue sauce. Grill for 4 to 5 minutes or until salmon is opaque and flakes easily when tested with a fork. Toast buns on the grill for the last minute.
3. Transfer salmon to toasted buns and top with slaw.

Nutrients per serving	
Calories	361
Total fat	18 g
Saturated fat	4 g
Cholesterol	75 mg
Sodium	516 mg
Carbohydrate	31 g
Fiber	4 g
Protein	35 g
Calcium	213 mg
Iron	1.8 mg

Cherry Tomato, Avocado and Cucumber Pitas

Makes 2 servings

✪ Great for Steps 1, 2, 3, 4 and 5

Nutrients per serving	
Calories	336
Total fat	12 g
Saturated fat	2 g
Cholesterol	0 mg
Sodium	535 mg
Carbohydrate	49 g
Fiber	13 g
Protein	9 g
Calcium	42 mg
Iron	3.0 mg

1	firm-ripe Hass avocado, diced	1
1 cup	halved cherry or grape tomatoes	250 mL
1 cup	diced seeded peeled cucumber	250 mL
½ tsp	ground cumin	2 mL
¼ tsp	fine sea salt	1 mL
1 tbsp	freshly squeezed lemon juice	15 mL
½ tsp	chipotle hot pepper sauce	2 mL
2	6-inch (15 cm) whole wheat pitas, tops split open	2

1. In a medium bowl, combine avocado, tomatoes, cucumber, cumin, salt, lemon juice and hot pepper sauce, gently tossing to coat. Stuff pitas with avocado mixture, dividing evenly.

Variation

Substitute ⅔ cup (150 mL) crumbled feta cheese or soft, mild goat cheese for the avocado.

Greek Salad Pitas

Makes 4 servings

✪ Great for Steps 1, 2, 3, 4 and 5

Nutrients per serving	
Calories	301
Total fat	8 g
Saturated fat	3 g
Cholesterol	17 mg
Sodium	482 mg
Carbohydrate	51 g
Fiber	9 g
Protein	13 g
Calcium	139 mg
Iron	3.3 mg

¼ tsp	fine sea salt	1 mL
⅛ tsp	freshly cracked black pepper	0.5 mL
1 tbsp	extra virgin olive oil	15 mL
1 tbsp	red wine vinegar	15 mL
1	small red bell pepper, finely chopped	1
1¼ cups	halved cherry or grape tomatoes	300 mL
1 cup	rinsed drained canned chickpeas	250 mL
1 cup	diced seeded peeled cucumber	250 mL
1 cup	chopped radishes	250 mL
½ cup	packed fresh mint leaves, chopped	125 mL
½ cup	crumbled feta cheese	125 mL
4	6-inch (15 cm) whole wheat pitas, tops split open	4

1. In a medium bowl, whisk together salt, pepper, oil and vinegar. Add red pepper, tomatoes, chickpeas, cucumber, radishes, mint and cheese, gently tossing to coat. Stuff pitas with salad mixture, dividing evenly.

Tunisian Tuna and Egg Salad Pitas

Makes 4 servings

✪ Great for Steps 1, 3, 4 and 5

The filling for this sandwich is known as salade méchouia, *arguably the most popular salad in Tunisia. Although the ingredients are familiar, the sum is exotic.*

Tip

To hard-cook eggs, place eggs in a saucepan large enough to hold them in a single layer. Add enough cold water to cover eggs by 1 inch (2.5 cm). Heat over high heat until water is just boiling. Remove from heat and cover pan. Let stand for about 12 minutes for large eggs (9 minutes for medium eggs; 15 minutes for extra-large eggs). Drain eggs and cool completely under cold running water or in a bowl of ice water. Refrigerate until ready to eat.

Nutrients per serving	
Calories	294
Total fat	6 g
Saturated fat	2 g
Cholesterol	103 mg
Sodium	529 mg
Carbohydrate	40 g
Fiber	6 g
Protein	21 g
Calcium	51 mg
Iron	3.5 mg

1/8 tsp	cayenne pepper	0.5 mL
2 tbsp	freshly squeezed lemon juice	30 mL
1 tbsp	extra virgin olive oil	15 mL
2	hard-cooked eggs (see tip, at left), cooled, peeled and coarsely chopped	2
1	can (6 oz/170 g) chunk light tuna in water, drained	1
1 cup	halved cherry tomatoes	250 mL
1/2 cup	chopped drained roasted red bell peppers	125 mL
2 tbsp	drained capers	30 mL
4	6-inch (15 cm) whole wheat pitas, tops split open	4
2 cups	packed arugula, roughly chopped	500 mL

1. In a medium bowl, whisk together cayenne, lemon juice and oil. Add eggs, tuna, tomatoes, roasted peppers and capers, gently tossing to flake tuna slightly and coat with dressing. Stuff pitas with tuna salad and arugula, dividing evenly.

Black Bean and Spinach Burritos

Makes 4 servings

✪ Great for Steps 1, 2, 3, 4 and 5

Who needs meat? The cumin- and cilantro-scented black bean filling for these burritos is hearty, satisfying and incredibly easy to prepare. Adding brown rice makes the burritos a complete meal — and completes the protein.

Tip

To streamline preparation time, use thawed frozen chopped onions in place of fresh. They are inexpensive and available in the frozen foods section of most supermarkets.

- **Preheat oven to 350°F (180°C)**

2 tsp	vegetable oil	10 mL
1 cup	chopped onion	250 mL
1	can (14 to 19 oz/398 to 540 mL) black beans, drained and rinsed	1
1½ cups	cooked long-grain brown rice (see page 438)	375 mL
2 tsp	ground cumin	10 mL
¼ tsp	fine sea salt	1 mL
⅓ cup	packed fresh cilantro leaves	75 mL
4	8-inch (20 cm) whole wheat tortillas, warmed	4
4 cups	packed baby spinach	1 L
½ cup	crumbled queso fresco or feta cheese	125 mL
1 cup	reduced-sodium salsa	250 mL

1. In a large skillet, heat oil over medium-high heat. Add onion and cook, stirring, for 5 to 6 minutes or until softened. Add beans, rice, cumin and salt; cook, stirring, for 1 minute. Stir in cilantro.
2. Top warmed tortillas with bean mixture, spinach and cheese, dividing evenly. Roll up like burritos, enclosing filling. Wrap tortillas individually in foil.
3. Bake in preheated oven for 20 minutes. Unwrap, cut in half and serve with salsa.

Nutrients per serving

Calories	318
Total fat	9 g
Saturated fat	3 g
Cholesterol	17 mg
Sodium	585 mg
Carbohydrate	63 g
Fiber	11 g
Protein	15 g
Calcium	178 mg
Iron	3.0 mg

Lentil, Mushroom and Kale Burritos

Makes 4 servings

✪ Great for Steps 1, 2, 3, 4 and 5

In this unconventional favorite, the deep, rich ensemble of lentils, mushrooms and kale is topped with gently assertive goat cheese and spicy salsa. Olé!

Tips

Look for canned lentils where canned beans are shelved, or in the health food section of the supermarket.

Unlike other greens, kale stems are so tough they are virtually inedible. Hence, they, along with the tougher part of the center rib, must be removed before cooking. To do so, lay a leaf upside down on a cutting board and use a paring knife to cut a V shape along both sides of the rib, cutting it and the stem free from the leaf.

Nutrients per serving	
Calories	316
Total fat	10 g
Saturated fat	3 g
Cholesterol	9 mg
Sodium	601 mg
Carbohydrate	55 g
Fiber	12 g
Protein	21 g
Calcium	254 mg
Iron	5.2 mg

2 tsp	extra virgin olive oil	10 mL
1	large bunch curly kale, stems and ribs removed, very thinly sliced crosswise (about 5 cups/1.25 L)	1
1 lb	cremini or button mushrooms, sliced	500 g
2 tsp	ground cumin	10 mL
1½ cups	drained canned lentils	375 mL
¾ cup	salsa	175 mL
4	10-inch (25 cm) whole wheat tortillas, warmed	4
½ cup	crumbled soft goat cheese	125 mL

1. In a large pot, heat oil over medium-high heat. Add kale, mushrooms and cumin; cook, stirring, for 5 minutes. Reduce heat to medium-low and cook, stirring, for 12 to 15 minutes or until kale is very wilted and mushrooms are browned. Add lentils and salsa; cook, stirring, for 3 minutes or until heated through.
2. Spoon lentil mixture down the center of each warmed tortilla, leaving a 2-inch (5 cm) border. Sprinkle with cheese. Roll up like burritos, enclosing filling, or like jelly rolls (ends open).

Superfood Spotlight

Lentils • Small, lens-shaped lentils — available dried and in cans — come in a variety of colors, including green, brown and red. Green and brown lentils tend to contain the highest levels of nutrients and fiber. Lentils are a very rich source of fiber, both insoluble and soluble, which helps protect against cancer and cardiovascular disease. They also contain plant chemicals called isoflavones, which may offer protection from cancer and coronary heart disease, and lignans, which have a mild estrogen-like effect that may lower the risk of cancer, minimize premenstrual syndrome and protect against osteoporosis. Lentils are also rich in B vitamins, folate and all major minerals, particularly iron and zinc.

California Vegetable Wraps

Makes 2 servings

✪ Great for Steps 1, 2, 3, 4 and 5

Nutrients per serving	
Calories	303
Total fat	9 g
Saturated fat	2 g
Cholesterol	0 mg
Sodium	578 mg
Carbohydrate	50 g
Fiber	11 g
Protein	14 g
Calcium	82 mg
Iron	3.0 mg

2	8-inch (20 cm) whole wheat tortillas	2
⅔ cup	hummus	150 mL
1 cup	sliced seedless cucumber	250 mL
1 cup	shredded carrot	250 mL
1 cup	shredded or chopped radishes	250 mL
½ cup	alfalfa sprouts	125 mL
1 tsp	red wine vinegar	5 mL
⅛ tsp	fine sea salt	0.5 mL
⅛ tsp	freshly ground black pepper	0.5 mL

1. Spread tortillas with hummus. Top with cucumber, carrot, radishes and sprouts, dividing evenly. Drizzle with vinegar and sprinkle with salt and pepper. Roll up like burritos, enclosing filling, or like jelly rolls (ends open).

Goat Cheese, Edamame and Roasted Pepper Wraps

Makes 4 servings

✪ Great for Steps 1, 2, 3, 4 and 5

Nutrients per serving	
Calories	260
Total fat	10 g
Saturated fat	4 g
Cholesterol	14 mg
Sodium	484 mg
Carbohydrate	25 g
Fiber	6 g
Protein	15 g
Calcium	87 mg
Iron	2.1 mg

1½ cups	frozen shelled edamame	375 mL
¼ cup	packed fresh basil leaves, chopped	60 mL
¼ tsp	fine sea salt	1 mL
2 tbsp	freshly squeezed lemon juice	30 mL
4	6-inch (15 cm) whole wheat tortillas	4
4 oz	mild creamy goat cheese, crumbled	125 g
½ cup	chopped drained roasted red bell peppers	125 mL

1. In a medium saucepan of boiling water, cook edamame for 15 to 20 minutes or until very tender. Drain and transfer to a small bowl. Add basil, salt and lemon juice. Mash with a fork.
2. Spread tortillas with edamame mixture. Top with cheese and roasted peppers, dividing evenly. Roll up like burritos, enclosing filling, or like jelly rolls (ends open).

Quinoa and Chickpea Wraps

Makes 2 servings

✪ Great for Steps 1, 2, 3, 4 and 5

Nutrients per serving	
Calories	315
Total fat	6 g
Saturated fat	1 g
Cholesterol	1 mg
Sodium	772 mg
Carbohydrate	68 g
Fiber	9 g
Protein	13 g
Calcium	89 mg
Iron	2.9 mg

1 tbsp	chopped fresh mint	15 mL
1/8 tsp	fine sea salt	0.5 mL
1/3 cup	nonfat plain Greek yogurt	75 mL
2	8-inch (20 cm) whole wheat tortillas	2
1 cup	rinsed drained canned chickpeas, coarsely mashed with a fork	250 mL
3/4 cup	cooked quinoa (see page 438), cooled	175 mL
1/4 cup	golden raisins, chopped	60 mL
1 tbsp	freshly squeezed lemon juice	15 mL

1. In a small bowl, whisk together mint, salt and yogurt.
2. Spread tortillas with yogurt mixture. Top with chickpeas, quinoa and raisins, dividing evenly. Sprinkle with lemon juice. Roll up like burritos, enclosing filling, or like jelly rolls (ends open).

Cashew Butter and Banana Wraps

Makes 4 servings

✪ Great for Steps 1, 2, 3, 4 and 5

Elvis was partial to peanut butter and banana sandwiches, but you needn't be a king (or The King) to love these wraps.

Nutrients per serving	
Calories	294
Total fat	9 g
Saturated fat	2 g
Cholesterol	0 mg
Sodium	350 mg
Carbohydrate	46 g
Fiber	4 g
Protein	6 g
Calcium	11 mg
Iron	1.2 mg

4	6-inch (15 cm) whole wheat tortillas	4
1/2 cup	unsweetened natural cashew butter or other nut butter	125 mL
8 tsp	liquid honey or brown rice syrup	40 mL
2	large firm-ripe bananas, sliced	2

1. Spread tortillas with cashew butter and honey. Top with bananas, dividing evenly. Roll up like jelly rolls (ends open).

Tempeh Fajita Wraps

Makes 4 servings

✪ Great for Steps 1, 3, 4 and 5

Nutrients per serving	
Calories	291
Total fat	11 g
Saturated fat	2 g
Cholesterol	0 mg
Sodium	449 mg
Carbohydrate	35 g
Fiber	5 g
Protein	17 g
Calcium	99 mg
Iron	2.8 mg

8 oz	tempeh	250 g
2 tsp	vegetable oil	10 mL
1	red bell pepper, thinly sliced	1
4	8-inch (20 cm) whole wheat tortillas, warmed	4
4 cups	packed baby spinach	1 L
1 cup	reduced-sodium chipotle salsa	250 mL

1. Cut tempeh in half crosswise, then cut each half lengthwise into six strips.
2. In a large skillet, heat oil over medium-high heat. Add tempeh and red pepper; cook, stirring, for 4 to 5 minutes or until pepper is softened.
3. Top warmed tortillas with tempeh mixture, spinach and salsa. Roll up like burritos, enclosing filling, or like jelly rolls (ends open).

Turkey, Kale and Cranberry Wraps

Makes 2 servings

✪ Great for Steps 1, 3, 4 and 5

Tip

Other greens, such as Swiss chard or spinach, may be used in place of the kale.

Nutrients per serving	
Calories	319
Total fat	7 g
Saturated fat	1 g
Cholesterol	35 mg
Sodium	518 mg
Carbohydrate	48 g
Fiber	6 g
Protein	43 g
Calcium	241 mg
Iron	5.3 mg

½ tsp	finely grated orange zest	2 mL
2 tbsp	freshly squeezed orange juice	30 mL
2 tsp	extra virgin olive oil	10 mL
½ tsp	Dijon mustard	2 mL
⅛ tsp	fine sea salt	0.5 mL
3 cups	very thinly sliced kale (tough stems and center ribs removed)	750 mL
¼ cup	dried cranberries or cherries, chopped	60 mL
2	10-inch (25 cm) whole wheat tortillas	2
8 oz	thinly sliced deli smoked turkey	250 g

1. In a medium bowl, whisk together orange zest, orange juice, oil, mustard and salt. Add kale and cranberries, tossing to combine.
2. Top tortillas with kale salad and turkey. Tightly roll up like jelly rolls. Cut wraps in half on the diagonal.

Smoked Turkey, Avocado and Mango Wraps

Makes 4 servings

✪ Great for Steps 1, 3, 4 and 5

Though pale green and delicate in flavor, avocados have no reason for humility. They are particularly rich in monounsaturated fat and potassium, and are a good source of folate. Here, they find tropical accord with sweet mango and smoky turkey in a delectable wrap.

Tip

Avocados do not ripen on the tree but rather after they have been harvested. To speed up the ripening process, place unripe avocados in a brown paper bag with an apple or banana for 2 to 3 days, until they are ripe.

1 tsp	mild curry powder	5 mL
Pinch	fine sea salt	Pinch
1⁄3 cup	nonfat plain Greek yogurt	75 mL
1 tsp	freshly squeezed lime juice	5 mL
1 tsp	agave nectar or liquid honey	5 mL
4	10-inch (25 cm) whole wheat tortillas	4
8 oz	thinly sliced smoked deli turkey	250 g
1	firm-ripe Hass avocado, thinly sliced	1
4 cups	thinly sliced romaine lettuce	1 L
1 cup	chopped firm-ripe mango	250 mL
1⁄2 cup	packed fresh cilantro leaves	125 mL

1. In a small bowl, whisk together curry powder, salt, yogurt, lime juice and agave nectar.
2. Spread tortillas with yogurt mixture. Top with turkey, avocado, romaine, mango and cilantro, dividing evenly. Roll up like burritos, enclosing filling, or like jelly rolls (ends open). Cut wraps in half crosswise.

Superfood Spotlight

Mangos • Mangos, grown throughout the tropics, are fruit superstars. Their orange flesh contains more beta carotene, which can protect against some cancers and heart disease, than almost any other fruit. They are also a valuable source of vitamin C and potassium and have high levels of pectin, a soluble fiber that helps reduce "bad" blood cholesterol. Further, unlike most other fruits, mangos contain a significant amount of the antioxidant vitamin E, which can boost the body's immune system and maintain healthy skin. Their medium-low glycemic index means they are a good choice for those watching their blood sugar, as they will help regulate blood sugar levels. Finally, mangos contain a special enzyme that can be a soothing digestive aid — and can also help tenderize meats.

Nutrients per serving	
Calories	300
Total fat	11 g
Saturated fat	2 g
Cholesterol	48 mg
Sodium	580 mg
Carbohydrate	34 g
Fiber	7 g
Protein	25 g
Calcium	61 mg
Iron	2.0 mg

Southeast Asian Roast Beef Wraps

Makes 4 servings

✪ Great for Steps 1, 3, 4 and 5

Nutrients per serving	
Calories	281
Total fat	10 g
Saturated fat	2 g
Cholesterol	31 mg
Sodium	574 mg
Carbohydrate	31 g
Fiber	6 g
Protein	21 g
Calcium	33 mg
Iron	2.4 mg

½ tsp	ground ginger	2 mL
3 tbsp	unsweetened natural peanut butter	45 mL
1 tbsp	freshly squeezed lime juice	15 mL
2 tsp	reduced-sodium tamari or soy sauce	10 mL
1 tsp	agave nectar or liquid honey	5 mL
1	red bell pepper, cut into thin strips	1
3 cups	shredded coleslaw mix (shredded cabbage and carrots)	750 mL
4	6-inch (15 cm) whole wheat tortillas	4
8 oz	sliced deli lean roast beef	250 g
⅓ cup	packed fresh cilantro leaves	75 mL

1. In a medium bowl, whisk together ginger, peanut butter, lime juice, tamari and agave nectar. Add red pepper and coleslaw mix, gently tossing to coat.
2. Top tortillas with coleslaw mixture, roast beef and cilantro, dividing evenly. Roll up like burritos, enclosing filling, or like jelly rolls (ends open).

Niçoise Salad Wraps

Makes 4 servings

✪ Great for Steps 1, 3, 4 and 5

Nutrients per serving	
Calories	270
Total fat	9 g
Saturated fat	2 g
Cholesterol	103 mg
Sodium	538 mg
Carbohydrate	26 g
Fiber	4 g
Protein	19 g
Calcium	45 mg
Iron	1.8 mg

¼ tsp	freshly cracked black pepper	1 mL
Pinch	fine sea salt	Pinch
1 tbsp	red wine vinegar	15 mL
1 tbsp	extra virgin olive oil	15 mL
¼ tsp	Dijon mustard	1 mL
1	can (6 oz/170 g) chunk light tuna in water, drained	1
¾ cup	halved cherry tomatoes	175 mL
⅓ cup	pitted brine-cured black olives (such as kalamata), quartered	75 mL
4	8-inch (20 cm) whole wheat tortillas	4
2	hard-cooked eggs (see tip, page 161), cooled and sliced crosswise	2
3 cups	chopped romaine lettuce	750 mL

1. In a medium bowl, whisk together pepper, salt, vinegar, oil and mustard. Add tuna, tomatoes and olives, gently tossing to flake tuna slightly and coat with dressing.
2. Top tortillas with tuna salad, eggs and lettuce. Roll up like burritos, enclosing filling, or like jelly rolls (ends open).

Portobello Pesto Burgers

Makes 4 servings

✪ Great for Steps 1, 2, 3, 4 and 5

Grilling is the name of the game for a vegetarian burger with plenty of personality and even more flavor. Stacked with meaty portobello mushrooms, roasted peppers and arugula, this is one meatless entrée that even chest-beating carnivores will devour and praise.

- **Preheat barbecue grill to medium-high**

1⁄4 cup	basil pesto	60 mL
1⁄4 cup	nonfat plain Greek yogurt	60 mL
4	large portobello mushrooms, stemmed and dark gills scraped out	4
	Nonstick cooking spray (preferably olive oil)	
1⁄8 tsp	fine sea salt	0.5 mL
1⁄8 tsp	freshly ground black pepper	0.5 mL
4	whole-grain hamburger buns, split	4
2 cups	packed arugula	500 mL
2⁄3 cup	drained roasted red bell peppers, cut into strips	150 mL

1. In a small bowl, whisk together pesto and yogurt. Set aside.
2. Lightly spray mushrooms with cooking spray and sprinkle with salt and pepper. Place mushrooms, rounded side up, on preheated barbecue and grill for 4 minutes. Turn mushrooms over. Grill for 4 to 5 minutes or until tender. Toast buns on the grill for the last minute.
3. Spread top halves of buns with pesto mixture. Transfer mushrooms to bottom halves and top with arugula and roasted peppers, dividing evenly. Cover with top halves, pressing down gently.

▶ Health Note

Mushrooms are an excellent source of potassium, a mineral that helps lower blood pressure and reduces the risk of stroke. They also provide 20% to 40% of the daily value of copper, a mineral that has cardio-protective properties.

Nutrients per serving	
Calories	207
Total fat	8 g
Saturated fat	1 g
Cholesterol	0 mg
Sodium	552 mg
Carbohydrate	29 g
Fiber	6 g
Protein	8 g
Calcium	89 mg
Iron	2.1 mg

Best Black Bean Burgers

Makes 4 servings

✪ Great for Steps 2, 3, 4 and 5

Black beans are a natural choice for vegetarian burgers. Their meaty texture stands up to being shaped into patties and takes deliciously to all of the favorite burger trappings. The Tex-Mex flavorings can be swapped out for the seasonings of your choice.

Tip

If you can only find larger 19-oz (540 mL) cans of beans, you will need about 1½ cans (3 cups/750 mL drained).

Variation

For vegan burgers, use 3 tbsp (45 mL) vegan mayonnaise alternative in place of the egg.

Nutrients per serving	
Calories	312
Total fat	8 g
Saturated fat	1 g
Cholesterol	45 mg
Sodium	592 mg
Carbohydrate	54 g
Fiber	13 g
Protein	16 g
Calcium	137 mg
Iron	4.3 mg

- **Food processor**

1	slice whole-grain bread	1
2	cans (each 14 to 15 oz/398 to 425 mL) black beans, drained and rinsed, divided	2
1	large egg	1
¼ cup	finely chopped fresh cilantro	60 mL
2 tsp	ground cumin	10 mL
1 tsp	dried oregano	5 mL
¼ tsp	cayenne pepper	1 mL
1 tbsp	extra virgin olive oil	15 mL
4	whole wheat hamburger buns, split and toasted	4

Suggested Accompaniments

Nonfat plain Greek yogurt

Salsa

Spinach leaves

1. In food processor, pulse bread into crumbs. Add half the beans, egg, cilantro, cumin, oregano and cayenne; pulse until a chunky purée forms.
2. Transfer purée to a medium bowl and stir in the remaining beans. Form into four ¾-inch (2 cm) thick patties.
3. In a large skillet, heat oil over medium heat. Add patties and cook for 4 minutes. Turn and cook for 3 to 4 minutes or until crispy on the outside and hot in the center.
4. Transfer patties to toasted buns. Top with any of the suggested accompaniments, as desired.

Spicy Chickpea Burgers

Makes 4 servings

✪ Great for Steps 2, 3, 4 and 5

This two-in-one indulgence combines the irresistible toppings of top-notch burgers — goat cheese and chiles — with the classic flavors of deep-fried falafels.

Tip

If you can only find larger 19-oz (540 mL) cans of chickpeas, you will need about 1½ cans (3 cups/750 mL drained).

- **Food processor**

1	can (14 to 15 oz/398 to 425 mL) chickpeas, drained and rinsed	1
1	can (4 oz /114 mL) diced mild green chiles	1
¾ cup	packed fresh cilantro or flat-leaf (Italian) parsley leaves	175 mL
1	large egg, lightly beaten	1
⅔ cup	fresh whole wheat bread crumbs	150 mL
1 tsp	ground cumin	5 mL
¾ tsp	hot smoked paprika	3 mL
½ tsp	fine sea salt	2 mL
2 tsp	extra virgin olive oil	10 mL
½ cup	crumbled soft goat cheese	125 mL
4	whole-grain hamburger buns, split and toasted	4

Suggested Accompaniments

Sliced tomatoes
Mesclun greens
Sliced cucumbers
Tahini

1. In food processor, combine chickpeas, chiles and cilantro; pulse until finely chopped.
2. Transfer chickpea mixture to a medium bowl and stir in egg, bread crumbs, cumin, paprika and salt. Form into four ¾-inch (2 cm) thick patties.
3. In a large skillet, heat oil over medium-low heat. Add patties and cook for 4 minutes. Turn and cook for 3 minutes. Top patties with goat cheese and cook for 1 minute or until patties are golden brown and hot in the center.
4. Transfer patties to toasted buns. Top with any of the suggested accompaniments, as desired.

Nutrients per serving	
Calories	325
Total fat	9 g
Saturated fat	4 g
Cholesterol	54 mg
Sodium	553 mg
Carbohydrate	48 g
Fiber	8 g
Protein	15 g
Calcium	100 mg
Iron	3.2 mg

Bulgur Burgers

Makes 4 servings

✪ Great for Steps 1, 2, 3, 4 and 5

These veggie burgers have great texture thanks to a combination of bulgur and red kidney beans. They get a power-up from hot smoked paprika and cumin, offset by luscious Greek yogurt and fresh spinach and tomato.

- **Food processor**

½ cup	fine or medium bulgur	125 mL
½ cup	boiling water	125 mL
3	cloves garlic, coarsely chopped	3
1 cup	rinsed drained canned red kidney beans	250 mL
¾ cup	lightly salted roasted sunflower seeds	175 mL
½ cup	packed fresh cilantro leaves	125 mL
2 tsp	ground cumin	10 mL
½ tsp	hot smoked paprika	2 mL
½ tsp	fine sea salt	2 mL
2 tsp	extra virgin olive oil	10 mL
4	multigrain English muffins, split and toasted	4
4	large tomato slices	4
2 cups	packed baby spinach	500 mL
¼ cup	nonfat plain Greek yogurt	60 mL

1. In a large bowl, combine bulgur and boiling water. Let stand for about 30 minutes or until water is absorbed. Fluff bulgur with a fork and cool to room temperature.
2. In food processor, combine cooled bulgur, garlic, beans, sunflower seeds, cilantro, cumin, paprika and salt; pulse until blended but still chunky. Form into four ¾-inch (2 cm) thick patties.
3. In a large skillet, heat oil over medium heat. Add patties and cook for 4 minutes. Turn and cook for 3 to 4 minutes or until crispy and hot in the center.
4. Transfer patties to toasted English muffins. Top with tomato, spinach and dollops of yogurt.

▶ Health Note

Sunflower seeds are a great natural source of potassium and phosphorus, as well as protein, iron and magnesium. A half cup (125 mL) of the seeds provides 7 g of dietary fiber, 15 g of protein and ample amounts of vitamin E and folate.

Nutrients per serving	
Calories	341
Total fat	10 g
Saturated fat	2 g
Cholesterol	0 mg
Sodium	530 mg
Carbohydrate	64 g
Fiber	14 g
Protein	19 g
Calcium	226 mg
Iron	5.4 mg

Texas BBQ Turkey Burgers

Makes 4 servings

✪ Great for Steps 3, 4 and 5

The addition of flavorful red beans and zesty barbecue sauce turns ground turkey into an amazing backyard burger worthy of its Texas moniker.

12 oz	lean ground turkey	375 g
1	large egg, lightly beaten	1
1 cup	rinsed drained canned red kidney beans, coarsely mashed with a fork	250 mL
1⁄3 cup	fresh whole wheat bread crumbs	75 mL
1⁄2 cup	finely chopped green onions	125 mL
1 tsp	ground cumin	5 mL
1⁄4 tsp	fine sea salt	1 mL
6 tbsp	barbecue sauce, divided	90 mL
2 tsp	vegetable oil	10 mL
4	multigrain English muffins, split and toasted	4
4	romaine or butter lettuce leaves	4
4	large tomato slices	4

1. In a large bowl, gently combine turkey, egg, beans, bread crumbs, green onions, cumin, salt and 4 tbsp (60 mL) of the barbecue sauce. Form into four 3⁄4-inch (2 cm) thick patties.
2. In a large nonstick pan, heat oil over medium heat. Add patties and cook for 6 minutes. Turn and cook for 6 to 7 minutes or until no longer pink inside.
3. Transfer patties to toasted English muffins. Top with romaine, tomato and the remaining barbecue sauce.

Variation

Substitute extra-lean ground beef or pork for the turkey.

Superfood Spotlight

Cumin • Small, brown cumin seeds are harvested from an herb belonging to the parsley family. Their flavor is warm and spicy but not too hot. The spice has been used since ancient times — the Romans used it as an appetizer and a digestive. Modern research has shown that, indeed, cumin stimulates the secretion of pancreatic enzymes necessary for efficient digestion and nutrient absorption. Currently cumin is being investigated for its antioxidant powers, and it may help to block cancer growth. The seeds are rich in iron. Cumin is an antiseptic, so an infusion of cumin seeds with honey makes an ideal drink for people with a sore throat.

Nutrients per serving	
Calories	364
Total fat	11 g
Saturated fat	2 g
Cholesterol	99 mg
Sodium	597 mg
Carbohydrate	56 g
Fiber	9 g
Protein	29 g
Calcium	331 mg
Iron	5.2 mg

Beef and Quinoa Power Burgers

Makes 4 servings

✪ Great for Steps 1, 3, 4 and 5

There are burgers and then there are burgers. *This is definitely one of the latter. This superfood variation takes the classic beef burger in an entirely new direction. And along with the incredibly delicious flavor, you also get complete protein from the quinoa, vitamin C from the tomatoes and substantial B vitamins from the spinach.*

Variation

Substitute lean ground turkey or extra-lean ground pork for the beef.

- **Food processor**

2⁄3 cup	quinoa, rinsed	150 mL
1 1⁄3 cups	water	325 mL
1 lb	extra-lean ground beef	500 g
1⁄2 cup	finely chopped green onions	125 mL
2 tsp	ground cumin	10 mL
1 tsp	fine sea salt	5 mL
1 tsp	extra virgin olive oil	5 mL
4	whole-grain hamburger buns, split and toasted	4
1⁄4 cup	hummus	60 mL
4	large tomato slices	4
2 cups	packed baby spinach or tender watercress sprigs	500 mL

1. In a medium saucepan, combine quinoa and water. Bring to a boil over medium-high heat. Reduce heat to low, cover and simmer for 15 to 18 minutes or until water is absorbed. Remove from heat and let cool to room temperature. Transfer to a large bowl.
2. In food processor, combine cooled quinoa, beef, green onions, cumin and salt; pulse until blended. Form into four 3⁄4-inch (2 cm) thick patties.
3. In a large skillet, heat oil over medium-high heat. Add patties and cook for 4 minutes. Turn and cook for 5 minutes or until no longer pink inside.
4. Spread top halves of buns with hummus. Transfer patties to bottom halves and top with tomato and spinach. Cover with top halves, pressing down gently.

Nutrients per serving	
Calories	386
Total fat	11 g
Saturated fat	3 g
Cholesterol	62 mg
Sodium	625 mg
Carbohydrate	45 g
Fiber	7 g
Protein	33 g
Calcium	912 mg
Iron	6.0 mg

Anytime Tuna Burgers

Makes 4 servings

✪ Great for Steps 1, 3, 4 and 5

Here, tender flakes of tuna are seasoned with Dijon mustard and green onions, lightly bound with egg and bread crumbs, then pan-fried until the cakes have a golden crust. Toasted English muffins, peppery watercress and sweet sliced tomatoes are all the accompaniment they need.

Tip

An equal amount of arugula or spinach leaves may be used in place of the watercress.

Nutrients per serving	
Calories	328
Total fat	7 g
Saturated fat	1 g
Cholesterol	116 mg
Sodium	417 mg
Carbohydrate	45 g
Fiber	6 g
Protein	32 g
Calcium	183 mg
Iron	4.8 mg

2	large eggs, lightly beaten	2
1½ tbsp	Dijon mustard	22 mL
2	cans (each 6 oz/170 g) chunk light tuna in water, drained	2
⅔ cup	packed fresh whole wheat bread crumbs	150 mL
½ cup	finely chopped green onions	125 mL
2 tsp	extra virgin olive oil	10 mL
4	multigrain English muffins, split and toasted	4
4	large tomato slices	4
2 cups	tender watercress sprigs	500 mL

1. In a medium bowl, whisk together eggs and mustard. Gently stir in tuna, bread crumbs and green onions, flaking tuna into small pieces. Form into four ¾-inch (2 cm) thick patties.
2. In a large skillet, heat oil over medium-high heat. Add patties and cook for 4 minutes. Turn and cook for 4 to 5 minutes or until browned and hot in the center.
3. Transfer patties to toasted English muffins. Top with tomato and watercress.

Thai Salmon Burgers

Makes 4 servings

✪ Great for Steps 1, 3, 4 and 5

These bravura burgers stimulate all the senses. Using canned salmon instead of fresh fillets simplifies matters significantly, making these easy (and affordable) enough for any night of the week.

Tips

Two tsp (10 mL) mild or medium curry powder may be used in place of the red curry paste.

For extra Thai flavor, add a few fresh basil or mint leaves (or both) with the mango and cucumber.

Nutrients per serving	
Calories	409
Total fat	18 g
Saturated fat	0 g
Cholesterol	0 mg
Sodium	280 mg
Carbohydrate	45 g
Fiber	6 g
Protein	39 g
Calcium	199 mg
Iron	4.8 mg

2 tsp	finely grated lime zest	10 mL
1⁄8 tsp	fine sea salt	0.5 mL
1 tbsp	Thai red curry paste	15 mL
1 tbsp	boiling water	15 mL
1	can (15 oz/425 g) wild Alaskan salmon, drained (skin removed, if necessary)	1
1	large egg white, lightly beaten	1
1⁄2 cup	fresh whole wheat bread crumbs	125 mL
1⁄2 cup	packed fresh cilantro leaves, chopped	125 mL
1⁄4 cup	finely chopped green onions	60 mL
1 tbsp	vegetable oil	15 mL
4	multigrain English muffins, split and toasted	4
3⁄4 cup	chopped ripe mango	175 mL
3⁄4 cup	chopped seeded peeled cucumber	175 mL

1. In a large bowl, whisk together lime zest, salt, curry paste and boiling water. Add salmon, egg white, bread crumbs, cilantro and green onions, gently tossing to combine. Form into four 3⁄4-inch (2 cm) thick patties.
2. In a large skillet, heat oil over medium heat. Add patties and cook for 4 minutes. Turn and cook for 3 to 4 minutes or until browned and hot in the center.
3. Transfer patties to toasted English muffins. Top with mango and cucumber.

Skillet Pizza Marinara

Makes 8 servings

✪ Great for Steps 1, 2, 4 and 5

Something special happens when you bake pizza in a deep skillet that always leaves people clamoring for more. Think of this recipe as a template for any number of healthy pizzas you can dream up — but when it comes to toppings, spinach is a terrific place to start.

Variation

Substitute 1½ cups (375 mL) sliced mushrooms for the spinach.

Nutrients per serving	
Calories	296
Total fat	10 g
Saturated fat	3 g
Cholesterol	16 mg
Sodium	587 mg
Carbohydrate	52 g
Fiber	8 g
Protein	15 g
Calcium	156 mg
Iron	2.9 mg

- **Preheat oven to 500°F (260°C)**
- **10-inch (25 cm) cast-iron skillet, sprayed with nonstick cooking spray (preferably olive oil)**

1 lb	Whole Wheat Pizza Dough (see recipe, page 481)	500 g
3 cups	packed baby spinach, coarsely chopped	750 mL
⅔ cup	reduced-sodium marinara sauce	150 mL
1¼ cups	shredded fontina or mozzarella cheese	300 mL
2 tbsp	freshly grated Parmesan cheese	30 mL

1. On a lightly floured work surface, roll dough into a 12-inch (30 cm) circle.
2. Press dough into bottom and up sides of prepared skillet. Top with spinach, then dollop with marinara sauce, spreading to cover (no need to cover entirely). Sprinkle with fontina and Parmesan.
3. Bake in preheated oven for 15 minutes. Reduce heat to 400°F (200°C). Bake for 8 to 11 minutes or until crust is golden brown. Let cool on a wire rack for 5 minutes.

Pizza Margherita

Makes 8 servings

✪ Great for Steps 1, 2, 4 and 5

More is often more, but not in the case of pizza Margherita, where restraint with the ingredients — good tomatoes, fresh mozzarella and verdant basil leaves — is definitely the key to success.

- **Preheat oven to 450°F (230°C)**
- **Large rimmed baking sheet, sprayed with nonstick cooking spray (preferably olive oil)**

1 lb	Whole Wheat Pizza Dough (see recipe, page 481)	500 g
1	clove garlic, minced	1
1/4 tsp	hot pepper flakes	1 mL
1 tbsp	extra virgin olive oil	15 mL
1	ball (about 6 oz/175 g) fresh mozzarella in water, drained and diced	1
2	plum (Roma) tomatoes, thinly sliced horizontally	2
1/4 cup	freshly grated Parmesan cheese	60 mL
1/3 cup	thinly sliced fresh basil	75 mL

1. On a lightly floured work surface, roll dough into a 14- by 10-inch (35 by 25 cm) oval. Transfer to prepared baking sheet.
2. In a small bowl, combine garlic, hot pepper flakes and oil. Brush over dough. Top with mozzarella, tomatoes and cheese.
3. Bake in preheated oven for 25 to 30 minutes or until crust is golden brown. Slide pizza onto a wire rack and let cool for 5 minutes. Top with basil.

Nutrients per serving	
Calories	300
Total fat	10 g
Saturated fat	3 g
Cholesterol	23 mg
Sodium	582 mg
Carbohydrate	51 g
Fiber	7 g
Protein	17 g
Calcium	202 mg
Iron	2.5 mg

Artichoke and Ricotta Pizza

Makes 8 servings

✪ Great for Steps 1, 2, 3, 4 and 5

Luscious, filling and ready in no time, this ricotta pizza finds a perfect complement of toppings with marinated artichokes and thinly sliced red onion.

Variation

Replace the artichokes with 1 cup (250 mL) drained roasted red bell peppers, thinly sliced, and 3 tbsp (45 mL) pitted brine-cured black olives, thinly sliced. In place of the artichoke marinade, drizzle the pizza with 1 tbsp (15 mL) extra virgin olive oil.

- **Preheat oven to 450°F (230°C)**
- **Large rimmed baking sheet, sprayed with nonstick cooking spray (preferably olive oil)**

1	jar (10 oz/284 mL) marinated artichoke hearts	1
1 lb	Whole Wheat Pizza Dough (see recipe, page 481)	500 g
1½ cups	nonfat ricotta cheese	375 mL
1 cup	thinly sliced red onion	250 mL
3 tbsp	freshly grated Parmesan cheese	45 mL
½ tsp	freshly cracked black pepper	2 mL

1. Drain artichoke hearts, reserving 2 tsp (10 mL) of the marinade. Coarsely chop artichokes.
2. On a lightly floured work surface, roll dough into a 14- by 10-inch (35 by 25 cm) oval. Transfer to prepared baking sheet.
3. Spread ricotta over dough, leaving a 1-inch (2.5 cm) border. Top with artichokes, red onion, Parmesan and pepper. Drizzle with the reserved marinade.
4. Bake in preheated oven for 25 to 30 minutes or until crust is golden brown. Slide pizza onto a wire rack and let cool for 5 minutes.

Nutrients per serving	
Calories	294
Total fat	9 g
Saturated fat	1 g
Cholesterol	7 mg
Sodium	601 mg
Carbohydrate	56 g
Fiber	7 g
Protein	19 g
Calcium	214 mg
Iron	2.8 mg

Greek Pizza

Makes 8 servings

✪ Great for Steps 1, 2, 4 and 5

A short list of ingredients and a few minutes are all it takes to put together this crisp, bubbly Grecian masterpiece. A quick flutter of fresh mint adds a final note of bright, pungent flavor.

- **Preheat oven to 450°F (230°C)**
- **Large rimmed baking sheet, sprayed with nonstick cooking spray (preferably olive oil)**

1 lb	Whole Wheat Pizza Dough (see recipe, page 481)	500 g
1	clove garlic, thinly sliced	1
1 cup	halved grape or cherry tomatoes	250 mL
1 cup	crumbled feta cheese	250 mL
3⁄4 cup	chopped red onion	175 mL
2 tsp	extra virgin olive oil	10 mL
1⁄4 cup	pitted brine-cured black olives (such as kalamata), coarsely chopped	60 mL
1⁄4 cup	packed fresh mint leaves, torn	60 mL

1. On a lightly floured work surface, roll dough into a 14- by 10-inch (35 by 25 cm) oval. Transfer to prepared baking sheet.
2. Arrange garlic, tomatoes, cheese and red onion on dough. Drizzle with oil.
3. Bake in preheated oven for 25 to 30 minutes or until crust is golden brown. Slide pizza onto a wire rack and let cool for 5 minutes. Top with olives and mint.

Superfood Spotlight

Mint • Mint has been used for thousands of years for both its flavor and its medicinal attributes. The three main types of mint commonly used are peppermint, spearmint and apple mint. The menthol oils they contain — particularly peppermint — are a natural remedy for indigestion, which is why mint tea is traditionally consumed after a rich meal. Menthol can also clear head and chest congestion during colds and flu and for people who suffer from allergic rhinitis. The oils are antibacterial and may help prevent *H. pylori*, which causes stomach ulcers, and food poisoning bugs salmonella and *E. coli* from multiplying. Some of the latest research on the healing powers of mint indicates that it contains phytonutrients that are able to help block the growth of certain cancers in animals.

Nutrients per serving

Calories	299
Total fat	10 g
Saturated fat	3 g
Cholesterol	15 mg
Sodium	606 mg
Carbohydrate	43 g
Fiber	6 g
Protein	12 g
Calcium	121 mg
Iron	2.3 mg

Asparagus and Goat Cheese Pizza

Makes 8 servings

✪ Great for Steps 1, 2, 4 and 5

Fresh asparagus, good-quality goat cheese, olive oil and lemon go a long way toward making this spring-inspired pizza truly memorable.

- **Preheat oven to 450°F (230°C)**
- **Large rimmed baking sheet, sprayed with nonstick cooking spray (preferably olive oil)**

1 lb	Whole Wheat Pizza Dough (see recipe, page 481)	500 g
6 oz	soft mild goat cheese, crumbled	175 g
2 tsp	finely grated lemon zest	10 mL
2 tbsp	freshly squeezed lemon juice	30 mL
1 tbsp	water	15 mL
1 lb	asparagus, trimmed and cut into 1-inch (2.5 cm) pieces	500 g
1 tbsp	extra virgin olive oil	15 mL
1/4 tsp	freshly cracked black pepper	1 mL

1. On a lightly floured work surface, roll dough into a 14- by 10-inch (35 by 25 cm) oval. Transfer to prepared baking sheet.
2. In a small bowl, combine goat cheese, lemon zest, lemon juice and water. Spread over dough, leaving a 1-inch (2.5 cm) border. Top with asparagus. Drizzle with oil and sprinkle with pepper.
3. Bake in preheated oven for 25 to 30 minutes or until crust is golden brown. Slide pizza onto a wire rack and let cool for 5 minutes.

▶ Health Note

Asparagus is high in folic acid, potassium, fiber, thiamin and vitamins A, B_6 and C. It also contains inulin, which helps to produce healthy bacteria in the intestinal tract and hinder digestion problems.

Nutrients per serving

Calories	289
Total fat	10 g
Saturated fat	3 g
Cholesterol	9 mg
Sodium	588 mg
Carbohydrate	53 g
Fiber	8 g
Protein	16 g
Calcium	65 mg
Iron	3.0 mg

Mushroom, Pepper and Arugula Pizza

Makes 8 servings

✪ Great for Steps 1, 2, 3, 4 and 5

Using whole wheat pizza dough you prepared ahead of time, you can make this incredible pizza just as fast as your favorite pizzeria could deliver one.

Tip

When selecting mushrooms, choose those with a fresh, smooth appearance, free from major blemishes and with a dry surface. Once home, keep mushrooms refrigerated; they're best when used within several days of purchase. When ready to use, gently wipe mushrooms with a damp cloth or soft brush to remove dirt. Alternatively, rinse them quickly with cold water, then immediately pat dry with paper towels.

Nutrients per serving	
Calories	276
Total fat	10 g
Saturated fat	2 g
Cholesterol	13 mg
Sodium	589 mg
Carbohydrate	54 g
Fiber	8 g
Protein	17 g
Calcium	165 mg
Iron	2.8 mg

- **Preheat oven to 450°F (230°C)**
- **Large rimmed baking sheet, sprayed with nonstick cooking spray (preferably olive oil)**

1 lb	Whole Wheat Pizza Dough (see recipe, page 481)	500 g
1/2 cup	reduced-sodium marinara sauce	125 mL
1	red bell pepper, sliced	1
8 oz	cremini or button mushrooms, sliced	250 g
1/2 cup	nonfat ricotta cheese	125 mL
1 cup	shredded part-skim mozzarella cheese	250 mL
1 cup	packed arugula, roughly chopped	250 mL
Pinch	fine sea salt	Pinch
1 tsp	extra virgin olive oil	5 mL

1. On a lightly floured work surface, roll dough into a 14- by 10-inch (35 by 25 cm) oval. Transfer to prepared baking sheet.
2. Spread sauce over dough, leaving a 1-inch (2.5 cm) border. Top with red pepper and mushrooms. Dollop with small spoonfuls of ricotta, then sprinkle with mozzarella.
3. Bake in preheated oven for 25 to 30 minutes or until crust is golden brown. Slide pizza onto a wire rack and let cool for 5 minutes.
4. In a small bowl, combine arugula, salt and oil. Scatter over pizza.

Superfood Spotlight

Bell Peppers • The bright colors of bell peppers signal that they contain high levels of carotenes for heart health and cancer protection, and are a rich source of vitamin C. Bell peppers come in a variety of colors, but red and orange bell peppers contain the highest levels of vitamin B_6 and carotenes. All bell peppers are extremely rich in vitamin C, with an average serving providing more than a day's recommended intake. In general, the deeper the color of the pepper, the more beneficial plant compounds it contains. These compounds include bioflavonoids, which protect against cancer, and phenols, which help block the action of cancer-causing chemicals in the body. Bell peppers also contain plant sterols, which may have an anticancer effect, and are an excellent source of vitamin E.

Pumpkin, Sausage and Smoked Gouda Pizza

Makes 8 servings

✪ Great for Steps 3, 4 and 5

Creamy, faintly sweet pumpkin purée works as a delectable and unique sauce for this autumnal pizza, setting it apart from its traditional tomato-based brethren.

Variations

You can use 1 cup (250 mL) thawed frozen winter squash purée (from a 12-oz/375 g package) in place of the pumpkin purée.

An equal amount of smoked Cheddar or smoked provolone cheese may be used in place of the Gouda.

Nutrients per serving	
Calories	287
Total fat	9 g
Saturated fat	3 g
Cholesterol	26 mg
Sodium	597 mg
Carbohydrate	52 g
Fiber	8 g
Protein	17 g
Calcium	176 mg
Iron	2.7 mg

- **Preheat oven to 450°F (230°C)**
- **Large rimmed baking sheet, sprayed with nonstick cooking spray (preferably olive oil)**

1 lb	Whole Wheat Pizza Dough (see recipe, page 481)	500 g
1 cup	pumpkin purée (not pie filling)	250 mL
1 tsp	dried rubbed sage	5 mL
1⁄4 tsp	fine sea salt	1 mL
1⁄8 tsp	freshly cracked black pepper	0.5 mL
2	links cooked chicken sausage, thinly sliced	2
1 1⁄4 cups	shredded smoked Gouda cheese	300 mL
1⁄4 cup	packed fresh parsley leaves, roughly chopped	60 mL

1. On a lightly floured work surface, roll dough into a 14- by 10-inch (35 by 25 cm) oval. Transfer to prepared baking sheet.
2. In a small bowl, whisk together pumpkin, sage, salt and pepper. Spread over dough, leaving a 1-inch (2.5 cm) border. Top with sausage and cheese.
3. Bake in preheated oven for 25 to 30 minutes or until crust is golden brown. Slide pizza onto a wire rack and let cool for 5 minutes. Sprinkle with parsley.

Meatless Main Dishes

One-Pot Eggplant, Mushroom and Potato Curry 250
Black Bean Chili–Topped Sweet Potatoes. 251
Chickpea Potato Masala 252
Koshari. 253
Spring Vegetable Tagine 254
Okra, Chickpea and Tomato Tagine 255
Spicy Punjabi Chickpeas with Mint Radish Raita 256
Grilled Eggplant with Chickpeas and Cashew Yogurt Sauce 257
Butternut Squash Farro with Chickpeas and Cranberries 258
White Bean Bajane with Thyme Barley 259
Speedy Southwest Black Bean and Quinoa Skillet 260
Sweet Potato and Spinach Curry with Quinoa 261
Delicata Squash with Quinoa Stuffing. 262
Quinoa-Stuffed Poblano Chiles. 263
Mushroom- and Bulgur-Stuffed Peppers. 264
Healthy Know-How: Macronutrients 101. 265
Thai Pumpkin and Brown Rice Risotto. 265
Barley Risotto with Asparagus and Lemon 266
Farro Risotto with Swiss Chard and Parmesan 267
Carrot and Feta Fritters with Minted Yogurt Sauce. 268
Quinoa Vegetable Cakes. 269
Cashew Oat Cakes with Spicy Tomato Sauce 270
Lentil Patties with Herbed Yogurt Sauce 271
Healthy Know-How: Top 10 Suggestions for Healthy Eating on a Budget . . 272

Portobello Pizzas 273
Broccoli and Spinach Enchiladas. 274
Winter Squash and Goat Cheese Enchiladas 275
Spinach Mushroom Quesadillas 276
Black Bean Tacos. 277
Eggplant Parmesan Melts 277
Seared Halloumi with Chickpea Salsa and Herbed Couscous. 278
Easy Ratatouille with Poached Eggs 279
Swiss Chard, Cherry Tomato and Ricotta Bake 280
Spanish Sweet Potato Tortilla with Roasted Pepper Sauce 281
Skillet-Roasted Cauliflower Omelet. 282
Greek Salad Frittata. 283
Persian Zucchini Frittata 284
Red Lentil Frittata 285
Quinoa, Mushroom and Green Onion Frittata 286
Spinach and Feta Crustless Quiche. 287
Crispy Baked Tofu 288
Tofu and Eggplant Stir-Fry. 289
Basil Coconut Tofu Curry. 290
Indian-Spiced Cauliflower, Spinach and Tofu Scramble 291
Stir-Fried Tofu with Bok Choy and Spinach 292
Quick Quinoa Stir-Fry with Vegetables and Tofu. 293
Tempeh with Moroccan Tomato Sauce 294
Thai Tempeh with Broccoli and Snow Peas. 295

One-Pot Eggplant, Mushroom and Potato Curry

Makes 4 servings

✪ Great for Steps 1, 2 and 4

Coconut milk ties this dish together, adding a tropical note and balancing the spices and heat from the curry paste. To be sure you're getting enough protein, serve over long-grain brown rice.

Tip

Use any variety of yellow-fleshed potatoes, such as Yukon gold.

Nutrients per serving	
Calories	251
Total fat	9 g
Saturated fat	4 g
Cholesterol	1 mg
Sodium	52 mg
Carbohydrate	41 g
Fiber	8 g
Protein	6 g
Calcium	50 mg
Iron	1.4 mg

1 tbsp	vegetable oil	15 mL
2 cups	cubed peeled yellow-fleshed potatoes (1/2-inch/1 cm cubes)	500 mL
1 1/4 cups	chopped onions	300 mL
1	eggplant, trimmed and cut into 1-inch (2.5 cm) cubes	1
12 oz	cremini or button mushrooms, halved (or quartered if large)	375 g
3/4 cup	reduced-sodium ready-to-use vegetable broth	175 mL
2 tbsp	Thai green curry paste	30 mL
1 1/2 tbsp	brown rice syrup or liquid honey	22 mL
1 cup	light coconut milk	250 mL
2 tbsp	freshly squeezed lime juice	30 mL
1/2 cup	packed fresh cilantro leaves, chopped, divided	125 mL

1. In a large saucepan, heat oil over medium-high heat. Add potatoes and onions; cook, stirring, for 5 minutes or until potatoes start to soften. Add eggplant and mushrooms; cook, stirring, for 5 minutes or until mushrooms release their liquid.
2. Stir in broth, curry paste and brown rice syrup. Bring to a boil. Reduce heat to medium-low, cover and simmer, stirring occasionally, for 15 to 20 minutes or until potatoes are tender. Stir in coconut milk, lime juice and half the cilantro; simmer, uncovered, stirring occasionally, for 5 minutes to heat through and blend the flavors. Serve sprinkled with the remaining cilantro.

Black Bean Chili–Topped Sweet Potatoes

Makes 2 servings

✪ Great for Steps 1, 2, 3 and 4

Whole baked sweet potatoes caramelize slightly in the oven, which gives them an additional dimension of subtle sweetness. A quick-as-can-be black bean chili — packed with protein, iron, folate and fiber — is an addictive topping that transforms them from side dish to main dish. Greek yogurt and cilantro add cooling and fresh finishing touches.

Tip

For an even faster entrée, substitute two 14-oz (398 mL) cans of vegetarian black bean chili, warmed, for the black bean and salsa chili prepared in step 2.

Nutrients per serving	
Calories	379
Total fat	2 g
Saturated fat	0 g
Cholesterol	0 mg
Sodium	536 mg
Carbohydrate	85 g
Fiber	18 g
Protein	17 g
Calcium	186 mg
Iron	4.6 mg

- **Preheat oven to 425°F (220°C)**
- **Rimmed baking sheet**

2	sweet potatoes (each about 12 oz/375 g)	2
1	can (14 to 19 oz/398 to 540 mL) black beans, drained and rinsed	1
1 tsp	ground cumin	5 mL
Pinch	cayenne pepper (optional)	Pinch
1½ cups	chunky chipotle salsa	375 mL
2 tbsp	nonfat plain Greek yogurt	30 mL
¼ cup	packed fresh cilantro leaves, chopped	60 mL

1. Prick sweet potatoes all over with a fork and place on baking sheet. Bake in preheated oven for about 1 hour or until tender.
2. Meanwhile, in a medium saucepan, combine beans, cumin, cayenne (if using) and salsa. Bring to a boil over medium-high heat. Reduce heat and simmer, stirring occasionally, for 5 to 10 minutes to blend the flavors.
3. Transfer sweet potatoes to dinner plates and let cool for 5 minutes. Slit each lengthwise, press to open, then spoon chili into the center. Top each with a dollop of yogurt and a sprinkle of cilantro.

Chickpea Potato Masala

Makes 6 servings

✪ Great for Steps 1, 2, 3 and 4

You might expect to find russet potatoes in a sensually spiced chickpea masala such as this, but I've used yellow-fleshed potatoes, such as Yukon gold, which hold their shape better after a long simmer.

Tips

To toast coconut, preheat oven to 300°F (150°C). Spread coconut in a thin, even layer on an ungreased baking sheet. Bake for 15 to 20 minutes, stirring every 5 minutes, until golden brown and fragrant. Transfer to a plate and let cool completely.

To be sure you're getting enough protein, serve over long-grain brown rice.

Nutrients per serving	
Calories	181
Total fat	6 g
Saturated fat	3 g
Cholesterol	0 mg
Sodium	503 mg
Carbohydrate	28 g
Fiber	6 g
Protein	6 g
Calcium	42 mg
Iron	1.9 mg

- **Blender**

3	cloves garlic	3
1	2-inch (5 cm) piece gingerroot, roughly chopped	1
1 tbsp	mild curry powder	15 mL
1½ tsp	ground cumin	7 mL
1 tsp	garam masala	5 mL
¾ tsp	fine sea salt	3 mL
2 cups	water, divided	500 mL
2 tsp	vegetable oil	10 mL
1½ cups	chopped onions	375 mL
1½ lbs	yellow-fleshed potatoes, peeled and cut into 1-inch (2.5 cm) cubes	750 g
1	can (14 to 19 oz/398 to 540 mL) chickpeas, drained and rinsed	1
1 cup	frozen petite peas, thawed	250 mL
½ cup	packed fresh cilantro leaves, chopped	125 mL
⅓ cup	unsweetened flaked coconut, toasted (see tip, at left)	75 mL

1. In blender, combine garlic, ginger, curry powder, cumin, garam masala, salt and ½ cup (125 mL) of the water; purée until smooth.
2. In a large saucepan, heat oil over medium-high heat. Add onions and cook, stirring occasionally, for 5 to 6 minutes or until softened. Add garlic purée and cook, stirring, for 1 minute or until thickened. Add potatoes, reduce heat and boil gently, stirring often, for about 10 minutes or until potatoes are barely tender.
3. Stir in chickpeas and the remaining water, scraping up any brown bits from bottom of pan. Increase heat to medium-high and bring to a boil. Reduce heat to medium-low, cover and simmer, stirring occasionally, for 16 to 20 minutes or until potatoes are tender. Add peas and simmer for 1 minute. Remove from heat and stir in cilantro and coconut.

▶ Health Note

Early research indicates that curcumin, a pigment found in turmeric, a common ingredient in yellow Indian curry powder and paste, may dissolve Alzheimer plaques and help fight cancer.

Koshari

Makes 6 servings

✪ Great for Steps 2, 3, 4 and 5

Koshari is to Egyptians what chili is to Americans. Made of lentils, rice, tomato sauce and a kick of spice, it is a fast-food staple offered by street vendors in cities such as Cairo. And what a great fast food: combining lentils with brown rice creates a complete protein, perfect for hours of energy. There are many variations of koshari, so tweak to your heart's content to make this basic recipe your own.

Tip

Crumbled feta cheese is similar to the Egyptian cheese *gibna beida*, a traditional topping for koshari.

Nutrients per serving	
Calories	295
Total fat	3 g
Saturated fat	0 g
Cholesterol	0 mg
Sodium	110 mg
Carbohydrate	55 g
Fiber	8 g
Protein	14 g
Calcium	55 mg
Iron	4.2 mg

1 cup	dried brown lentils, rinsed	250 mL
2 cups	water	500 mL
1 cup	whole wheat macaroni	250 mL
3 cups	cooked long-grain brown rice (see page 438)	750 mL
1 tbsp	ground cumin	15 mL
1/4 tsp	cayenne pepper	1 mL
1	jar (26 oz/700 mL) reduced-sodium chunky marinara sauce	1

Suggested Accompaniments

Chopped fresh mint
Chopped fresh parsley
Crumbled feta cheese

1. In a large saucepan, combine lentils and 2 cups (500 mL) water. Bring to a boil over medium-high heat. Reduce heat and simmer, stirring occasionally, for 40 to 45 minutes or until very tender.
2. Meanwhile, in a large pot of boiling water, cook macaroni until al dente. Drain and add to lentils.
3. Stir in rice, cumin, cayenne and marinara sauce; simmer, stirring occasionally, for 10 minutes.
4. Serve in bowls, with any of the suggested accompaniments, as desired.

Variation

For a less traditional but even higher-protein version of koshari, substitute 3 cups (750 mL) cooked quinoa for the brown rice.

Spring Vegetable Tagine

Makes 4 servings

✪ Great for Steps 1, 2, 3 and 4

A hearty yet refined mingling of sweet and spicy, this easy Moroccan-inspired meal is reason enough to keep peas — both protein-rich chickpeas and vitamin-packed spring peas — in the pantry and freezer. Serve with whole wheat couscous or quinoa.

Tip

Other varieties of tender squash, such as yellow crookneck or small pattypan, may be used in place of the zucchini.

Nutrients per serving	
Calories	247
Total fat	5 g
Saturated fat	1 g
Cholesterol	0 mg
Sodium	492 mg
Carbohydrate	42 g
Fiber	9 g
Protein	9 g
Calcium	89 mg
Iron	3.3 mg

1 tbsp	extra virgin olive oil	15 mL
2 cups	chopped onions	500 mL
2 tsp	ground cumin	10 mL
1 tsp	ground cinnamon	5 mL
1 tsp	ground coriander	5 mL
3	small zucchini, trimmed and diced	3
1	can (14 to 15 oz/398 to 425 mL) diced tomatoes, with juice	1
1	can (14 to 19 oz/398 to 540 mL) chickpeas, drained and rinsed	1
1/4 cup	golden or dark raisins	60 mL
1 cup	reduced-sodium ready-to-use vegetable broth	250 mL
1 cup	frozen petite peas, thawed	250 mL
1/2 cup	packed fresh cilantro leaves, chopped, divided	125 mL

1. In a large saucepan, heat oil over medium-high heat. Add onions and cook, stirring, for 6 to 8 minutes or until softened. Add cumin, cinnamon and coriander; cook, stirring, for 30 seconds.
2. Stir in zucchini, tomatoes with juice, chickpeas, raisins and broth. Bring to a boil. Reduce heat to medium-low, cover and simmer, stirring occasionally, for 10 minutes or until zucchini is tender. Stir in peas and half the cilantro; simmer for 1 minute. Serve sprinkled with the remaining cilantro.

Superfood Spotlight

Peas • Whether freshly picked or bought frozen, peas are a rich source of a variety of nutrients. They are particularly high in vitamin C, folate and vitamin B_3, and their very high lutein and zeaxanthin content means that they help protect the eyes from macular degeneration. The B vitamins they contain may help protect the bones from osteoporosis and help to decrease the risk of strokes by keeping levels of the amino acid homocysteine low in the blood. Because they are high in protein, peas are useful for vegetarians. In addition, their high fiber content partly comprises pectin, a jellylike substance that helps lower "bad" blood cholesterol and may help prevent heart and arterial disease.

Okra, Chickpea and Tomato Tagine

Makes 6 servings

✪ Great for Steps 1, 2, 3 and 4

Stir-frying the okra until crisp and brown before simmering it with spiced tomatoes and chickpeas unlocks its succulence. To be sure you're getting enough protein, serve with quinoa or whole wheat couscous.

Tip

An equal amount of fresh flat-leaf (Italian) parsley leaves may be used in place of the cilantro.

Nutrients per serving	
Calories	155
Total fat	4 g
Saturated fat	1 g
Cholesterol	0 mg
Sodium	517 mg
Carbohydrate	24 g
Fiber	6 g
Protein	5 g
Calcium	95 mg
Iron	1.5 mg

4 tsp	extra virgin olive oil, divided	20 mL
1 lb	fresh or thawed frozen okra, trimmed and cut into ½-inch (1 cm) slices	500 g
½ tsp	fine sea salt, divided	2 mL
1	large red bell pepper, finely chopped	1
1¼ cups	chopped onions	300 mL
3	cloves garlic, minced	3
1½ tsp	ground cumin	7 mL
1 tsp	hot smoked paprika	5 mL
1 tsp	ground ginger	5 mL
1	can (14 to 15 oz/398 to 425 mL) diced tomatoes, with juice	1
1	can (14 to 19 oz/398 to 540 mL) chickpeas, drained and rinsed	1
1 cup	packed fresh cilantro leaves, chopped, divided	250 mL
½ cup	reduced-sodium ready-to-use vegetable or chicken broth	125 mL

1. In a large saucepan, heat half the oil over medium-high heat. Add okra and half the salt; cook, stirring, for 12 to 15 minutes or until browned. Transfer to a plate.
2. In the same pan, heat the remaining oil over medium-high heat. Add red pepper and onions; cook, stirring, for 6 to 8 minutes or until softened. Add garlic, cumin, paprika, ginger and the remaining salt; cook, stirring, for 30 seconds.
3. Stir in tomatoes with juice, chickpeas, half the cilantro and broth. Bring to a boil. Reduce heat to medium-low, cover, leaving lid ajar, and simmer, stirring once or twice, for 10 minutes. Return okra to the pan and simmer for 3 minutes to heat through and blend the flavors. Serve sprinkled with the remaining cilantro.

Spicy Punjabi Chickpeas with Mint Radish Raita

Makes 4 servings

✪ Great for Steps 1, 2, 3 and 4

This classic Punjabi dish, called masaledar chholay, *is a typical offering for Sunday lunch. A spoonful of tangy raita on top amplifies the tug-of-war between mild and bold in the dish. Serve it with brown basmati rice.*

Tip

For a milder raita, use an equal amount of chopped seeded cucumber in place of the radishes.

Nutrients per serving	
Calories	193
Total fat	4 g
Saturated fat	0 g
Cholesterol	0 mg
Sodium	561 mg
Carbohydrate	30 g
Fiber	6 g
Protein	10 g
Calcium	104 mg
Iron	2.4 mg

- **Blender**

4	cloves garlic	4
1	jalapeño pepper, seeded and roughly chopped	1
1	1-inch (2.5 cm) piece gingerroot, roughly chopped	1
1 cup	water	250 mL
2 tsp	vegetable oil	10 mL
1½ cups	chopped onions	375 mL
½ tsp	fine sea salt, divided	2 mL
1 tbsp	ground cumin	15 mL
1½ tsp	ground coriander	7 mL
1	can (14 to 15 oz/398 to 425 mL) diced tomatoes, with juice	1
1	can (14 to 19 oz/398 to 540 mL) chickpeas, drained and rinsed	1
¾ cup	chopped red radishes	175 mL
¼ cup	packed fresh mint leaves, chopped	60 mL
¾ cup	nonfat plain Greek yogurt	175 mL
2 tsp	freshly squeezed lime juice	10 mL

1. In blender, combine garlic, jalapeño, ginger and water; purée until smooth.
2. In a large skillet, heat oil over medium-high heat. Add onions and half the salt; cook, stirring, for 5 to 6 minutes or until softened. Add cumin and coriander; cook, stirring, for 30 seconds.
3. Stir in garlic purée, tomatoes with juice and chickpeas. Reduce heat and simmer, stirring occasionally, for 8 to 10 minutes or until thickened.
4. In a small bowl, combine radishes, mint, the remaining salt, yogurt and lime juice. Serve alongside the chickpea mixture.

Grilled Eggplant with Chickpeas and Cashew Yogurt Sauce

Makes 4 servings

✪ Great for Steps 1, 2, 3 and 4

This beautifully balanced dish draws its inspiration from the Punjabi region of India, where it is common to serve main dishes with a savory nut and yogurt sauce.

Tip

Look for roasted cashews lightly seasoned with sea salt.

Nutrients per serving	
Calories	298
Total fat	8 g
Saturated fat	1 g
Cholesterol	1 mg
Sodium	507 mg
Carbohydrate	49 g
Fiber	15 g
Protein	13 g
Calcium	159 mg
Iron	2.9 mg

- **Preheat barbecue grill to medium-high**

2 tsp	extra virgin olive oil	10 mL
1½ cups	chopped onions	375 mL
2½ tsp	garam masala	12 mL
½ tsp	fine sea salt, divided	2 mL
1	can (14 to 15 oz/398 to 425 mL) diced tomatoes, with juice	1
1	can (14 to 19 oz/398 to 540 mL) chickpeas, drained and rinsed	1
⅓ cup	water	75 mL
1 tbsp	freshly squeezed lemon juice	15 mL
2	large eggplants, trimmed and cut crosswise into ½-inch (1 cm) thick slices	2
	Nonstick cooking spray (preferably olive oil)	
2	cloves garlic, mashed (see tip, page 121)	2
⅓ cup	packed fresh mint leaves, chopped	75 mL
¼ cup	lightly salted roasted cashews, finely chopped	60 mL
1 cup	nonfat plain yogurt	250 mL

1. In a large skillet, heat oil over medium-high heat. Add onions and cook, stirring, for 5 to 6 minutes or until softened. Add garam masala and half the salt; cook, stirring, for 30 seconds.
2. Stir in tomatoes with juice, chickpeas and water. Bring to a boil. Reduce heat to medium-low, cover and simmer, stirring occasionally, for 10 minutes. Stir in lemon juice.
3. Meanwhile, spray eggplant slices with cooking spray and sprinkle with the remaining salt. Place on preheated barbecue and grill, turning once, for 4 to 5 minutes per side or until tender and deep golden brown on both sides.
4. In a small bowl, combine garlic, mint, cashews and yogurt.
5. Arrange grilled eggplant slices on a warm platter and top with chickpea mixture. Drizzle with some of the cashew yogurt sauce and serve the remainder alongside.

Butternut Squash Farro with Chickpeas and Cranberries

Makes 6 servings

✪ Great for Steps 1, 2, 3, 4 and 5

Who says main dishes have to be conventional? Here, meat moves aside to put nutty farro, toothsome chickpeas and sweet butternut squash front and center. A lemony yogurt pulls it all together. While this combination of flavors and textures is decidedly brand new, mixing different grains, beans and reduced-fat dairy products is a longstanding option for creating complete proteins in vegetarian meals.

Tip

Dried currants, raisins or dried cherries may be used in place of the cranberries.

Nutrients per serving	
Calories	340
Total fat	5 g
Saturated fat	1 g
Cholesterol	1 mg
Sodium	533 mg
Carbohydrate	67 g
Fiber	14 g
Protein	11 g
Calcium	117 mg
Iron	2.5 mg

- **Preheat oven to 400°F (200°C)**
- **Large rimmed baking sheet, lined with foil and sprayed with nonstick cooking spray (preferably olive oil)**

1 cup	nonfat plain yogurt	250 mL
1 tbsp	freshly squeezed lemon juice	15 mL
1	large red onion, cut into 1-inch (2.5 cm) chunks	1
4 cups	cubed butternut squash (½-inch/1 cm cubes)	1 L
4 tsp	extra virgin olive oil, divided	20 mL
1½ cups	semi-pearled farro	375 mL
1	can (14 to 19 oz/398 to 540 mL) chickpeas, drained and rinsed	1
3	cloves garlic, minced	3
2 tsp	ground cumin	10 mL
1 tsp	fine sea salt	5 mL
½ cup	packed fresh cilantro leaves, chopped	125 mL
¼ cup	dried cranberries, chopped	60 mL

1. In a small bowl, whisk together yogurt and lemon juice. Cover and refrigerate until ready to use.
2. On prepared baking sheet, toss red onion and squash with half the oil. Spread out in a single layer. Roast in preheated oven for 20 to 25 minutes, stirring once or twice, until vegetables are golden brown and tender.
3. Meanwhile, in a large pot of boiling water, cook farro for 25 to 30 minutes or until al dente. Drain well.
4. In the same pot, heat the remaining oil over medium-high heat. Add chickpeas and cook, stirring, for 5 minutes. Add garlic, cumin and salt; cook, stirring, for 1 minute. Add roasted vegetables and cooked farro; cook, stirring, for 2 minutes or until heated through. Serve topped with cilantro, cranberries and lemon yogurt.

White Bean Bajane with Thyme Barley

Makes 6 servings

✪ Great for Steps 1, 2, 3, 4 and 5

Bajane is a Provençal term for the midday meal, but you are more likely to make this satisfying dish for a weeknight repast.

Tip

For the white beans, you could use Great Northern beans, cannellini (white kidney) beans or white pea (navy) beans.

1 cup	pearl barley	250 mL
3 tsp	dried thyme, divided	15 mL
3¾ cups	reduced-sodium ready-to-use vegetable broth, divided	925 mL
2 tsp	extra virgin olive oil	10 mL
2½ cups	sliced fennel bulb, fronds reserved (about 1 large)	625 mL
2 cups	chopped onions	500 mL
4	cloves garlic, minced	4
½ tsp	fine sea salt	2 mL
¼ tsp	freshly cracked black pepper	1 mL
1	can (14 to 19 oz/398 to 540 mL) white beans, drained and rinsed	1
8 cups	packed baby spinach (about 8 oz/250 g)	2 L
1 cup	drained roasted red bell peppers, coarsely chopped	250 mL
2 tsp	finely grated lemon zest	10 mL
1 tbsp	freshly squeezed lemon juice	15 mL

1. In a medium saucepan, combine barley, 1 tsp (5 mL) of the thyme and 2¾ cups (675 mL) of the broth. Bring to a boil over high heat. Reduce heat to medium-low, cover and simmer for 35 to 40 minutes or until barley is tender and liquid is absorbed.
2. Meanwhile, in a large saucepan, heat oil over medium-high heat. Add sliced fennel and onions; cook, stirring, for 6 to 8 minutes or until softened. Add garlic, the remaining thyme, salt and pepper; cook, stirring, for 30 seconds.
3. Stir the remaining broth into the fennel mixture. Bring to a boil. Add beans, spinach, roasted peppers, lemon zest and lemon juice. Reduce heat and simmer, stirring once or twice, for 5 minutes or until spinach is wilted and flavors are blended.
4. Chop enough of the fennel fronds to measure 2 tbsp (30 mL).
5. Divide barley among bowls, top with bean mixture and sprinkle with fennel fronds.

Nutrients per serving	
Calories	254
Total fat	2 g
Saturated fat	0 g
Cholesterol	0 mg
Sodium	542 mg
Carbohydrate	51 g
Fiber	13 g
Protein	10 g
Calcium	102 mg
Iron	3.1 mg

Speedy Southwest Black Bean and Quinoa Skillet

Makes 4 servings

✪ Great for Steps 2, 3, 4 and 5

This colorful one-pot main dish returns quinoa to its Central American roots in a matter of minutes.

1 cup	quinoa, rinsed	250 mL
1 tsp	ground cumin	5 mL
¼ tsp	fine sea salt	1 mL
2 cups	water	500 mL
1¼ cups	chipotle salsa, divided	300 mL
1	can (14 to 19 oz/398 to 540 mL) black beans, drained and rinsed	1
1 cup	frozen corn kernels	250 mL
½ cup	chopped green onions	125 mL
¼ cup	packed fresh cilantro leaves, chopped	60 mL

Suggested Accompaniments

Warm corn tortillas or whole wheat tortillas

Crumbled queso fresco

Roasted pumpkin seeds

1. In a large skillet, combine quinoa, cumin, salt, water and ½ cup (125 mL) of the salsa. Bring to a boil over high heat. Reduce heat to medium-low, cover and simmer, stirring once or twice, for 11 to 13 minutes or until most (but not all) of the liquid is absorbed.
2. Stir in beans, corn and green onions. Cover and simmer, without stirring, for 7 to 10 minutes or until liquid is absorbed. Remove from heat and stir in cilantro and the remaining salsa. Serve with any of the suggested accompaniments, as desired.

Superfood Spotlight

Black Beans • Shiny, oval black beans are an inexpensive addition to the diet. Nutritionally, they are high in the indigestible portion of the plant known as insoluble fiber, which can reduce cholesterol. Their extremely high magnesium content means they are an excellent food for people at risk of developing or suffering from heart disease — an optimum intake of magnesium is linked with a reduced risk of various heart problems. Black beans are also rich in antioxidant compounds called anthocyanins, flavonoids that can help prevent cancer and blood clots. The darker the bean's seed coat, the higher its level of antioxidant activity. In addition, black beans are an excellent source of minerals and folate.

Nutrients per serving	
Calories	285
Total fat	3 g
Saturated fat	0 g
Cholesterol	0 mg
Sodium	520 mg
Carbohydrate	51 g
Fiber	8 g
Protein	12 g
Calcium	70 mg
Iron	3.9 mg

Sweet Potato and Spinach Curry with Quinoa

Makes 4 servings

✪ Great for Steps 1, 2, 3, 4 and 5

If you've never had sweet potatoes in a curry dish before, you'll be surprised by how well they take to bold spices. Creamy coconut milk and earthy quinoa stealthily round out the interplay of sweet and umami that will have you savoring every last bite.

1 cup	quinoa, rinsed	250 mL
$3\frac{1}{2}$ cups	water, divided	875 mL
2 tsp	vegetable oil	10 mL
1	large onion, thinly sliced	1
2 tbsp	mild curry powder	30 mL
$\frac{1}{8}$ tsp	cayenne pepper (optional)	0.5 mL
2 tsp	reduced-sodium tamari or soy sauce	10 mL
2 lbs	sweet potatoes, peeled and cut into 1-inch (2.5 cm) chunks	1 kg
1	can (14 oz/398 mL) light coconut milk	1
8 cups	packed baby spinach (about 8 oz/250 g)	2 L
1 tbsp	freshly squeezed lime juice	15 mL

1. In a medium saucepan, combine quinoa and 2 cups (500 mL) of the water. Bring to a boil over medium-high heat. Reduce heat to low, cover and simmer for 15 to 18 minutes or until water is absorbed.
2. Meanwhile, in a large saucepan, heat oil over medium-high heat. Add onion and cook, stirring, for 6 to 8 minutes or until softened. Add curry powder, cayenne (if using) and tamari; cook, stirring, for 30 seconds.
3. Stir in sweet potatoes and the remaining water. Bring to a boil. Reduce heat and boil for 12 minutes. Add coconut milk, reduce heat and simmer, stirring occasionally, for 3 to 7 minutes or until sweet potatoes are tender. Stir in spinach and lime juice; simmer for 1 minute or until spinach is wilted. Serve with quinoa.

Nutrients per serving	
Calories	446
Total fat	12 g
Saturated fat	7 g
Cholesterol	0 mg
Sodium	251 mg
Carbohydrate	76 g
Fiber	13 g
Protein	12 g
Calcium	143 mg
Iron	5.7 mg

Delicata Squash with Quinoa Stuffing

Makes 4 servings

✪ Great for Steps 1, 2, 3, 4 and 5

Delicata squash at its seasonal best lends subtle sweetness and rich, mellow flavor to a protein-, vitamin- and antioxidant-rich stuffing of quinoa, peppery arugula and tart cranberries.

Tip

Acorn squash may be used in place of the delicata squash.

Nutrients per serving	
Calories	300
Total fat	8 g
Saturated fat	1 g
Cholesterol	0 mg
Sodium	489 mg
Carbohydrate	48 g
Fiber	6 g
Protein	14 g
Calcium	116 mg
Iron	4.5 mg

- **Preheat oven to 350°F (180°C)**
- **Large rimmed baking sheet**

2	delicata squash (each about 1 lb/500 g), halved lengthwise and seeded	2
	Nonstick cooking spray (preferably olive oil)	
3/4 tsp	fine sea salt, divided	3 mL
2 cups	water	500 mL
1 cup	quinoa, rinsed	250 mL
1/3 cup	dried cranberries, chopped	75 mL
1/4 tsp	freshly cracked black pepper	1 mL
1 tbsp	white wine vinegar	15 mL
2 tsp	liquid honey or agave nectar	10 mL
2 cups	packed arugula, roughly chopped	500 mL
1/2 cup	packed fresh mint leaves, chopped	125 mL
1/4 cup	lightly salted roasted almonds, chopped (optional)	60 mL

1. Lightly spray cut sides of squash with cooking spray. Sprinkle with 1/4 tsp (1 mL) of the salt. Place cut side down on baking sheet. Bake in preheated oven for 40 to 45 minutes or until tender.
2. Meanwhile, in a medium saucepan, combine water and quinoa. Bring to a boil over medium-high heat. Reduce heat to low, cover and simmer for 10 minutes. Stir in cranberries, cover and simmer for 5 to 8 minutes or until water is absorbed.
3. In a large bowl, whisk together the remaining salt, pepper, vinegar and honey. Add quinoa mixture, arugula and mint, gently tossing to combine.
4. Fill squash cavities with quinoa mixture. Sprinkle with almonds, if desired.

Quinoa-Stuffed Poblano Chiles

Makes 4 servings

✪ Great for Steps 1, 2, 3, 4 and 5

In Central America, poblanos are typically stuffed with rice, meat or a combination of the two. Here, quinoa substitutes, which is perfectly fitting (as well as scrumptious), given its Andean pedigree.

Variations

For a thicker sauce, use canned tomato purée in place of the tomato juice.

An equal amount of another grain, such as long-grain brown rice, millet, bulgur or barley, may be used in place of the quinoa (see Cooking Whole Grains, page 438).

Nutrients per serving	
Calories	291
Total fat	9 g
Saturated fat	4 g
Cholesterol	14 mg
Sodium	585 mg
Carbohydrate	36 g
Fiber	5 g
Protein	13 g
Calcium	96 mg
Iron	4.3 mg

- **Preheat oven to 350°F (180°C)**
- **9-inch (23 cm) square glass baking dish or metal baking pan**

3/4 cup	quinoa, rinsed	175 mL
1 1/2 cups	water	375 mL
2 tsp	vegetable oil	10 mL
4	cloves garlic, minced	4
1	small red bell pepper, chopped	1
1 cup	chopped green onions	250 mL
2 tsp	minced seeded jalapeño pepper	10 mL
1 1/2 tsp	ground cumin	7 mL
3/4 tsp	fine sea salt	3 mL
1/2 cup	packed fresh cilantro leaves, chopped	125 mL
2 tbsp	freshly squeezed lime juice	30 mL
4	poblano chile peppers, cut in half lengthwise and seeded	4
2 cups	reduced-sodium tomato juice	500 mL
4 oz	soft goat cheese, crumbled	125 g

1. In a medium saucepan, combine quinoa and water. Bring to a boil over medium-high heat. Reduce heat to low, cover and simmer for 15 to 18 minutes or until water is absorbed.
2. Meanwhile, in a large skillet, heat oil over medium-high heat. Add garlic, red pepper, green onions, jalapeño, cumin and salt; cook, stirring, for 5 to 6 minutes or until pepper is slightly softened. Remove from heat and stir in cooked quinoa, cilantro and lime juice.
3. Place poblano halves, cut side up, in baking dish. Spoon about 1/3 cup (75 mL) quinoa mixture into each half. Pour tomato juice into dish (do not pour on top of poblanos).
4. Cover and bake in preheated oven for 20 minutes. Sprinkle poblanos with goat cheese. Bake, uncovered, for 10 to 14 minutes or until tomato juice is bubbling and poblanos are softened. Serve, spooning tomato juice over poblanos.

Mushroom- and Bulgur-Stuffed Peppers

Makes 6 servings

✪ Great for Steps 1, 2, 4 and 5

You can't go wrong with stuffed peppers for supper, especially when they're enlivened with fire-roasted tomatoes, mushrooms and Parmesan cheese. Bulgur becomes irresistible when it soaks up the flavors from the pepper shells as well as the herbs and sautéed mushrooms in the stuffing.

Tip

The carotenes in bell peppers are made more available to the body if the peppers are cooked and eaten with a little oil. If you eat peppers raw in a salad, drizzle them with some olive oil to help absorption.

Nutrients per serving	
Calories	181
Total fat	3 g
Saturated fat	1 g
Cholesterol	7 mg
Sodium	384 mg
Carbohydrate	34 g
Fiber	7 g
Protein	9 g
Calcium	121 mg
Iron	2.5 mg

- **Preheat oven to 350°F (180°C)**
- **13- by 9-inch (33 by 23 cm) glass baking dish**

1 cup	fine or medium bulgur	250 mL
1 cup	boiling water	250 mL
6	red or green bell peppers	6
1 tsp	extra virgin olive oil	5 mL
1 lb	cremini or button mushrooms, chopped	500 g
1 cup	packed fresh flat-leaf (Italian) parsley leaves, chopped	250 mL
2 tsp	dried oregano	10 mL
1	can (14 to 15 oz/398 to 425 mL) fire-roasted tomatoes, with juice	1
1/4 tsp	fine sea salt	1 mL
1/4 cup	freshly grated Parmesan cheese	60 mL

1. In a medium bowl, combine bulgur and boiling water. Let stand for about 30 minutes or until water is absorbed.
2. Cut tops off bell peppers, setting the tops aside. Pull out and discard seeds and membranes.
3. In a large skillet, heat oil over medium-high heat. Add mushrooms and cook, stirring, for 4 to 5 minutes or until tender. Add parsley and oregano; cook, stirring, for 1 minute. Add cooked bulgur, tomatoes with juice and salt; cook, stirring, for 3 minutes.
4. Spoon about 3/4 cup (175 mL) of the bulgur mixture into each bell pepper. Top each with 2 tsp (10 mL) cheese. Place stuffed peppers in baking dish, tucking tops beside peppers.
5. Bake in preheated oven for 25 to 30 minutes or until peppers are soft. Serve, replacing pepper tops on each stuffed pepper.

Variation

An equal amount of another grain, such as long-grain brown rice, millet, quinoa or barley, may be used in place of the bulgur (see Cooking Whole Grains, page 438).

Healthy Know-How

Macronutrients 101

Nutrients are substances found in food that the body needs for growth, metabolism and other functions. Macronutrients are nutrients that provide calories or energy. "Macro" means large, and these nutrients are needed in large amounts. There are three macronutrients: carbohydrate, protein and fat. The amount of calories that each of these provides varies: carbohydrate provides 4 calories per gram; protein provides 4 calories per gram; fat provides 9 calories per gram.

So, if the Nutrition Facts label on a product says 12 g of carbohydrate, 0 g of fat and 0 g of protein per serving, you know the food has about 48 calories per serving (12 g of carbohydrate multiplied by 4 calories per gram = 48 calories).

Besides carbohydrate, protein and fat, the only other substance that provides calories is alcohol. Alcohol provides 7 calories per gram. Alcohol, however, is not a macronutrient because we do not need it for survival.

Thai Pumpkin and Brown Rice Risotto

Makes 4 servings

✪ Great for Steps 2, 4 and 5

This riff on risotto uses brown rice and adds exotic flair. To up the protein, stir in 2 cups (500 mL) rinsed drained canned chickpeas with the pumpkin.

Nutrients per serving	
Calories	177
Total fat	8 g
Saturated fat	3 g
Cholesterol	1 mg
Sodium	98 mg
Carbohydrate	25 g
Fiber	3 g
Protein	4 g
Calcium	28 mg
Iron	1.5 mg

1⅔ cups	reduced-sodium vegetable or chicken broth	400 mL
½ cup	light coconut milk	125 mL
1 tbsp	brown rice syrup or liquid honey	15 mL
2 tbsp	Thai red or green curry paste	30 mL
1 cup	brown basmati rice or other long-grain brown rice	250 mL
½ cup	packed fresh cilantro leaves, chopped, divided	125 mL
¾ cup	pumpkin purée (not pie filling)	175 mL
2 tbsp	freshly squeezed lime juice	30 mL
¼ cup	lightly salted roasted cashews, chopped	60 mL

1. In a medium saucepan, whisk together broth, coconut milk, brown rice syrup and curry paste. Bring to a boil over medium-high heat. Stir in rice. Reduce heat to low, cover and simmer for 45 to 50 minutes or until liquid is absorbed.
2. Stir in half the cilantro, pumpkin and lime juice; simmer, uncovered, stirring occasionally, for 1 to 2 minutes or until heated through. Serve sprinkled with cashews and the remaining cilantro.

Barley Risotto with Asparagus and Lemon

Makes 4 servings

✪ Great for Steps 1, 2, 4 and 5

Here, the bright flavors of lemon, basil and asparagus play against the earthiness of barley and onions.

2 tsp	extra virgin olive oil	10 mL
1 cup	finely chopped onion	250 mL
1 cup	pearl barley	250 mL
½ cup	dry white wine	125 mL
4 cups	reduced-sodium ready-to-use vegetable broth, divided	1 L
1 lb	asparagus, trimmed and cut into 1-inch (2.5 cm) pieces	500 g
1 cup	frozen petite peas, thawed	250 mL
½ cup	packed fresh basil leaves, chopped, divided	125 mL
¼ cup	freshly grated Parmesan cheese	60 mL
1 tsp	finely grated lemon zest	5 mL
2 tbsp	freshly squeezed lemon juice	30 mL

1. In a large saucepan, heat oil over medium-high heat. Add onion and barley; cook, stirring, for 5 to 6 minutes or until onion is softened. Add wine and cook, stirring, for 3 to 5 minutes or until liquid is evaporated.
2. Stir in 2 cups (500 mL) of the broth. Bring to a boil, stirring often. Reduce heat and simmer, stirring occasionally, for about 20 minutes or until liquid is absorbed. Add the remaining broth and simmer, stirring occasionally, for about 20 minutes or until barley is tender and mixture is creamy (there should still be some liquid).
3. Stir in asparagus and simmer, stirring occasionally, for 4 to 5 minutes or until tender. Stir in peas, half the basil, cheese, lemon zest and lemon juice; simmer for 1 minute or until heated through. Serve sprinkled with the remaining basil.

Superfood Spotlight

Barley • Barley is a grain with a rich, slightly nutty flavor and a chewy texture that is akin to al dente pasta. It provides a very high level of fiber, including soluble fiber, as well as a fiber-like compound called lignan, which may protect against breast cancer, other hormone-dependent cancers and heart disease. It also has very high levels of selenium, which may significantly reduce the risk of a range of cancers, most notably colon cancer. Unusually for a grain, barley also contains lutein and zeaxanthin, which help to protect eyesight and eye health.

Nutrients per serving	
Calories	345
Total fat	6 g
Saturated fat	2 g
Cholesterol	10 mg
Sodium	430 mg
Carbohydrate	57 g
Fiber	15 g
Protein	12 g
Calcium	183 mg
Iron	2.8 mg

Farro Risotto with Swiss Chard and Parmesan

Makes 4 servings

✪ Great for Steps 1, 2, 4 and 5

This farro risotto ("farrotto") has all of the richness and satisfaction you'd expect from traditional risotto, but is so easy and good for you that you needn't wait for a special occasion to savor it.

1	large bunch Swiss chard	1
4 tsp	extra virgin olive oil, divided	20 mL
4	cloves garlic, minced	4
1/2 tsp	fine sea salt	2 mL
1/4 tsp	freshly ground black pepper	1 mL
2 cups	chopped onions	500 mL
1	can (14 to 15 oz/398 to 425 mL) diced tomatoes, with juice	1
1 cup	semi-pearled farro	250 mL
2 tsp	dried Italian seasoning	10 mL
2 cups	reduced-sodium ready-to-use vegetable broth	500 mL
1/2 cup	freshly grated Parmesan cheese	125 mL

1. Trim off tough stems from Swiss chard and chop tender stems. Thinly slice leaves crosswise. You should have about 5 cups (1.25 L) leaves and tender stems.
2. In a large saucepan, heat half the oil over medium-high heat. Add Swiss chard and cook, stirring, for 3 to 4 minutes or until just wilted. Add garlic, salt and pepper; cook, stirring, for 30 seconds. Transfer to a bowl.
3. In the same pan, heat the remaining oil over medium-high heat. Add onions and cook, stirring, for 6 to 8 minutes or until softened.
4. Stir in tomatoes with juice, farro, Italian seasoning and broth. Bring to a boil. Reduce heat and simmer, stirring often, for 25 to 30 minutes or until liquid is nearly absorbed. Remove from heat and stir in Swiss chard mixture and cheese.

Nutrients per serving	
Calories	333
Total fat	9 g
Saturated fat	3 g
Cholesterol	20 mg
Sodium	550 mg
Carbohydrate	55 g
Fiber	11 g
Protein	11 g
Calcium	270 mg
Iron	2.4 mg

Carrot and Feta Fritters with Minted Yogurt Sauce

Makes 4 servings

✪ Great for Steps 1, 2, 3, 4 and 5

You'll be thinking about these zingy fritters long after you've forked up the last bite. A combination of sweet carrots, tangy feta and the exotic aroma of garam masala, paired with a cooling minted yogurt sauce that cuts right through the richness, these irresistible fritters are vegetarian fare reinvented.

Tip

Other tender greens, such as arugula, watercress sprigs or spinach may be used in place of the mesclun.

Nutrients per serving	
Calories	239
Total fat	9 g
Saturated fat	4 g
Cholesterol	108 mg
Sodium	420 mg
Carbohydrate	25 g
Fiber	5 g
Protein	11 g
Calcium	226 mg
Iron	3.7 mg

- **Preheat oven to 200°F (100°C)**
- **Small rimmed baking sheet**

½ cup	packed fresh mint leaves, chopped	125 mL
¾ tsp	fine sea salt, divided	3 mL
½ cup	nonfat plain yogurt	125 mL
½ cup	whole wheat pastry flour	125 mL
1 tsp	garam masala	5 mL
¼ tsp	baking powder	1 mL
2	large eggs	2
2 cups	finely shredded carrots	500 mL
1 cup	chopped green onions	250 mL
½ cup	crumbled feta cheese	125 mL
2 tbsp	water	30 mL
4 tsp	vegetable oil, divided	20 mL
8 cups	mesclun (mixed baby lettuce)	2 L

1. In a small bowl, whisk together mint, a pinch of the salt and yogurt. Refrigerate until ready to use.
2. In a large bowl, whisk together flour, garam masala, baking powder and the remaining salt. Whisk in eggs, carrots, green onions, cheese and water.
3. In a large skillet, heat half the oil over medium-high heat. Scoop batter into the pan by ¼ cup (60 mL) dollops, flattening them slightly with the back of a spoon. Cook, turning once, for 2 to 3 minutes per side or until golden brown on both sides and hot in the center. Transfer to baking sheet and keep warm in preheated oven. Repeat with the remaining oil and batter, adjusting heat as necessary between batches.
4. Divide mesclun among four plates and top with fritters. Serve with minted yogurt sauce.

Quinoa Vegetable Cakes

Makes 4 servings

✪ Great for Steps 1, 2, 3, 4 and 5

As easy to prepare as pancakes, but with a flavor all their own, these delicious little cakes get a touch of Greece from garlic, yogurt and dill.

Tip

To prepare 3 cups (750 mL) cooked quinoa, combine 1 cup (250 mL) quinoa and 2 cups (500 mL) water in a medium saucepan. Bring to a boil over medium-high heat. Reduce heat to low, cover and simmer for 15 to 18 minutes or until water is absorbed. Let cool completely.

Nutrients per serving	
Calories	208
Total fat	3 g
Saturated fat	1 g
Cholesterol	46 mg
Sodium	389 mg
Carbohydrate	36 g
Fiber	6 g
Protein	12 g
Calcium	240 mg
Iron	5.3 mg

- **Preheat oven to 400°F (200°C)**
- **Large rimmed baking sheet, sprayed with nonstick cooking spray (preferably olive oil)**

2	cloves garlic, minced	2
1	package (10 oz/300 g) frozen chopped spinach, thawed and squeezed dry	1
3 cups	cooked quinoa (see tip, at left), cooled	750 mL
3⁄4 cup	finely shredded carrots	175 mL
1⁄2 cup	finely chopped green onions	125 mL
1⁄4 cup	whole wheat flour	60 mL
1 tbsp	dried Italian seasoning	15 mL
1 tsp	baking powder	5 mL
1⁄2 tsp	fine sea salt	2 mL
1⁄2 tsp	freshly ground black pepper	2 mL
1	large egg, lightly beaten	1
1 tbsp	chopped fresh dill	15 mL
1 cup	nonfat plain yogurt	250 mL
1 tbsp	freshly squeezed lemon juice	15 mL

1. In a large bowl, combine garlic, spinach, quinoa, carrots, green onions, flour, Italian seasoning, baking powder, salt, pepper and egg.
2. Scoop 8 equal mounds of quinoa mixture onto prepared baking sheet. Flatten to 1⁄2-inch (1 cm) thickness with a spatula.
3. Bake in preheated oven for 15 minutes. Turn cakes over and bake for 8 to 12 minutes or until golden brown and hot in the center.
4. In a small bowl, whisk together dill, yogurt and lemon juice.
5. Serve warm quinoa cakes with yogurt sauce drizzled on top or served alongside.

Cashew Oat Cakes with Spicy Tomato Sauce

Makes 4 servings

✪ Great for Steps 1, 2, 3, 4 and 5

Chopped cashews give these meaty oat cakes a rich, nutty flavor. Roasted cashews deliver the most flavor, but raw cashews work well too, so use whichever you prefer.

Tip

Look for roasted cashews lightly seasoned with sea salt.

Nutrients per serving	
Calories	350
Total fat	14 g
Saturated fat	3 g
Cholesterol	100 mg
Sodium	402 mg
Carbohydrate	45 g
Fiber	6 g
Protein	14 g
Calcium	205 mg
Iron	4.2 mg

- **Preheat oven to 200°F (100°C)**
- **Small rimmed baking sheet**

2 cups	skim milk or plain almond milk	500 mL
1¾ cups	large-flake (old-fashioned) rolled oats	425 mL
¾ tsp	fine sea salt	3 mL
¼ tsp	freshly cracked black pepper	1 mL
4 tsp	extra virgin olive oil, divided	20 mL
1¼ cups	chopped onions	300 mL
1 cup	finely shredded carrots	250 mL
3 tbsp	lightly salted roasted cashews, chopped	45 mL
½ cup	packed fresh flat-leaf (Italian) parsley leaves, chopped	125 mL
2	large eggs, lightly beaten	2
1½ cups	reduced-sodium marinara sauce	375 mL
¼ tsp	hot pepper flakes	1 mL

1. In a medium saucepan, bring milk to a boil over medium-high heat. Stir in oats, salt and pepper. Remove from heat and let stand, covered, for 15 minutes.
2. In a large skillet, heat 2 tsp (10 mL) of the oil over medium-high heat. Add onions and cook, stirring, for 5 to 6 minutes or until softened. Add carrots and cashews; cook, stirring, for 2 to 3 minutes or until carrot is softened. Transfer to a large bowl and stir in oat mixture, parsley and eggs. Wipe skillet clean.
3. In a small saucepan, combine marinara sauce and hot pepper flakes. Warm over low heat, stirring often, until heated through. Cover and keep warm.
4. Meanwhile, shape oat mixture into 8 equal balls. In the same skillet, heat 1 tsp (5 mL) of the oil over medium heat. Place 4 oat balls in skillet and flatten with a spatula to about ½-inch (1 cm) thickness. Cook, turning once, for 3 to 5 minutes per side or until golden brown on both sides and hot in the center. Transfer to baking sheet and keep warm in preheated oven. Repeat with the remaining oil and oat balls, adjusting heat between batches as necessary. Serve oat cakes with warm sauce.

Lentil Patties with Herbed Yogurt Sauce

Makes 6 servings

✪ Great for Steps 1, 2, 3, 4 and 5

Earthy red lentils, sweet carrots and vibrant cumin are the stars of these crispy-creamy patties. A drizzle of lemony herbed yogurt heightens the wow factor.

Tips

I recommend red lentils for this recipe because they cook so quickly, but if green or brown lentils are what's on hand, use either instead. Just be sure to cook them until very tender (see Cooking Legumes, page 436).

The patties can be prepared through step 4, covered and refrigerated overnight.

Nutrients per serving	
Calories	306
Total fat	5 g
Saturated fat	1 g
Cholesterol	61 mg
Sodium	379 mg
Carbohydrate	47 g
Fiber	10 g
Protein	20 g
Calcium	138 mg
Iron	4.7 mg

- **Large rimmed baking sheet, lined with foil and sprayed with nonstick cooking spray**

1½ cups	dried red lentils, rinsed	375 mL
4 cups	water	1 L
1 tbsp	extra virgin olive oil	15 mL
1 cup	finely chopped onion	250 mL
1½ cups	finely shredded carrots	375 mL
3	cloves garlic, minced	3
1½ tsp	ground cumin	7 mL
¾ tsp	fine sea salt	3 mL
⅛ tsp	cayenne pepper	0.5 mL
¾ cup	fresh whole wheat bread crumbs	175 mL
¾ cup	packed fresh flat-leaf (Italian) parsley leaves, divided	175 mL
2	large eggs, lightly beaten	2
	Nonstick cooking spray	
1 cup	nonfat plain yogurt	250 mL
1 tbsp	freshly squeezed lemon juice	15 mL
8 cups	mesclun (mixed baby lettuce)	2 L

1. In a medium saucepan, combine lentils and water. Bring to a boil over medium-high heat. Reduce heat and simmer for about 22 minutes or until very tender but not mushy. Drain and let cool completely.
2. Preheat broiler, with rack set 4 to 6 inches (10 to 15 cm) from the heat source.
3. In a large skillet, heat oil over medium-high heat. Add onion and cook, stirring, for 5 to 6 minutes or until softened. Add carrots and cook, stirring, for 2 to 3 minutes or until softened. Add garlic, cumin, salt and cayenne; cook, stirring, for 30 seconds.
4. In a large bowl, combine cooled lentils, onion mixture, bread crumbs, half the parsley and eggs. Shape into 12 balls. Place balls on prepared baking sheet and flatten with a spatula to about ½-inch (1 cm) thickness. Spray tops with cooking spray.
5. Broil patties, turning once, for 3 to 4 minutes per side or until golden brown on both sides and hot in the center.
6. Meanwhile, in a small bowl, whisk together the remaining parsley, yogurt and lemon juice.
7. Divide mesclun among four plates and top with lentil patties. Drizzle with yogurt sauce.

Healthy Know-How

Top 10 Suggestions for Healthy Eating on a Budget

1. **Eat less meat.** Shifting meat away from the center of the plate, or eating it only once or twice a week, is a quick way to cut costs. You can also make soups, stews, chilis and casseroles that extend smaller amounts of meat with whole grains, beans and vegetables.
2. **Emphasize grains and legumes.** Grains and legumes are inexpensive and pack a nutritional power punch. Plus, they give meals a heft that most people rely on meat for. When time is especially short, canned beans and frozen brown rice can bring a meal together in minutes.
3. **Buy in bulk.** Buying food in bulk can save a lot of money. You can purchase grains, pastas, dried fruits, nuts, flours, spices and herbs in the bulk aisles of grocery and natural foods stores, choosing an amount of each that works for your household.
4. **Make smart choices in organic produce.** It's not realistic for most people to buy organic produce all of the time — it is not always available, and the cost is often prohibitive. Use the Dirty Dozen list on page 25 to guide your choices: buy organic Dirty Dozen items whenever possible; for all other produce, stick with the regular produce bins.
5. **Eat seasonally.** Seasonal foods taste better, are more nutritious and don't need to be shipped in from half a world away! They often cost less as well: they are typically on sale at the supermarket and in abundance at the farmers' market. Plan ahead and stock up on fruits and vegetables in their natural season, then freeze them for the off-season.
6. **Preserve it when it's cheap.** If you have enough storage space, try canning, drying or freezing fresh fruits and vegetables. All of these preserving methods are excellent ways to cash in on seasonal foods that are lower in cost but higher in taste and nutrition. (Also take advantage of sales on non-perishable healthy foods. If your favorite cereal is on for a great price, buy extra.)
7. **Use dry milk powder and frozen vegetables in recipes.** Keep a box of dry milk powder in the pantry for use in recipes and save your fluid milk for drinking. Similarly, use inexpensive (but still healthful) frozen vegetables in soups, casseroles and chilis; save fresh vegetables for salads, side dishes and eating out of hand.
8. **Make extra for the freezer.** Prepare a double batch of pasta or whole grains for a main meal, then freeze the extras in individual portions. With a bit of marinara sauce, fresh vegetables or cheese, the leftovers make an excellent starting point for a quick lunch.
9. **Prepare meats and poultry yourself.** Ready-to-cook meats and poultry (such as marinated meats and boneless skinless chicken) cost more for less product. Buy your meats and poultry plain, and skin, bone and season them yourself.
10. **Skip processed foods.** Empty calories still leave you hungry for real food. Most processed foods — like candy, chips and soda — are simply fillers that you can gradually wean yourself off of purchasing and eating.

Portobello Pizzas

Makes 4 servings

✪ Great for Steps 1, 2, 3 and 4

The meaty robustness of portobellos makes a delicious "crust" in this addictive spin on pizza.

Tip

When selecting mushrooms, choose those with a fresh, smooth appearance, free from major blemishes and with a dry surface. Once home, keep mushrooms refrigerated; they're best when used within several days of purchase. When ready to use, gently wipe mushrooms with a damp cloth or soft brush to remove dirt. Alternatively, rinse them quickly with cold water, then immediately pat dry with paper towels.

Nutrients per serving	
Calories	217
Total fat	10 g
Saturated fat	5 g
Cholesterol	48 mg
Sodium	436 mg
Carbohydrate	8 g
Fiber	1 g
Protein	15 g
Calcium	253 mg
Iron	1.2 mg

- **Preheat oven to 500°F (260°C)**
- **Large rimmed baking sheet, lined with foil and sprayed with nonstick cooking spray (preferably olive oil)**

4	extra-large portobello mushrooms	4
2 tbsp	balsamic vinegar	30 mL
2 tbsp	basil pesto	30 mL
1½ cups	shredded smoked provolone or mozzarella cheese	375 mL
½ cup	chopped drained marinated artichoke hearts	125 mL
¼ cup	turkey pepperoni slices or soy pepperoni slices, coarsely chopped	60 mL
2 tbsp	chopped pitted brine-cured black olives (such as kalamata) (optional)	30 mL

1. Remove stems from mushrooms. Chop stems and set aside. Using a spoon, gently scoop out black gills on underside of mushroom caps. Discard gills. Place mushrooms, hollow side down, on prepared baking sheet.
2. In a small bowl, whisk together vinegar and pesto. Brush over tops of mushrooms. Bake in preheated oven for 5 to 7 minutes or until tender.
3. Meanwhile, in a medium bowl, combine chopped mushroom stems, cheese, artichokes, pepperoni and olives (if using).
4. Turn mushrooms over on baking sheet and fill caps with cheese mixture. Bake for 7 to 10 minutes or until filling is melted and bubbly.

▶ Health Note

Early research indicates that beneficial bacteria and nutrients found within mushrooms' cell walls may strengthen the body's defenses against disease.

Broccoli and Spinach Enchiladas

Makes 8 servings

✪ Great for Steps 1, 2, 3, 4 and 5

This California-inspired variation on classic Mexican fare is my idea of rich, delicious comfort food at its best. Broccoli and spinach are the perfect vegetables for balancing the tangy cheese and earthy whole wheat tortillas.

Tip

Nonfat ricotta cheese can be used in place of the cottage cheese.

Nutrients per serving	
Calories	284
Total fat	10 g
Saturated fat	4 g
Cholesterol	16 mg
Sodium	502 mg
Carbohydrate	34 g
Fiber	6 g
Protein	15 g
Calcium	215 mg
Iron	2.4 mg

- **Preheat oven to 350°F (180°C)**
- **9-inch (23 cm) square glass baking dish or metal baking pan, sprayed with nonstick cooking spray**

2 tsp	extra virgin olive oil	10 mL
1¼ cups	chopped onions	300 mL
1	package (10 oz/300 g) frozen chopped spinach, thawed and squeezed dry	1
1 cup	finely chopped broccoli	250 mL
1 tsp	ground cumin	5 mL
1½ cups	picante sauce, divided	375 mL
1 cup	nonfat cottage cheese	250 mL
1 cup	shredded sharp (old) white Cheddar cheese, divided	250 mL
8	8-inch (20 cm) whole wheat tortillas, warmed	8

1. In a large skillet, heat oil over medium heat. Add onions and cook, stirring, for 6 to 8 minutes or until softened. Add spinach, broccoli, cumin and ⅓ cup (75 mL) of the picante sauce; cook, stirring, for 1 minute. Remove from heat and stir in cottage cheese and ⅓ cup (75 mL) of the Cheddar.
2. Spoon about ⅓ cup (75 mL) of the spinach mixture down the center of each warmed tortilla. Roll up like a cigar and place, seam side down, in prepared baking dish. Spoon the remaining picante sauce over top.
3. Cover and bake in preheated oven for 20 to 25 minutes or until heated through. Sprinkle with the remaining Cheddar. Bake, uncovered, for 5 minutes or until cheese is bubbly.

Winter Squash and Goat Cheese Enchiladas

Makes 4 servings

✪ Great for Steps 2, 3, 4 and 5

This dish takes everyday frozen winter squash and with little effort — and no tricks — turns it into an unexpectedly sophisticated and delicious filling for enchiladas.

Tip

For the white beans, you could use Great Northern beans, cannellini (white kidney) beans or white pea (navy) beans.

- **Preheat oven to 350°F (180°C)**
- **13- by 9-inch (33 by 23 cm) glass baking dish, sprayed with nonstick cooking spray (preferably olive oil)**

1	can (14 to 19 oz/398 to 540 mL) white beans, drained and rinsed	1
1 cup	thawed frozen winter squash or canned pumpkin purée (not pie filling)	250 mL
2 tsp	ground cumin, divided	10 mL
1½ cups	chipotle salsa, divided	375 mL
1½ cups	reduced-sodium tomato juice	375 mL
12	6-inch (15 cm) corn tortillas, warmed	12
4 oz	mild goat cheese, crumbled	125 g
½ cup	thinly sliced green onions	125 mL

1. In a medium saucepan, combine beans, squash, half the cumin and ½ cup (125 mL) of the salsa. Using a fork, coarsely mash some of the beans. Cook, stirring, over medium heat for 5 to 6 minutes to heat through and blend the flavors.
2. In a medium bowl, whisk together tomato juice, the remaining salsa and the remaining cumin. Spread 1 cup (250 mL) of the sauce in bottom of prepared baking dish.
3. Lay tortillas on work surface. Spoon about ¼ cup (60 mL) of the filling down the center of each warmed tortilla. Roll up like a cigar and place, seam side down, in baking dish. Top with the remaining sauce.
4. Cover and bake in preheated oven for 20 minutes. Sprinkle with goat cheese and green onions. Bake, uncovered, for 10 to 15 minutes or until cheese is melted and sauce is bubbly.

▶ Health Note

Research reveals that milled yellow corn products — such as cornmeal, grits and the corn flour used to make corn tortillas — are rich in the carotenoids zeaxanthin and lutein, two antioxidants that protect the eyes and skin against UV damage.

Nutrients per serving	
Calories	323
Total fat	3 g
Saturated fat	0 g
Cholesterol	0 mg
Sodium	698 mg
Carbohydrate	64 g
Fiber	12 g
Protein	11 g
Calcium	99 mg
Iron	2.9 mg

Spinach Mushroom Quesadillas

Makes 4 servings

✪ Great for Steps 1, 2, 4 and 5

A squeeze of lime unites all of the flavors in these newfangled quesadillas.

Tip

When selecting mushrooms, choose those with a fresh, smooth appearance, free from major blemishes and with a dry surface. Once home, keep mushrooms refrigerated; they're best when used within several days of purchase. When ready to use, gently wipe mushrooms with a damp cloth or soft brush to remove dirt. Alternatively, rinse them quickly with cold water, then immediately pat dry with paper towels.

Nutrients per serving	
Calories	392
Total fat	12 g
Saturated fat	13 g
Cholesterol	59 mg
Sodium	473 mg
Carbohydrate	39 g
Fiber	6 g
Protein	25 g
Calcium	565 mg
Iron	3.7 mg

- **Preheat oven to 400°F (200°C)**
- **Large rimmed baking sheet, sprayed with nonstick cooking spray (preferably olive oil)**

2 tsp	vegetable oil	10 mL
1 cup	thinly sliced onions	250 mL
8 oz	cremini or button mushrooms, thinly sliced	250 g
1	package (10 oz/300 g) frozen chopped spinach, thawed and squeezed dry	1
1/8 tsp	fine sea salt	0.5 mL
1 tbsp	freshly squeezed lime juice	15 mL
4	10-inch (25 cm) whole wheat tortillas	4
2 cups	shredded pepper Jack cheese	500 mL
	Nonstick cooking spray (preferably olive oil)	

1. In a large skillet, heat oil over medium-high heat. Add onions and cook, stirring, for 6 to 8 minutes or until softened. Add mushrooms and cook, stirring occasionally, for 4 to 5 minutes or until tender. Add spinach, salt and lime juice; cook, stirring, for 1 minute or until warmed through.
2. Place 2 tortillas on prepared baking sheet. Divide spinach mixture between tortillas, spreading to cover. Sprinkle with cheese. Top with the remaining tortillas, pressing down gently. Lightly spray with cooking spray.
3. Bake in preheated oven for 10 to 12 minutes or until cheese is melted and tortillas are golden brown. Transfer to cutting board and cut each quesadilla into quarters.

Black Bean Tacos

Makes 4 servings

✪ Great for Steps 1, 2, 3, 4 and 5

Nutrients per serving	
Calories	287
Total fat	3 g
Saturated fat	0 g
Cholesterol	0 mg
Sodium	456 mg
Carbohydrate	54 g
Fiber	7 g
Protein	10 g
Calcium	74 mg
Iron	1.6 mg

1	can (14 to 19 oz/398 to 540 mL) black beans, drained and rinsed	1
1½ cups	chipotle salsa	375 mL
¼ tsp	ground cumin	1 mL
½ cup	nonfat plain Greek yogurt	125 mL
1 tbsp	freshly squeezed lime juice	15 mL
8	6-inch (15 cm) corn tortillas, warmed	8
2 cups	shredded coleslaw mix (shredded cabbage and carrots)	500 mL
½ cup	packed fresh cilantro leaves	125 mL

1. In a large skillet, combine beans and salsa. Using a fork, partially mash the beans. Cook, stirring, over medium heat for 4 to 5 minutes or until heated through.
2. Meanwhile, in a small bowl, whisk together cumin, yogurt and lime juice.
3. Fill warmed tortillas with bean mixture, coleslaw, cilantro and dollops of lime yogurt.

Eggplant Parmesan Melts

Makes 6 servings

✪ Great for Steps 1, 2 and 4

Tip

Serve with crusty whole-grain bread.

Nutrients per serving	
Calories	180
Total fat	9 g
Saturated fat	5 g
Cholesterol	23 mg
Sodium	396 mg
Carbohydrate	19 g
Fiber	11 g
Protein	10 g
Calcium	235 mg
Iron	0.9 mg

- **Preheat oven to 400°F (200°C)**
- **Large rimmed baking sheet, sprayed with nonstick cooking spray (preferably olive oil)**

2	large eggplants (each about 2 lbs/1 kg), trimmed and cut crosswise into ½-inch (1 cm) thick slices	2
	Nonstick cooking spray	
½ tsp	fine sea salt, divided	2 mL
4	tomatoes, sliced	4
1	ball (about 6 oz/175 g) fresh mozzarella in water, drained and diced	1
2 tbsp	freshly grated Parmesan cheese	30 mL
½ cup	packed fresh basil leaves, torn	125 mL

1. Lightly spray both sides of eggplant slices with cooking spray. Place on prepared baking sheet and sprinkle with half the salt. Bake in preheated oven for 25 to 30 minutes or until softened.
2. Arrange tomato slices on top of eggplant slices. Sprinkle with mozzarella, Parmesan and the remaining salt. Bake for 5 to 8 minutes or until cheese is melted. Top with basil.

Seared Halloumi with Chickpea Salsa and Herbed Couscous

Makes 4 servings

✪ Great for Steps 1, 2, 3, 4 and 5

Halloumi, a firm, mild Cypriot cheese popular in Greece — and becoming increasingly so in the U.S. and Canada — can be cooked directly on a grill or in a skillet. The outside will get brown and crisp; the inside will be soft and melted.

1 cup	reduced-sodium ready-to-use vegetable broth	250 mL
1 cup	whole wheat couscous	250 mL
1	can (14 to 19 oz/398 to 540 mL) chickpeas, drained and rinsed	1
1½ cups	cherry or grape tomatoes, quartered	375 mL
¼ tsp	cayenne pepper	1 mL
4 tsp	extra virgin olive oil, divided	20 mL
2 tsp	sherry vinegar or red wine vinegar	10 mL
8 oz	Halloumi cheese, cut into 4 thick slices	250 g
½ cup	packed fresh mint leaves, chopped	125 mL
½ cup	packed fresh cilantro leaves, chopped	125 mL

1. In a small saucepan, bring broth to a boil over medium-high heat. Remove from heat and whisk in couscous. Cover and let stand for 5 minutes.
2. Meanwhile, in a medium bowl, combine chickpeas, tomatoes, cayenne, half the oil and vinegar.
3. In a large skillet, heat the remaining oil over medium-high heat. Add cheese and cook, turning once, for 2 to 3 minutes per side or until golden brown on both sides.
4. Fluff couscous with a fork, then gently stir in mint and cilantro. Divide couscous among plates and top with grilled cheese and chickpea salsa.

Nutrients per serving	
Calories	408
Total fat	13 g
Saturated fat	7 g
Cholesterol	29 mg
Sodium	504 mg
Carbohydrate	55 g
Fiber	11 g
Protein	23 g
Calcium	143 mg
Iron	4.0 mg

Easy Ratatouille with Poached Eggs

Makes 4 servings

✪ Great for Steps 1, 2 and 4

Only in summer, when vegetables are so full of flavor, could a one-dish dinner like ratatouille seem so special. A gentle simmer, fresh basil and a small amount of olive oil are all that's needed to enhance the vegetables' natural goodness. But some crusty whole-grain bread alongside, to mop up every last bit of juice, isn't a bad idea.

2 tsp	extra virgin olive oil	10 mL
3	cloves garlic, minced	3
1	large red bell pepper, coarsely chopped	1
1½ cups	chopped onions	375 mL
2 tsp	dried herbes de Provence or Italian seasoning	10 mL
2	small zucchini, cut into 1-inch (2.5 cm) cubes	2
1	eggplant (about 1½ lbs/750 g), trimmed and cut into 1-inch (2.5 cm) cubes	1
1	can (14 to 15 oz/398 to 425 mL) diced tomatoes, with juice	1
½ tsp	fine sea salt	2 mL
1¼ cups	water	300 mL
2 tsp	balsamic vinegar	10 mL
4	large eggs	4
⅛ tsp	freshly ground black pepper	0.5 mL
¾ cup	packed fresh basil leaves, torn	175 mL

1. In a large skillet, heat oil over medium-high heat. Add garlic, red pepper, onions and herbes de Provence; cook, stirring, for 6 to 8 minutes or until onions are softened. Add zucchini and eggplant; cook, stirring, for 5 minutes or until softened.
2. Add tomatoes with juice, salt and water. Bring to a boil. Reduce heat to low, cover and simmer, stirring occasionally, for 20 minutes. Uncover and simmer, stirring occasionally, for 15 to 20 minutes or until reduced and thickened. Stir in vinegar.
3. Make four holes in the ratatouille for the eggs. Crack an egg into each hole and season with pepper. Cover and cook for 2 to 5 minutes or until eggs are set as desired. Serve sprinkled with basil.

Nutrients per serving	
Calories	205
Total fat	7 g
Saturated fat	2 g
Cholesterol	180 mg
Sodium	536 mg
Carbohydrate	25 g
Fiber	8 g
Protein	11 g
Calcium	86 mg
Iron	2.4 mg

Swiss Chard, Cherry Tomato and Ricotta Bake

Makes 4 servings

✪ Great for Steps 1, 2, 3 and 4

A touch of nutmeg adds just the right nuance to Swiss chard and cherry tomatoes in this easily assembled dish that is at once show-stopping and approachable.

Tips

You can use 2 cups (500 mL) diced plum (Roma) tomatoes in place of the cherry tomatoes.

An equal amount of kale, spinach or regular Swiss chard may be used in place of the red Swiss chard.

Nutrients per serving	
Calories	126
Total fat	5 g
Saturated fat	2 g
Cholesterol	15 mg
Sodium	435 mg
Carbohydrate	8 g
Fiber	2 g
Protein	12 g
Calcium	334 mg
Iron	1.0 mg

- **9-inch (23 cm) glass baking pan, sprayed with nonstick cooking spray (preferably olive oil)**

2 tsp	extra virgin olive oil	10 mL
1	large bunch red Swiss chard, ribs removed, leaves thinly sliced crosswise (about 5 cups/1.25 L)	1
2	cloves garlic, minced	2
1⁄2 tsp	fine sea salt	2 mL
1⁄2 tsp	ground nutmeg	2 mL
4	large eggs, beaten	4
1 cup	nonfat ricotta cheese	250 mL
4 tbsp	freshly grated Parmesan cheese, divided	60 mL
1⁄4 tsp	freshly cracked black pepper	1 mL
2 cups	cherry or grape tomatoes, halved	500 mL

1. In a large skillet, heat oil over medium-high heat. Add Swiss chard and cook, stirring, for 5 to 6 minutes or until wilted and tender. Add garlic and cook, stirring, for 1 minute. Remove from heat. Press chard against side of pan with a wooden spoon to release juices. Drain and discard juices. Stir in salt and nutmeg. Let cool to room temperature.
2. Preheat oven to 400°F (200°C).
3. In a medium bowl, combine eggs, ricotta, half the Parmesan and pepper. Stir in Swiss chard mixture.
4. Spread ricotta mixture evenly in prepared baking pan. Scatter tomatoes evenly over top. Sprinkle with the remaining Parmesan.
5. Bake for 12 to 17 minutes or until golden and set at the center. Let cool on a wire rack for at least 10 minutes before cutting. Serve warm or let cool completely.

Spanish Sweet Potato Tortilla with Roasted Pepper Sauce

Makes 4 servings

✪ Great for Steps 1, 2 and 4

In this addictive twist on the Spanish-style frittata known as a tortilla, sweet potatoes are subbed in for regular potatoes. Both the sauce and the tortilla may be made in advance — both taste just right at room temperature.

Tip

An equal amount of coarsely shredded peeled yellow-fleshed potatoes can be used in place of the sweet potatoes.

Nutrients per serving	
Calories	257
Total fat	10 g
Saturated fat	2 g
Cholesterol	270 mg
Sodium	215 mg
Carbohydrate	29 g
Fiber	4 g
Protein	12 g
Calcium	88 mg
Iron	3.3 mg

- **Preheat broiler, with rack set 4 to 6 inches (10 to 15 cm) from the heat source**
- **Blender**
- **Large ovenproof skillet**

1	jar (12 oz/340 mL) roasted red bell peppers, drained	1
1	clove garlic, minced	1
1 tsp	sweet smoked paprika	5 mL
3⁄4 tsp	ground cumin	3 mL
	Fine sea salt	
2 tbsp	water	30 mL
2 tsp	sherry vinegar or white wine vinegar	10 mL
6	large eggs	6
1 tbsp	extra virgin olive oil	15 mL
4 cups	coarsely shredded peeled sweet potatoes (about 2 medium)	1 L
1 cup	chopped green onions	250 mL

1. In blender, combine roasted peppers, garlic, paprika, cumin, a pinch of salt, water and vinegar; purée until smooth. Set aside.
2. In a medium bowl, whisk together eggs and 1 tsp (5 mL) salt.
3. In ovenproof skillet, heat oil over medium-high heat. Add sweet potatoes and cook, stirring, for 8 to 10 minutes or until softened. Add green onions and egg mixture, gently shaking pan to distribute eggs. Reduce heat to medium and cook for about 8 minutes, gently shaking pan every minute, until eggs are almost set.
4. Place skillet under the preheated broiler and broil for 1 to 2 minutes or until lightly browned. Slide out of the pan onto a cutting board and cut into wedges. Serve with roasted pepper sauce.

Skillet-Roasted Cauliflower Omelet

Makes 4 servings

✪ Great for Steps 1, 2 and 4

Zesty feta and the fresh, grassy flavor of parsley bring out cauliflower's best, turning this otherwise simple weeknight omelet into a fine-dining experience.

5	large eggs	5
1/4 tsp	fine sea salt	1 mL
1/4 tsp	freshly cracked black pepper	1 mL
2 tsp	extra virgin olive oil	10 mL
3 cups	coarsely chopped cauliflower florets	750 mL
2	cloves garlic, minced	2
1/2 cup	crumbled feta cheese	125 mL
1/4 cup	packed fresh flat-leaf (Italian) parsley leaves	60 mL

1. In a large bowl, whisk together eggs, salt and pepper. Set aside.
2. In a large skillet, heat oil over medium-high heat. Add cauliflower and cook, stirring, for 7 to 10 minutes or until browned and tender. Reduce heat to medium, add garlic and cook, stirring, for 30 seconds.
3. Pour egg mixture over cauliflower. Cook, lifting edges to allow uncooked eggs to run underneath and shaking skillet occasionally to loosen omelet, for 4 to 5 minutes or until almost set. Slide out onto a large plate.
4. Invert skillet over omelet and, using pot holders, firmly hold plate and skillet together. Invert omelet back into skillet and cook for 1 to 2 minutes to set eggs. Slide out onto plate and sprinkle with cheese and parsley.

▶ Health Note

Cauliflower may be pale, but it's powerful. A 1-cup (250 mL) serving offers a high level of fiber, 14% of the body's daily folate needs and nearly a day's worth of vitamin C.

Nutrients per serving	
Calories	212
Total fat	15 g
Saturated fat	5 g
Cholesterol	242 mg
Sodium	498 mg
Carbohydrate	7 g
Fiber	2 g
Protein	12 g
Calcium	148 mg
Iron	1.9 mg

Greek Salad Frittata

Makes 4 servings

✪ Great for Steps 1, 2 and 4

The classic ingredients of Greek salad — cherry tomatoes, red onion, olives and feta — enliven everyday eggs in this bright, beautiful frittata.

Tip

You can use 1⁄4 cup (60 mL) packed fresh dill, chopped, in place of the parsley.

Nutrients per serving	
Calories	281
Total fat	17 g
Saturated fat	6 g
Cholesterol	377 mg
Sodium	515 mg
Carbohydrate	13 g
Fiber	3 g
Protein	17 g
Calcium	191 mg
Iron	3.4 mg

- **Preheat broiler**
- **Large ovenproof skillet**

8	large eggs	8
3⁄4 cup	packed fresh parsley leaves, roughly chopped	175 mL
1⁄4 tsp	fine sea salt	1 mL
1⁄4 tsp	freshly cracked black pepper	1 mL
1 tbsp	extra virgin olive oil	15 mL
1 1⁄2 cups	coarsely chopped red onion	375 mL
2 cups	cherry tomatoes, halved	500 mL
1⁄3 cup	pitted brine-cured black olives (such as kalamata), coarsely chopped	75 mL
1⁄2 cup	crumbled feta cheese	125 mL

1. In a large bowl, whisk together eggs, parsley, salt and pepper. Set aside.
2. In ovenproof skillet, heat oil over medium-high heat. Add red onion and cook, stirring, for 6 to 8 minutes or until softened. Add tomatoes and olives; cook, stirring, for 1 to 2 minutes or until tomatoes begin to soften slightly.
3. Reduce heat to medium and pour in egg mixture. Cook for about 2 minutes, gently shaking pan to distribute eggs as they begin to set, until slightly set but still slightly runny. Sprinkle with cheese.
4. Place skillet under preheated broiler and broil for 5 to 6 minutes or until puffed and golden. Cut into wedges and serve straight from the pan.

Persian Zucchini Frittata

Makes 4 servings

✪ Great for Steps 1, 2 and 4

If you're hankering for a new spin on eggs, consider kuku kadoo, *the Persian version of the familiar frittata. Fresh herbs and pungent garlic give way to tender zucchini, bound together by turmeric- and ginger-scented eggs.*

- **Preheat oven to 400°F (200°C)**
- **9-inch (23 cm) square glass baking dish, sprayed with nonstick cooking spray (preferably olive oil)**

2 tsp	extra virgin olive oil	10 mL
2	zucchini, halved lengthwise and cut into 1/4-inch (0.5 cm) thick slices	2
1 1/2 cups	chopped onions	375 mL
2	cloves garlic, minced	2
2 tsp	minced gingerroot	10 mL
1 1/2 tbsp	whole wheat flour	22 mL
1 tsp	ground turmeric	5 mL
1/2 tsp	fine sea salt	2 mL
1/4 tsp	baking soda	1 mL
6	large eggs	6
1/3 cup	packed fresh parsley leaves, chopped	75 mL

1. In a large skillet, heat oil over medium-high heat. Add zucchini and onions; cook, stirring, for 6 to 8 minutes or until softened. Add garlic, ginger, flour, turmeric, salt and baking soda; cook, stirring, for 1 minute. Let cool slightly.
2. In a large bowl, whisk together eggs and parsley. Add zucchini mixture, stirring to combine. Spread evenly in prepared baking dish.
3. Bake in preheated oven for 25 to 30 minutes or until just set. Let cool on a wire rack for at least 10 minutes before cutting. Serve warm or let cool completely.

Nutrients per serving

Calories	172
Total fat	9 g
Saturated fat	2 g
Cholesterol	270 mg
Sodium	440 mg
Carbohydrate	11 g
Fiber	2 g
Protein	11 g
Calcium	65 mg
Iron	2.2 mg

Red Lentil Frittata

Makes 6 servings

✪ Great for Steps 3 and 4

Goat cheese makes a tangy counterpoint for the Middle Eastern flavors — cumin, lentils and roasted red bell peppers — in this easy, inspired frittata.

Tip

An equal amount of green or brown lentils may be used in place of the red lentils. See Cooking Legumes, page 436, as these lentils require a longer cooking time.

- **9-inch (23 cm) glass baking dish, sprayed with nonstick cooking spray (preferably olive oil)**

1/2 cup	dried red lentils, rinsed	125 mL
2 cups	water	500 mL
8	large eggs	12
1	clove garlic, minced	1
1 1/2 tsp	ground cumin	7 mL
3/4 tsp	fine sea salt	3 mL
1/4 tsp	freshly cracked black pepper	1 mL
1 cup	chopped drained roasted red bell peppers	250 mL
1/2 cup	packed fresh cilantro leaves, chopped	125 mL
2 oz	soft goat cheese, crumbled	60 g

1. In a medium saucepan, combine lentils and water. Bring to a boil over medium-high heat. Reduce heat and simmer for about 22 minutes or until very tender but not mushy. Drain and let cool slightly.
2. Preheat oven to 375°F (190°C).
3. In a large bowl, whisk together eggs, garlic, cumin, salt and pepper. Stir in cooked lentils, roasted peppers, cilantro and cheese. Spread evenly in prepared baking dish.
4. Bake in preheated oven for 25 to 30 minutes or until golden brown, puffed and set at the center. Let cool on a wire rack for at least 10 minutes before cutting. Serve warm or let cool completely.

Nutrients per serving	
Calories	192
Total fat	8 g
Saturated fat	3 g
Cholesterol	245 mg
Sodium	383 mg
Carbohydrate	13 g
Fiber	3 g
Protein	15 g
Calcium	63 mg
Iron	2.6 mg

Quinoa, Mushroom and Green Onion Frittata

Makes 4 servings

✪ Great for Steps 1, 2, 3, 4 and 5

In this redesigned version of an Italian classic, nutty quinoa joins salty Parmesan and sautéed mushrooms to give the eggs a satisfying undercurrent of umami.

Tip

To prepare 1½ cups (375 mL) cooked quinoa, combine ½ cup (125 mL) quinoa and 1 cup (250 mL) water in a medium saucepan. Bring to a boil over medium-high heat. Reduce heat to low, cover and simmer for 15 to 18 minutes or until water is absorbed. Let cool completely.

Nutrients per serving	
Calories	382
Total fat	13 g
Saturated fat	4 g
Cholesterol	190 mg
Sodium	587 mg
Carbohydrate	47 g
Fiber	5 g
Protein	23 g
Calcium	170 mg
Iron	5.2 mg

- **Preheat oven to 350°F (180°C)**
- **8-inch (20 cm) square glass baking dish, sprayed with nonstick cooking spray (preferably olive oil)**

4	large eggs	4
4	large egg whites	4
½ tsp	fine sea salt	2 mL
¼ tsp	freshly ground black pepper	1 mL
2 tsp	extra virgin olive oil	10 mL
8 oz	cremini or button mushrooms, sliced	250 g
1½ cups	chopped green onions	375 mL
1½ cups	cooked quinoa (see tip, at left), cooled	375 mL
¼ cup	freshly grated Parmesan cheese	60 mL

1. In a large bowl, whisk together eggs, egg whites, salt and pepper. Set aside.
2. In a large skillet, heat oil over medium-high heat. Add mushrooms and green onions; cook, stirring, for 5 to 7 minutes or until softened. Stir in quinoa and cook, stirring, for 1 minute. Spread mixture in prepared baking dish.
3. Pour egg mixture over quinoa mixture. Sprinkle with cheese.
4. Bake in preheated oven for 23 to 28 minutes or until golden and set. Let cool on a wire rack for at least 10 minutes before cutting. Serve warm or let cool completely.

Spinach and Feta Crustless Quiche

Makes 8 servings

✪ Great for Steps 2, 3 and 4

One of the easiest, most convenient and most economical dinners you can throw together on any given weeknight, this creamy quiche is pure comfort food.

- **Preheat oven to 350°F (180°C)**
- **Blender**
- **9-inch (23 cm) glass pie plate, sprayed with nonstick cooking spray (preferably olive oil)**

4	large eggs	4
1	container (16 oz/500 g) nonfat cottage cheese	1
1	package (10 oz/300 g) frozen chopped spinach, thawed and squeezed dry	1
1¼ cups	finely chopped green onions	300 mL
1 cup	crumbled feta cheese	250 mL
⅛ tsp	freshly ground black pepper	0.5 mL
3 tbsp	toasted wheat germ	45 mL

1. In blender, combine eggs and cottage cheese; purée until smooth.
2. Transfer purée to a medium bowl and stir in spinach, green onions, cheese and pepper. Spread evenly in prepared pie plate.
3. Bake in preheated oven for 25 minutes. Sprinkle with wheat germ and bake for 10 to 15 minutes or until golden brown and set.

▶ Health Note

The eggs and spinach in this easy quiche are more than a delicious duo: the combination is also a perfect way to add lutein to your diet. Lutein, a carotenoid thought to help prevent age-related macular degeneration and cataracts, is present in even higher amounts in eggs than in green vegetables such as spinach. But according to a recent study in the *Journal of Nutrition*, eating the two ingredients ensemble is an excellent way to maximize lutein absorption.

Nutrients per serving	
Calories	159
Total fat	7 g
Saturated fat	4 g
Cholesterol	110 mg
Sodium	512 mg
Carbohydrate	8 g
Fiber	2 g
Protein	16 g
Calcium	216 mg
Iron	2.2 mg

Crispy Baked Tofu

Makes 4 servings

✪ Great for Step 3

Golden brown and crispy, this quick and easy baked tofu can be used in any recipe that calls for purchased baked tofu. You can also use it as a substitute for chicken in any recipe or nibble it as a snack.

- **Large rimmed baking sheet, lined with parchment paper**

16 oz	extra-firm tofu, drained	500 g
	Nonstick cooking spray	

1. Wrap tofu in four or five layers of paper towels. Place on a dinner plate. Cover with a second dinner plate. Place two or three heavy cans on top. Let drain for 30 minutes. Remove cans, plates and paper towels. Repeat process once more.
2. Preheat oven to 400°F (200°C).
3. Cut tofu into 1-inch (2.5 cm) cubes. Spray all sides with cooking spray, then arrange in single layer on prepared baking sheet.
4. Bake in preheated oven for 20 minutes. Turn cubes with a spatula and bake for 18 to 22 minutes or until golden brown and crispy.

Tip

The tofu can be tossed with a small amount of almost any herb or spice after spraying and before baking.

Storage Tip

Store cooled tofu cubes in an airtight container in the refrigerator for up to 5 days.

Nutrients per serving	
Calories	111
Total fat	6 g
Saturated fat	0 g
Cholesterol	0 mg
Sodium	34 mg
Carbohydrate	3 g
Fiber	2 g
Protein	11 g
Calcium	237 mg
Iron	2.3 mg

Tofu and Eggplant Stir-Fry

Makes 4 servings

✪ Great for Steps 1, 2, 3 and 4

This quick-to-the-table tofu and eggplant dish couldn't be simpler or more satisfying. Serve over brown rice.

Tip

An equal amount of fresh cilantro or mint leaves may be used in place of the basil.

Nutrients per serving	
Calories	230
Total fat	12 g
Saturated fat	1 g
Cholesterol	1 mg
Sodium	263 mg
Carbohydrate	20 g
Fiber	7 g
Protein	13 g
Calcium	264 mg
Iron	3.0 mg

4 tsp	vegetable oil, divided	20 mL
16 oz	extra-firm tofu, drained, cut into 1-inch (2.5 cm) pieces and patted dry	500 g
3	cloves garlic, minced	3
1	red bell pepper, sliced	1
1 lb	eggplant, trimmed and cut into 3- by 1-inch (7.5 by 2.5 cm) strips	500 g
1/4 cup	hoisin sauce	60 mL
2 tbsp	water	30 mL
1/4 cup	packed fresh basil leaves, thinly sliced	60 mL

1. In a large skillet, heat half the oil over medium-high heat. Add tofu and cook, stirring, for 4 to 6 minutes or until browned. Using a slotted spoon, transfer tofu to a plate.
2. In the same skillet, heat the remaining oil over medium-high heat. Add garlic, red pepper and eggplant; cook, stirring, for 8 to 10 minutes or until softened. Return tofu to the pan and add hoisin and water; cook, stirring, for 2 to 3 minutes or until heated through. Remove from heat and stir in basil.

Basil Coconut Tofu Curry

Makes 6 servings

✪ Great for Steps 1, 2, 3 and 4

This recipe disproves the notion that tofu is boring and bland; here, it is vibrant with Southeast Asian flavors that satisfy on every level. To be sure you're getting enough protein, serve over brown jasmine rice.

Tip

To save time, you can replace the fresh green beans with a thawed 16-oz (454 g) package of frozen cut green beans.

1 tbsp	cornstarch	15 mL
2 cups	reduced-sodium ready-to-use vegetable broth, divided	500 mL
2 tsp	vegetable oil	10 mL
4 cups	green beans, trimmed and cut into 1-inch (2.5 cm) pieces	1 L
1½ cups	sliced onions	375 mL
2 tbsp	Thai green curry paste	30 mL
16 oz	extra-firm tofu, drained and cut into ½-inch (1 cm) cubes	500 g
1	can (14 oz/398 mL) light coconut milk	1
1 cup	packed fresh basil leaves, torn	250 mL
2 tbsp	freshly squeezed lime juice	30 mL
1 tsp	reduced-sodium tamari or soy sauce	5 mL

1. In a small bowl, whisk together cornstarch and 2 tbsp (30 mL) of the broth until smooth. Set aside.
2. In a large skillet, heat oil over medium-high heat. Add green beans and onions; cook, stirring, for 6 to 8 minutes or until onions are softened. Reduce heat to medium and add curry paste; cook, stirring, for 1 minute.
3. Stir in cornstarch mixture, tofu, coconut milk and the remaining broth. Reduce heat and simmer, stirring occasionally, for 6 to 8 minutes or until vegetables are tender and sauce is slightly thickened. Stir in basil, lime juice and tamari.

Nutrients per serving	
Calories	202
Total fat	11 g
Saturated fat	5 g
Cholesterol	1 mg
Sodium	108 mg
Carbohydrate	15 g
Fiber	4 g
Protein	9 g
Calcium	23 mg
Iron	2.5 mg

Indian-Spiced Cauliflower, Spinach and Tofu Scramble

Makes 4 servings

✪ Great for Steps 1, 2, 3 and 4

The multiple layers of flavor in this 30-minute, one-pot meal are hypnotizing.

Tip

For a milder dish, use an equal amount of mild curry powder in place of the hot curry powder.

Nutrients per serving	
Calories	145
Total fat	6 g
Saturated fat	1 g
Cholesterol	0 mg
Sodium	408 mg
Carbohydrate	14 g
Fiber	5 g
Protein	12 g
Calcium	102 mg
Iron	3.6 mg

16 oz	firm tofu, drained and crumbled	500 g
2 tsp	vegetable oil	10 mL
2 cups	small cauliflower florets	500 mL
2	cloves garlic, minced	2
1 tbsp	minced gingerroot	15 mL
1¼ tsp	hot curry powder	6 mL
1 tsp	ground cumin	5 mL
½ tsp	ground coriander	2 mL
½ tsp	fine sea salt	2 mL
8 cups	packed baby spinach (about 8 oz/250 g)	2 L

1. Spread tofu on paper towels and let drain for 15 minutes.
2. Meanwhile, in a large skillet, heat oil over medium-high heat. Add cauliflower and cook, stirring, for 10 to 12 minutes or until browned. Add garlic, ginger, curry powder, cumin, coriander and salt; cook, stirring, for 30 seconds.
3. Stir in drained tofu and cook, stirring, for 2 minutes or until heated through. Add spinach and cook, stirring, for 2 to 3 minutes or until wilted.

Stir-Fried Tofu with Bok Choy and Spinach

Makes 4 servings

✪ Great for Steps 1, 2, 3 and 4

This meaty yet meat-free stir-fry — a hearty mix of bok choy, spinach and tofu — gets a boost from toasted sesame oil and tart rice vinegar.

Tip

Choose unseasoned rice vinegar; seasoned rice vinegar has added salt and sugar.

4 tbsp	reduced-sodium tamari or soy sauce, divided	60 mL
4 tsp	toasted sesame oil, divided	20 mL
4 tsp	unseasoned rice vinegar, divided	20 mL
16 oz	extra-firm tofu, drained	500 g
2 tsp	vegetable oil	10 mL
2	cloves garlic, finely chopped	2
1 cup	sliced green onions	250 mL
2 tbsp	chopped gingerroot	30 mL
6 cups	sliced bok choy (about 1 medium head)	1.5 L
8 cups	packed baby spinach (about 8 oz/250 g)	2 L

1. In a small bowl, whisk together half the tamari, half the sesame oil and $\frac{1}{2}$ tsp (2 mL) of the vinegar. Set aside.
2. Cut tofu into 1-inch (2.5 cm) cubes. Press between a double layer of paper towels to remove excess moisture.
3. In a large saucepan, heat vegetable oil over medium-high heat. Add tofu and cook, stirring, for 3 to 4 minutes or until golden. Transfer to a medium bowl and add tamari mixture, tossing to combine.
4. In the same saucepan, heat the remaining sesame oil over medium heat. Add garlic, green onions and ginger; cook, stirring, for 30 seconds. Add bok choy, the remaining tamari and the remaining vinegar; cook, stirring, for 2 to 3 minutes or until bok choy is wilted. Add spinach and cook, stirring, for 1 to 2 minutes or until wilted. Add tofu mixture and cook, stirring, for 1 minute or until heated through.

Superfood Spotlight

Ginger • For thousands of years, ginger has been considered a healthy food, and recent research has borne this out. The main active compounds are terpenes and gingerols, which have anticancer properties and have been shown to destroy colon, ovarian and rectal cancer cells. Gingerols also have a powerful anti-inflammatory action, and ginger has been shown to improve pain and swelling in up to 75% of people with arthritis, as well as improving mobility. In addition, ginger may ease migraine tension and has long been used as a remedy for nausea and to aid digestion, relaxing the intestines and helping to eliminate flatulence.

Nutrients per serving

Calories	223
Total fat	14 g
Saturated fat	1 g
Cholesterol	0 mg
Sodium	479 mg
Carbohydrate	14 g
Fiber	5 g
Protein	15 g
Calcium	388 mg
Iron	5.8 mg

Quick Quinoa Stir-Fry with Vegetables and Tofu

Makes 4 servings

✪ Great for Steps 2, 3, 4 and 5

Quinoa is a mild, slightly sweet grain with hints of corn, nuts and grass. Here, it's studded with assorted vegetables and sesame seeds, creating a substantial stir-fry worthy of its billing as a main course.

Tip

To prepare 4 cups (1 L) cooked quinoa, combine 1⅓ cups (325 mL) quinoa and 2⅔ cups (650 mL) water in a medium saucepan. Bring to a boil over medium-high heat. Reduce heat to low, cover and simmer for 15 to 18 minutes or until water is absorbed. Let cool completely, then transfer to an airtight container and refrigerate until chilled.

Nutrients per serving	
Calories	313
Total fat	9 g
Saturated fat	1 g
Cholesterol	0 mg
Sodium	361 mg
Carbohydrate	46 g
Fiber	7 g
Protein	16 g
Calcium	175 mg
Iron	6.1 mg

2 tsp	vegetable oil, divided	10 mL
8 oz	extra-firm tofu, drained, cut into 1-inch (2.5 cm) cubes and patted dry	250 g
12 oz	frozen stir-fry vegetables, thawed and patted dry	375 g
3	cloves garlic, minced	3
1 tbsp	minced gingerroot	15 mL
4 cups	cooked quinoa (see tip, at left), chilled	1 L
⅓ cup	thinly sliced green onions	75 mL
¼ cup	teriyaki sauce	60 mL
1 tbsp	toasted sesame seeds (see tip, page 426)	15 mL

1. In a large skillet, heat half the oil over medium-high heat. Add tofu and cook, stirring, for 3 to 4 minutes or until golden. Using a slotted spoon, transfer tofu to a plate.
2. In the same skillet, heat the remaining oil over medium-high heat. Add stir-fry vegetables and cook, stirring, for 2 minutes. Add garlic and ginger; cook, stirring, for 30 seconds. Return tofu to the pan and add quinoa, green onions and teriyaki sauce; cook, stirring, for 2 to 3 minutes or until well coated and warmed through. Serve sprinkled with sesame seeds.

▶ Health Note

Once a revered food staple of the ancient Incas, quinoa (pronounced *KEEN-wah*) is packed with high-quality protein. In fact, at as much as 20% protein, it has more protein than any other whole grain. Add to that a good dose of B vitamins, iron, calcium, potassium, magnesium and vitamin E, and it's easy to see why quinoa flies out of the bulk bins at health food stores.

Tempeh with Moroccan Tomato Sauce

Makes 4 servings

✪ Great for Steps 3 and 4

This Moroccan-sauced tempeh dish gets brilliant color and lively flavor from an easy tomato topping. Serve with whole wheat couscous or quinoa.

Tips

Any other variety of tempeh may be used in place of the five-grain tempeh.

Moroccan tomato sauce is also delicious with cooked chicken breasts, white fish fillets or tofu.

- **Blender or food processor**

1 cup	packed fresh flat-leaf (Italian) parsley leaves	250 mL
1½ tsp	ground cumin	7 mL
1½ tsp	sweet paprika or sweet smoked paprika	7 mL
½ tsp	dried oregano	2 mL
¼ tsp	ground ginger	1 mL
⅛ tsp	fine sea salt	0.5 mL
⅛ tsp	freshly ground black pepper	0.5 mL
¾ cup	tomato purée	175 mL
1 tbsp	freshly squeezed lemon juice	15 mL
8 oz	five-grain tempeh	250 g
2 tsp	extra virgin olive oil	10 mL

1. In blender, combine parsley, cumin, paprika, oregano, ginger, salt, pepper, tomato purée and lemon juice; purée until smooth.
2. In a small saucepan, heat tomato mixture over medium-low heat, stirring occasionally, for 4 to 5 minutes or until warmed through.
3. Meanwhile, cut tempeh in half crosswise, then cut each half lengthwise into 6 strips.
4. In a large skillet, heat oil over medium-high heat. Add tempeh strips and cook, turning once, for 4 to 5 minutes or until golden and warmed through. Serve with tomato sauce.

Nutrients per serving	
Calories	190
Total fat	7 g
Saturated fat	1 g
Cholesterol	1 mg
Sodium	102 mg
Carbohydrate	21 g
Fiber	7 g
Protein	10 g
Calcium	98 mg
Iron	3.3 mg

Thai Tempeh with Broccoli and Snow Peas

Makes 4 servings

✪ Great for Steps 1, 2, 3 and 4

Noodles often own the spotlight in Thai cooking, but this easy, satay-inspired stir-fry is equally worthy of the limelight. Serve over brown rice.

2	cloves garlic, minced	2
2 tsp	ground ginger	10 mL
1/8 tsp	cayenne pepper	0.5 mL
1/2 cup	light coconut milk	125 mL
1/3 cup	reduced-sodium ready-to-use vegetable or chicken broth	75 mL
3 tbsp	unsweetened natural peanut butter or other nut butter	45 mL
2 tbsp	reduced-sodium tamari or soy sauce	30 mL
2 tbsp	freshly squeezed lime juice	30 mL
2 tbsp	brown rice syrup or liquid honey	30 mL
2 tsp	vegetable oil	10 mL
8 oz	tempeh, cut into 1/2-inch (1 cm) strips	250 g
2 cups	snow peas, trimmed	500 mL
2 cups	small broccoli florets	500 mL
1/2 cup	packed fresh cilantro leaves, chopped	125 mL

1. In a small bowl, whisk together garlic, ginger, cayenne, coconut milk, broth, peanut butter, tamari, lime juice and brown rice syrup.
2. In a large skillet, heat oil over medium-high heat. Add tempeh and cook, stirring, for 1 minute. Add snow peas and broccoli; cook, stirring, for 1 to 2 minutes or until tender-crisp. Add peanut sauce, reduce heat and simmer, stirring once or twice, for 2 to 3 minutes or until sauce is slightly thickened. Serve sprinkled with cilantro.

Nutrients per serving	
Calories	313
Total fat	17 g
Saturated fat	4 g
Cholesterol	0 mg
Sodium	344 mg
Carbohydrate	26 g
Fiber	3 g
Protein	17 g
Calcium	114 mg
Iron	2.8 mg

Poultry and Lean Meat Main Dishes

Chicken with Sautéed Apples and Swiss Chard 298
Greek Chicken with Cherry Tomatoes and Feta 299
Chicken with Cherry Tomato and Avocado Salsa 300
Spicy Skillet Chicken with Avocado Mango Salsa 301
Miso Chicken with Crunchy Herb Salad 302
Thai Chicken and Basil 303
Broccoli, Asparagus and Chicken Stir-Fry 304
Spicy Chicken, Spinach and Peanut Stir-Fry 305
Stir-Fried Tangerine Chicken 306
Chicken Souvlaki 307
Chicken Shwarma 308
Japanese Sesame Chicken Skewers 309
Chicken and Zucchini Spiedini with Salsa Verde 310
Cuban Chicken with Black Beans and Brown Rice 311
Jamaican Chicken Couscous 312
Pineapple Mint Chicken 313
Chicken Biryani 314
Spring Vegetable Chicken Quinoa 315
Chicken and Black Bean Chilaquiles 316
Chicken Sausage and Black-Eyed Peas 317
Turkey Sausage with Mustard Greens and Kidney Beans 318

Turkey Sausage, Spinach and Chickpea Ragù 319
Stuffed Swiss Chard Leaves 320
Asian Lettuce Wraps 321
Moroccan-Spiced Ground Turkey with Apricot Couscous 322
Roasted Pork Tenderloin with Pear Slaw 323
Healthy Know-How: Protein 101 324
Honey Mustard Pork Tenderloin with Mustard Greens 325
Chipotle Maple Pork with Sweet Potato and Spinach Hash 326
Sautéed Pork Chops with Balsamic Onions, Kale and Cherries 327
Korean Sesame Soy Pork with Quick Kimchi Slaw 328
Stir-Fried Pork and Peppers with Buckwheat Noodles 329
Thai-Style Pork with Brown Jasmine Rice 330
Cuban Braised Beef with Brown Rice and Mango 331
Grilled Steak with Arugula and Parmesan 332
Japanese Ginger Beef Bowls 333
Grilled Steak Tacos with Avocado and Cumin Lime Slaw 334
Picadillo 335
Quick Beef Ragù with Spaghetti Squash 336
Spiced Beef Keema with Chickpeas and Green Peas 337
Persian Ground Beef Kebabs 338
Middle Eastern Meatballs with Feta Sauce 339

Chicken with Sautéed Apples and Swiss Chard

Makes 4 servings

✪ Great for Steps 1, 3 and 4

Welcome the first chill of autumn with this hearty dish. The possibilities for variation are broad — for example, spinach for the Swiss chard, pears for the apples or lean pork chops for the chicken.

1	large bunch red Swiss chard	1
4	boneless skinless chicken breasts (each about 4 oz/125 g)	4
1/2 tsp	fine sea salt, divided	2 mL
1/4 tsp	freshly ground black pepper	1 mL
2 tsp	vegetable oil	10 mL
2	cloves garlic, minced	2
1	large tart-sweet apple (such as Braeburn or Gala), sliced	1
1/2 cup	unsweetened apple juice	125 mL
1 tbsp	Dijon mustard	15 mL

1. Trim stems and center ribs from Swiss chard and chop stems and ribs. Thinly slice the leaves crosswise (to measure about 5 cups/1.25 L).
2. Sprinkle chicken with half the salt and the pepper. In a large skillet, heat oil over medium-high heat. Add chicken and cook, turning once, for 4 to 5 minutes per side or until browned on both sides. Transfer to a plate.
3. Add garlic, apple, the remaining salt, apple juice and mustard to the skillet. Bring to a boil over medium-high heat. Stir in Swiss chard stems and leaves. Reduce heat and simmer, stirring occasionally, for 5 minutes. Return chicken and any accumulated juices to pan. Simmer, stirring occasionally, for 3 to 4 minutes or until no longer pink inside.

Superfood Spotlight

Chicken Breasts • A portion of lean chicken contains nearly half a day's recommended intake of protein for an adult woman, plus a whole day's intake of niacin (vitamin B_3), which is involved in repairing DNA. Lean chicken also makes a large contribution to our intake of minerals, including iron, potassium and the antioxidant zinc. It is especially rich in selenium, a mineral that is often lacking in our diets and that plays a role in thyroid metabolism and has strong anticancer action.

Nutrients per serving	
Calories	217
Total fat	5 g
Saturated fat	0 g
Cholesterol	66 mg
Sodium	608 mg
Carbohydrate	14 g
Fiber	1 g
Protein	29 g
Calcium	17 mg
Iron	2.0 mg

Greek Chicken with Cherry Tomatoes and Feta

Makes 4 servings

✪ Great for Steps 1, 3 and 4

Chicken breasts, workhorses of the weekday dinner world, take on Mediterranean style when accentuated with the flavors of Greece: tomatoes, olives, feta and mint.

2 cups	cherry or grape tomatoes, halved	500 mL
½ cup	packed fresh mint leaves, thinly sliced	125 mL
½ cup	crumbled feta cheese	125 mL
⅓ cup	pitted brine-cured black olives (such as kalamata), roughly chopped	75 mL
3 tsp	extra virgin olive oil, divided	15 mL
½ tsp	fine sea salt, divided	2 mL
½ tsp	freshly cracked black pepper, divided	2 mL
4	boneless skinless chicken breasts (each about 4 oz/125 g)	4

1. In a medium bowl, combine tomatoes, mint, feta, olives, 1 tsp (5 mL) of the oil, half the salt and half the pepper. Let stand until ready to serve.
2. Sprinkle chicken with the remaining salt and pepper. In a large skillet, heat the remaining oil over medium-high heat. Add chicken and cook, turning once, for 5 to 6 minutes per side or until no longer pink inside. Serve with tomato mixture.

Tip

Any leftover tomato mixture can be tucked into a whole wheat pita (perhaps with some spinach leaves or shredded lettuce) for a quick sandwich.

Variation

Replace the tomatoes with a 12-oz (340 mL) jar of roasted red bell peppers, drained and coarsely chopped.

Nutrients per serving	
Calories	254
Total fat	11 g
Saturated fat	4 g
Cholesterol	83 mg
Sodium	630 mg
Carbohydrate	6 g
Fiber	2 g
Protein	32 g
Calcium	117 mg
Iron	2.4 mg

Chicken with Cherry Tomato and Avocado Salsa

Makes 4 servings

✪ Great for Steps 1, 3 and 4

A simple cherry tomato and avocado salsa is served with chicken that's been quickly seared to tender perfection. Enjoy the free time that follows.

Tip

Any leftover salsa can be tucked into a whole wheat pita (perhaps with some spinach leaves or shredded lettuce) for a quick sandwich.

Nutrients per serving	
Calories	257
Total fat	12 g
Saturated fat	1 g
Cholesterol	66 mg
Sodium	561 mg
Carbohydrate	8 g
Fiber	4 g
Protein	29 g
Calcium	12 mg
Iron	2.2 mg

1	small firm-ripe Hass avocado, diced	1
1 cup	cherry or grape tomatoes, quartered	250 mL
1/4 cup	chopped green onions	60 mL
1/4 cup	packed fresh cilantro leaves, chopped	60 mL
1 tbsp	minced seeded jalapeño pepper	15 mL
1/2 tsp	fine sea salt, divided	2 mL
1 tbsp	freshly squeezed lime juice	15 mL
1/4 tsp	freshly cracked black pepper	1 mL
2 tsp	vegetable oil	10 mL
4	boneless skinless chicken breasts (each about 4 oz/125 g)	4

1. In a medium bowl, combine avocado, tomatoes, green onions, cilantro, jalapeño, half the salt, and lime juice.
2. Sprinkle chicken with the remaining salt and pepper. In a large skillet, heat oil over medium-high heat. Add chicken and cook, turning once, for 5 to 6 minutes per side or until an instant-read thermometer inserted in the thickest part of the breast registers 165°F (74°C). Serve with avocado salsa.

Spicy Skillet Chicken with Avocado Mango Salsa

Makes 4 servings

✪ Great for Steps 1, 3 and 4

Avocados and mangos are great superfoods to add to any meal. Creamy avocados are rich in heart-healthy monounsaturated fat, fiber and vitamin E; sweet, tropical mangos add vitamins A and C.

Tip

Any leftover salsa can be tucked into a whole wheat pita (perhaps with some spinach leaves or shredded lettuce) for a quick sandwich.

1	small firm-ripe Hass avocado, diced	1
1 cup	diced mango	250 mL
1/4 cup	packed fresh cilantro leaves, chopped	60 mL
3/4 tsp	chipotle chile powder, divided	3 mL
1/2 tsp	fine sea salt, divided	2 mL
2 tbsp	freshly squeezed lime juice	30 mL
1 tsp	agave nectar or liquid honey	5 mL
4	boneless skinless chicken breasts (each about 4 oz/125 g)	4
3/4 tsp	ground cumin	3 mL
2 tsp	vegetable oil	10 mL

1. In a small bowl, combine avocado, mango, cilantro, 1/4 tsp (1 mL) of the chipotle chile powder, half the salt, lime juice and agave nectar.
2. Sprinkle chicken with cumin, the remaining chile powder and the remaining salt. In a large skillet, heat oil over medium-high heat. Add chicken and cook, turning once, for 5 to 6 minutes per side or until an instant-read thermometer inserted in the thickest part of the breast registers 165°F (74°C). Serve with avocado mango salsa.

Nutrients per serving	
Calories	282
Total fat	12 g
Saturated fat	1 g
Cholesterol	66 mg
Sodium	548 mg
Carbohydrate	14 g
Fiber	4 g
Protein	29 g
Calcium	17 mg
Iron	2.3 mg

Miso Chicken with Crunchy Herb Salad

Makes 4 servings

✪ Great for Steps 1, 3 and 4

A miso-sesame paste smeared on everyday chicken breasts leads to a captivating new take on a weeknight standby; a zesty, crunchy herb salad adds harmonic balance.

Variations

Substitute spinach or tender watercress sprigs for the mesclun.

Replace the cilantro with ¼ cup (60 mL) packed fresh mint leaves.

Nutrients per serving	
Calories	222
Total fat	9 g
Saturated fat	1 g
Cholesterol	66 mg
Sodium	592 mg
Carbohydrate	5 g
Fiber	1 g
Protein	30 g
Calcium	28 mg
Iron	2.2 mg

1 tbsp	minced gingerroot	15 mL
2 tbsp	yellow miso	30 mL
3 tsp	toasted sesame oil, divided	15 mL
3 tsp	unseasoned rice vinegar, divided	15 mL
1 tsp	Asian chili-garlic sauce	5 mL
4	boneless skinless chicken breasts (each about 4 oz/125 g)	4
3 cups	mesclun (mixed baby lettuce)	750 mL
1 cup	chopped celery	250 mL
½ cup	packed fresh cilantro leaves	125 mL
¼ cup	chopped fresh chives	60 mL
⅛ tsp	fine sea salt	0.5 mL
2 tsp	vegetable oil	10 mL

1. In a shallow dish, whisk together ginger, miso, 1½ tsp (7 mL) of the sesame oil, 2 tsp (10 mL) of the vinegar and chili-garlic sauce. Add chicken and turn to coat. Cover and refrigerate for 1 to 2 hours.
2. When ready to serve, in a medium bowl, combine mesclun, celery, cilantro, chives, salt, the remaining sesame oil and the remaining vinegar. Toss to combine.
3. In a large skillet, heat vegetable oil over medium-high heat. Remove chicken from marinade, discarding marinade, and add to skillet. Cook, turning once, for 5 to 6 minutes per side or until an instant-read thermometer inserted in the thickest part of the breast registers 165°F (74°C). Serve with herb salad.

▶ Health Note

Sesame oil is an excellent source of polyunsaturated fatty acids — including omega-3, omega-6 and omega-9 — which aid in the prevention and treatment of chronic diseases such as coronary heart disease, hypertension, diabetes and arthritis. It has also been shown to help lower blood pressure, increase good cholesterol, decrease bad cholesterol and help maintain normal blood pressure levels.

Thai Chicken and Basil

Makes 4 servings

✪ Great for Steps 1, 3 and 4

Tip

If chicken breast cutlets are not available, use 1 lb (500 g) chicken breasts and cut them into cutlets. Place one breast on a cutting board. With one hand flat on top, use a large, sharp knife in the other hand to cut the breast in half horizontally. Separate the chicken into two slices. Place a sheet of waxed paper on top of a cutting board. Place one of the chicken slices on the waxed paper, then lay another piece of waxed paper on top. Pound the chicken with a meat mallet or rolling pin until it is an even 1/4 inch (0.5 cm) thick throughout the whole piece. Repeat with the second slice and the remaining chicken breasts.

Nutrients per serving	
Calories	210
Total fat	5 g
Saturated fat	0 g
Cholesterol	66 mg
Sodium	598 mg
Carbohydrate	11 g
Fiber	2 g
Protein	29 g
Calcium	35 mg
Iron	2.1 mg

1 tbsp	fish sauce (nam pla)	15 mL
1 tbsp	freshly squeezed lime juice	15 mL
2 tsp	brown rice syrup or liquid honey	10 mL
2 tsp	vegetable oil	10 mL
1 1/2 cups	thinly sliced onions	375 mL
1 lb	chicken breast cutlets, cut crosswise into 1/2-inch (1 cm) wide strips	500 g
2	cloves garlic, thinly sliced	2
1/4 tsp	hot pepper flakes	1 mL
1/4 cup	water	60 mL
1 cup	packed fresh basil leaves, torn	250 mL

1. In a small bowl or cup, whisk together fish sauce, lime juice and brown rice syrup.
2. In a large skillet, heat oil over medium-high heat. Add onions and cook, stirring, for 5 minutes or until slightly softened. Add chicken, garlic and hot pepper flakes; cook, stirring, for 2 to 3 minutes or until chicken is browned on all sides.
3. Stir in fish sauce mixture and water; cook, stirring, for 2 to 3 minutes or until sauce is slightly thickened and chicken is no longer pink inside. Remove from heat and stir in basil. Let stand for 1 minute or until basil is wilted.

Superfood Spotlight

Basil • Basil is perhaps best known as the main ingredient in the Italian sauce pesto, but it has been a component of Indian and Mediterranean cuisines for thousands of years. It has also long been used in traditional herbal medicine as a remedy for indigestion, nausea and stomachache. Basil is mildly sedative and contains strongly antioxidant flavonoid compounds. Volatile oils in the leaves contain chemicals that fight food poisoning bacteria, as well as the chemical eugenol, an anti-inflammatory similar to aspirin that can help relieve the pain of arthritis and may ease irritable bowel syndrome. An infusion of basil oil can even be used as an insect repellent and to offer relief from stings.

Broccoli, Asparagus and Chicken Stir-Fry

Makes 4 servings

✪ Great for Steps 1, 3 and 4

No take-out food comes close to rivaling a simple, homemade stir-fry — especially when intensely flavorful hoisin sauce is added to the mix.

Tip

You can also use chicken or turkey breast cutlets, cut into thin strips, in place of the chicken breasts.

2 tbsp	toasted sesame oil, divided	30 mL
3	cloves garlic, minced	3
1 lb	asparagus, trimmed and cut into 1-inch (2.5 cm) pieces	500 g
2 cups	small broccoli florets	500 mL
½ cup	reduced-sodium ready-to-use chicken or vegetable broth, divided	125 mL
1 lb	boneless skinless chicken breasts, cut into thin strips	500 g
¼ tsp	fine sea salt	1 mL
⅛ tsp	cayenne pepper	0.5 mL
½ cup	chopped green onions	125 mL
¼ cup	hoisin sauce	60 mL

1. In a large skillet, heat half the oil over medium-high heat. Add garlic and cook, stirring, for 30 seconds. Add asparagus, broccoli and half the broth; cover and cook for about 3 minutes or until vegetables are tender-crisp. Transfer vegetable mixture to a bowl.
2. Sprinkle chicken with salt and cayenne. In the same skillet, heat the remaining oil over medium-high heat. Add chicken and green onions; cook, stirring, for 3 to 4 minutes or until chicken is no longer pink inside. Return vegetable mixture to the pan and add the remaining broth and hoisin; cook, stirring, for 1 minute.

Nutrients per serving	
Calories	271
Total fat	10 g
Saturated fat	1 g
Cholesterol	61 mg
Sodium	552 mg
Carbohydrate	17 g
Fiber	4 g
Protein	30 g
Calcium	51 mg
Iron	2.8 mg

Spicy Chicken, Spinach and Peanut Stir-Fry

Makes 4 servings

✪ Great for Steps 1, 3 and 4

A final sprinkling of peanuts adds both body and crunch to this filling stir-fry. The basil and ginger add hits of freshness and heat, respectively, as well as vivid flavor.

Tip

Look for roasted peanuts lightly seasoned with sea salt.

1 tbsp	vegetable oil	15 mL
2	large red bell peppers, thinly sliced	2
1 lb	boneless skinless chicken breasts, cut into thin strips	500 g
6	green onions, trimmed and cut into 2-inch (5 cm) pieces	6
3 tbsp	minced gingerroot	45 mL
8 cups	packed spinach leaves (about 6 oz/175 g)	2 L
3 tbsp	reduced-sodium tamari or soy sauce	45 mL
2 tbsp	unseasoned rice vinegar	30 mL
1 tbsp	brown rice syrup or liquid honey	15 mL
1 tbsp	Asian chile-garlic sauce	15 mL
1 cup	packed fresh basil leaves	250 mL
$\frac{1}{3}$ cup	lightly salted roasted peanuts	75 mL

1. In a large skillet, heat oil over medium-high heat. Add red peppers and cook, stirring, for 5 to 6 minutes or until slightly softened. Add chicken, green onions and ginger; cook, stirring, for 2 minutes.
2. Add half the spinach, tamari, vinegar, brown rice syrup and chile-garlic sauce; cook, stirring, for 1 minute or until spinach is wilted. Add the remaining spinach and basil; cook, stirring, for 1 minute or until spinach is wilted and chicken is no longer pink inside. Serve sprinkled with peanuts.

Superfood Spotlight

Spinach • Spinach is a powerhouse of health benefits. Its many flavonoid compounds act as antioxidants, fighting against stomach, skin, breast, prostate and other cancers. Spinach is also rich in carotenes (which protect eyesight) and vitamin K (which boosts bone strength and may help prevent osteoporosis). In addition, spinach contains peptides, aspects of protein that have been shown to lower blood pressure. Its relatively high vitamin E content may help protect the brain from cognitive decline as we age.

Nutrients per serving

Calories	306
Total fat	12 g
Saturated fat	1 g
Cholesterol	60 mg
Sodium	589 mg
Carbohydrate	19 g
Fiber	6 g
Protein	32 g
Calcium	86 mg
Iron	4.6 mg

Stir-Fried Tangerine Chicken

Makes 4 servings

✪ Great for Steps 3 and 4

Tangerines have an impressive tart-sweet citrus flavor that is both distinctive and extraordinarily delicious in this easily assembled stir-fry.

Tip

If you can't find tangerines, use orange zest and juice instead.

1 lb	boneless skinless chicken breasts, cut into thin strips	500 g
1/4 tsp	fine sea salt	1 mL
1/4 tsp	freshly cracked black pepper	1 mL
2 tsp	vegetable oil	10 mL
1 tbsp	minced gingerroot	15 mL
1 tsp	finely grated tangerine zest	5 mL
1/4 cup	freshly squeezed tangerine juice	60 mL
3 tbsp	orange marmalade	45 mL
3 tbsp	reduced-sodium tamari or soy sauce	45 mL
1 tbsp	freshly squeezed lime juice	15 mL
1/2 cup	thinly sliced green onions	125 mL

1. Sprinkle chicken with salt and pepper. In a large skillet, heat oil over medium-high heat. Add chicken and cook, stirring, for 3 minutes.
2. Stir in ginger, tangerine zest, tangerine juice, marmalade and tamari. Bring to a boil, stirring constantly. Boil, stirring, for 1 minute or until sauce is slightly thickened and chicken is no longer pink inside. Remove from heat and stir in lime juice. Serve sprinkled with green onions.

▸ Health Note

Tangerines have an abundance of impressive nutrients, notably vitamins A and C, which can stop free radicals from damaging oxygen cells. They also contain tangeritin, a flavonoid that appears to be extremely potent against several types of breast cancer.

Nutrients per serving	
Calories	208
Total fat	5 g
Saturated fat	0 g
Cholesterol	60 mg
Sodium	607 mg
Carbohydrate	15 g
Fiber	0 g
Protein	26 g
Calcium	12 mg
Iron	2.1 mg

Chicken Souvlaki

Makes 4 servings

✪ Great for Steps 1, 3, 4 and 5

You can hold the pickles, ketchup and mustard on hamburgers and hot dogs, but when it comes to Greek fast food — like this quick, easy and addictively delicious chicken souvlaki — don't skip the onions. In their many layers are multiple phytonutrients that studies indicate can help lower cholesterol and ward off cancer. Plus, due to their high vitamin C content, onions can even help fight the common cold. More souvlaki with onions, please!

Tip

An equal amount of diced tomatoes may be used in place of the cherry tomatoes.

Nutrients per serving	
Calories	400
Total fat	7 g
Saturated fat	1 g
Cholesterol	60 mg
Sodium	598 mg
Carbohydrate	50 g
Fiber	8 g
Protein	37 g
Calcium	75 mg
Iron	4.3 mg

1 cup	shredded seeded peeled cucumber	250 mL
1/4 cup	packed fresh flat-leaf (Italian) parsley	60 mL
1 tsp	fine sea salt, divided	5 mL
2/3 cup	nonfat plain Greek yogurt	150 mL
1 tsp	finely grated lemon zest	5 mL
2 tsp	freshly squeezed lemon juice	10 mL
2 tsp	extra virgin olive oil	10 mL
1	red bell pepper, thinly sliced	1
1 1/2 cups	sliced onions	375 mL
1 lb	boneless skinless chicken breasts, cut into thin strips	500 g
2	cloves garlic, minced	2
1 tsp	dried oregano	5 mL
1/4 tsp	freshly cracked black pepper	1 mL
4	6-inch (15 cm) whole wheat pitas, warmed	4
1 1/2 cups	halved cherry or grape tomatoes	375 mL

1. In a small bowl, combine cucumber, parsley, 1/4 tsp (1 mL) of the salt, yogurt, lemon zest and lemon juice. Cover and refrigerate until ready to use.
2. In a large skillet, heat oil over medium-high heat. Add red pepper and onions; cook, stirring, for 6 to 8 minutes or until softened. Add chicken, garlic, oregano, pepper and the remaining salt; cook, stirring, for 5 to 6 minutes or until chicken is no longer pink inside.
3. Place a warmed pita on each dinner plate. Arrange chicken on pitas, along with cherry tomatoes and yogurt sauce.

Chicken Shwarma

Makes 4 servings

✪ Great for Steps 1, 3, 4 and 5

At once exotic and homey, this Middle Eastern chicken dish has warming spices that delight the palate and, according to some of the newest laboratory research, may help heal the body. For example, turmeric (a primary ingredient in many Indian yellow curry powder and paste blends) contains a compound called curcumin, which has been shown to protect the eyes from free radicals, one of the leading causes of cataracts.

Nutrients per serving	
Calories	414
Total fat	10 g
Saturated fat	1 g
Cholesterol	60 mg
Sodium	621 mg
Carbohydrate	45 g
Fiber	6 g
Protein	37 g
Calcium	73 mg
Iron	4.9 mg

- **Six 10-inch (25 cm) metal skewers, or wooden skewers soaked in warm water for 30 minutes**

4	cloves garlic, minced	4
2 tsp	mild curry powder	10 mL
1½ tsp	ground cumin	7 mL
1½ tsp	ground ginger	7 mL
¾ tsp	fine sea salt, divided	3 mL
3 tbsp	freshly squeezed lemon juice, divided	45 mL
2 tsp	extra virgin olive oil	10 mL
1 lb	boneless skinless chicken breasts, cut into thin strips	500 g
⅔ cup	nonfat plain Greek yogurt	150 mL
2 tbsp	tahini	30 mL
4	6-inch (15 cm) whole wheat pitas	4
1 cup	chopped romaine lettuce	250 mL
1	large tomato, sliced	1

1. In a large bowl, whisk together garlic, curry powder, cumin, ginger, ½ tsp (2 mL) of the salt, 2 tbsp (30 mL) of the lemon juice, and oil. Add chicken and toss to coat. Let stand for 20 minutes.
2. Meanwhile, preheat barbecue grill to medium-high.
3. In a small bowl, whisk together yogurt, tahini, the remaining lemon juice and the remaining salt. Cover and refrigerate until ready to use.
4. Remove chicken from marinade, discarding marinade, and thread chicken onto skewers. Grill for 3 to 5 minutes per side or until chicken is no longer pink inside. Transfer to a plate.
5. Place pitas on grill and warm for 1 minute per side.
6. Place a pita on each dinner plate. Remove chicken from skewers and place on pitas, along with lettuce and tomato. Drizzle with yogurt sauce.

Japanese Sesame Chicken Skewers

Makes 4 servings

✪ Great for Steps 1, 3 and 4

A riff on a Japanese classic, this easy version of chicken teriyaki gets a boost of fresh flavor and bold red color from red peppers. Serve with brown rice.

Tip

To toast sesame seeds, place up to 3 tbsp (45 mL) seeds in a medium skillet set over medium heat. Cook, shaking the skillet, for 3 to 5 minutes or until seeds are golden brown and fragrant. Let cool completely before use.

Nutrients per serving	
Calories	225
Total fat	6 g
Saturated fat	0 g
Cholesterol	60 mg
Sodium	577 mg
Carbohydrate	11 g
Fiber	1 g
Protein	28 g
Calcium	21 mg
Iron	2.2 mg

- **Six 10-inch (25 cm) metal skewers, or wooden skewers soaked in warm water for 30 minutes**

1 tbsp	minced gingerroot	15 mL
1⁄4 cup	mirin or sherry	60 mL
1⁄4 cup	reduced-sodium tamari or soy sauce	60 mL
1 tsp	toasted sesame oil	5 mL
1 lb	boneless skinless chicken breasts, cut into 1-inch (2.5 cm) strips	500 g
1	large red bell pepper, cut into 1-inch (2.5 cm) pieces	1
2 tbsp	toasted sesame seeds (see tip, at left)	30 mL

1. In a large bowl, whisk together ginger, mirin, tamari and sesame oil. Add chicken and toss to coat. Let stand for 15 minutes.
2. Meanwhile, preheat barbecue grill to medium-high.
3. Remove chicken from marinade, reserving marinade. Alternately thread chicken and red pepper onto skewers.
4. In a small saucepan, bring reserved marinade to a boil over medium-high heat. Boil until reduced by about half. Brush skewers with marinade.
5. Grill skewers for 3 to 5 minutes per side, brushing occasionally with marinade, until chicken is no longer pink inside. Serve sprinkled with sesame seeds.

▶ Health Note

A quick spell on the grill does more than just enhance the flavor of a bell pepper — it also releases the beta carotene from the pepper's fiber cells.

Chicken and Zucchini Spiedini with Salsa Verde

Makes 4 servings

✪ Great for Steps 1, 3 and 4

Both chicken and zucchini have a natural affinity for the grill. Case in point, chicken spiedini, the Italian version of kebabs. A quick, emerald blender sauce enriches the flavor of the kebabs and boosts your health in one fell swoop: this briny, grassy and citrusy salsa verde is a vitamin C superstar, thanks to the fresh parsley and lemon.

Tip

Other tender summer squash, such as crookneck or pattypan, may be used in place of the zucchini.

Nutrients per serving	
Calories	175
Total fat	6 g
Saturated fat	1 g
Cholesterol	60 mg
Sodium	620 mg
Carbohydrate	4 g
Fiber	1 g
Protein	26 g
Calcium	27 mg
Iron	2.5 mg

- **Preheat barbecue grill to medium-high**
- **Blender or food processor**
- **Six 10-inch (25 cm) metal skewers, or wooden skewers soaked in warm water for 30 minutes**

Salsa Verde

1	clove garlic	1
1 cup	packed fresh flat-leaf (Italian) parsley leaves	250 mL
2 tbsp	drained capers	30 mL
1 tsp	finely grated lemon zest	5 mL
3 tbsp	water	45 mL
2 tbsp	freshly squeezed lemon juice	30 mL
1 tbsp	extra virgin olive oil	15 mL

Spiedini

1 lb	boneless skinless chicken breasts, cut into 1-inch (2.5 cm) cubes	500 g
3	zucchini, cut crosswise into 1-inch (2.5 cm) slices	3
	Nonstick cooking spray (preferably olive oil)	
½ tsp	fine sea salt	2 mL
¼ tsp	freshly ground black pepper	1 mL

1. *Salsa:* In blender, combine garlic, parsley, capers, lemon zest, water, lemon juice and oil; purée until smooth.
2. *Spiedini:* Thread chicken and zucchini onto skewers. Spray with cooking spray and sprinkle with salt and pepper. Grill on preheated barbecue for 3 to 5 minutes per side or until chicken is no longer pink inside. Serve with salsa.

Cuban Chicken with Black Beans and Brown Rice

Makes 4 servings

✪ Great for Steps 3, 4 and 5

With nutrients ranging from protein and fiber to isoflavones, black beans can power you through the busiest days and, in the case of this Cuban-inspired main dish, do so with tremendous flavor and flair.

2 tsp	extra virgin olive oil	10 mL
1 cup	chopped onion	250 mL
1 lb	boneless skinless chicken breasts, cut into 1-inch (2.5 cm) cubes	500 g
4	cloves garlic, minced	4
2½ tsp	ground cumin	12 mL
1½ tsp	dried oregano	7 mL
½ tsp	fine sea salt	2 mL
½ tsp	freshly cracked black pepper	2 mL
1	can (14 to 19 oz/398 to 540 mL) black beans, drained and rinsed	1
1	can (14 to 15 oz/398 to 425 mL) diced tomatoes, with juice	1
1 tbsp	finely grated orange zest	15 mL
¼ cup	freshly squeezed orange juice	60 mL
3 cups	hot cooked long-grain brown rice (see page 438)	750 mL

1. In a large skillet, heat oil over medium-high heat. Add onion and cook, stirring, for 5 minutes or until slightly softened. Add chicken, garlic, cumin, oregano, salt and pepper; cook, stirring, for 4 minutes or until chicken is browned on all sides.
2. Stir in beans, tomatoes with juice, orange zest and orange juice. Reduce heat and simmer, stirring occasionally, for 5 to 7 minutes or until sauce is slightly thickened and chicken is no longer pink inside.
3. Divide rice among four shallow bowls and top with chicken mixture.

Nutrients per serving	
Calories	459
Total fat	7 g
Saturated fat	1 g
Cholesterol	60 mg
Sodium	646 mg
Carbohydrate	62 g
Fiber	9 g
Protein	36 g
Calcium	98 mg
Iron	4.5 mg

Jamaican Chicken Couscous

Makes 6 servings

✪ Great for Steps 3, 4 and 5

Ready-made spice blends are a busy home cook's best friend. Here, Jamaican jerk seasoning transports chicken and couscous down to the island in a matter of minutes.

Variation

Substitute dried cranberries, dark raisins or chopped dried apricots for the golden raisins.

1 lb	boneless skinless chicken breasts, cut into 1-inch (2.5 cm) cubes	500 g
1 tbsp	salt-free dry Jamaican jerk seasoning	15 mL
1/2 tsp	fine sea salt	2 mL
1 tbsp	vegetable oil	15 mL
1 cup	reduced-sodium ready-to-use chicken or vegetable broth	250 mL
1 tbsp	finely grated orange zest	15 mL
1 cup	freshly squeezed orange juice	250 mL
1 1/4 cups	whole wheat couscous	300 mL
1/2 cup	golden raisins	125 mL
2/3 cup	thinly sliced green onions	150 mL
2 tbsp	sliced toasted almonds	30 mL

1. In a large sealable plastic bag, combine chicken, jerk seasoning and salt, shaking to coat chicken.
2. In a large skillet, heat oil over medium-high heat. Add chicken and cook, stirring, for 6 to 8 minutes or until no longer pink inside.
3. Stir in broth, orange zest and orange juice. Bring to a boil. Stir in couscous and raisins. Remove from heat, cover and let stand for 5 minutes. Fluff couscous with a fork. Serve sprinkled with green onions and almonds.

Nutrients per serving	
Calories	335
Total fat	6 g
Saturated fat	0 g
Cholesterol	40 mg
Sodium	456 mg
Carbohydrate	48 g
Fiber	6 g
Protein	24 g
Calcium	41 mg
Iron	3.1 mg

Pineapple Mint Chicken

Makes 4 servings

✪ Great for Steps 1, 3 and 4

Match a relaxed weekend day with an equally laid-back supper: spiced lemon chicken, a pineapple-mint pan sauce and but one skillet to clean. Serve with whole wheat couscous or brown rice.

Tip

A pineapple is ripe enough to eat when a leaf is easily pulled from the top. To prepare pineapple, cut off the leafy top and a small layer of the base, then slice off the tough skin and "eyes." Cut the flesh into slices, then remove the chewy central core from each slice.

1 tsp	ground cardamom	5 mL
1 tsp	finely grated lemon zest	5 mL
1/2 tsp	fine sea salt	2 mL
1/4 tsp	freshly ground black pepper	1 mL
1 lb	boneless skinless chicken breasts, cut into 1-inch (2.5 cm) cubes	500 g
2 tsp	vegetable oil	10 mL
1 cup	chopped onion	250 mL
2 cups	coarsely chopped fresh or thawed frozen pineapple	500 mL
1/2 cup	unsweetened pineapple juice	125 mL
1/4 cup	reduced-sodium ready-to-use chicken or vegetable broth	60 mL
1/2 cup	packed fresh mint leaves, chopped	125 mL

1. In a small bowl, combine cardamom, lemon zest, salt and pepper. Sprinkle over chicken.
2. In a large skillet, heat oil over medium-high heat. Add onion and cook, stirring, for 5 to 6 minutes or until softened. Push onion to sides of pan and add chicken; cook, stirring, for 2 to 3 minutes or until white all over.
3. Stir in pineapple, pineapple juice and broth. Increase heat to high and bring to a boil. Reduce heat and simmer, stirring occasionally, for 4 to 5 minutes, scraping up brown bits on bottom of pan, until sauce is thickened and chicken is no longer pink inside. Serve sprinkled with mint.

Nutrients per serving	
Calories	280
Total fat	5 g
Saturated fat	0 g
Cholesterol	60 mg
Sodium	492 mg
Carbohydrate	33 g
Fiber	3 g
Protein	27 g
Calcium	44 mg
Iron	2.4 mg

Chicken Biryani

Makes 4 servings

✪ Great for Steps 1, 3, 4 and 5

The preparation for this version of chicken biryani — a favorite Punjabi chicken dish from northern India — may not be strictly traditional, but the resulting flavor is. Raisins are a key ingredient, offsetting the spice and heat of the dish with a delicate sweetness.

Tip

Look for roasted pistachios lightly seasoned with sea salt.

2 tsp	vegetable oil	10 mL
1 cup	chopped onion	250 mL
3	cloves garlic, minced	3
2 tbsp	minced gingerroot	30 mL
2 tsp	garam masala	10 mL
2 tsp	ground cumin	10 mL
3/4 tsp	fine sea salt	3 mL
1/8 tsp	cayenne pepper	0.5 mL
1 lb	boneless skinless chicken breasts, cut into 1-inch (2.5 cm) cubes	500 g
1	can (14 to 15 oz/398 to 425 mL) petite diced tomatoes, with juice	1
1 cup	brown basmati or other long-grain brown rice	250 mL
1/3 cup	golden raisins	75 mL
1 3/4 cups	reduced-sodium ready-to-use chicken broth	425 mL
3/4 cup	water	175 mL
1/4 cup	packed fresh cilantro leaves, chopped	60 mL
2 tbsp	freshly squeezed lime juice	30 mL
1/4 cup	chopped lightly salted roasted pistachios	60 mL

1. In a large skillet, heat oil over medium-high heat. Add onion and cook, stirring, for 5 to 6 minutes or until softened. Add garlic, ginger, garam masala, cumin, salt and cayenne; cook, stirring, for 1 minute. Add chicken and cook, stirring, for 3 to 5 minutes or until browned on all sides.
2. Stir in tomatoes with juice, rice, raisins, broth and water. Bring to a boil. Reduce heat to low, cover and simmer, stirring occasionally, for 40 to 45 minutes or until rice is tender. Stir in cilantro and lime juice. Serve sprinkled with pistachios.

▸ Health Note

Raisins are high in fiber, rich in iron and a good source of potassium, a mineral that has been shown to lower high blood pressure.

Nutrients per serving	
Calories	353
Total fat	9 g
Saturated fat	1 g
Cholesterol	60 mg
Sodium	645 mg
Carbohydrate	36 g
Fiber	4 g
Protein	31 g
Calcium	60 mg
Iron	3.6 mg

Spring Vegetable Chicken Quinoa

Makes 6 servings

✪ Great for Steps 1, 3, 4 and 5

Quinoa adds a stick-to-the-ribs earthiness to this chicken dish, while peas, asparagus and lemon render it just right for spring.

Tip

An equal amount of fresh mint or cilantro leaves may be used in place of the parsley.

1 tbsp	extra virgin olive oil	15 mL
6	green onions, thinly sliced crosswise, white and green parts separated	6
1 cup	quinoa, rinsed	250 mL
2 tsp	finely grated lemon zest	10 mL
3/4 tsp	fine sea salt	3 mL
1/2 tsp	freshly cracked black pepper	2 mL
2 cups	water	500 mL
1 lb	asparagus, trimmed and cut into 1/2-inch (1 cm) pieces	500 g
2 cups	diced cooked chicken breast	500 mL
2/3 cup	frozen petite peas, thawed	150 mL
1 tbsp	freshly squeezed lemon juice	15 mL
1/4 cup	packed fresh flat-leaf (Italian) parsley leaves, chopped	60 mL

1. In a medium saucepan, heat oil over medium-high heat. Add white parts of green onions and cook, stirring, for 2 to 3 minutes or until softened.
2. Stir in quinoa, lemon zest, salt, pepper and water. Bring to a boil. Reduce heat to low, cover and simmer for 11 minutes. Stir in asparagus, cover and simmer for 4 to 5 minutes or until liquid is absorbed and quinoa and asparagus are tender.
3. Remove from heat and stir in chicken, peas and lemon juice. Cover and let stand for 2 minutes to warm through. Stir in parsley and green parts of green onions.

Nutrients per serving	
Calories	253
Total fat	6 g
Saturated fat	1 g
Cholesterol	40 mg
Sodium	525 mg
Carbohydrate	27 g
Fiber	5 g
Protein	24 g
Calcium	56 mg
Iron	3.3 mg

Chicken and Black Bean Chilaquiles

Makes 6 servings

✪ Great for Steps 1, 3, 4 and 5

Once a way to make use of stale tortillas, chilaquiles are so good that it wasn't long before people simply started using fresh tortillas so they could enjoy this meal anytime.

- **Preheat oven to 450°F (230°C)**
- **9-inch (23 cm) glass baking dish, sprayed with nonstick cooking spray (preferably olive oil)**

1 tsp	vegetable oil	5 mL
1 cup	thinly sliced onion	250 mL
4	cloves garlic, minced	4
2 cups	diced or shredded cooked chicken breast	500 mL
1½ tsp	ground cumin	7 mL
1	can (14 to 19 oz/398 to 540 mL) black beans, drained and rinsed	1
1	can (10 oz/284 mL) diced tomatoes with chiles, with juice	1
1 cup	reduced-sodium ready-to-use chicken broth	250 mL
15	6-inch (15 cm) corn tortillas, cut into 1-inch (2.5 cm) strips	15
½ cup	crumbled queso fresco or feta cheese	125 mL

1. In a large skillet, heat oil over medium-high heat. Add onion and cook, stirring, for 5 to 6 minutes or until softened. Add garlic, chicken and cumin; cook, stirring, for 1 minute. Remove from heat and stir in beans.
2. In a medium bowl, combine tomatoes with juice and broth.
3. Arrange half the tortilla strips in bottom of prepared baking dish. Layer half the chicken mixture over tortillas. Top with the remaining tortillas and chicken mixture. Pour tomato mixture evenly over top. Sprinkle with cheese.
4. Bake in preheated oven for 12 to 15 minutes or until tortillas are lightly browned and cheese is melted.

▶ Health Note

Corn tortillas are more than just a convenient and inexpensive ingredient. Research has determined that corn increases the absorption of iron by up to 50%, making it a good aid in preventing iron-deficiency anemia. In addition, the American Institute for Cancer Research includes corn and corn tortillas on a list of foods that lower the risk of cancer and promote overall health.

Nutrients per serving	
Calories	340
Total fat	7 g
Saturated fat	2 g
Cholesterol	29 mg
Sodium	478 mg
Carbohydrate	51 g
Fiber	6 g
Protein	16 g
Calcium	106 mg
Iron	1.9 mg

Chicken Sausage and Black-Eyed Peas

Makes 6 servings

✪ Great for Steps 1, 3 and 4

This quick and hearty dish is an ode to hoppin' john, the traditional Southern dish eaten for the New Year to bring good luck. It is pure comfort food, and a powerhouse of nutrients thanks to the antioxidant-rich mustard greens and high-protein, high-fiber black-eyed peas. Chili wishes it could be this delicious and nutritious.

Tip

One pound (500 g) of chopped trimmed fresh mustard greens may be used in place of the frozen greens. After adding the greens in step 2, boil, without stirring, for 4 to 5 minutes or until greens are wilted but not yet tender. Continue with step 2.

Nutrients per serving	
Calories	276
Total fat	12 g
Saturated fat	4 g
Cholesterol	65 mg
Sodium	639 mg
Carbohydrate	24 g
Fiber	7 g
Protein	16 g
Calcium	146 mg
Iron	2.9 mg

2 tsp	vegetable oil	10 mL
12 oz	fully cooked chicken sausages, thinly sliced crosswise	375 g
1 cup	chopped onion	250 mL
3	cloves garlic, minced	3
1 tsp	dried thyme	5 mL
1/2 tsp	fine sea salt	2 mL
1/8 tsp	cayenne pepper	0.5 mL
1 cup	reduced-sodium ready-to-use vegetable or chicken broth	250 mL
1	package (10 oz/300 g) frozen chopped mustard greens	1
2	cans (each 14 to 19 oz/398 to 540 mL) black-eyed peas, drained and rinsed	2

1. In a large pot, heat oil over medium-high heat. Add sausages and onion; cook, stirring, for about 5 minutes or until sausages are browned and onions are slightly softened. Add garlic, thyme, salt and cayenne; cook, stirring, for 30 seconds.
2. Stir in broth and bring to a boil. Add mustard greens and boil, without stirring, for 2 to 3 minutes or until greens are thawed. Stir to combine. Add black-eyed peas. Reduce heat to low, cover and simmer, stirring occasionally, for 10 to 15 minutes or until greens are tender.

Turkey Sausage with Mustard Greens and Kidney Beans

Makes 6 servings

✪ Great for Steps 1, 3 and 4

Nuggets of sausage lend some meatball action to this hearty one-pot supper that's chock-full of antioxidant-rich mustard greens and dark red kidney beans.

Tip

Two pounds (1 kg) of chopped trimmed fresh mustard greens may be used in place of the frozen greens. After adding the greens in step 2, boil, without stirring, for 4 to 5 minutes or until greens are wilted but not yet tender. Continue with step 2.

2 tsp	extra virgin olive oil	10 mL
1½ lbs	Italian turkey sausage (bulk or casings removed)	750 g
2	large onions, quartered	2
2	cans (each 14 to 19 oz/398 to 540 mL) dark red kidney beans, drained and rinsed	2
2 tsp	ground cumin	10 mL
½ tsp	freshly cracked black pepper	2 mL
¾ cup	reduced-sodium ready-to-use chicken or vegetable broth	175 mL
2	packages (each 10 oz/300 g) frozen chopped mustard greens	2
1 tsp	red wine vinegar	5 mL

1. In a large pot, heat oil over medium-high heat. Add sausage and cook, breaking it up with a spoon, for 6 to 8 minutes or until no longer pink. Add onions and cook, stirring occasionally and breaking onions up with spoon, for 8 to 10 minutes or until softened.
2. Stir in beans, cumin, pepper and broth. Bring to a boil and boil for 2 minutes. Add mustard greens and boil, without stirring, for 2 to 3 minutes or until greens are thawed. Stir to combine. Reduce heat to low, cover and simmer, stirring occasionally, for 10 to 15 minutes or until greens are tender.

Superfood Spotlight

Kidney Beans • Dark red kidney beans are an invaluable pantry staple, as they are high in good-quality protein and minerals, all for cents on the dollar. An average portion of kidney beans contains at least a quarter of a day's iron needs, to help prevent anemia and increase energy levels, while their zinc content helps boost the immune system and maintain fertility. The high amount of insoluble fiber helps prevent colon cancer, and the total fiber content helps people with diabetes or insulin resistance regulate blood sugar levels.

Nutrients per serving	
Calories	382
Total fat	11 g
Saturated fat	5 g
Cholesterol	67 mg
Sodium	694 mg
Carbohydrate	38 g
Fiber	13 g
Protein	31 g
Calcium	233 mg
Iron	15.8 mg

Turkey Sausage, Spinach and Chickpea Ragù

Makes 6 servings

✪ Great for Steps 1, 3 and 4

This hearty ragù gets its heft from Italian turkey sausage and chickpeas. With the addition of a heap of superfood spinach — loaded with carotenoids, vitamin C, calcium, iron and folate — it's as healthy as it is stick-to-the-ribs good. Serve with crusty whole-grain bread.

Variation

An equal amount of white beans (such as Great Northern or cannellini) may be used in place of the chickpeas.

Nutrients per serving	
Calories	285
Total fat	10 g
Saturated fat	3 g
Cholesterol	33 mg
Sodium	636 mg
Carbohydrate	33 g
Fiber	10 g
Protein	20 g
Calcium	205 mg
Iron	9.8 mg

2 tsp	extra virgin olive oil	10 mL
1½ cups	chopped onions	375 mL
12 oz	Italian turkey sausage (bulk or casings removed)	375 g
¼ tsp	fine sea salt	1 mL
⅛ tsp	cayenne pepper	0.5 mL
¼ cup	tomato paste	60 mL
2	cans (each 14 to 19 oz/398 to 540 mL) chickpeas, drained and rinsed	2
1¼ cups	reduced-sodium ready-to-use vegetable or chicken broth	300 mL
2	packages (each 10 oz/300 g) frozen spinach	2

1. In a large pot, heat oil over medium-high heat. Add onions and cook, stirring, for 5 to 6 minutes or until softened. Add sausage and cook, breaking it up with a spoon, for 6 to 8 minutes or until no longer pink. Add salt, cayenne and tomato paste; cook, stirring, for 1 minute.
2. Stir in chickpeas and broth. Bring to a boil. Add spinach and cook, without stirring, for 2 minutes or until spinach is thawed. Stir to combine. Reduce heat to low, cover and simmer, stirring occasionally, for 5 minutes.

Stuffed Swiss Chard Leaves

Makes 4 servings

✪ Great for Steps 1, 3, 4 and 5

Any variety of Swiss chard will work in this dish, but use rainbow chard if you can. It has the familiar mineral quality of spinach, but with hints of beet thanks to the red- or orange-hued ribs. Here, the mild, sea-salty leaves work in perfect contrast to a rustic filling of sausage, marinara sauce and Parmesan cheese.

Tip

Any variety of Swiss chard leaves may be used in this recipe.

1 lb	Italian turkey sausage (bulk or casings removed)	500 g
1	large egg, beaten	1
1 cup	fresh whole wheat bread crumbs	250 mL
½ cup	finely chopped onion	125 mL
2 tsp	dried Italian seasoning	10 mL
8	large Swiss chard leaves, tough stems removed	8
1½ cups	reduced-sodium ready-to-use beef or vegetable broth	375 mL
1	jar (26 oz/700 mL) reduced-sodium marinara sauce	1
⅓ cup	freshly grated Parmesan cheese	75 mL

1. In a large bowl, gently combine sausage, egg, bread crumbs, onion and Italian seasoning. Form into eight 3-inch (7.5 cm) oblong portions.
2. Place Swiss chard leaves on a work surface, underside of leaves facing up. Place a portion of sausage mixture in the center of each leaf. Tuck in ends, then tightly roll leaf around filling.
3. Place rolls, seam side down, in a large skillet. Pour in broth, cover and bring to a boil over high heat. Reduce heat and simmer, stirring occasionally, for 8 to 10 minutes or until no longer pink inside. Discard broth.
4. Meanwhile, in a medium saucepan, warm marinara sauce over medium heat, stirring often.
5. Serve rolls topped with marinara sauce and sprinkled with cheese.

Nutrients per serving	
Calories	381
Total fat	12 g
Saturated fat	7 g
Cholesterol	74 mg
Sodium	697 mg
Carbohydrate	38 g
Fiber	7 g
Protein	29 g
Calcium	252 mg
Iron	17.1 mg

Asian Lettuce Wraps

Makes 4 servings

✪ Great for Steps 1, 3, 4 and 5

This so-easy supper is a balanced blend of piquant ginger-garlic sauce, turkey, aromatic rice and an assortment of tender-crisp vegetables. The sum total is handheld satisfaction.

2 tsp	vegetable oil	10 mL
1 lb	lean ground turkey	500 g
5	cloves garlic, minced	5
2 tbsp	minced gingerroot	30 mL
1⁄4 cup	hoisin sauce	60 mL
1⁄4 cup	water	60 mL
12	butter lettuce leaves	12
2 1⁄4 cups	hot cooked brown jasmine rice (see page 438)	650 mL
1 cup	shredded carrots	250 mL
1 cup	mung bean sprouts	250 mL
1⁄2 cup	packed fresh mint or cilantro leaves	125 mL

1. In a large skillet, heat oil over medium-high heat. Add turkey and cook, breaking it up with a spoon, for 5 to 6 minutes or until no longer pink. Add garlic and ginger; cook, stirring, for 30 seconds.
2. Stir in hoisin sauce and water. Reduce heat and simmer, stirring occasionally, for 6 to 8 minutes or until thickened.
3. Place lettuce leaves on a work surface, underside of leaves facing up. Spoon rice down the center of each leaf, then top with turkey mixture, carrots, bean sprouts and mint. Tuck in ends, then tightly roll leaf around filling.

▸ Health Note

You can increase the health benefits you receive from garlic by letting it stand for about 15 minutes after mincing it. Researchers at the American Institute for Cancer Research found that when chopped, minced or crushed garlic was allowed to stand before it was cooked or combined with acidic ingredients (such as vinegar or lemon juice in a salad dressing), more of its cancer-fighting compounds were preserved.

Nutrients per serving	
Calories	362
Total fat	11 g
Saturated fat	3 g
Cholesterol	66 mg
Sodium	338 mg
Carbohydrate	40 g
Fiber	4 g
Protein	27 g
Calcium	59 mg
Iron	3.5 mg

Moroccan-Spiced Ground Turkey with Apricot Couscous

Makes 4 servings

✪ Great for Steps 1, 3, 4 and 5

White meat turkey is one of the leanest meat protein sources. In addition, it is high in nutrients, notably heart-healthy niacin, selenium, vitamins B_6 and B_{12} and zinc. Here, it co-stars with a quick apricot couscous and vibrant spices that will transport you to Morocco with the first bite.

Tip

Other dried fruit, such as dark or golden raisins, cranberries or currants may be used in place of the apricots.

2 tsp	extra virgin olive oil	10 mL
1	small red bell pepper, chopped	1
1 cup	chopped onion	250 mL
1 lb	ground turkey breast	500 g
1½ tsp	ground ginger	7 mL
1 tsp	ground cumin	5 mL
½ tsp	ground cinnamon	2 mL
½ tsp	fine sea salt, divided	2 mL
⅛ tsp	cayenne pepper	0.5 mL
1	can (14 to 15 oz/398 to 425 mL) petite diced tomatoes, with juice	1
⅔ cup	packed fresh cilantro leaves, chopped, divided	150 mL
1 cup	whole wheat couscous	250 mL
1⅓ cups	boiling water	325 mL
¼ cup	chopped dried apricots	60 mL

1. In a large skillet, heat oil over medium-high heat. Add red pepper and onion; cook, stirring, for 6 to 8 minutes or until softened. Add turkey, ginger, cumin, cinnamon, half the salt, and cayenne; cook, breaking turkey up with a spoon, for 5 to 6 minutes or until turkey is no longer pink.
2. Stir in tomatoes with juice and bring to a boil. Reduce heat and simmer, stirring once or twice, for 5 minutes. Stir in half the cilantro.
3. Meanwhile, in a small bowl, combine couscous, the remaining salt and boiling water. Cover with a plate and let stand for 5 minutes or until liquid is absorbed. Fluff with a fork. Stir in apricots.
4. Serve turkey mixture over couscous, sprinkled with the remaining cilantro.

Nutrients per serving	
Calories	424
Total fat	11 g
Saturated fat	3 g
Cholesterol	52 mg
Sodium	496 mg
Carbohydrate	53 g
Fiber	9 g
Protein	33 g
Calcium	60 mg
Iron	4.7 mg

Roasted Pork Tenderloin with Pear Slaw

Makes 4 servings

✪ Great for Steps 1, 3 and 4

Pork and pears make a very fine couple. Napa cabbage adds a fresh crunch, as well as fiber.

Nutrients per serving	
Calories	223
Total fat	8 g
Saturated fat	2 g
Cholesterol	81 mg
Sodium	398 mg
Carbohydrate	10 g
Fiber	2 g
Protein	27 g
Calcium	61 mg
Iron	1.7 mg

- **Preheat oven to 400°F (200°C)**
- **Large ovenproof skillet**

1/2 tsp	fine sea salt, divided	2 mL
1/2 tsp	freshly ground black pepper, divided	2 mL
2 tbsp	cider vinegar	30 mL
4 tsp	extra virgin olive oil, divided	20 mL
1 tbsp	liquid honey	15 mL
1 tsp	Dijon mustard	5 mL
1	firm-ripe Bosc pear, cut into very thin wedges	1
4 cups	thinly sliced napa cabbage	1 L
1/2 cup	thinly sliced green onions	125 mL
1 lb	pork tenderloin, trimmed	500 g

1. In a large bowl, whisk together half the salt, half the pepper, vinegar, half the oil, honey and mustard. Add pear, cabbage and green onions, gently tossing to combine. Set aside.
2. Sprinkle pork with the remaining salt and pepper. In ovenproof skillet, heat the remaining oil over medium-high heat. Add pork and cook, turning several times, for 3 to 4 minutes or until browned all over.
3. Transfer skillet to preheated oven and roast for 12 to 14 minutes or until an instant-read thermometer inserted in the thickest part of the tenderloin registers 145°F (63°C) for medium-rare, or until desired doneness. Let rest for at least 5 minutes before slicing. Serve with slaw.

▸ Health Note

Pears contain vitamin C, potassium, a good amount of fiber and antioxidants with anticancer and antibacterial properties. They are less likely than many other fruits to produce an adverse or allergic response, which makes them particularly useful as a first fruit for young children.

Healthy Know-How

Protein 101

According to the Dietary Reference Intakes published by the USDA, 10% to 35% of calories should come from protein. Most North Americans get plenty of protein and easily meet this need by consuming a balanced diet. Protein is needed for:

- Growth (especially important for children, teens and pregnant women)
- Tissue repair
- Immune function
- Making essential hormones and enzymes
- Energy when carbohydrate is not available
- Preserving lean muscle mass

Protein is found in meats, poultry, fish, meat substitutes, cheese, milk, nuts and legumes, and in smaller quantities in starchy foods and vegetables. When we eat these foods, our body breaks down the protein into amino acids (the building blocks of protein). Some amino acids are essential, which means we need to get them from food; others are nonessential, which means the body can make them. Protein from animal sources contains all of the essential amino acids. With the exception of quinoa, plant sources of protein do not contain all of the essential amino acids and need to be combined with complementary protein sources to form a "complete protein."

Honey Mustard Pork Tenderloin with Mustard Greens

Makes 4 servings

✪ Great for Steps 1, 3 and 4

The salty-sweet and tangy elements in this fantastic entrée support the earthy, spicy flavor of the mustard greens. Sautéing the greens separately from the other elements in the dish means that they're cooked perfectly before they get a quick drizzle of the sauce.

- **Preheat oven to 375°F (190°C)**
- **Broiler pan, sprayed with nonstick cooking spray (preferably olive oil)**

1 lb	pork tenderloin, trimmed	500 g
1/4 tsp	fine sea salt	1 mL
1 1/4 cups	reduced-sodium ready-to-use chicken or vegetable broth, divided	300 mL
3 tbsp	liquid honey	45 mL
2 tbsp	whole-grain mustard, divided	30 mL
2 tbsp	sherry vinegar or white wine vinegar	30 mL
6 cups	packed torn trimmed mustard greens	1.5 L

1. Place pork on prepared pan and sprinkle with salt. Bake in preheated oven for 25 to 30 minutes or until an instant-read thermometer inserted in the thickest part of the tenderloin registers 145°F (63°C) for medium-rare, or until desired doneness. Let rest for 10 minutes, then cut into 1/4-inch (0.5 cm) thick slices.
2. Meanwhile, in a small saucepan, combine 1 cup (250 mL) of the broth, honey, 1 tbsp (15 mL) of the mustard and vinegar. Bring to a boil over medium-high heat. Reduce heat and boil gently, stirring occasionally, for 10 minutes or until thickened. Remove from heat.
3. In a large skillet, combine mustard greens, the remaining broth and the remaining mustard. Cover and cook over medium heat, stirring occasionally, for 7 to 8 minutes or until greens are just tender.
4. Serve pork with greens, drizzling both with honey-mustard sauce.

▶ Health Note

Mustard greens are one of the most nutritious green leafy vegetables, rich in vitamin A, carotenes, vitamin K and flavonoid antioxidants.

Nutrients per serving	
Calories	219
Total fat	3 g
Saturated fat	1 g
Cholesterol	74 mg
Sodium	317 mg
Carbohydrate	21 g
Fiber	3 g
Protein	27 g
Calcium	97 mg
Iron	2.7 mg

Chipotle Maple Pork with Sweet Potato and Spinach Hash

Makes 4 servings

✪ Great for Steps 1, 3 and 4

Standard pork tenderloin pales in the face of this delicious, spicy-sweet dish. Its spiciness is easily varied: just add more or less chipotle chile powder to suit your taste.

Tip

If you can't find chipotle chile powder, you can use an equal amount of hot smoked paprika.

Nutrients per serving	
Calories	324
Total fat	8 g
Saturated fat	2 g
Cholesterol	81 mg
Sodium	488 mg
Carbohydrate	35 g
Fiber	6 g
Protein	30 g
Calcium	91 mg
Iron	3.4 mg

- **Preheat oven to 400°F (200°C)**
- **Large ovenproof skillet**

1 lb	pork tenderloin, trimmed	500 g
1 tsp	chipotle chile powder	5 mL
1/2 tsp	fine sea salt, divided	2 mL
4 tsp	extra virgin olive oil, divided	20 mL
1 cup	chopped onion	250 mL
2	sweet potatoes (about 1 lb/500 g total), peeled and shredded	2
6 cups	packed baby spinach (about 6 oz/175 g), chopped	1.5 L
2 tbsp	pure maple syrup	30 mL

1. Sprinkle pork with chipotle chile powder and half the salt. In ovenproof skillet, heat 2 tsp (10 mL) of the oil over medium-high heat. Add pork and cook, turning several times, for 3 to 4 minutes or until browned all over.
2. Transfer skillet to preheated oven and roast for 12 to 14 minutes or until an instant-read thermometer inserted in the thickest part of the tenderloin registers 145°F (63°C) for medium-rare, or until desired doneness. Let rest for at least 5 minutes before slicing.
3. Meanwhile, in a large skillet, heat the remaining oil over medium-high heat. Add onion and cook, stirring, for 2 minutes. Add sweet potatoes and the remaining salt; cook, stirring, for 8 to 10 minutes or until sweet potatoes are tender. Add spinach and maple syrup; cook, stirring, for 1 to 2 minutes or until spinach is just wilted. Serve with pork.

Sautéed Pork Chops with Balsamic Onions, Kale and Cherries

Makes 4 servings

✪ Great for Steps 1, 3 and 4

Pork chops and kale revel in a sweet-tart sauce of balsamic vinegar, onions and cherries infused with the piquant flavor of freshly cracked black pepper.

Tip

Unlike other greens, kale stems are so tough they are virtually inedible. Hence, they, along with the tougher part of the center rib, must be removed before cooking. To do so, lay a leaf upside down on a cutting board and use a paring knife to cut a V shape along both sides of the rib, cutting it and the stem free from the leaf.

4	boneless pork loin chops (each about 6 oz/175 g)	4
½ tsp	fine sea salt, divided	2 mL
½ tsp	freshly cracked black pepper, divided	2 mL
4 tsp	extra virgin olive oil, divided	20 mL
1	small red onion, cut into ¼-inch (0.5 cm) thick rings	1
1	large bunch curly kale, stems and ribs removed, leaves very thinly sliced crosswise (about 5 cups/1.25 L)	1
¼ cup	dried cherries or cranberries, chopped	60 mL
¼ cup	balsamic vinegar	60 mL
2 tsp	liquid honey	10 mL

1. Sprinkle pork with half the salt and half the pepper. In a large skillet, heat half the oil over medium-high heat. Add pork and cook, turning once, for 5 to 6 minutes per side or until just a hint of pink remains inside. Transfer to a plate and tent with foil to keep warm.
2. In the same skillet, heat the remaining oil over medium-high heat. Add red onion and cook, stirring, for 3 minutes. Add kale, cherries, vinegar, honey and the remaining salt and pepper; cook, stirring, for 2 minutes. Reduce heat to low, cover and simmer, stirring occasionally, for 8 to 10 minutes or until kale is tender. Serve with pork.

Nutrients per serving	
Calories	322
Total fat	9 g
Saturated fat	2 g
Cholesterol	94 mg
Sodium	436 mg
Carbohydrate	21 g
Fiber	2 g
Protein	39 g
Calcium	190 mg
Iron	4.4 mg

Korean Sesame Soy Pork with Quick Kimchi Slaw

Makes 4 servings

✪ Great for Steps 1, 3 and 4

Salty-sweet meats and tangy kimchi are a classic Korean pairing. Here, the kimchi is a quick and nutritious slaw: the cabbage in the mix has phytochemicals that researchers believe may ward off disease. Further, cabbage may lower cholesterol nearly as much as oat bran.

Tip

Choose unseasoned rice vinegar over seasoned rice vinegar, which has added sugar and salt.

Nutrients per serving	
Calories	259
Total fat	10 g
Saturated fat	2 g
Cholesterol	74 mg
Sodium	606 mg
Carbohydrate	21 g
Fiber	2 g
Protein	26 g
Calcium	49 mg
Iron	2.6 mg

Kimchi Slaw

2 tbsp	unseasoned rice vinegar	30 mL
1 tbsp	reduced-sodium tamari or soy sauce	15 mL
2 tsp	Asian chile-garlic sauce	10 mL
1 tsp	sesame oil	5 mL
4 cups	shredded coleslaw mix (shredded cabbage and carrots)	1 L
½ cup	chopped green onions	125 mL

Sesame Soy Pork

2 tsp	ground ginger	10 mL
¼ cup	reduced-sodium tamari or soy sauce	60 mL
2 tbsp	Asian chile-garlic sauce	30 mL
2 tbsp	brown rice syrup or liquid honey	30 mL
2 tbsp	sesame oil	30 mL
1 lb	pork tenderloin, trimmed and cut crosswise into very thin slices	500 g
2 tbsp	sesame seeds, toasted (optional)	30 mL

1. *Slaw:* In a large bowl, whisk together vinegar, tamari, chile-garlic sauce and oil. Add coleslaw and green onions, gently tossing to combine. Cover and refrigerate until ready to serve.
2. *Pork:* In a medium bowl, whisk together ginger, tamari, chile-garlic sauce, brown rice syrup and oil. Add pork and toss to coat. Cover and refrigerate for 15 minutes.
3. Remove half the pork slices from marinade, shaking off excess. In a large skillet, cook pork over medium-high heat, stirring, for 2 to 4 minutes or until browned on all sides and just a hint of pink remains inside pork. Transfer to a plate. Repeat with the remaining pork, discarding marinade. Return all pork to skillet and cook, stirring, until heated through.
4. Serve pork with slaw and garnish with sesame seeds, if desired.

Stir-Fried Pork and Peppers with Buckwheat Noodles

Makes 4 servings

✪ Great for Steps 1, 3, 4 and 5

If the mention of pork brings to mind plain chops, this flavorful stir-fry, with its luscious peanut sauce, crisp red peppers and bed of buckwheat noodles, will be a delicious surprise. The dish is packed with protein and fiber, which means even a small serving — think leftovers for lunch the following day — will leave you satisfied for hours.

Variation

Replace the pork with an equal amount of boneless skinless chicken breasts, cut into thin strips.

Nutrients per serving	
Calories	373
Total fat	8 g
Saturated fat	1 g
Cholesterol	74 mg
Sodium	607 mg
Carbohydrate	42 g
Fiber	5 g
Protein	32 g
Calcium	38 mg
Iron	3.4 mg

6 oz	soba (buckwheat) noodles	175 g
1 lb	pork tenderloin, trimmed	500 g
2 tsp	toasted sesame oil	10 mL
1 tbsp	minced gingerroot	15 mL
1 tbsp	Asian chile-garlic sauce	15 mL
1	large red bell pepper, cut into very thin strips	1
1⁄4 cup	reduced-sodium ready-to-use vegetable or chicken broth	60 mL
1 1⁄2 tbsp	reduced-sodium tamari or soy sauce	22 mL
1 tbsp	unsweetened natural peanut butter or other nut butter	15 mL
1 tbsp	brown rice syrup or liquid honey	15 mL
6	green onions, trimmed and cut into 2-inch (5 cm) pieces	6

1. In a large pot of boiling salted water, cook soba noodles according to package directions until tender. Drain.
2. Meanwhile, cut pork crosswise into 1⁄2-inch (1 cm) thick slices. Place slices cut side down and cut into 1⁄2-inch (1 cm) wide strips.
3. In a large skillet, heat oil over medium-high heat. Add pork, ginger and chile-garlic sauce; cook, stirring, for 2 minutes. Add red pepper and cook, stirring, for 2 minutes.
4. Stir in broth, tamari, peanut butter and brown rice syrup. Reduce heat and simmer, stirring, for 1 minute or until sauce is slightly thickened and just a hint of pink remains inside pork. Stir in green onions. Serve over noodles.

Thai-Style Pork with Brown Jasmine Rice

Makes 4 servings

✪ Great for Steps 1, 3, 4 and 5

A simple, four-ingredient sauce makes a perfect finish for the pork and peppers in this weeknight- and wallet-friendly stir-fry.

Variation

Substitute lean ground turkey or chicken for the pork.

3 tbsp	fish sauce (nam pla)	45 mL
2 tbsp	freshly squeezed lime juice	30 mL
1½ tbsp	Asian chile-garlic sauce	22 mL
1 tbsp	brown rice syrup or liquid honey	15 mL
2 tsp	vegetable oil	10 mL
1 lb	extra-lean ground pork	500 g
1	large red bell pepper, chopped	1
1 cup	packed fresh basil leaves, torn	250 mL
3 cups	hot cooked brown jasmine rice (see page 438)	750 mL

1. In a small bowl, combine fish sauce, lime juice, chile-garlic sauce and brown rice syrup.
2. In a large skillet, heat oil over medium-high heat. Add pork and red pepper; cook, breaking pork up with a spoon, for 5 to 6 minutes or until pork is no longer pink. Drain off any fat. Add fish sauce mixture and basil; cook, stirring, for 30 seconds or until basil is wilted. Serve over rice.

Nutrients per serving	
Calories	409
Total fat	11 g
Saturated fat	3 g
Cholesterol	79 mg
Sodium	630 mg
Carbohydrate	43 g
Fiber	3 g
Protein	40 g
Calcium	62 mg
Iron	2.4 mg

Cuban Braised Beef with Brown Rice and Mango

Makes 4 servings

✪ Great for Steps 1, 3, 4 and 5

Adding fruit to main dishes is common in Caribbean cuisine, and it's a tradition worth adopting, as it's a great way to hit your five-a-day fruit goal. Here, mango's natural sweetness adds balance to braised beef and brightens the spicy and herbal aromatics from the chili powder and oregano.

2 tsp	vegetable oil	10 mL
1 lb	eye of round beef roast, trimmed and cut into 1-inch (2.5 cm) pieces	500 g
1	red bell pepper, thinly sliced	1
¼ tsp	fine sea salt	1 mL
2	cans (each 10 oz/284 mL) diced tomatoes with chiles, with juice	2
1 tbsp	chili powder	15 mL
2 tsp	ground cumin	10 mL
1 tsp	ground oregano	5 mL
¼ tsp	freshly cracked black pepper	1 mL
3 cups	hot cooked long-grain brown rice (see page 438)	750 mL
1 cup	diced firm-ripe mango	250 mL
½ cup	packed fresh cilantro leaves, chopped	125 mL

1. In a large saucepan, heat oil over medium-high heat. Add beef, red pepper and salt; cook, stirring, for 5 to 6 minutes or until beef is browned on all sides.
2. Stir in tomatoes with juice, chili powder, cumin, oregano and pepper. Bring to a boil. Reduce heat to low, cover and simmer, stirring occasionally, for 1½ to 2 hours or until beef is fork-tender.
3. Divide rice among four bowls and spoon beef over top. Top with mango and cilantro.

Superfood Spotlight

Oregano • According to tests carried out by the U.S. Department of Agriculture, oregano — both fresh and dried — has more antioxidant activity than any other herb. It has demonstrated 42 times more antioxidant activity than apples, 12 times more than oranges and 4 times more than blueberries. Its volatile oils include thymol and carvacrol, which have both been shown to strongly inhibit the growth of bacteria, including *Staphylococcus aureus*. Oregano is also a good source of several nutrients, including calcium, potassium, iron and magnesium. It is high in dietary fiber and may help lower "bad" cholesterol.

Nutrients per serving	
Calories	424
Total fat	10 g
Saturated fat	3 g
Cholesterol	68 mg
Sodium	487 mg
Carbohydrate	51 g
Fiber	6 g
Protein	31 g
Calcium	72 mg
Iron	4.6 mg

Grilled Steak with Arugula and Parmesan

Makes 4 servings

✪ Great for Steps 1, 3 and 4

This dish embodies what's wonderful about grilling: in a short amount of time, a few simple ingredients are easily transformed into a fabulous, fuss-free dinner sure to please all. While almost any fresh greens may accompany the steak, the peppery bite of arugula is especially flavorful.

- **Preheat barbecue grill to medium-high**

12 oz	boneless beef top loin (strip loin) or top sirloin steak, trimmed	375 g
	Nonstick cooking spray	
1/2 tsp	fine sea salt, divided	2 mL
1/2 tsp	freshly cracked black pepper, divided	2 mL
1 tbsp	extra virgin olive oil	15 mL
1 tsp	freshly squeezed lemon juice	5 mL
1 tsp	balsamic vinegar	5 mL
4 cups	packed arugula	1 L
1/4 cup	shaved Parmesan cheese	60 mL

1. Pat steak dry with paper towels. Lightly spray with cooking spray and sprinkle with half the salt and half the pepper. Grill on preheated barbecue, turning once, for 5 to 6 minutes per side for medium-rare, or to desired doneness. Transfer to a cutting board and let rest for 5 minutes.
2. Meanwhile, in a small bowl, whisk together oil, lemon juice, vinegar and the remaining salt and pepper.
3. Divide arugula among four dinner plates. Thinly slice steak and arrange on top of arugula. Drizzle with dressing and scatter cheese over top.

▶ Health Note

Arugula is a great source of vitamins C, A and K, as well as bioflavonoids, iron and potassium.

Nutrients per serving	
Calories	252
Total fat	13 g
Saturated fat	7 g
Cholesterol	85 mg
Sodium	480 mg
Carbohydrate	1 g
Fiber	0 g
Protein	22 g
Calcium	154 mg
Iron	1.7 mg

Japanese Ginger Beef Bowls

Makes 4 servings

✪ Great for Steps 1, 3, 4 and 5

This aromatic one-bowl dinner features a classic combination of Japanese flavors, but the spicy, ginger-infused sauce is what sets the dish apart.

Tip

Placing the steak in the freezer for 15 minutes makes it easier to slice.

12 oz	boneless beef top loin (strip loin) or top sirloin steak, trimmed	375 g
2 tbsp	minced gingerroot	30 mL
2/3 cup	reduced-sodium ready-to-use beef or vegetable broth	150 mL
1/3 cup	mirin or sherry	75 mL
3 tbsp	reduced-sodium tamari or soy sauce	45 mL
1 tbsp	brown rice syrup or liquid honey	15 mL
2 tsp	Asian chile-garlic sauce	10 mL
2 cups	thinly sliced onions	500 mL
3 cups	hot cooked short- or medium-grain brown rice (see page 438)	750 mL
1/3 cup	thinly sliced green onions	75 mL

1. Wrap steak in foil and place in the freezer for 15 minutes.
2. Meanwhile, in a small saucepan, whisk together ginger, broth, mirin, tamari, brown rice syrup and chile-garlic sauce. Bring to a boil over medium-high heat. Add onions, reduce heat and simmer for 5 to 7 minutes or until softened.
3. Remove steak from freezer and remove foil. Using a very sharp knife, slice steak as thinly as possible across the grain. Add to the pan and cook for 2 to 3 minutes or until just cooked through.
4. Divide rice among four bowls. Top with beef mixture and sprinkle with green onions.

▶ Health Note

Ginger has phytonutrients that act as inhibitors, meaning it may play a useful role in preventing the growth or spread of cancer cells, a subject of major scientific research.

Nutrients per serving	
Calories	401
Total fat	14 g
Saturated fat	6 g
Cholesterol	75 mg
Sodium	120 mg
Carbohydrate	53 g
Fiber	4 g
Protein	24 g
Calcium	60 mg
Iron	2.3 mg

Grilled Steak Tacos with Avocado and Cumin Lime Slaw

Makes 4 servings

✪ Great for Steps 1, 3, 4 and 5

Here, steak rubbed with chipotle chile powder gets even more alluring smokiness from the grill. Luscious and nutritious avocado, crisp coleslaw — high in vitamin C and elevated with a quick, creamy cumin lime dressing — and ready-made salsa complete the transformation from ordinary to extraordinary.

Tip

The steak may be broiled instead of grilled. Preheat broiler and spray a broiler pan with nonstick cooking spray. Place steak on prepared pan. Broil, turning once, for 6 to 8 minutes for medium-rare, or until desired doneness.

Nutrients per serving	
Calories	496
Total fat	23 g
Saturated fat	7 g
Cholesterol	75 mg
Sodium	596 mg
Carbohydrate	53 g
Fiber	11 g
Protein	30 g
Calcium	86 mg
Iron	2.6 mg

- **Preheat barbecue grill to medium-high**

1	clove garlic, minced	1
1 tsp	ground cumin	5 mL
1/2 tsp	fine sea salt, divided	2 mL
3 tbsp	nonfat plain Greek yogurt	45 mL
3 tbsp	freshly squeezed lime juice	45 mL
4 cups	shredded coleslaw mix (shredded cabbage and carrots)	1 L
12 oz	boneless beef top loin (strip loin) or top sirloin steak, trimmed	375 g
1 tsp	chipotle chile powder	5 mL
8	6-inch (15 cm) whole wheat flour tortillas, warmed	8
1	small firm-ripe Hass avocado, sliced	1
1/2 cup	salsa	125 mL

1. In a medium bowl, whisk together garlic, cumin, half the salt, yogurt and lime juice. Add coleslaw, gently tossing to combine. Let stand for 10 minutes.
2. Meanwhile, sprinkle steak with chipotle chile powder and the remaining salt. Grill on preheated barbecue, turning once, for 6 to 8 minutes for medium-rare, or until desired doneness. Transfer to a cutting board. Let rest for 5 minutes, then thinly slice across the grain.
3. Fill warm tortillas with steak and top with slaw, avocado and salsa.

Picadillo

Makes 4 servings

✪ Great for Steps 1, 3 and 4

If ever there was an easy dinner to brighten winter's gloom, picadillo — a spicy Mexican ground beef dish — is it. The fresh cilantro is a must, providing bright contrast to the spicy beef and salty-sweet flavors from the olives and raisins. Diced eggs provide color as well as nutrition, specifically protein, carotenoids and vitamins B, A and D. Just be sure to use a good-quality salsa to marry the ingredients with the best flavor.

1 lb	extra-lean ground beef	500 g
1/3 cup	golden raisins, chopped	75 mL
1 1/4 tsp	ground cumin	6 mL
1 1/2 cups	salsa	375 mL
2	large hard-cooked eggs (see tip, page 161), peeled and chopped	2
1/2 cup	packed fresh cilantro leaves, chopped	125 mL
1/3 cup	chopped pimiento-stuffed green olives	75 mL
1	small head Boston or butter lettuce, leaves separated	1

1. In a large skillet, cook beef over medium-high heat, breaking it up with a spoon, for 5 to 6 minutes or until no longer pink. Drain off any fat. Add raisins, cumin and salsa; reduce heat and simmer, stirring occasionally, for 5 minutes. Remove from heat and stir in eggs, cilantro and olives.
2. Place lettuce leaves on a work surface, underside of leaves facing up. Spoon beef mixture down the center of each leaf. Tuck in ends, then tightly roll leaf around filling.

Superfood Spotlight

Lettuce • There are dozens of different types of lettuce available in stores and to buy as seeds. When making your choices, keep in mind that varieties that are dark green or have red tinges contain more carotenes and vitamin C than paler lettuces. Romaine lettuce, for example, has five times as much vitamin C as iceberg lettuce. The more vibrant heads also contain good amounts of folate, potassium and iron. Lettuce is high in fiber, very low in calories and low on the glycemic index.

Nutrients per serving	
Calories	250
Total fat	10 g
Saturated fat	4 g
Cholesterol	92 mg
Sodium	403 mg
Carbohydrate	15 g
Fiber	1 g
Protein	28 g
Calcium	61 mg
Iron	4.0 mg

Quick Beef Ragù with Spaghetti Squash

Makes 4 servings

✪ Great for Steps 1, 3 and 4

In this enlightened take on everyone's favorite bowl of spaghetti, strands of squash replace the noodles to delicious effect.

1	spaghetti squash (about 2 lbs/1 kg)	1
1 lb	extra-lean ground beef	500 g
½ cup	packed fresh basil leaves, chopped, divided	125 mL
1½ cups	reduced-sodium marinara sauce	375 mL
¼ cup	water	60 mL
¼ tsp	fine sea salt	1 mL
1 tbsp	extra virgin olive oil	15 mL
¼ cup	freshly grated Parmesan cheese	60 mL

1. Pierce squash all over with a fork. Place on a paper towel in the microwave. Microwave on Medium-High (70%) for 13 to 15 minutes or until soft. Let cool for 5 to 10 minutes.
2. Meanwhile, in a large skillet, cook beef over medium-high heat, breaking it up with a spoon, for 5 to 6 minutes or until no longer pink. Drain off any fat. Add half the basil, marinara sauce and water. Reduce heat and simmer, stirring occasionally, for 10 minutes or until thickened.
3. Cut squash in half, remove seeds and scoop out pulp. Transfer pulp to a bowl and, using a fork, rake into strands. Add salt and oil, tossing to coat.
4. Divide squash among four plates and top with beef ragù, cheese and the remaining basil.

▶ Health Note

Spaghetti squash is a good source of heart-healthy niacin, vitamin B_6, pantothenic acid, potassium and manganese, and a very good source of dietary fiber and vitamin C.

Tip

The spaghetti squash may also be prepared in the oven. Preheat oven to 325°F (160°C) and lightly spray a small rimmed baking sheet with nonstick cooking spray (preferably olive oil). Cut squash in half lengthwise and remove seeds. Place squash, cut side down, on prepared baking sheet and bake for 35 to 40 minutes or until a knife is easily inserted. Let cool for 5 to 10 minutes, then scoop out pulp and proceed with step 3.

Nutrients per serving	
Calories	346
Total fat	14 g
Saturated fat	5 g
Cholesterol	72 mg
Sodium	386 mg
Carbohydrate	21 g
Fiber	3 g
Protein	28 g
Calcium	182 mg
Iron	4.2 mg

Spiced Beef Keema with Chickpeas and Green Peas

Makes 4 servings

✪ Great for Steps 1, 3 and 4

Keema, a spicy dish made with minced or ground lamb or beef, is a classic Indian entrée. The addition of tender petite peas and toothsome chickpeas contributes intriguing textures and both subtly sweet (petite peas) and nutty (chickpeas) flavors. Serve with whole wheat naan to complete the dinner with ease and style.

2 tsp	vegetable oil	10 mL
1½ cups	chopped onions	375 mL
2 tbsp	minced gingerroot	30 mL
12 oz	extra-lean ground beef	375 g
2 tsp	mild curry powder	10 mL
1 tsp	garam masala	5 mL
½ tsp	ground cumin	2 mL
¼ tsp	fine sea salt	1 mL
⅛ tsp	cayenne pepper	0.5 mL
1	can (14 to 19 oz/398 to 540 mL) chickpeas, drained and rinsed	1
2	cans (each 10 oz/284 mL) diced tomatoes with chiles, with juice	2
1 cup	frozen petite peas, thawed	250 mL
½ cup	packed fresh cilantro leaves, chopped	125 mL
1 tbsp	freshly squeezed lime juice	15 mL

1. In a large skillet, heat oil over medium-high heat. Add onions and cook, stirring, for 5 to 6 minutes or until slightly softened. Add ginger and cook, stirring, for 1 minute. Add beef and cook, breaking it up with a spoon, for 5 to 6 minutes or until no longer pink. Drain off any fat. Add curry powder, garam masala, cumin, salt and cayenne; cook, stirring, for 30 seconds.
2. Add chickpeas and tomatoes with juice. Bring to a boil. Reduce heat and simmer, stirring occasionally, for 5 minutes to blend the flavors. Add peas and cook for 1 minute to warm through. Stir in cilantro and lime juice.

Nutrients per serving	
Calories	345
Total fat	11 g
Saturated fat	3 g
Cholesterol	52 mg
Sodium	597 mg
Carbohydrate	33 g
Fiber	8 g
Protein	28 g
Calcium	77 mg
Iron	4.6 mg

Persian Ground Beef Kebabs

Makes 4 servings

✪ Great for Steps 1, 3 and 4

These Persian-inspired kebabs make a delicious change of pace from the usual ground beef dishes. The combination of spices and herbs — vitamin C–packed cilantro and mint — is nothing short of addictive. Preparing accompaniments is as simple as opening a container of plain nonfat yogurt and warming whole wheat pita bread.

Tip

The kebabs can be broiled instead of grilled. Preheat broiler and place kebabs on a broiler tray sprayed with nonstick cooking spray. Broil for 6 to 10 minutes, turning once halfway through, until no longer pink inside.

Nutrients per serving	
Calories	210
Total fat	10 g
Saturated fat	4 g
Cholesterol	87 mg
Sodium	392 mg
Carbohydrate	3 g
Fiber	1 g
Protein	26 g
Calcium	28 mg
Iron	2.7 mg

- **Preheat barbecue grill to medium-high**
- **Eight 10-inch (25 cm) metal skewers, or wooden skewers soaked in warm water for 30 minutes**

1 lb	extra-lean ground beef	500 g
1	large egg	1
2⁄3 cup	grated onion	150 mL
2⁄3 cup	packed fresh cilantro leaves, chopped	150 mL
1⁄3 cup	packed fresh mint leaves, chopped	75 mL
1 tsp	ground coriander	5 mL
1⁄2 tsp	ground ginger	2 mL
1⁄2 tsp	ground cinnamon	2 mL
1⁄2 tsp	fine sea salt	2 mL
1⁄4 tsp	freshly ground black pepper	1 mL

1. In a large bowl, gently combine beef, egg, onion, cilantro, mint, coriander, ginger, cinnamon, salt and pepper.
2. Divide meat mixture into 8 portions. Form each portion around a skewer, shaping the meat into a 6- by 1-inch (15 by 2.5 cm) cylinder around the skewer.
3. Grill kebabs on preheated barbecue, turning once or twice, for 6 to 10 minutes or until no longer pink inside.

Middle Eastern Meatballs with Feta Sauce

Makes 4 servings

✪ Great for Steps 3, 4 and 5

Attention, mint: please step away from the desserts. Here, the vibrant herb shows off its versatility — and its Middle Eastern side. Serve these meatballs with brown rice or quinoa.

- **Preheat oven to 400°F (200°C)**
- **Food processor**
- **Large rimmed baking sheet, sprayed with nonstick cooking spray (preferably olive oil)**

1/4 cup	fine or medium bulgur	60 mL
1/4 cup	boiling water	60 mL
1/2 cup	crumbled feta cheese	125 mL
1/4 cup	nonfat plain yogurt	60 mL
1/2 tsp	freshly cracked black pepper, divided	2 mL
1	can (14 to 19 oz/398 to 540 mL) chickpeas, drained and rinsed	1
8 oz	extra-lean ground beef	250 g
2/3 cup	packed fresh mint leaves, chopped	150 mL
1/2 tsp	fine sea salt	2 mL

1. In a medium bowl, combine bulgur and boiling water. Let stand for 30 minutes or until water is absorbed.
2. Meanwhile, in a small bowl, mash cheese with the back of a fork until smooth. Stir in yogurt and half the pepper. Refrigerate until ready to use.
3. In food processor, pulse chickpeas until coarsely chopped. Transfer to a large bowl and add bulgur, beef, mint, salt and the remaining pepper. Gently combine until mixture holds together. Form into 16 meatballs and arrange on prepared baking sheet.
4. Bake in preheated oven for 14 to 18 minutes or until no longer pink inside. Serve with feta sauce.

▸ Health Note

Mint is rich in vitamins A, C and B_{12}, thiamine, folic acid and riboflavin, and has been used for centuries to aid digestion.

Nutrients per serving	
Calories	271
Total fat	10 g
Saturated fat	5 g
Cholesterol	52 mg
Sodium	606 mg
Carbohydrate	24 g
Fiber	5 g
Protein	22 g
Calcium	145 mg
Iron	2.7 mg

Fish and Seafood Main Dishes

Grilled Striped Bass with Kiwi and Cucumber Salsa 342
Seared Striped Bass with Broccoli and Almond Quinoa 343
Black Cod with Fresh Herb Sauce 344
Healthy Know-How: Food Allergies and Sensitivities 101 345
Grilled Black Cod with North African Salsa 346
Ginger Soy Cod 347
Cod Poached in Tapenade Tomato Broth 347
Cod with Roasted Tomatoes and Edamame Mash 348
Herbed Cod Cakes 349
Whole Grain–Crusted Fish Sticks 350
Foil-Roasted Halibut and Asparagus 351
Halibut with Beets and Beet Greens 352
Halibut with Coconut Lime Sauce 353
Broiled Mahi Mahi with Red Pepper Harissa 354
Grilled Salmon with Mustard Maple Vinaigrette 355
Oven-BBQ Salmon with Fresh Corn Basil Relish 356
Spice-Crusted Salmon with Mint Raita 357
Seared Salmon with Fresh Pineapple Salsa 358
Hoisin Salmon 358
Seared Salmon with Warm Lentil and Arugula Salad 359

Thai Red Curry–Glazed Salmon 360
Swedish Salmon, Asparagus and Potato Omelet 361
Salmon Cakes with Buttermilk Dressing and Mixed Greens 362
Lemon Dill Tilapia in Foil 363
Mediterranean Grilled Tilapia and Whole Wheat Couscous 364
Garam Masala–Spiced Tilapia with Watermelon Salsa 365
Grilled Tilapia Tacos with Mango Salsa 366
Chipotle Tilapia Tacos with Pineapple 367
Broiled Herbed Trout Fillets 368
Baked Trout with Shiitake Mushrooms and Ginger 369
Tuna with Farro and Fennel 370
Tuna and Asparagus Frittata 371
Spicy Tuna Cakes with Lemony Spinach 372
Provençal Poached Sea Scallops 373
Shrimp and Asparagus Stir-Fry 374
Greek Grilled Shrimp with Feta and Dill 375
Moroccan-Spiced Shrimp 376
Cannellini Beans with Shrimp and Roasted Peppers 377
Couscous Paella with Shrimp and Chicken Sausage 378
One-Pan Shrimp Pilau 379

Grilled Striped Bass with Kiwi and Cucumber Salsa

Makes 4 servings

✪ Great for Steps 1, 3 and 4

Fresh salsas are not only fun to eat, they also preserve the nutrients of the ingredients by keeping them free from heat. This salsa, made with fresh kiwi, cucumber and lemon, is perfectly harmonious with the gently spiced bass.

Tip

Cod, halibut or any other firm white fish fillets may be used in place of the bass.

Nutrients per serving	
Calories	201
Total fat	4 g
Saturated fat	1 g
Cholesterol	100 mg
Sodium	299 mg
Carbohydrate	14 g
Fiber	2 g
Protein	28 g
Calcium	50 mg
Iron	1.5 mg

- **Preheat barbecue grill to medium-high**

1½ cups	diced kiwifruit	375 mL
½ cup	diced seeded peeled cucumber	125 mL
¼ cup	packed fresh cilantro leaves, chopped	60 mL
1 tbsp	minced seeded jalapeño pepper	15 mL
2 tbsp	freshly squeezed lemon juice	30 mL
2 tsp	agave nectar or liquid honey	10 mL
4	skinless striped bass fillets (each about 5 oz/150 g)	4
	Nonstick cooking spray	
¼ tsp	fine sea salt	1 mL
¼ tsp	freshly cracked black pepper	1 mL
⅛ tsp	ground allspice	0.5 mL

1. In a medium bowl, combine kiwi, cucumber, cilantro, jalapeño, lemon juice and agave nectar. Cover and refrigerate until ready to use.
2. Lightly spray both sides of fish with cooking spray. Sprinkle with salt, pepper and allspice. Grill on preheated barbecue, turning once, for about 5 minutes per side or until fish is opaque and flakes easily when tested with a fork. Serve topped with kiwi and cucumber salsa.

Seared Striped Bass with Broccoli and Almond Quinoa

Makes 4 servings

✪ Great for Steps 1, 3, 4 and 5

Striped bass gets a smoky edge, while broccoli seems like something new in the part modern, part rustic, thoroughly satisfying side, dolled up with quinoa and golden raisins.

Tips

Look for roasted almonds lightly seasoned with sea salt. If using unsalted roasted almonds (or toasted almonds), add 1/8 tsp (0.5 mL) fine sea salt to the recipe.

Cod, halibut or any other firm white fish fillets may be used in place of the bass.

Nutrients per serving	
Calories	369
Total fat	11 g
Saturated fat	2 g
Cholesterol	90 mg
Sodium	403 mg
Carbohydrate	38 g
Fiber	5 g
Protein	32 g
Calcium	89 mg
Iron	4.4 mg

1 cup	quinoa, rinsed	250 mL
1/2 tsp	fine sea salt, divided	2 mL
1 2/3 cups	water	400 mL
2 1/2 cups	broccoli florets, finely chopped	625 mL
3 tbsp	golden raisins, chopped	45 mL
1/2 cup	thinly sliced green onions	125 mL
1/4 cup	lightly salted roasted almonds, chopped	60 mL
4	skinless striped bass fillets (each about 5 oz/150 g)	4
1/2 tsp	sweet or hot smoked paprika	2 mL
2 tsp	extra virgin olive oil	10 mL

1. In a medium saucepan, combine quinoa, half the salt, and water. Bring to a boil over medium-high heat. Reduce heat to low, cover and simmer for 12 minutes. Stir in broccoli and raisins; cover and simmer for 3 to 6 minutes or until water is absorbed. Remove from heat and stir in green onions and almonds.
2. Meanwhile, sprinkle fish with paprika and the remaining salt. In a large skillet, heat oil over medium-high heat. Add fish and cook, turning once, for 3 to 4 minutes per side or until fish is opaque and flakes easily when tested with a fork. Serve with quinoa.

Black Cod with Fresh Herb Sauce

Makes 4 servings

✪ Great for Steps 1, 3 and 4

Firm, meaty black cod fillets stand up beautifully to a fresh sauce fragrant with herbs.

Tips

An equal amount of chopped green onions (green parts only) may be used in place of the chives.

Sea bass, halibut, cod or any other firm white fish fillets may be used in place of the black cod.

- **Preheat broiler, with rack set 4 to 6 inches (10 to 15 cm) from the heat source**
- **Blender or food processor**
- **Broiler pan, sprayed with nonstick cooking spray (preferably olive oil)**

1/2 cup	packed fresh basil leaves	125 mL
1/2 cup	packed fresh flat-leaf (Italian) parsley leaves	125 mL
3 tbsp	coarsely chopped fresh chives	45 mL
3 tbsp	reduced-sodium ready-to-use vegetable broth	45 mL
2 tbsp	freshly squeezed lemon juice	30 mL
5 tsp	extra virgin olive oil, divided	25 mL
4	skin-on black cod (sablefish) fillets (each about 5 oz/150 g and 1 inch/2.5 cm thick)	4
1/4 tsp	fine sea salt	1 mL

1. In blender, combine basil, parsley, chives, broth, lemon juice and 3 tsp (15 mL) of the oil; purée until smooth. Set aside.
2. Place fish, skin side down, on prepared pan. Brush with the remaining oil and sprinkle with salt. Broil for 6 to 8 minutes or until fish is opaque and flakes easily when tested with a fork. Serve with sauce spooned over top.

Nutrients per serving	
Calories	301
Total fat	25 g
Saturated fat	5 g
Cholesterol	61 mg
Sodium	256 mg
Carbohydrate	2 g
Fiber	1 g
Protein	17 g
Calcium	96 mg
Iron	2.3 mg

Healthy Know-How

Food Allergies and Sensitivities 101

Food Allergies

An allergic reaction can occur anytime a person is introduced to something new. If the body perceives the new substance as a threat, the immune system produces antibodies to fight it off. Reactions tend to occur soon after the food is eaten, or when the person comes into contact with the food, and the symptoms can range from mild to severe. Some of the more common symptoms include the following:

- Breathing problems and throat tightening
- Swelling of eyes, lips and/or tongue
- Sneezing and wheezing
- Rashes or hives
- Persistent diarrhea or abdominal pain
- Vomiting

Some of the most common foods that trigger an allergic reaction are:

- Cow's milk and dairy products
- Eggs
- Fish and shellfish
- Peanuts
- Tree nuts (walnuts, pecans, etc.)
- Citrus fruits and berries
- Soy
- Wheat

Food Sensitivities

The symptoms of food sensitivities, or food intolerances, can be similar to those caused by food allergies, but are much milder; moreover, they are not allergies because the body does not produce antibodies. Sensitivities can be triggered by foods a person has trouble digesting, such as milk, wheat or soy, or food additives and preservatives. Some of the more common sensitivity symptoms include the following:

- Eczema, skin rashes and hives
- Runny nose or sudden congestion
- Dark circles under eyes or puffy red eyes
- Bloating, diarrhea or excessive gas

If you suspect any type of food allergy or sensitivity, consult with your doctor immediately.

Grilled Black Cod with North African Salsa

Makes 4 servings

✪ Great for Steps 1, 3 and 4

Accompanying broiled black cod with an intensely flavored, North African–inspired salsa takes a straightforward fish to an exotic place.

Tip

Sea bass, halibut, cod or any other firm white fish fillets may be used in place of the black cod.

Nutrients per serving

Calories	325
Total fat	25 g
Saturated fat	5 g
Cholesterol	61 mg
Sodium	310 mg
Carbohydrate	8 g
Fiber	1 g
Protein	17 g
Calcium	66 mg
Iron	2.4 mg

- **Preheat broiler, with rack set 4 to 6 inches (10 to 15 cm) from the heat source**
- **Broiler pan, sprayed with nonstick cooking spray (preferably olive oil)**

2/3 cup	chopped drained roasted red bell peppers	150 mL
1/4 cup	chopped pitted brine-cured black olives (such as kalamata)	60 mL
1/4 cup	chopped red onion	60 mL
1/4 cup	packed fresh mint leaves, chopped	60 mL
2 tbsp	golden raisins, chopped	30 mL
2 tbsp	freshly squeezed lemon juice, divided	30 mL
4 tsp	extra virgin olive oil, divided	20 mL
1/2 tsp	ground cumin	2 mL
1/4 tsp	ground cinnamon	1 mL
1/4 tsp	cayenne pepper	1 mL
4	skin-on black cod (sablefish) fillets (each about 5 oz/150 g)	4
1/4 tsp	fine sea salt	1 mL

1. In a medium bowl, combine roasted peppers, olives, red onion, mint, raisins and half the lemon juice.
2. In a small skillet, heat half the oil over medium heat. Add cumin, cinnamon and cayenne; cook, stirring, for about 1 minute or until fragrant. Stir into red pepper salsa. Set aside.
3. Place fish, skin side down, on prepared pan. Sprinkle the top with the remaining lemon juice, then brush with the remaining oil. Sprinkle with salt. Broil for 6 to 8 minutes or until fish is opaque and flakes easily when tested with a fork. Serve with salsa spooned over top.

Ginger Soy Cod

Makes 4 servings

✪ Great for Steps 1, 3 and 4

Nutrients per serving	
Calories	121
Total fat	1 g
Saturated fat	0 g
Cholesterol	46 mg
Sodium	362 mg
Carbohydrate	4 g
Fiber	1 g
Protein	24 g
Calcium	38 mg
Iron	1.1 mg

2 tbsp	minced gingerroot	30 mL
3 tbsp	unseasoned rice vinegar	45 mL
2 tbsp	reduced-sodium tamari or soy sauce	30 mL
4	skinless Pacific cod fillets (each about 5 oz/150 g)	4
6	green onions, trimmed and cut into 2-inch (5 cm) pieces	6

1. In a large skillet, combine ginger, vinegar and tamari. Add fish and bring to a boil over medium-high heat. Reduce heat to low, cover and simmer for 5 to 7 minutes or until fish is almost opaque. Scatter green onions over fish. Cover and simmer for 1 to 2 minutes or until fish is opaque and flakes easily when tested with a fork.

Cod Poached in Tapenade Tomato Broth

Makes 4 servings

✪ Great for Steps 1, 3 and 4

Poaching is one of the easiest ways to cook fish.

Nutrients per serving	
Calories	212
Total fat	2 g
Saturated fat	0 g
Cholesterol	65 mg
Sodium	645 mg
Carbohydrate	6 g
Fiber	1 g
Protein	33 g
Calcium	44 mg
Iron	1.7 mg

1	can (14 to 15 oz/398 to 425 mL) diced tomatoes with Italian seasonings, with juice	1
2 tbsp	drained capers	30 mL
½ tsp	hot pepper flakes	2 mL
¾ cup	dry white wine	175 mL
½ cup	water	125 mL
4	skinless Pacific cod fillets (each about 6 oz/175 g)	4
¼ cup	chopped pitted brine-cured black olives (such as kalamata)	60 mL
¼ cup	packed fresh flat-leaf (Italian) parsley leaves, chopped	60 mL

1. In a large skillet, combine tomatoes with juice, capers, hot pepper flakes, wine and water. Bring to a boil over medium-high heat. Reduce heat and simmer, stirring occasionally, for 2 minutes.
2. Add fish to skillet. Reduce heat to low, cover and simmer for 5 to 6 minutes or until fish is opaque and flakes easily when tested with a fork. Serve topped with olives and parsley.

Cod with Roasted Tomatoes and Edamame Mash

Makes 4 servings

✪ Great for Steps 1, 3 and 4

I'm all for simple dishes in which every ingredient speaks for itself. Sometimes, though, it's nice to have a dish remind you how ingredients can become even more special when they interact. This cod, tomato and edamame dish is just such a reminder — you don't taste the parts, just the gorgeous cod with a green freshness from the edamame mash. You'll want some good crusty bread to soak up every last drop of the incredibly flavorful roasted cherry tomatoes.

Tip

Sea bass, halibut or any other firm white fish fillets may be used in place of the cod.

Nutrients per serving	
Calories	266
Total fat	5 g
Saturated fat	1 g
Cholesterol	65 mg
Sodium	453 mg
Carbohydrate	14 g
Fiber	6 g
Protein	41 g
Calcium	86 mg
Iron	2.8 mg

- **Preheat oven to 400°F (200°C)**
- **Large rimmed baking sheet, lined with foil and sprayed with nonstick cooking spray (preferably olive oil)**
- **Food processor**

3 cups	cherry or grape tomatoes	750 mL
	Nonstick cooking spray (preferably olive oil)	
1 tsp	fine sea salt, divided	5 mL
4	skinless Pacific cod fillets (each about 6 oz/175 g)	4
1/4 tsp	freshly cracked black pepper	1 mL
2 cups	frozen shelled edamame or frozen lima beans	500 mL
1	clove garlic	1
1/2 cup	packed fresh basil leaves	125 mL
1/2 cup	reduced-sodium ready-to-use chicken or vegetable broth	125 mL
1 tsp	finely grated lemon zest	5 mL
3 tbsp	freshly squeezed lemon juice	45 mL

1. Place tomatoes on prepared baking sheet. Lightly spray with cooking spray and sprinkle with 1/4 tsp (1 mL) of the salt. Roast in preheated oven for 5 minutes or until skins begin to burst.
2. Lightly spray both sides of fish with cooking spray, then sprinkle with pepper and 1/4 tsp (1 mL) salt. Place fish on baking sheet with tomatoes. Roast for 7 to 10 minutes or until fish is opaque and flakes easily when tested with a fork.
3. Meanwhile, in a medium saucepan of boiling water, cook edamame for 4 to 6 minutes or until tender. Drain.
4. In food processor, combine cooked edamame, garlic, basil, the remaining salt, broth, lemon zest and lemon juice; pulse until blended into a thick purée.
5. Serve fish with tomatoes and their juices and edamame mash.

Herbed Cod Cakes

Makes 4 servings

✪ Great for Steps 1, 3, 4 and 5

Flaky cod, treated like a crab cake, brings a bit of the New England seaside to your kitchen.

Tip

Sea bass, halibut or any other firm white fish fillets may be used in place of the cod.

Nutrients per serving	
Calories	233
Total fat	12 g
Saturated fat	2 g
Cholesterol	90 mg
Sodium	439 mg
Carbohydrate	7 g
Fiber	1 g
Protein	23 g
Calcium	20 mg
Iron	1.2 mg

- **Preheat oven to 400°F (200°C)**
- **9-inch (23 cm) glass baking dish, sprayed with nonstick cooking spray (preferably olive oil)**

1 lb	skinless Pacific cod fillets	500 g
4 tsp	extra virgin olive oil, divided	20 mL
1	large egg, lightly beaten	1
1/3 cup	fresh whole wheat bread crumbs	75 mL
1/4 cup	packed fresh flat-leaf (Italian) parsley leaves, chopped	60 mL
1/4 cup	thinly sliced green onions	60 mL
1/4 tsp	fine sea salt	1 mL
2 tbsp	olive oil mayonnaise	30 mL
2 tbsp	Dijon mustard	30 mL
1 tbsp	freshly squeezed lemon juice	15 mL
1/4 tsp	hot pepper sauce	1 mL

1. Place fish in prepared baking dish. Brush both sides of fish with half the oil. Bake in preheated oven for 7 to 10 minutes or until fish is opaque and flakes easily when tested with a fork. Let cool completely, then pat dry with paper towels. Flake fish into small pieces.
2. In a large bowl, gently combine flaked fish, egg, bread crumbs, parsley, green onions, salt, mayonnaise, mustard, lemon juice and hot pepper sauce until ingredients just hold together. Form into eight 1/2-inch (1 cm) thick patties.
3. In a large skillet, heat the remaining oil over medium-high heat. Add patties and cook, turning once, for 2 to 3 minutes per side or until golden brown on both sides and hot in the center.

Whole Grain–Crusted Fish Sticks

Makes 4 servings

✪ Great for Steps 1, 3, 4 and 5

Cod fillet strips stay tender and moist when baked in a crunchy crust of flax seeds and whole-grain cracker crumbs. Full disclosure to your children of the good-for-you-ingredients is not required.

Tip

The fish sticks can be prepared through step 2 and frozen. Wrap the fish sticks in plastic wrap, then foil, completely enclosing them, and freeze for up to 3 months. When ready to bake, unwrap the frozen fish sticks (do not thaw), place on prepared baking sheet and bake at 450°F (230°C) for 18 to 22 minutes, turning once halfway through, until coating is golden brown and fish is opaque and flakes easily when tested with a fork.

Nutrients per serving	
Calories	263
Total fat	7 g
Saturated fat	1 g
Cholesterol	73 mg
Sodium	316 mg
Carbohydrate	11 g
Fiber	3 g
Protein	37 g
Calcium	42 mg
Iron	1.2 mg

- **Preheat oven to 450°F (230°C)**
- **Large rimmed baking sheet, sprayed with nonstick cooking spray (preferably olive oil)**

1¾ cups	whole-grain cracker crumbs	425 mL
3 tbsp	ground flax seeds (flaxseed meal)	45 mL
1 tbsp	Old Bay seasoning	15 mL
2	large eggs	2
1½ lbs	skinless Pacific cod fillets, cut into 3-inch (7.5 cm) strips	750 g

1. In a shallow dish, combine cracker crumbs, flax seeds and Old Bay seasoning.
2. In another shallow dish, beat eggs. Dip fish strips in egg, shaking off excess, then in cracker mixture, pressing to adhere and shaking off excess. Place on prepared baking sheet. Discard any excess cracker mixture and egg.
3. Bake in preheated oven for 12 to 16 minutes, turning once halfway through, until coating is golden brown and fish is opaque and flakes easily when tested with a fork.

Foil-Roasted Halibut and Asparagus

Makes 4 servings

✪ Great for Steps 1, 3 and 4

Favorite springtime ingredients — asparagus, tarragon and citrus — join forces in this foil-roasted main dish, whose complex flavors belie its incredible ease of preparation (and cleanup).

Tips

Sea bass, cod or any other firm white fish fillets may be used in place of the halibut.

Four 12-inch (30 cm) squares of parchment paper may be used in place of the foil. To seal the packets, fold the parchment over the fish and asparagus, then fold and crimp the edges tightly to enclose the filling completely.

Nutrients per serving	
Calories	200
Total fat	6 g
Saturated fat	1 g
Cholesterol	40 mg
Sodium	243 mg
Carbohydrate	7 g
Fiber	3 g
Protein	29 g
Calcium	89 mg
Iron	1.5 mg

- **Preheat oven to 400°F (200°C)**
- **Four 12-inch (30 cm) squares foil**
- **Large rimmed baking sheet**

	Nonstick cooking spray (preferably olive oil)	
4	skinless Pacific halibut fillets (each about 5 oz/150 g)	4
1 tbsp	minced fresh tarragon	15 mL
2 tsp	finely grated orange zest	10 mL
1⁄4 tsp	fine sea salt	1 mL
1⁄4 tsp	freshly cracked black pepper	1 mL
1 lb	thin asparagus spears, trimmed and cut into 1-inch (2.5 cm) pieces	500 g
1⁄4 cup	freshly squeezed orange juice	60 mL
1 tbsp	extra virgin olive oil	15 mL

1. Place foil squares on a work surface and spray with cooking spray. Top each square with a fish fillet and sprinkle with tarragon, orange zest, salt and pepper. Arrange asparagus around each fillet, then drizzle fish and asparagus with orange juice and oil. Fold foil over fish and asparagus, crimping edges tightly to seal. Place packets on baking sheet.
2. Bake in preheated oven for 13 to 15 minutes or until fish is opaque and flakes easily when tested with a fork. Slide packets onto plates.

Halibut with Beets and Beet Greens

Makes 4 servings

✪ Great for Steps 1, 3 and 4

Fresh halibut has a mild flavor of the sea, and fresh beets and their vibrant greens make a breathtaking accompaniment. A quick gremolata of orange zest, garlic and parsley simultaneously unites the dish's components and elevates the final result.

Tips

Sea bass, cod or any other firm white fish fillets may be used in place of the halibut.

The beets may be roasted instead of microwaved. Preheat oven to 400°F (200°C). Wrap each beet in foil. Place beets directly on oven rack and roast for 1½ hours or until fork-tender. Let cool slightly, then peel and slice beets.

Nutrients per serving	
Calories	290
Total fat	11 g
Saturated fat	2 g
Cholesterol	51 mg
Sodium	157 mg
Carbohydrate	12 g
Fiber	3 g
Protein	36 g
Calcium	110 mg
Iron	2.7 mg

- **Preheat oven to 450°F (230°C)**
- **Large rimmed baking sheet, sprayed with nonstick cooking spray (preferably olive oil)**

Gremolata

1	clove garlic, minced	1
½ cup	packed fresh flat-leaf (Italian) parsley leaves, chopped	125 mL
1 tbsp	finely grated orange zest	15 mL

4	beets (about 2 inches/5 cm in diameter), with green tops attached	4
½ cup	thinly sliced shallots	125 mL
½ tsp	fine sea salt, divided	2 mL
6 tsp	extra virgin olive oil, divided	30 mL
4	skinless Pacific halibut fillets (each about 5 oz/150 g)	4

1. *Gremolata:* In a small bowl, combine garlic, parsley and orange zest. Set aside.
2. Trim leaves and stems from beets, reserving leaves and tender portion of stems, and scrub beets. Rinse and spin-dry beet greens and tender stems, then coarsely chop and set aside.
3. Place beets in a medium microwave-safe bowl and add enough water to cover halfway. Cover and microwave on High for 8 to 10 minutes or until just tender. Uncover, drain and let cool slightly. Peel beets and cut into ¼-inch (0.5 cm) slices.
4. In the same bowl, combine sliced beets, shallots, half the salt, 1 tbsp (15 mL) of the gremolata and 2 tsp (10 mL) of the oil. Spread in a single layer on half of the prepared baking sheet.
5. Toss beet greens with 2 tsp (10 mL) oil. Mound on other side of baking sheet.
6. Sprinkle fish with the remaining salt and place on top of the beet greens. Brush fish with the remaining oil and sprinkle with 2 tbsp (30 mL) gremolata.
7. Roast in preheated oven for about 8 minutes or until fish is opaque and flakes easily when tested with a fork.
8. Divide fish, greens and beets among plates. Sprinkle with the remaining gremolata.

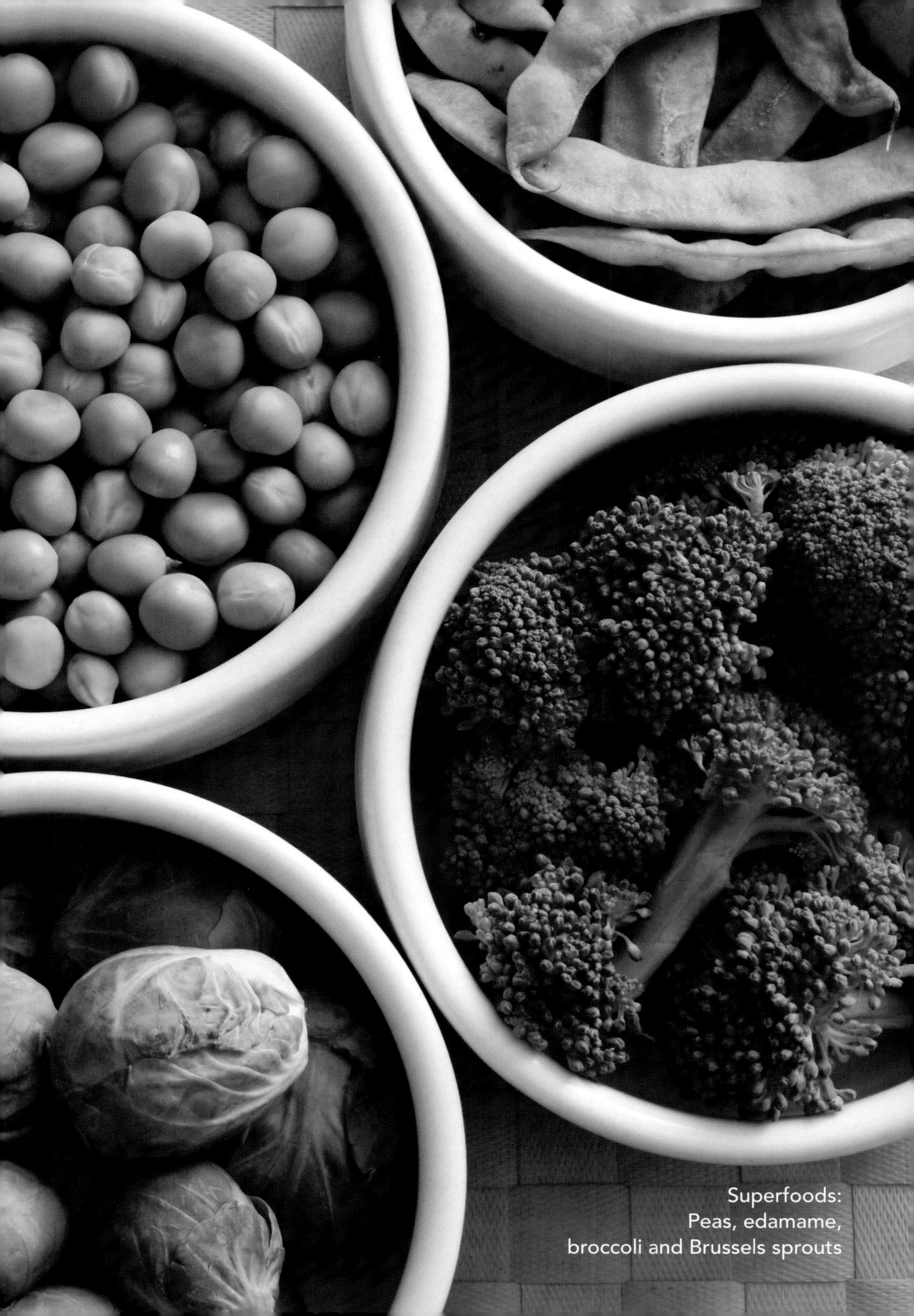

Superfoods:
Peas, edamame,
broccoli and Brussels sprouts

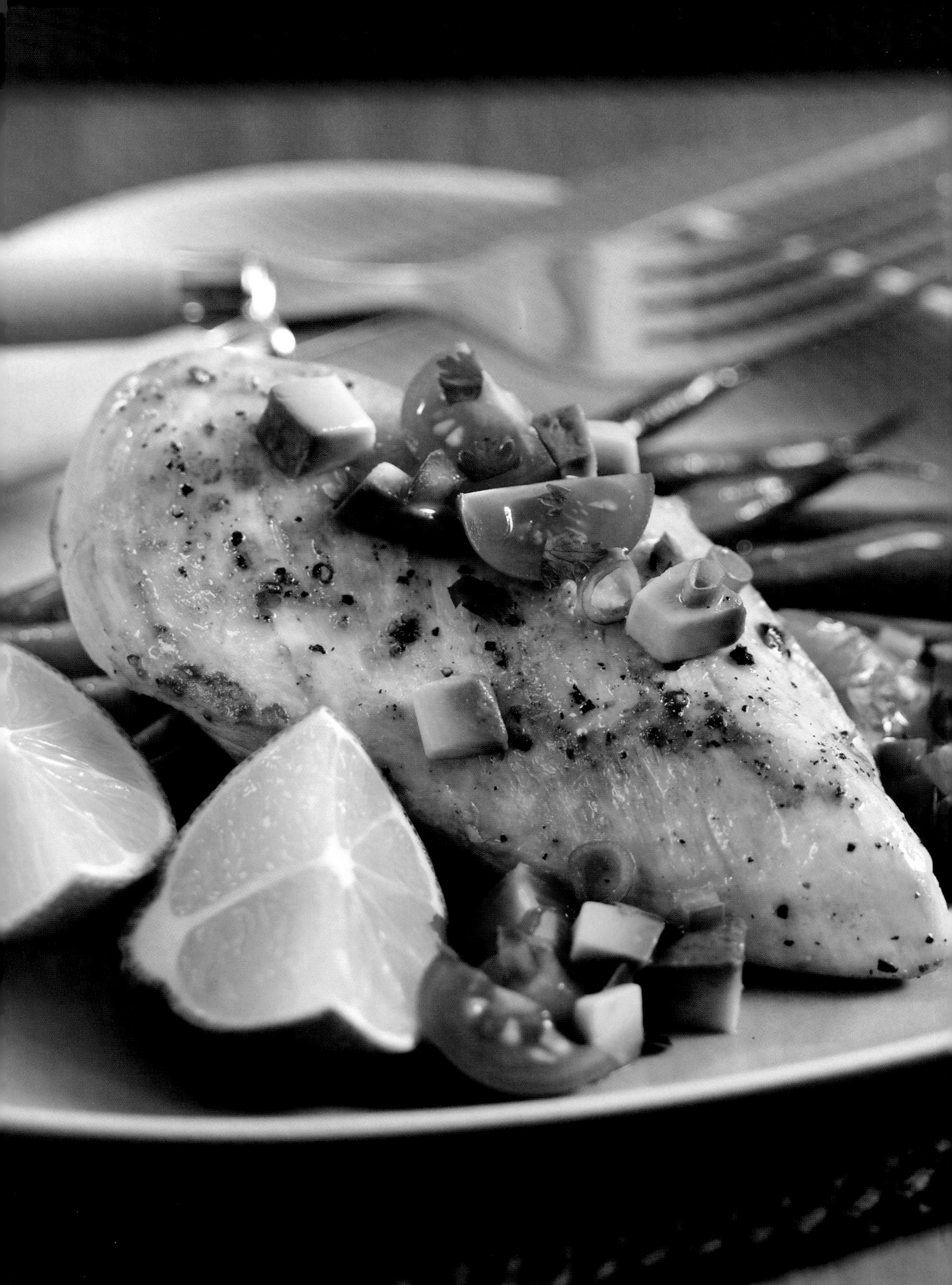

Chicken with Cherry Tomato and Avocado Salsa (page 300)

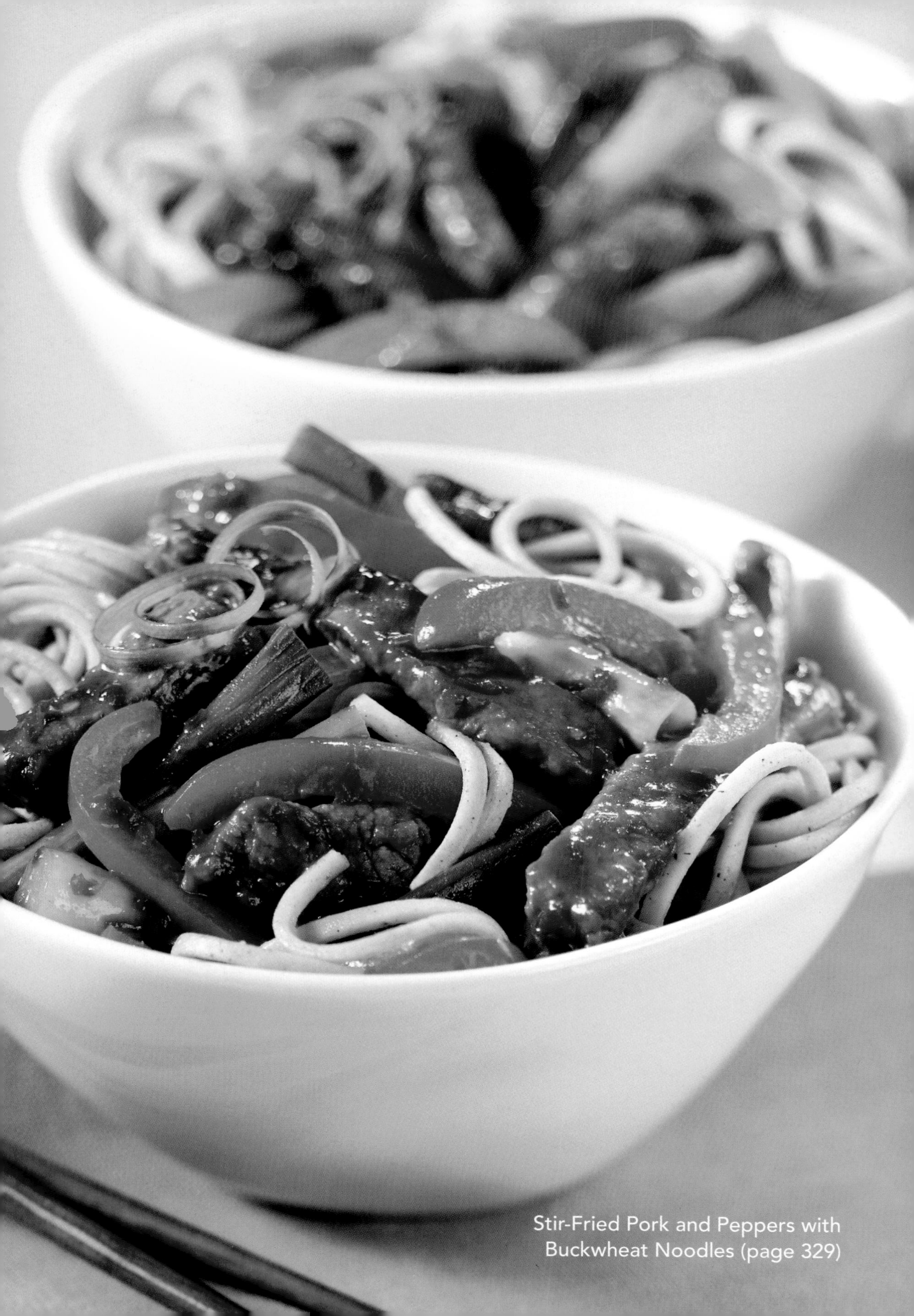

Stir-Fried Pork and Peppers with Buckwheat Noodles (page 329)

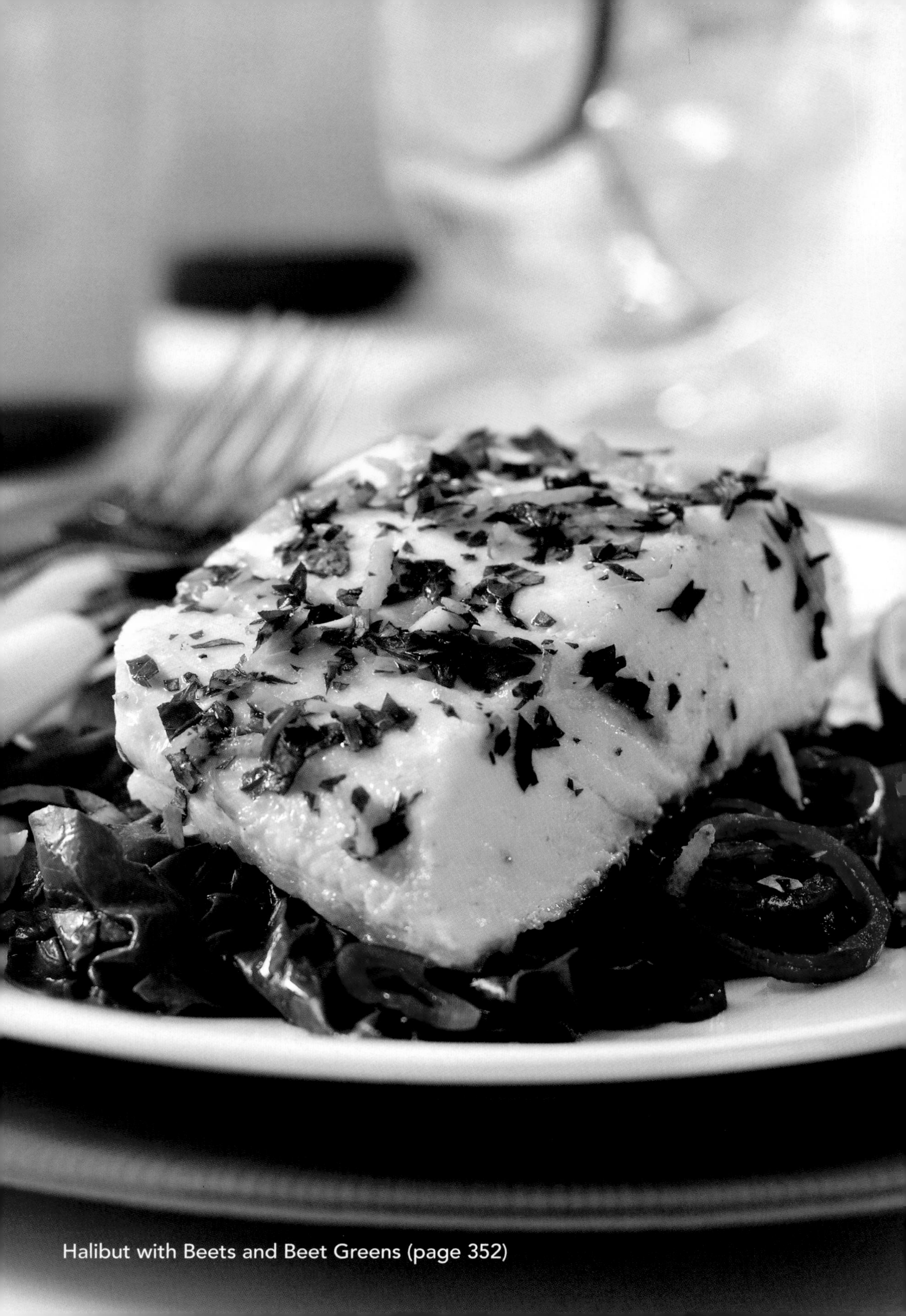

Halibut with Beets and Beet Greens (page 352)

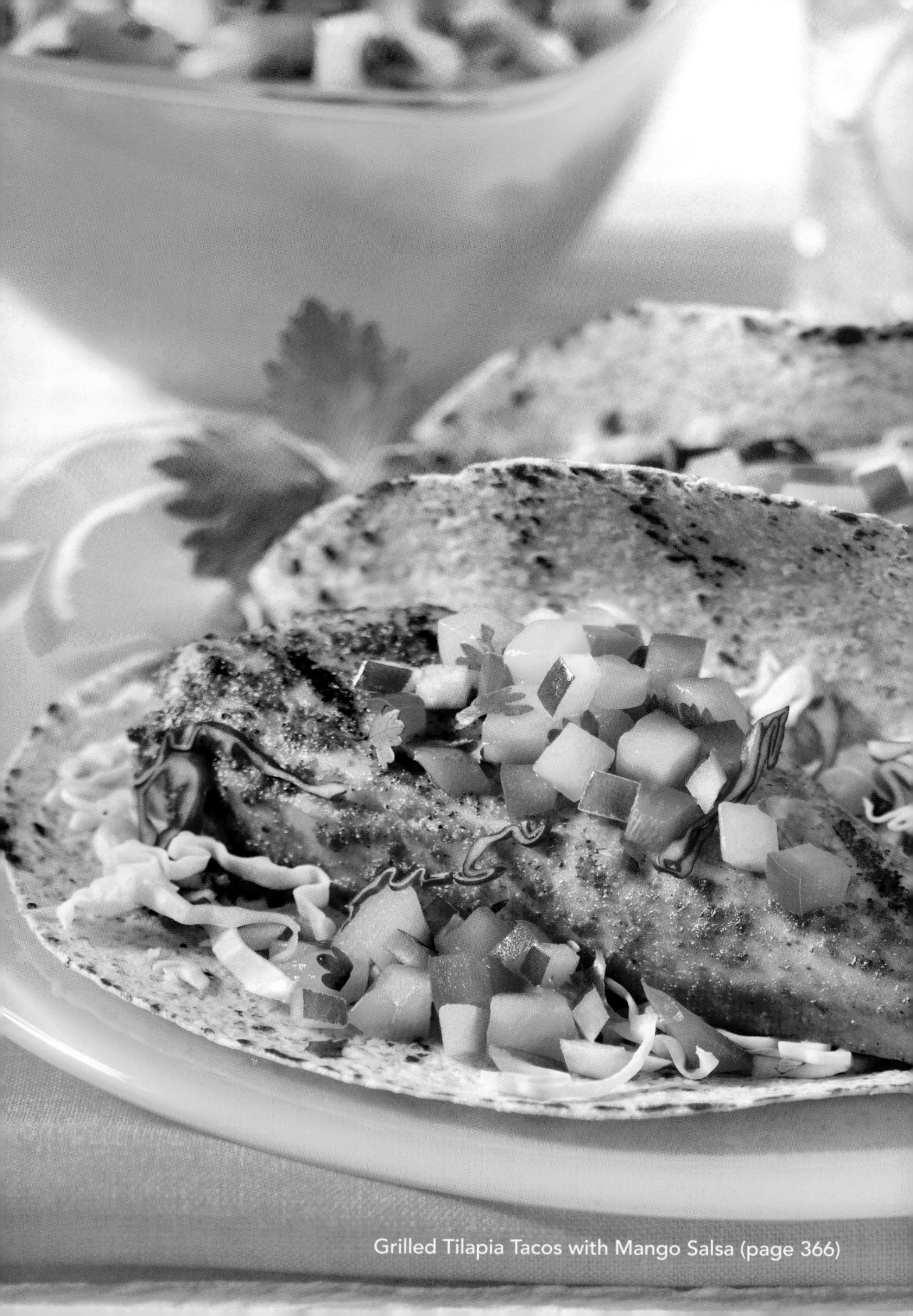
Grilled Tilapia Tacos with Mango Salsa (page 366)

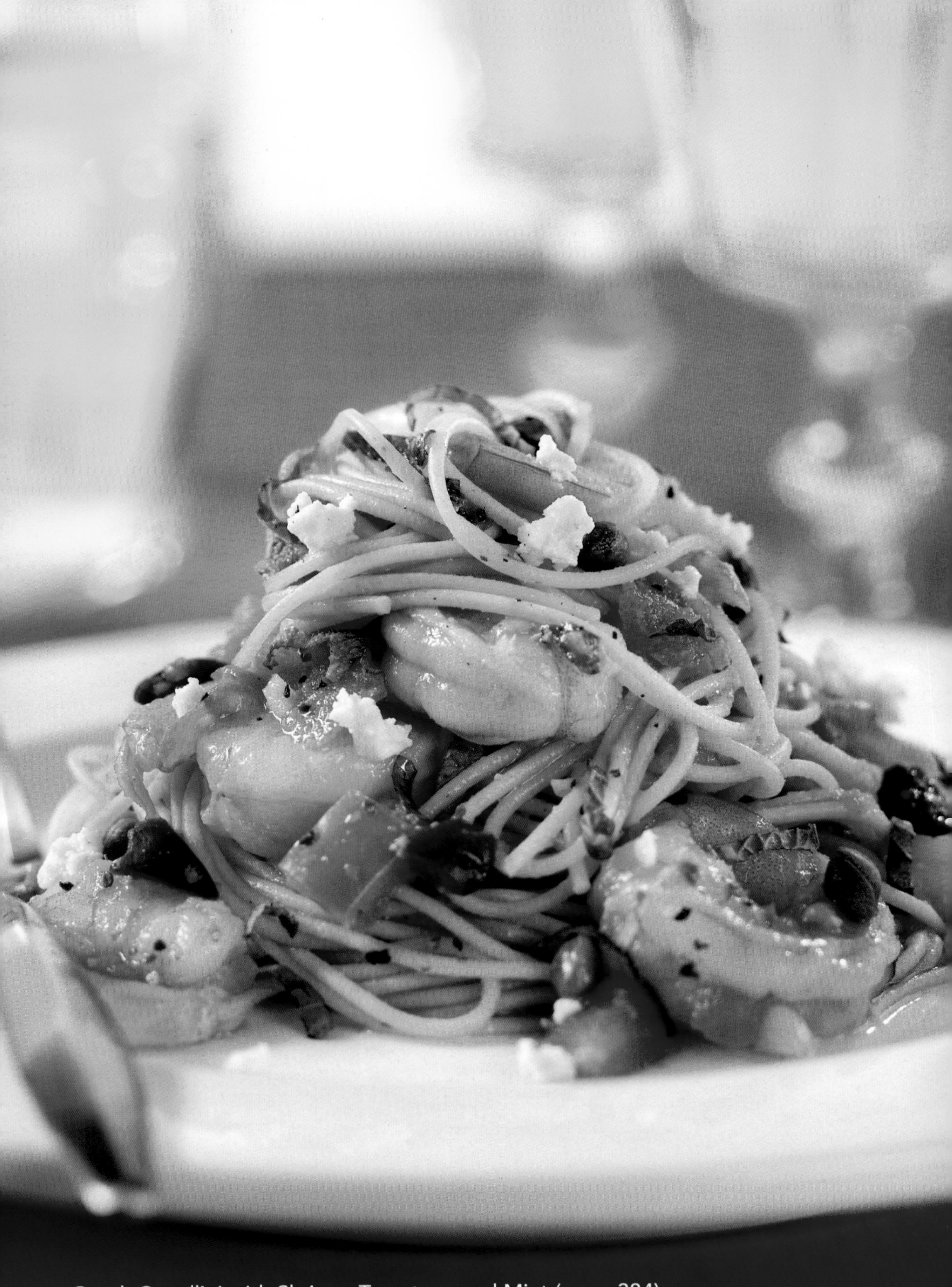

Greek Capellini with Shrimp, Tomatoes and Mint (page 384)

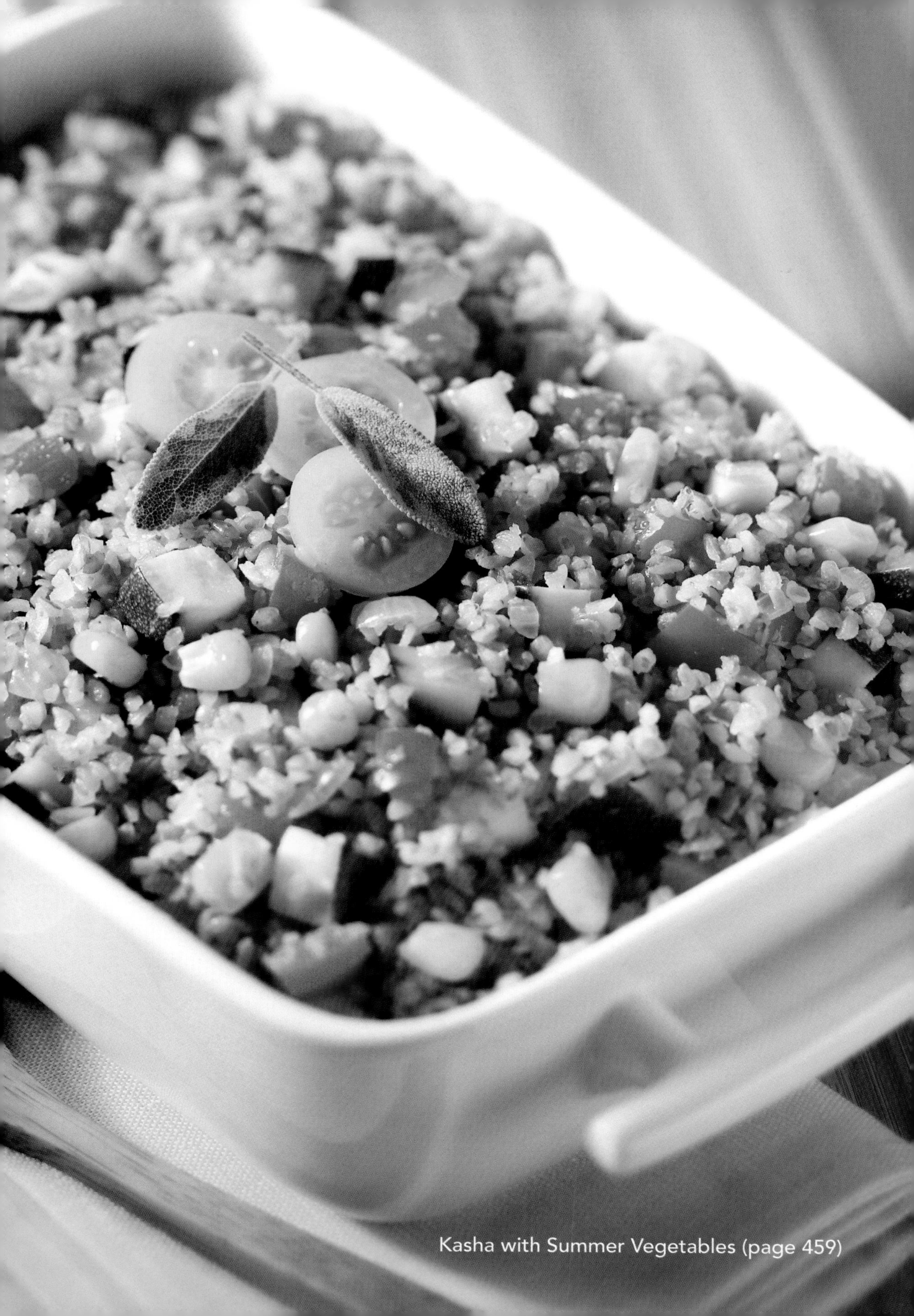
Kasha with Summer Vegetables (page 459)

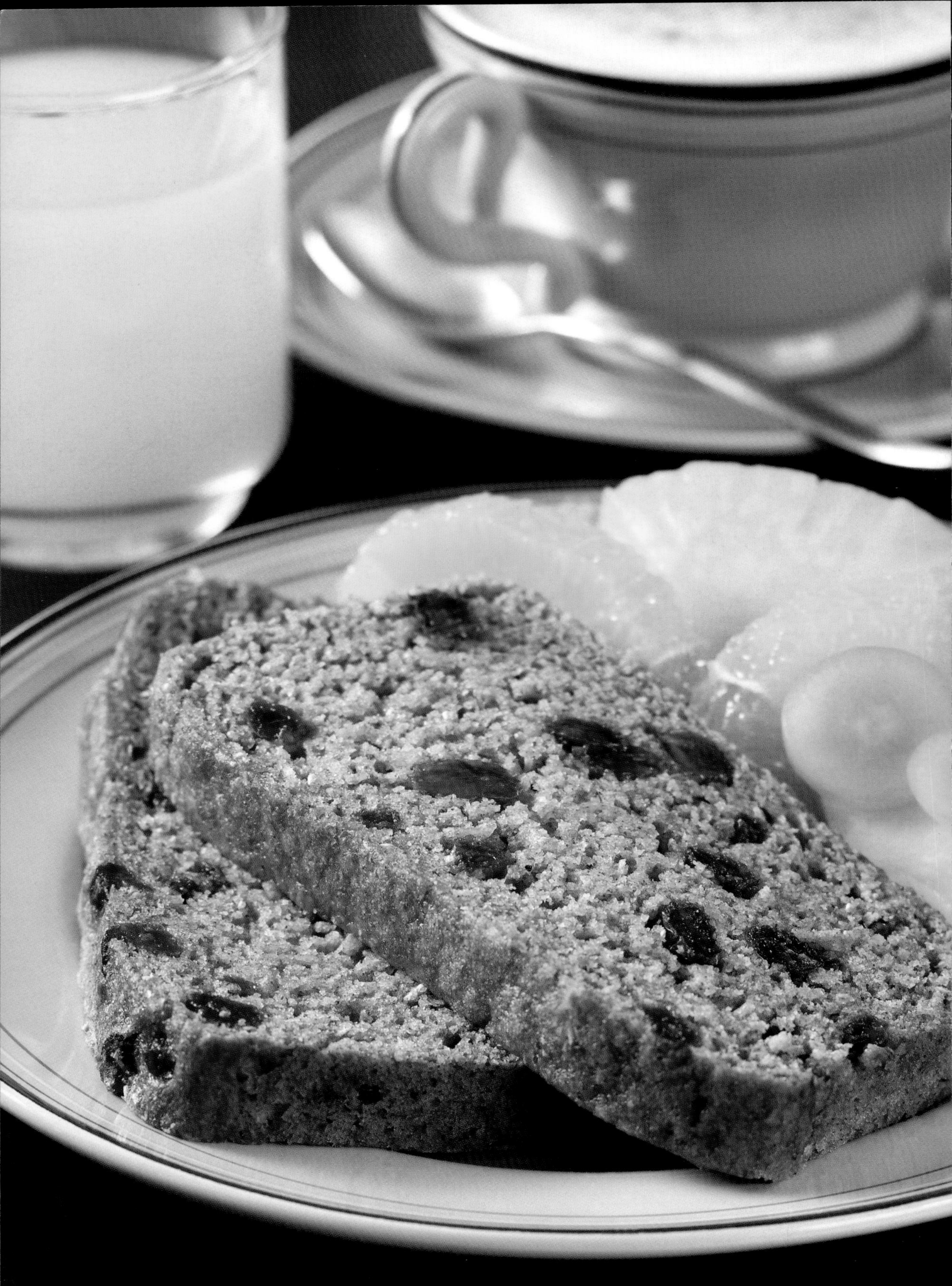

Cranberry, Orange and Agave Bread (page 476)

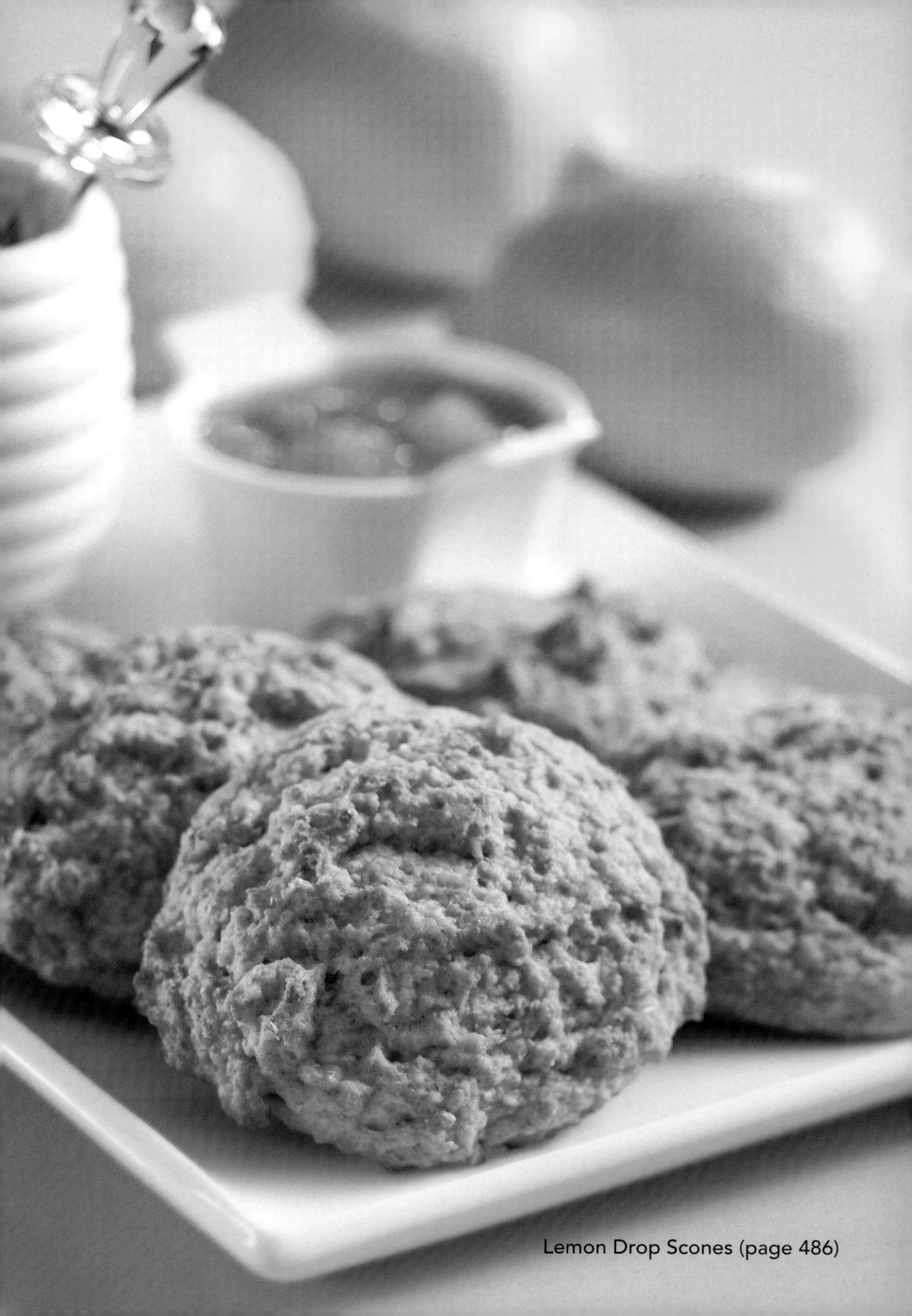

Lemon Drop Scones (page 486)

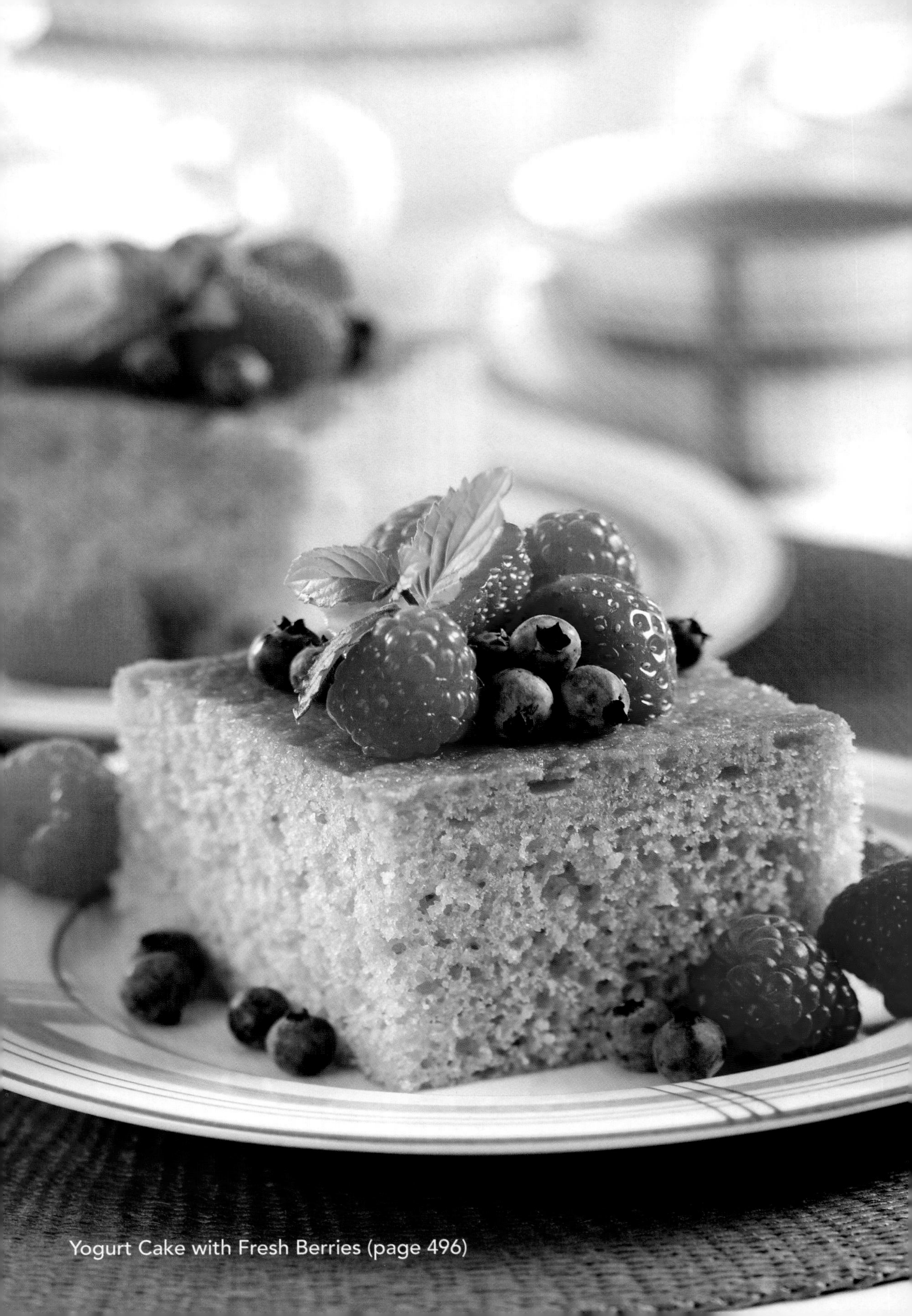

Yogurt Cake with Fresh Berries (page 496)

Fresh Ginger Gingerbread (page 500)
with Minted Fruit Salad (page 507)

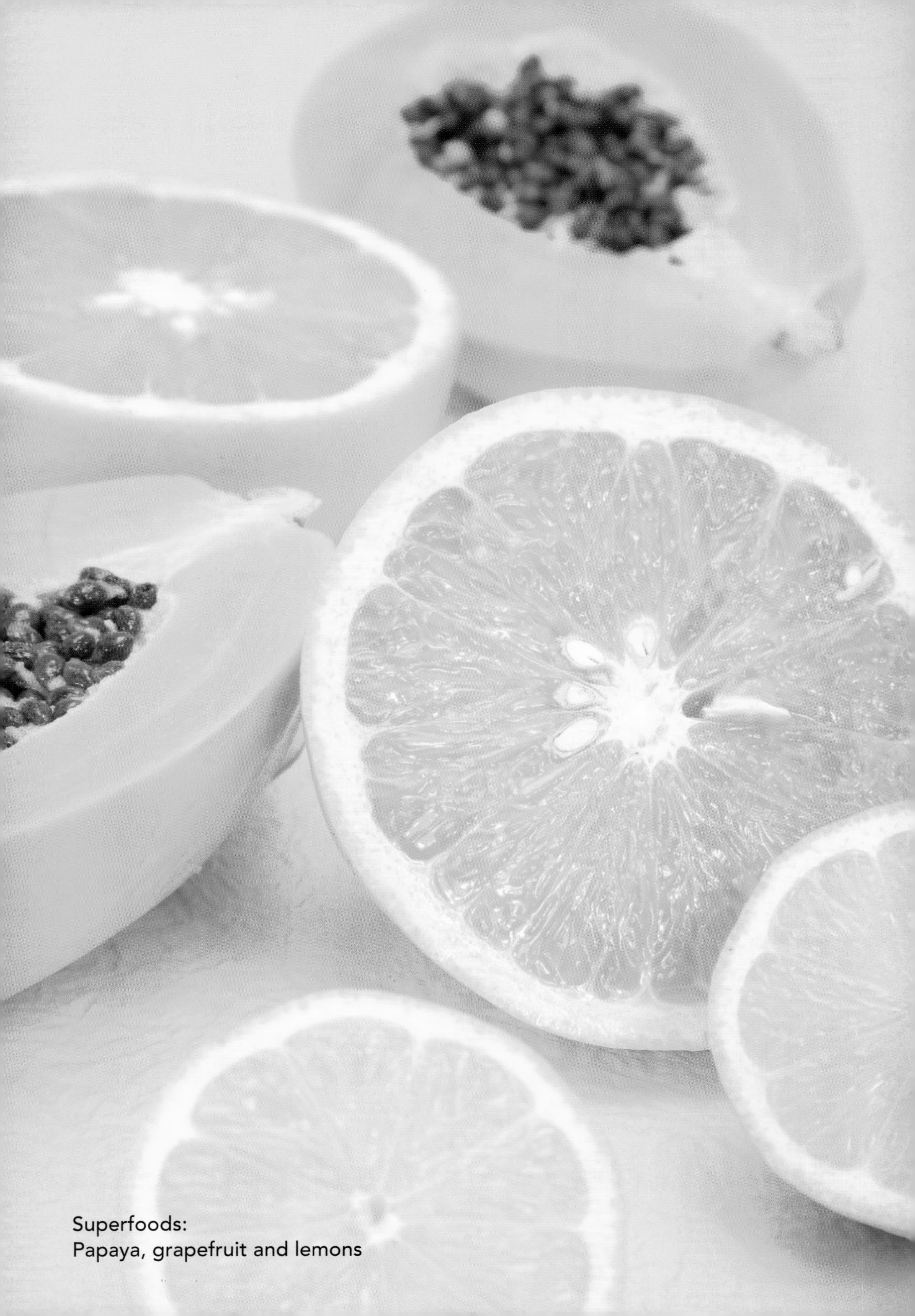

Superfoods:
Papaya, grapefruit and lemons

Halibut with Coconut Lime Sauce

Makes 4 servings

✪ Great for Steps 1, 3 and 4

Highly prized for its firm, mild flesh, halibut is well worth the occasional splurge at the fish counter. Here, it heads to the islands in a splendid ginger- and lime-infused coconut sauce.

Tip

Sea bass, cod or any other firm white fish fillets may be used in place of the halibut.

- **Preheat oven to 350°F (180°C)**
- **9-inch (23 cm) glass baking dish, sprayed with nonstick cooking spray (preferably olive oil)**

1 tsp	vegetable oil	5 mL
2	cloves garlic, minced	2
1 tbsp	minced gingerroot	15 mL
1/2 tsp	fine sea salt	2 mL
1/8 tsp	cayenne pepper	0.5 mL
1/2 cup	light coconut milk	125 mL
1 tsp	grated lime zest	5 mL
2 tbsp	freshly squeezed lime juice	30 mL
4	skinless Pacific halibut fillets (each about 5 oz/150 g)	4
1/2 cup	packed fresh cilantro leaves, chopped	125 mL

1. In a medium skillet, heat oil over medium heat. Add garlic and ginger; cook, stirring, for 2 minutes. Add salt, cayenne, coconut milk, lime zest and lime juice; reduce heat and simmer, stirring occasionally, for 5 minutes.
2. Place fish in prepared baking dish and spoon coconut sauce over top. Bake in preheated oven for 13 to 16 minutes or until fish is opaque and flakes easily when tested with a fork.
3. Place a fillet on each plate and spoon sauce over top. Sprinkle with cilantro.

Superfood Spotlight

Cilantro • Cilantro has a reputation for being high on the list of healing herbs. Research has shown that, when cilantro was added to the diet of diabetic mice, it helped stimulate their secretion of insulin and lowered their blood sugar. The leaves contain the compound dodecenal, which tests show is twice as effective at killing salmonella bacteria as some antibiotics. In addition, eight other antibiotic compounds were isolated from the plant. Cilantro has also been shown to lower "bad" cholesterol and increase "good" cholesterol. It is a good source of several nutrients, including potassium and calcium, and contains high levels of lutein and zeaxanthin, which help protect our eyes and eyesight.

Nutrients per serving

Calories	149
Total fat	5 g
Saturated fat	2 g
Cholesterol	61 mg
Sodium	441 mg
Carbohydrate	2 g
Fiber	0 g
Protein	24 g
Calcium	16 mg
Iron	0.3 mg

Broiled Mahi Mahi with Red Pepper Harissa

Makes 4 servings

✪ Great for Steps 1, 3 and 4

Mahi mahi, like cod, is mild in flavor yet meaty in texture. Here, it embraces the roasted sweetness of bell peppers, whose rich flavor is offset by smoky paprika and pungent garlic.

Tips

According to the Monterey Bay Aquarium Seafood Watch, U.S.-caught mahi mahi, in comparison to mahi mahi caught in other regions, is abundant, well managed and caught in an environmentally friendly way.

Sea bass, cod, halibut or any other firm white fish fillets may be used in place of the mahi mahi.

Nutrients per serving	
Calories	218
Total fat	7 g
Saturated fat	1 g
Cholesterol	51 mg
Sodium	269 mg
Carbohydrate	3 g
Fiber	1 g
Protein	34 g
Calcium	83 mg
Iron	1.7 mg

- **Preheat broiler, with rack set 4 to 6 inches (10 to 15 cm) from the heat source**
- **Blender**
- **Broiler pan, sprayed with nonstick cooking spray (preferably olive oil)**

1	jar (8 oz/227 mL) roasted red bell peppers, drained	1
1	clove garlic	1
3⁄4 tsp	hot smoked paprika	3 mL
1⁄2 tsp	ground cumin	2 mL
1⁄4 tsp	ground coriander	1 mL
3 tbsp	reduced-sodium ready-to-use vegetable broth	45 mL
4	skinless mahi mahi or Pacific halibut fillets (each about 5 oz/150 g)	4
1 tbsp	extra virgin olive oil	15 mL
1⁄4 tsp	fine sea salt	1 mL
1⁄4 tsp	freshly cracked black pepper	1 mL

1. In blender, combine roasted peppers, garlic, paprika, cumin, coriander and broth; purée until smooth. Set aside.
2. Place fish on prepared pan. Brush both sides with oil and sprinkle with salt and pepper. Broil, turning once, for about 4 minutes per side or until fish is opaque and flakes easily when tested with a fork. Serve with red pepper harissa.

Grilled Salmon with Mustard Maple Vinaigrette

Makes 4 servings

✪ Great for Steps 1, 3 and 4

With a nod to the Pacific Northwest, this super-quick mustard and maple glaze keeps the salmon fillets incredibly moist. A peppery bed of fresh watercress balances and brightens all.

Tip

According to the Monterey Bay Aquarium Seafood Watch, some of the best choices for wild salmon are those caught in Alaska, British Columbia, California, Oregon and Washington. Compared with salmon caught in other regions, these options are abundant, well managed and caught in an environmentally friendly way.

Nutrients per serving	
Calories	274
Total fat	17 g
Saturated fat	4 g
Cholesterol	63 mg
Sodium	308 mg
Carbohydrate	5 g
Fiber	0 g
Protein	26 g
Calcium	79 mg
Iron	0.4 mg

- **Preheat barbecue grill to medium-high**

1 tbsp	cider vinegar	15 mL
1 tbsp	pure maple syrup	15 mL
1 tbsp	extra virgin olive oil	15 mL
2 tsp	whole-grain Dijon mustard	10 mL
4	skinless wild salmon fillets (each about 5 oz/150 g)	4
	Nonstick cooking spray (preferably olive oil)	
1/4 tsp	fine sea salt	1 mL
1/4 tsp	freshly cracked black pepper	1 mL
4 cups	packed watercress sprigs	1 L

1. In a small bowl or cup, whisk together vinegar, maple syrup, oil and mustard. Set aside.
2. Lightly spray both sides of fish with cooking spray, then sprinkle with salt and pepper. Grill on preheated barbecue, turning once, for 3 to 4 minutes per side or until fish is opaque and flakes easily when tested with a fork.
3. Divide watercress among four dinner plates. Top with salmon and drizzle fish and watercress with vinaigrette.

Oven-BBQ Salmon with Fresh Corn Basil Relish

Makes 4 servings

✪ Great for Steps 1, 3 and 4

Your eyes aren't playing tricks on you: this gorgeous salmon emerged from your oven, not your grill. Together with the fresh corn basil relish (which coaxes out the natural richness of the fish), the dish is a beautiful union between land and sea.

Tip

If wild salmon is unavailable, look for U.S.-farmed salmon (such as Coho, Sake or Silver), which is farmed in an environmentally friendly way.

Nutrients per serving	
Calories	299
Total fat	15 g
Saturated fat	4 g
Cholesterol	63 mg
Sodium	312 mg
Carbohydrate	13 g
Fiber	1 g
Protein	26 g
Calcium	139 mg
Iron	0.4 mg

- **Preheat oven to 500°F (260°C)**
- **Small rimmed baking sheet, sprayed with nonstick cooking spray (preferably olive oil)**

1 tsp	vegetable oil	5 mL
1 cup	fresh or thawed frozen corn kernels	250 mL
1⁄4 cup	finely chopped red onion	60 mL
1⁄8 tsp	fine sea salt	0.5 mL
2 tsp	freshly squeezed lemon juice	10 mL
1⁄4 cup	packed fresh basil leaves, chopped	60 mL
4	skinless wild salmon fillets (each about 5 oz/150 g)	4
1⁄4 cup	barbecue sauce	60 mL

1. In a large skillet, heat oil over medium-high heat. Add corn, red onion and salt; cook, stirring, for 2 minutes. Transfer to a small bowl and stir in lemon juice. Let cool, then stir in basil just before serving.
2. Place fish, skinned side down, on prepared baking sheet. Generously brush with barbecue sauce. Bake in preheated oven for 7 to 11 minutes or until fish is opaque and flakes easily when tested with a fork. Serve with corn relish.

Spice-Crusted Salmon with Mint Raita

Makes 4 servings

✪ Great for Steps 1, 3 and 4

A minted, tart yogurt raita gives sprightliness to robustly spiced salmon.

Tips

According to the Monterey Bay Aquarium Seafood Watch, some of the best choices for wild salmon are those caught in Alaska, British Columbia, California, Oregon and Washington. Compared with salmon caught in other regions, these options are abundant, well managed and caught in an environmentally friendly way.

If wild salmon is unavailable, look for U.S.-farmed salmon (such as Coho, Sake or Silver), which is farmed in an environmentally friendly way.

Nutrients per serving	
Calories	263
Total fat	16 g
Saturated fat	4 g
Cholesterol	63 mg
Sodium	427 mg
Carbohydrate	4 g
Fiber	1 g
Protein	26 g
Calcium	85 mg
Iron	0.6 mg

1	clove garlic, minced	1
1/4 cup	packed fresh mint leaves, chopped	60 mL
2 tsp	minced gingerroot	10 mL
1/2 tsp	fine sea salt, divided	2 mL
1/2 cup	nonfat plain yogurt	125 mL
3 tsp	freshly squeezed lime juice, divided	15 mL
1 tsp	fennel seeds	5 mL
1 tsp	coriander seeds	5 mL
4	skin-on wild salmon fillets (each about 5 oz/150 g)	4
	Nonstick cooking spray	
1/4 tsp	freshly cracked black pepper	1 mL
2 tsp	vegetable oil	10 mL
4	lime wedges	4

1. In a small bowl, whisk together garlic, mint, ginger, a pinch of the salt, yogurt and 1 tsp (5 mL) of the lime juice. Cover and refrigerate until ready to use.
2. In a sealable plastic bag, combine fennel seeds and coriander seeds. Seal and, using a mallet or rolling pin, crush seeds.
3. Lightly spray skinless side of fish with cooking spray. Sprinkle with crushed seeds, pepper and the remaining salt. In a large skillet, heat oil over medium-high heat. Add fish, seed side down, and cook, turning once, for about 3 to 4 minutes per side or until fish is opaque and flakes easily when tested with a fork. Drizzle with the remaining lime juice. Serve seed side up, with lime wedges and mint raita.

Seared Salmon with Fresh Pineapple Salsa

Makes 4 servings

✪ Great for Steps 1, 3 and 4

Nutrients per serving	
Calories	292
Total fat	15 g
Saturated fat	4 g
Cholesterol	63 mg
Sodium	240 mg
Carbohydrate	13 g
Fiber	1 g
Protein	25 g
Calcium	44 mg
Iron	0.5 mg

1 cup	diced fresh pineapple (see tip, page 367)	250 mL
2 tbsp	chopped fresh mint	30 mL
2 tsp	minced gingerroot	10 mL
2 tbsp	orange marmalade	30 mL
1 tbsp	freshly squeezed lime juice	15 mL
4	skinless wild salmon fillets (each about 5 oz/150 g)	4
2 tsp	vegetable oil	10 mL
1/4 tsp	fine sea salt	1 mL
1/8 tsp	cayenne pepper	0.5 mL

1. In a small bowl, combine pineapple, mint, ginger, orange marmalade and lime juice. Set aside.
2. Brush both sides of fish with oil and sprinkle with salt and cayenne. Heat a large skillet over medium-high heat. Add fish and cook, turning once, for 3 to 4 minutes per side or until fish is opaque and flakes easily when tested with a fork. Serve with pineapple salsa.

Hoisin Salmon

Makes 4 servings

✪ Great for Steps 1, 3 and 4

Nutrients per serving	
Calories	264
Total fat	13 g
Saturated fat	4 g
Cholesterol	63 mg
Sodium	282 mg
Carbohydrate	9 g
Fiber	0 g
Protein	25 g
Calcium	36 mg
Iron	0.7 mg

- **Preheat broiler, with rack set 4 to 6 inches (10 to 15 cm) from the heat source**
- **Broiler pan, sprayed with nonstick cooking spray (preferably olive oil)**

3 tbsp	hoisin sauce	45 mL
2 tsp	liquid honey or agave nectar	10 mL
1 tsp	hot Chinese mustard or Dijon mustard	5 mL
1/2 tsp	unseasoned rice vinegar	2 mL
4	skinless wild salmon fillets (each about 5 oz/150 g)	4
1/3 cup	thinly sliced green onions	75 mL

1. In a small cup, whisk together hoisin sauce, honey, mustard and vinegar.
2. Place fish on prepared pan and brush both sides with half the hoisin mixture, coating evenly. Broil for 5 to 8 minutes, basting once with the remaining sauce, until fish is opaque and flakes easily when tested with a fork. Serve sprinkled with green onions.

Seared Salmon with Warm Lentil and Arugula Salad

Makes 4 servings

✪ Great for Steps 1, 3 and 4

Vive la France: *A lovely lentil and arugula salad, with a mustardy vinaigrette for verve, makes this simple pan-cooked fish taste deep and complex.*

Tip

According to the Monterey Bay Aquarium Seafood Watch, some of the best choices for wild salmon are those caught in Alaska, British Columbia, California, Oregon and Washington. Compared with salmon caught in other regions, these options are abundant, well managed and caught in an environmentally friendly way.

4 cups	water	1 L
1 cup	dried green lentils, rinsed	250 mL
3/4 tsp	fine sea salt, divided	3 mL
1/2 tsp	freshly cracked black pepper, divided	2 mL
4 tsp	extra virgin olive oil, divided	20 mL
1 tbsp	red wine vinegar	15 mL
1 tsp	Dijon mustard	5 mL
1 tsp	liquid honey	5 mL
4	skinless wild salmon fillets (each about 5 oz/150 g)	4
3 cups	packed arugula, roughly chopped	750 mL
1/2 cup	packed fresh flat-leaf (Italian) parsley leaves, chopped	125 mL
1/3 cup	finely chopped red onion	75 mL

1. In a medium saucepan, bring water to a boil over high heat. Add lentils, reduce heat and simmer for about 30 minutes or until tender but not mushy. Drain.
2. In a medium bowl, combine cooked lentils, 1/2 tsp (2 mL) of the salt, half the pepper, half the oil, vinegar, mustard and honey. Let cool slightly.
3. Meanwhile, sprinkle both sides of fish with the remaining salt and pepper. In a large skillet, heat the remaining oil over medium-high heat. Add fish and cook, turning once, for 3 to 4 minutes per side or until fish is opaque and flakes easily when tested with a fork.
4. To the lentil mixture, add arugula, parsley and red onion, gently tossing to combine. Serve with salmon.

Superfood Spotlight

Salmon • Much of the salmon we eat today is farmed rather than wild. Although wild salmon tends to contain less fat and a little more of some nutrients, the two types are broadly comparable. Salmon is a major source of fish oils, which provide protection against heart disease, blood clots, stroke, high blood pressure, high blood cholesterol, Alzheimer's disease, depression and certain skin conditions. Salmon is also an excellent source of selenium, which protects against cancer, as well as protein, niacin, vitamin B_{12}, magnesium and vitamin B_6.

Nutrients per serving	
Calories	432
Total fat	19 g
Saturated fat	5 g
Cholesterol	63 mg
Sodium	528 mg
Carbohydrate	31 g
Fiber	8 g
Protein	36 g
Calcium	90 mg
Iron	3.7 mg

Thai Red Curry–Glazed Salmon

Makes 4 servings

✪ Great for Steps 1, 3 and 4

Broiling salmon gives it a light golden crust and a flaky, moist center. The texture is made all the more memorable when it's paired with bold Thai red curry paste, fresh lime juice and mint.

Tips

If wild salmon is unavailable, look for U.S.-farmed salmon (such as Coho, Sake or Silver), which is farmed in an environmentally friendly way.

An equal amount of cilantro leaves may be used in place of the mint.

Nutrients per serving	
Calories	273
Total fat	17 g
Saturated fat	5 g
Cholesterol	63 mg
Sodium	248 mg
Carbohydrate	4 g
Fiber	0 g
Protein	25 g
Calcium	38 mg
Iron	0.6 mg

- **Preheat broiler, with rack set 4 to 6 inches (10 to 15 cm) from the heat source**
- **Broiler pan, sprayed with nonstick cooking spray (preferably olive oil)**

1/4 tsp	fine sea salt	1 mL
1 tbsp	Thai red curry paste	15 mL
1 tbsp	vegetable oil	15 mL
2 tsp	agave nectar or liquid honey	10 mL
4	skinless wild salmon fillets (each about 5 oz/150 g)	4
1 1/2 tbsp	freshly squeezed lime juice	22 mL
1/4 cup	packed fresh mint leaves, chopped	60 mL

1. In a small bowl, whisk together salt, curry paste, oil and agave nectar until smooth.
2. Place fish on prepared pan and brush both sides with curry mixture, coating evenly. Broil for 5 to 8 minutes or until fish is opaque and flakes easily when tested with a fork. Serve drizzled with lime juice and sprinkled with mint.

Swedish Salmon, Asparagus and Potato Omelet

Makes 6 servings

✪ Great for Steps 1, 3 and 4

This is a simplified version of laxpudding (salmon pudding), which is based on the traditional Swedish housewife's firm conviction that a good dinner provides an excellent basis for the next day's lunch. With a little salmon, some eggs and a few potatoes, you can go a long way.

Tip

Other varieties of waxy potatoes may be used in place of the red-skinned potatoes.

Nutrients per serving	
Calories	314
Total fat	11 g
Saturated fat	3 g
Cholesterol	246 mg
Sodium	769 mg
Carbohydrate	17 g
Fiber	3 g
Protein	36 g
Calcium	100 mg
Iron	2.8 mg

- **Preheat broiler, with rack set 4 to 6 inches (10 to 15 cm) from the heat source**
- **Large ovenproof skillet**

12 oz	red-skinned potatoes (3 to 4 medium), cut into 1⁄2-inch (1 cm) cubes	375 g
8 oz	asparagus, trimmed and cut into 1⁄2-inch (1 cm) pieces	250 g
6	large eggs, lightly beaten	6
3	large egg whites, lightly beaten	3
1⁄2 tsp	fine sea salt	2 mL
1⁄4 tsp	freshly ground black pepper	1 mL
2 tsp	extra virgin olive oil	10 mL
1	small red bell pepper, chopped	1
1 cup	chopped onion	250 mL
1	can (15 oz/425 g) wild Alaskan salmon, drained and flaked (skin removed, if necessary)	1
3 tbsp	chopped fresh dill	45 mL

1. Place potatoes in a medium saucepan and cover with cold water. Bring to a boil over medium-high heat. Boil for about 7 minutes or until just tender. Add asparagus and cook for 30 seconds. Drain and set aside.
2. In a medium bowl, whisk together eggs, egg whites, salt and pepper. Set aside.
3. In ovenproof skillet, heat oil over medium-high heat. Add red pepper and onion; cook, stirring, for 6 to 8 minutes or until softened. Add potato mixture and cook, stirring, for 5 minutes. Add salmon and dill; cook, stirring, for 1 minute.
4. Pour in egg mixture, reduce heat to low and cook, stirring occasionally, for about 5 minutes or until eggs begin to set but are still wet on top. Cook, without stirring, for 5 minutes.
5. Place skillet under the preheated broiler and broil for 2 to 3 minutes or until golden and set at center. Let cool for at least 15 minutes before serving.

Salmon Cakes with Buttermilk Dressing and Mixed Greens

Makes 4 servings

✪ Great for Steps 1, 3, 4 and 5

Here, pantry-friendly canned salmon gets the patty-cake treatment. Accompanying the cakes is a fresh bed of baby lettuce and a pleasingly Southern buttermilk dressing. Enjoy, y'all.

Variation

Other tender greens or lettuces, such as arugula, spinach, watercress sprigs or torn butter lettuce, may be used in place of the mesclun.

5 tbsp	finely sliced green onions, divided	75 mL
	Fine sea salt	
1⁄2 cup	buttermilk	125 mL
3 tsp	Dijon mustard, divided	15 mL
2 tsp	freshly squeezed lemon juice	10 mL
1⁄2 cup	fresh whole wheat bread crumbs	125 mL
1⁄4 tsp	freshly ground black pepper	1 mL
2	large egg whites, beaten	2
1	can (15 oz/425 g) wild Alaskan salmon, drained and flaked (skin removed, if necessary)	1
4 tsp	extra virgin olive oil, divided	20 mL
8 cups	mesclun (mixed baby lettuce)	2 L

1. In a small bowl, whisk together 1 tbsp (15 mL) of the green onions, 1⁄8 tsp (0.5 mL) salt, buttermilk, 1 tsp (5 mL) of the mustard, and lemon juice. Set aside.
2. In a large bowl, gently combine bread crumbs, the remaining green onions, 1⁄4 tsp (1 mL) salt, pepper, egg whites, salmon and the remaining mustard. Form into eight 3⁄4-inch (2 cm) thick patties.
3. In a large skillet, heat half the oil over medium-high heat. Add half the patties and cook, turning once, for 5 to 6 minutes per side or until golden brown on both sides and hot in the center. Transfer to a plate and tent with foil to keep warm. Repeat with the remaining oil and patties.
4. Divide mesclun among four plates. Top each with 2 salmon cakes and drizzle with some of the dressing. Pass the remaining dressing at the table.

Nutrients per serving	
Calories	337
Total fat	13 g
Saturated fat	3 g
Cholesterol	101 mg
Sodium	607 mg
Carbohydrate	13 g
Fiber	2 g
Protein	43 g
Calcium	144 mg
Iron	3.6 mg

Lemon Dill Tilapia in Foil

Makes 4 servings

✪ Great for Steps 1, 3 and 4

Sometimes, the plainest, simplest dishes are the best. It doesn't get easier or more tasty than foil packets of tilapia with lemon, dill, parsley and olive oil!

Tip

Other mild, lean white fish, such as orange roughy, snapper, cod, tilefish or striped bass, may be used in place of the tilapia.

- **Preheat oven to 375°F (190°C)**
- **Four 12-inch (30 cm) squares foil**
- **Large rimmed baking sheet**

2	lemons, each cut into 6 slices	2
4	skinless farmed tilapia fillets (each about 6 oz/175 g)	4
1/2 tsp	fine sea salt, divided	2 mL
1/2 tsp	freshly cracked black pepper, divided	2 mL
1/2 cup	shredded carrot	125 mL
2 tbsp	chopped fresh dill	30 mL
2 tbsp	chopped fresh flat-leaf (Italian) parsley	30 mL
2 tsp	extra virgin olive oil	10 mL

1. Place foil squares on a work surface. Place 3 lemon slices in an overlapping line down the center of each square. Top each with a fish fillet and sprinkle with half the salt and half the pepper. Top with equal amounts of carrot, dill and parsley. Drizzle with oil and sprinkle with the remaining salt and pepper. Fold foil over fish and vegetables, crimping edges tightly to seal. Place packets on baking sheet.
2. Bake in preheated oven for 18 to 22 minutes or until fish is opaque and flakes easily when tested with a fork. Slide packets onto plates.

Superfood Spotlight

Lemons • All parts of the lemon contain valuable nutrients and antioxidants. Lemons are a particularly good source of vitamin C. The plant compound antioxidants include limonene, an oil found in the peel of the lemon that may help prevent breast and other cancers and lower "bad" blood cholesterol, and rutin, which has been found to strengthen veins and prevent fluid retention. Lemons stimulate the taste buds and may be useful for people with a poor appetite.

Nutrients per serving	
Calories	202
Total fat	5 g
Saturated fat	1 g
Cholesterol	88 mg
Sodium	452 mg
Carbohydrate	4 g
Fiber	2 g
Protein	35 g
Calcium	35 mg
Iron	1.2 mg

Mediterranean Grilled Tilapia and Whole Wheat Couscous

Makes 4 servings

✪ Great for Steps 1, 3, 4 and 5

Aromatic without being spicy, this tilapia dish has a touch of the exotic but will please traditionalists, too. The couscous hits notes of earthy, briny, sweet and salty, and the tilapia is wonderfully delicious with a bit of char from the grill.

2	cloves garlic, minced	2
1 tsp	minced fresh rosemary	5 mL
1/2 tsp	fine sea salt, divided	2 mL
1/4 tsp	freshly cracked black pepper	1 mL
2 tbsp	freshly squeezed lemon juice	30 mL
1 tbsp	extra virgin olive oil	15 mL
4	skinless farmed tilapia fillets (each about 6 oz/175 g)	4
1 cup	whole wheat couscous	250 mL
1 cup	boiling water	250 mL
1/3 cup	packed fresh flat-leaf (Italian) parsley leaves, chopped	75 mL
2 tbsp	chopped sun-dried tomatoes	30 mL
1 tbsp	minced pitted brine-cured black olives (such as kalamata)	15 mL

1. In a shallow dish, whisk together garlic, rosemary, half the salt, pepper, lemon juice and oil. Add tilapia and turn to coat. Let stand for 15 minutes.
2. Meanwhile, preheat barbecue grill to medium-high.
3. In a medium bowl, combine couscous, the remaining salt and boiling water. Cover with a plate and let stand for 5 minutes. Fluff with a fork. Stir in parsley, sun-dried tomatoes and olives.
4. Grill tilapia for 2 to 3 minutes per side or until fish is opaque and flakes easily when tested with a fork. Serve with couscous.

Tip

According to the Monterey Bay Aquarium Seafood Watch, U.S.- and Canadian-farmed tilapia are the best choices because the supplies are abundant, well managed and farmed in an environmentally friendly way. A good alternative is tilapia farmed in Brazil, Costa Rica, Honduras or Ecuador.

Nutrients per serving	
Calories	381
Total fat	7 g
Saturated fat	2 g
Cholesterol	88 mg
Sodium	495 mg
Carbohydrate	40 g
Fiber	7 g
Protein	43 g
Calcium	52 mg
Iron	3.0 mg

Garam Masala–Spiced Tilapia with Watermelon Salsa

Makes 4 servings

✪ Great for Steps 1, 3 and 4

Garam masala reinvents farm-raised tilapia, balancing the slightly sweet fillets with warming spices and exotic flair. The boldly flavored fish is made even more magical when it's paired with a harmonizing watermelon salsa.

Tip

Other mild, lean white fish, such as orange roughy, snapper, cod, tilefish or striped bass, may be used in place of the tilapia.

2 cups	cubed seedless watermelon (1/4-inch/0.5 cm cubes)	500 mL
1/2 cup	chopped red onion	125 mL
1/4 cup	packed fresh mint leaves, chopped	60 mL
1/2 tsp	fine sea salt, divided	2 mL
1/8 tsp	cayenne pepper	0.5 mL
1 tbsp	freshly squeezed lime juice	15 mL
1 tsp	agave nectar or liquid honey	5 mL
4	skinless farmed tilapia fillets (each about 6 oz/175 g)	4
1 1/2 tsp	garam masala	7 mL
2 tsp	vegetable oil	10 mL

1. In a medium bowl, combine watermelon, red onion, mint, half the salt, cayenne, lime juice and agave nectar. Cover and refrigerate until ready to use.
2. Sprinkle both sides of fish with garam masala and the remaining salt. In a large skillet, heat oil over medium-high heat. Add fish and cook, turning once, for 2 to 3 minutes per side or until fish is opaque and flakes easily when tested with a fork. Serve with watermelon salsa.

Superfood Spotlight

Melons • Melons contain over 92% water, so they can help prevent fluid retention and balance sodium in the body while also keeping the kidneys working well. All melons are rich in vitamin B_6 and potassium, and several varieties are high in bioflavonoids, which have anti-aging properties and help fight cancer and heart disease. Further, all melons are high in soluble fiber, which contributes to arterial health and can lower "bad" blood cholesterol. Watermelon is a particularly good source of lycopene (which protects against prostate cancer) and also contains citrulline, an amino acid that aids blood flow to muscles, improving their function during exercise.

Nutrients per serving

Calories	223
Total fat	5 g
Saturated fat	1 g
Cholesterol	88 mg
Sodium	445 mg
Carbohydrate	11 g
Fiber	1 g
Protein	36 g
Calcium	32 mg
Iron	1.3 mg

Grilled Tilapia Tacos with Mango Salsa

Makes 4 servings

✪ Great for Steps 1, 3, 4 and 5

This dish showcases tilapia's outdoorsy side and the bright, fresh flavor of early summer mangos in tropical tacos that are perfect for lunch with friends or a light dinner eaten al fresco. Brushing the delicate fillets with a spiced lime vinaigrette seals in their juices and intensifies the flavor of the tacos.

Tip

According to the Monterey Bay Aquarium Seafood Watch, U.S.- and Canadian-farmed tilapia are the best choices because the supplies are abundant, well managed and farmed in an environmentally friendly way. A good alternative is tilapia farmed in Brazil, Costa Rica, Honduras or Ecuador.

Nutrients per serving	
Calories	370
Total fat	9 g
Saturated fat	2 g
Cholesterol	88 mg
Sodium	579 mg
Carbohydrate	34 g
Fiber	5 g
Protein	41 g
Calcium	52 mg
Iron	1.7 mg

- **Preheat barbecue grill to medium-high**

Salsa

1 cup	chopped fresh or thawed frozen mango	250 mL
1/2 cup	chopped red bell pepper	125 mL
1/2 cup	packed fresh cilantro leaves, chopped	125 mL
1/4 cup	finely chopped red onion	60 mL
1/4 tsp	fine sea salt	1 mL
1 tbsp	freshly squeezed lime juice	15 mL

Tacos

1 tsp	ground cumin	5 mL
1/2 tsp	chili powder	2 mL
1/4 tsp	fine sea salt	1 mL
1 tbsp	freshly squeezed lime juice	15 mL
2 tsp	vegetable oil	10 mL
4	skinless farmed tilapia fillets (each about 6 oz/175 g)	4
4	8-inch (20 cm) whole wheat tortillas, warmed	4
2 cups	shredded purple or green cabbage	500 mL

1. *Salsa:* In a small bowl, combine mango, red pepper, cilantro, red onion, salt and lime juice.
2. *Tacos:* In a small cup, whisk together cumin, chili powder, salt, lime juice and oil. Brush on both sides of fish, coating evenly.
3. Grill fish on preheated barbecue, turning once, for 2 to 3 minutes per side or until fish is opaque and flakes easily when tested with a fork. Flake fish into small pieces.
4. Fill warmed tortillas with fish, cabbage and salsa.

Chipotle Tilapia Tacos with Pineapple

Makes 4 servings

✪ Great for Steps 1, 3, 4 and 5

A refined rethinking of a taqueria favorite provides a quick-to-the-table, imaginative way to serve tilapia.

Tips

A pineapple is ripe enough to eat when a leaf is easily pulled from the top. To prepare a pineapple, cut off the leafy top and a small layer of the base, then slice off the tough skin and "eyes." Cut the flesh into slices, then remove the chewy central core from each slice. Cut each slice into dice.

Thawed frozen diced pineapple may be used in place of the fresh pineapple.

Variation

Substitute diced mango for the pineapple.

Nutrients per serving	
Calories	351
Total fat	5 g
Saturated fat	1 g
Cholesterol	88 mg
Sodium	356 mg
Carbohydrate	39 g
Fiber	4 g
Protein	38 g
Calcium	45 mg
Iron	1.5 mg

- **Preheat broiler, with rack set 4 to 6 inches (10 to 15 cm) from the heat source**
- **Broiler pan, sprayed with nonstick cooking spray (preferably olive oil)**

4	skinless farmed tilapia fillets (each about 6 oz/175 g)	4
	Nonstick cooking spray	
3/4 tsp	chipotle chile powder	3 mL
1/2 tsp	ground cumin	2 mL
1/4 tsp	fine sea salt	1 mL
8	6-inch (15 cm) corn tortillas, warmed	8
2 cups	shredded coleslaw mix (shredded cabbage and carrots)	500 mL
1 cup	diced fresh pineapple (see tip, at left)	250 mL
1/2 cup	packed fresh cilantro leaves	125 mL
4	lime wedges	4

1. Place fish on prepared pan. Lightly spray both sides of fish with cooking spray, then sprinkle with chipotle chile powder, cumin and salt. Broil for 4 to 6 minutes or until fish is opaque and flakes easily when tested with a fork. Flake fish into small pieces.
2. Fill warmed tortillas with fish, coleslaw, pineapple and cilantro. Serve with lime wedges.

Broiled Herbed Trout Fillets

Makes 4 servings

✪ Great for Steps 1, 3 and 4

Butterflied trout fillets enhanced by a fresh herb dressing cook quickly under the broiler, delivering a light, satisfying entrée.

Tip

Other mild, lean white fish, such as orange roughy, snapper, cod, tilefish or striped bass, may be used in place of the trout.

- **Preheat broiler, with rack set 4 to 6 inches (10 to 15 cm) from the heat source**
- **Broiler pan, sprayed with nonstick cooking spray (preferably olive oil)**

1	clove garlic, minced	1
1 tbsp	minced fresh flat-leaf (Italian) parsley	15 mL
1 tbsp	minced fresh chives	15 mL
2 tsp	minced fresh oregano	10 mL
1/2 tsp	fine sea salt	2 mL
1/4 tsp	freshly cracked black pepper	1 mL
1 tbsp	extra virgin olive oil	15 mL
1 tbsp	freshly squeezed lemon juice	15 mL
4	skin-on trout fillets (each about 6 oz/175 g)	4

1. In a medium bowl, whisk together garlic, parsley, chives, oregano, salt, pepper, oil and lemon juice.
2. Place fish, skin side down, on prepared pan. Generously brush with dressing. Broil for 4 to 6 minutes or until fish is opaque and flakes easily when tested with a fork.

Nutrients per serving	
Calories	216
Total fat	10 g
Saturated fat	2 g
Cholesterol	145 mg
Sodium	422 mg
Carbohydrate	1 g
Fiber	0 g
Protein	30 g
Calcium	41 mg
Iron	0.7 mg

Baked Trout with Shiitake Mushrooms and Ginger

Makes 4 servings

✪ Great for Steps 1, 3 and 4

Trout travels to Japan: mushrooms and ginger are phenomenal flavorings for delicate trout in this ultra-streamlined dish.

Tips

Other mild, lean white fish, such as orange roughy, snapper, cod, tilefish or striped bass, may be used in place of the trout.

Other mushrooms, such as button or cremini, may be used in place of the shiitake mushrooms.

Nutrients per serving	
Calories	225
Total fat	9 g
Saturated fat	2 g
Cholesterol	145 mg
Sodium	419 mg
Carbohydrate	5 g
Fiber	1 g
Protein	31 g
Calcium	46 mg
Iron	1.2 mg

- **Preheat oven to 400°F (200°C)**
- **Large rimmed baking sheet, lined with foil and sprayed with nonstick cooking spray (preferably olive oil)**

4	skin-on trout fillets (each about 6 oz/175 g)	4
1/4 tsp	fine sea salt	1 mL
1/8 tsp	freshly ground black pepper	0.5 mL
3	cloves garlic, thinly sliced	3
8 oz	shiitake mushrooms, stems removed, caps thinly sliced	250 g
1/2 cup	thinly sliced green onions	125 mL
2 tsp	minced gingerroot	10 mL
4 tsp	reduced-sodium tamari or soy sauce	20 mL
2 tsp	toasted sesame oil	10 mL

1. Place fish, skin side down, on prepared baking sheet. Sprinkle with salt and pepper.
2. In a medium bowl, combine garlic, mushrooms, green onions, ginger, tamari and sesame oil. Spoon over fish.
3. Bake in preheated oven for 15 to 18 minutes or until fish is opaque and flakes easily when tested with a fork.

▶ Health Note

Trout contains energizing B vitamins and brain-enhancing omega-3 fatty acids.

Tuna with Farro and Fennel

Makes 4 servings

✪ Great for Steps 1, 3, 4 and 5

Although it may sound like an unusual pairing, the toothsome flavor and texture of farro really complements the meaty flavor of tuna. The richness is balanced by pleasantly licorice fennel, delicate yet deep-flavored, plus green olives and lemon.

Tip

The nutrients in carrots are more available to the body when the carrots are cooked. Further, combining carrots with a small amount of fat (e.g., olive oil, vegetable oil or butter) during cooking helps the body absorb the carotenes.

Nutrients per serving	
Calories	335
Total fat	7 g
Saturated fat	1 g
Cholesterol	8 mg
Sodium	531 mg
Carbohydrate	52 g
Fiber	12 g
Protein	19 g
Calcium	88 mg
Iron	2.3 mg

1	can (6 oz/170 g) oil-packed tuna	1
2	cloves garlic, minced	2
1	small bulb fennel, chopped, fronds reserved	1
1 cup	chopped carrots	250 mL
1 cup	chopped onion	250 mL
6 cups	water	1.5 L
1 cup	semi-pearled farro or pearl barley	250 mL
2 cups	packed arugula or tender watercress sprigs, roughly chopped	500 mL
1⁄3 cup	pitted green olives, coarsely chopped	75 mL
1⁄4 tsp	fine sea salt	1 mL
2 tbsp	freshly squeezed lemon juice	30 mL

1. Drain tuna, reserving 2 tsp (10 mL) oil. Flake tuna with a fork and set aside.
2. In a medium saucepan, heat the reserved tuna oil over medium heat. Add garlic, fennel, carrots and onion; cook, stirring, for 6 to 8 minutes or until softened. Transfer to a bowl.
3. In the same pan, bring water to a boil. Add farro and cook for 25 to 30 minutes or until tender. Drain well and return to the pan.
4. Chop enough of the reserved fennel fronds to measure 2 tbsp (30 mL). To the farro, add chopped fronds, tuna, vegetable mixture, arugula, olives, salt and lemon juice; cook, stirring, over medium heat until warmed through.

Superfood Spotlight

Tuna • Tuna is an excellent source of protein and is especially rich in B vitamins, selenium and magnesium. A small portion contains around 20% of your daily vitamin E needs. Although most types of tuna contain fewer essential omega-3 fats than some other oily fishes, they still provide a good amount of EPA and DHA fats. DHA is particularly effective at keeping our hearts and brains healthy and in good working order. Just one portion of tuna can provide the recommended 1.4 g of these fats per week.

Tuna and Asparagus Frittata

Makes 4 servings

✪ Great for Steps 1, 3 and 4

Here, eggs and canned tuna respectively escape their scrambled and sandwich clichés to find new expression in a dinnertime frittata. Tender pieces of asparagus add freshness and balance.

Tip

You can use any type of milk you have on hand, but for a lower-fat dish overall, opt for lower-fat or skim (nonfat) milk.

Variation

Replace the asparagus with 1 large red bell pepper, chopped.

- **Preheat oven to 350°F (180°C)**
- **8-inch (20 cm) square or round glass baking dish, sprayed with nonstick cooking spray (preferably olive oil)**

1 tsp	extra virgin olive oil	5 mL
1½ cups	sliced trimmed asparagus	375 mL
6	large eggs	6
1 cup	milk	250 mL
2 tsp	dried Italian seasoning	10 mL
¼ tsp	fine sea salt	1 mL
¼ tsp	freshly cracked black pepper	1 mL
1	can (6 oz/170 g) water-packed tuna, drained and flaked with a fork	1

1. In a large skillet, heat oil over medium-high heat. Add asparagus and cook, stirring, for 5 to 6 minutes or until softened. Remove from heat.
2. In a large bowl, beat eggs, milk, Italian seasoning, salt and pepper. Stir in asparagus and tuna. Pour into prepared baking dish.
3. Bake in preheated oven for 30 to 35 minutes or until golden, slightly puffed and set at the center. Let cool for 5 minutes, then cut into squares or wedges.

Nutrients per serving	
Calories	201
Total fat	8 g
Saturated fat	2 g
Cholesterol	284 mg
Sodium	328 mg
Carbohydrate	7 g
Fiber	1 g
Protein	24 g
Calcium	132 mg
Iron	3.1 mg

Spicy Tuna Cakes with Lemony Spinach

Makes 4 servings

✪ Great for Steps 1, 3, 4 and 5

In this simple, fresh-tasting dish, flavorful pantry ingredients boost canned tuna to dinner-worthy status, while an easy spinach and lemon sauté gives it fast flair.

Variation

An equal amount of mesclun, arugula or tender watercress sprigs may be used in place of the spinach.

Nutrients per serving	
Calories	223
Total fat	7 g
Saturated fat	1 g
Cholesterol	15 mg
Sodium	451 mg
Carbohydrate	12 g
Fiber	3 g
Protein	27 g
Calcium	39 mg
Iron	3.0 mg

- **Preheat oven to 200°F (100°C)**
- **Rimmed baking sheet, lined with foil**

2	cans (each 6 oz/170 g) oil-packed tuna	2
1/2 cup	fresh whole wheat bread crumbs	125 mL
1/3 cup	finely chopped green onions	75 mL
2 tsp	finely grated lemon zest, divided	10 mL
1/4 tsp	cayenne pepper	1 mL
1	large egg	1
1 tsp	Dijon mustard	5 mL
6 cups	packed baby spinach (about 6 oz/175 g)	1.5 L
1/8 tsp	fine sea salt	0.5 mL
1 1/2 tbsp	freshly squeezed lemon juice	22 mL

1. Drain tuna, reserving 4 tsp (20 mL) oil. Flake tuna with a fork and set both aside.
2. In a medium bowl, gently combine bread crumbs, green onions, half the lemon zest, cayenne, egg and mustard. Gently stir in tuna. Form into eight 1/2-inch (1 cm) thick patties.
3. In a large skillet, heat 1 tsp (5 mL) of the reserved tuna oil over medium heat. Add half the patties and cook, turning once, for 4 to 5 minutes per side or until golden brown on both sides and hot in the center. Transfer to a plate and tent with foil to keep warm. Repeat with another 1 tsp (5 mL) oil and the remaining patties.
4. In the same skillet, heat the remaining tuna oil over medium heat. Add spinach, the remaining lemon zest and salt; cook, stirring, for 2 to 3 minutes or until wilted. Drizzle with lemon juice.
5. Divide spinach among four plates and top each with 2 tuna cakes.

Provençal Poached Sea Scallops

Makes 4 servings

✪ Great for Steps 1, 3 and 4

You could hardly serve scallops better than to combine them with the classic flavors of Provence.

Tip

Leeks trap dirt and sand in their layers as they grow, so it is very important to clean them thoroughly. Use a sharp knife to cut off the root end and the dark green, woody part of the stalk. Slice the white and pale green parts of the leek in half lengthwise, then thinly slice crosswise (or as directed in your recipe). Place sliced leeks in a medium bowl and fill bowl with water. Gently swish leeks with your hand to remove any dirt embedded in the layers. Drain leeks, shaking off excess water, then pat dry with paper towels.

Nutrients per serving	
Calories	268
Total fat	9 g
Saturated fat	1 g
Cholesterol	60 mg
Sodium	561 mg
Carbohydrate	11 g
Fiber	2 g
Protein	31 g
Calcium	81 mg
Iron	1.5 mg

4 tsp	extra virgin olive oil, divided	20 mL
4	carrots, cut into thin strips	4
2	large leeks (white and light green parts only), cut into thin strips	2
2 tsp	dried herbes de Provence or Italian seasoning	10 mL
1/2 cup	dry white wine	125 mL
1/2 cup	water	125 mL
1 1/2 lbs	large sea scallops, side muscles removed	750 g
1/4 tsp	fine sea salt	1 mL
2	cloves garlic, finely chopped	2
1 cup	packed fresh flat-leaf (Italian) parsley leaves, chopped	250 mL
2 tbsp	chopped toasted walnuts	30 mL

1. In a large skillet, heat half the oil over medium-high heat. Add carrots and leeks; cook, stirring, for 2 minutes.
2. Stir in herbes de Provence, wine and water. Bring to a boil. Place scallops on top of vegetables and sprinkle with salt. Reduce heat to low, cover and simmer for 5 to 8 minutes or until scallops are firm and opaque.
3. Transfer scallops to four shallow dinner bowls. Stir garlic, parsley, walnuts and the remaining oil into vegetable mixture, then spoon over scallops.

Superfood Spotlight

Scallops • Scallops are an excellent source of vitamin B_{12}, which is needed by the body to deactivate homocysteine, a chemical that can damage blood vessel walls. High homocysteine levels are also linked with osteoporosis. A recent study found that osteoporosis occurred more frequently among women whose vitamin B_{12} status was deficient. In addition, a high intake of vitamin B_{12} has also been shown to be protective against colon cancer. Scallops are also a very good source of magnesium, and a regular intake helps build bone, release energy, regulate nerves and keep the heart healthy.

Shrimp and Asparagus Stir-Fry

Makes 4 servings

✪ Great for Steps 1, 3 and 4

You're going to love this stir-fry, with its sea-salty-sweet shrimp and crisp vegetables — so much so, you may swear off takeout. Serve it over brown rice.

2	cloves garlic, minced	2
1½ tsp	ground ginger	7 mL
½ tsp	cornstarch	2 mL
3 tbsp	mirin or sherry	45 mL
3 tbsp	reduced-sodium tamari or soy sauce	45 mL
2 tbsp	brown rice syrup or liquid honey	30 mL
1 tbsp	toasted sesame oil	15 mL
1	small red bell pepper, cut into 1-inch (2.5 cm) pieces	1
12 oz	asparagus, trimmed and cut into 1-inch (2.5 cm) pieces	375 g
¼ tsp	hot pepper flakes	1 mL
6	green onions, trimmed and cut into 1-inch (2.5 cm) pieces	6
1 lb	medium-large shrimp, peeled and deveined	500 g
¼ cup	water	60 mL

1. In a small bowl, whisk together garlic, ginger, cornstarch, mirin, tamari, brown rice syrup and sesame oil.
2. In a large skillet, heat garlic mixture over medium-high heat. Add red pepper, asparagus and hot pepper flakes; cook, stirring, for 2 minutes or until vegetables are slightly softened. Add green onions, shrimp and water; cook, stirring, for 2 to 3 minutes or until shrimp are pink, firm and opaque. Serve immediately.

▸ Health Note

A 4-oz (125 g) serving of shrimp has a mere 120 calories but supplies 23 g of protein, as well as omega-3 fatty acids and selenium, an antioxidant linked to lower rates of colon and lung cancer. Plus, researchers at Rockefeller University in New York City have determined that eating 10 oz (300 g) of shrimp daily can raise your HDL ("good") cholesterol by about 12%.

Nutrients per serving	
Calories	264
Total fat	6 g
Saturated fat	1 g
Cholesterol	172 mg
Sodium	508 mg
Carbohydrate	24 g
Fiber	4 g
Protein	27 g
Calcium	117 mg
Iron	5.8 mg

Greek Grilled Shrimp with Feta and Dill

Makes 4 servings

✪ Great for Steps 1, 3 and 4

Lemon, dill and feta is a flavor trio that flatters shrimp, and somehow, with the added grill flavor, the effect is tripled here. Serve over whole wheat couscous.

- **Preheat barbecue grill to medium-high**
- **Six 10-inch (25 cm) metal skewers, or wooden skewers soaked in warm water for 30 minutes**

1/2 cup	crumbled feta cheese	125 mL
1 tbsp	minced fresh dill	15 mL
1/4 tsp	freshly cracked black pepper	1 mL
2 tbsp	freshly squeezed lemon juice	30 mL
1 tbsp	extra virgin olive oil	15 mL
1 lb	large shrimp, peeled and deveined	500 g
	Nonstick cooking spray (preferably olive oil)	
1/4 tsp	fine sea salt	1 mL

1. In a small bowl, combine cheese, dill, pepper, lemon juice and oil. Set aside.
2. Thread shrimp onto skewers. Spray with cooking spray and sprinkle with salt. Grill on preheated barbecue, turning once, for 2 to 3 minutes per side or until shrimp are pink, firm and opaque. Serve with feta sauce spooned over top.

Nutrients per serving	
Calories	214
Total fat	10 g
Saturated fat	4 g
Cholesterol	207 mg
Sodium	509 mg
Carbohydrate	3 g
Fiber	0 g
Protein	28 g
Calcium	158 mg
Iron	3.2 mg

Moroccan-Spiced Shrimp

Makes 4 servings

✪ Great for Steps 1, 3, 4 and 5

Here, shrimp is emboldened with warm Moroccan spices, tart citrus and sweet currants.

Variation

Substitute an equal amount of quinoa or bulgur for the couscous (see Cooking Whole Grains, page 438, for cooking instructions).

1 cup	whole wheat couscous	250 mL
½ tsp	fine sea salt, divided	2 mL
1 cup	boiling water	250 mL
2 tsp	extra virgin olive oil	10 mL
1	red bell pepper, chopped	1
1¼ cups	chopped onions	300 mL
2 tsp	ground cumin	10 mL
1 tsp	ground cinnamon	5 mL
⅛ tsp	cayenne pepper	0.5 mL
1	can (28 oz/796 mL) whole tomatoes, drained and roughly chopped	1
¼ cup	currants or chopped raisins	60 mL
1 lb	large shrimp, peeled and deveined	500 g
2 tbsp	freshly squeezed lemon juice	30 mL
½ cup	packed fresh cilantro or flat-leaf (Italian) parsley leaves, chopped	125 mL

1. In a medium bowl, combine couscous, half the salt and boiling water. Cover with a plate and let stand for 5 minutes. Fluff with a fork.
2. Meanwhile, in a large skillet, heat oil over medium-high heat. Add red pepper, onions and the remaining salt; cook, stirring, for 6 to 8 minutes or until softened. Add cumin, cinnamon and cayenne; cook, stirring, for 30 seconds.
3. Stir in tomatoes and currants. Bring to a boil. Add shrimp, reduce heat and simmer, stirring occasionally, for 2 to 3 minutes or until shrimp are pink, firm and opaque. Stir in lemon juice.
4. Divide couscous among four shallow bowls. Top with shrimp mixture and sprinkle with cilantro.

Nutrients per serving	
Calories	396
Total fat	5 g
Saturated fat	1 g
Cholesterol	172 mg
Sodium	620 mg
Carbohydrate	63 g
Fiber	12 g
Protein	33 g
Calcium	148 mg
Iron	5.3 mg

Cannellini Beans with Shrimp and Roasted Peppers

Makes 4 servings

✪ Great for Steps 1, 3 and 4

Just what everyone wants on a cool evening — tender shrimp, sweet roasted peppers and creamy cannellini beans are the mouthwatering trinity at the core of this warm bowl of dinner goodness.

Tip

If you can only find larger 19-oz (540 mL) cans of beans, you will need about 1½ cans (3 cups/750 mL drained).

3 tsp	extra virgin olive oil, divided	15 mL
12 oz	medium shrimp, peeled and deveined	375 g
4	cloves garlic, minced	4
2	cans (each 14 to 15 oz/398 to 425 mL) cannellini (white kidney) beans, drained and rinsed	2
½ cup	reduced-sodium ready-to-use chicken or vegetable broth	125 mL
1	jar (12 oz/340 mL) roasted red bell peppers, drained and coarsely chopped	1
¾ cup	packed fresh basil leaves, thinly sliced, divided	175 mL

1. In a large skillet, heat 2 tsp (10 mL) of the oil over medium-high heat. Add shrimp and cook, stirring, for 2 to 3 minutes or until pink, firm and opaque. Transfer to a plate and tent with foil to keep warm.
2. In the same skillet, heat the remaining oil over medium-high heat. Add garlic and cook, stirring, for 30 seconds. Add ¼ cup (60 mL) of the beans and the broth. Mash beans with a fork. Add the remaining beans and roasted peppers. Bring to a boil. Reduce heat and simmer, stirring occasionally, for 3 minutes. Stir in half the basil.
3. Serve beans topped with shrimp and the remaining basil.

Nutrients per serving	
Calories	337
Total fat	5 g
Saturated fat	1 g
Cholesterol	143 mg
Sodium	540 mg
Carbohydrate	40 g
Fiber	11 g
Protein	33 g
Calcium	174 mg
Iron	5.9 mg

Couscous Paella with Shrimp and Chicken Sausage

Makes 6 servings

✪ Great for Steps 1, 3, 4 and 5

Paella aficionados will flip for this faster, healthier rendition, seasoned with smoked paprika and oregano. The shrimp and sausage are mainstays, and the peppers and peas are de rigueur extras.

2 tsp	extra virgin olive oil	10 mL
1	small red bell pepper, cut into ½-inch (1 cm) pieces	1
1 cup	chopped onion	250 mL
2	links cooked lower-fat chicken sausages (about 8 oz/250 g total), diced	2
2	cloves garlic, minced	2
1 tsp	sweet smoked paprika	5 mL
1 tsp	dried oregano	5 mL
1 cup	reduced-sodium ready-to-use chicken or vegetable broth	250 mL
8 oz	medium shrimp, peeled and deveined	250 g
1 cup	whole wheat couscous	250 mL
¾ cup	frozen petite peas, thawed	175 mL
½ cup	packed fresh flat-leaf (Italian) parsley leaves, chopped	125 mL
2 tbsp	freshly squeezed lemon juice	30 mL

1. In a large skillet, heat oil over medium-high heat. Add red pepper and onion; cook, stirring, for 6 to 8 minutes or until softened. Add sausage, garlic, paprika and oregano; cook, stirring, for 2 minutes.
2. Stir in broth and bring to a boil. Remove from heat and stir in shrimp, couscous and peas. Cover and let stand for 5 minutes or until liquid is absorbed and shrimp are pink, firm and opaque. Fluff couscous with a fork. Stir in parsley and lemon juice.

▸ Health Note

Whole wheat pasta — including couscous — has a lower glycemic index than whole wheat bread, which means it won't cause blood sugar spikes. In general, 1 cup (250 mL) of whole wheat pasta has triple the fiber of regular pasta, so it's very satisfying.

Nutrients per serving	
Calories	252
Total fat	4 g
Saturated fat	1 g
Cholesterol	72 mg
Sodium	416 mg
Carbohydrate	38 g
Fiber	7 g
Protein	18 g
Calcium	67 mg
Iron	3.8 mg

One-Pan Shrimp Pilau

Makes 4 servings

✪ Great for Steps 1, 3, 4 and 5

This Indian-spiced riff on traditional rice pilaf gets multiple layers of texture (shrimp, peas, peppers and rice) and flavor (curry powder, lime and cilantro) without any fussy steps or ingredients.

2 tsp	vegetable oil	10 mL
1	small red bell pepper, chopped	1
1 cup	chopped onion	250 mL
1 cup	long-grain brown rice	250 mL
1½ tbsp	mild curry powder	22 mL
1 tsp	ground cumin	5 mL
2½ cups	reduced-sodium ready-to-use chicken or vegetable broth	625 mL
8 oz	fully cooked deveined peeled medium shrimp	250 g
1 cup	frozen petite peas, thawed	250 mL
¾ cup	packed fresh cilantro leaves, chopped	175 mL
2 tbsp	freshly squeezed lime juice	30 mL

1. In a large skillet, heat oil over medium-high heat. Add red pepper and onion; cook, stirring, for 6 to 8 minutes or until softened. Add rice, curry powder and cumin; cook, stirring, for 1 minute.
2. Stir in broth and bring to a boil. Reduce heat to low, cover and simmer for 40 to 45 minutes or until liquid is absorbed. Stir in shrimp, peas, cilantro and lime juice; cook, stirring, for 1 to 2 minutes or until warmed through.

Superfood Spotlight

Brown Rice • Although white rice contains few nutrients other than starch, brown rice has several nutritional benefits. Regular consumption of brown rice and other whole grains has been shown to help prevent heart disease, diabetes and some cancers. It is a good source of fiber, which can help reduce cholesterol levels in the blood and keep blood sugar levels even. Brown rice also contains some protein and is a good source of several B vitamins and minerals, particularly selenium and magnesium.

Nutrients per serving	
Calories	214
Total fat	4 g
Saturated fat	1 g
Cholesterol	95 mg
Sodium	216 mg
Carbohydrate	26 g
Fiber	6 g
Protein	17 g
Calcium	86 mg
Iron	3.6 mg

Multigrain Pasta and Noodles

Red Pepper Pesto Capellini. 382
Capellini with Watercress, Carrots and Almonds. 383
Greek Capellini with Shrimp, Tomatoes and Mint. 384
Kamut Ditalini with Broccoli Rabe, Pesto and White Beans 385
Farfalle with Swiss Chard, White Beans and Walnuts 386
Farfalle with Tuna and Tomatoes. 387
Butternut Squash Fettuccine 388
Fusilli with Chickpeas, Tomatoes, Feta and Herbs 389
Falafel Fusilli with Spinach and Feta 390
Fusilli with Red Lentils, Spinach and Feta 391
Broccoli Rabe and Chicken Sausage Fusilli. 392
Healthy Know-How: What Is the Glycemic Index? 393
Gemelli with Wilted Mustard Greens 393
Multigrain Gemelli with Beets, Beet Greens and Goat Cheese 394
Gemelli with Ricotta, Peas and Lemon 395
Roasted Vegetable Linguine 396
Multigrain Linguine with Clam Sauce 397
Carrot Macaroni and Cheese. 398
Multigrain Macaroni with Zucchini, Greek Yogurt and Romano 399
Moussaka Macaroni. 400
Whole Wheat Orzo with Swiss Chard and Pecans. 401
Healthy Know-How: Nutrition Tips for Kids. 402
Asparagus Penne with Goat Cheese. 403
Penne with Hummus, Smoked Paprika and Chickpeas 404
Penne with Chicken Sausage, Mustard and Basil 405
Chicken Sausage, Arugula and Tomato Penne 406

Turkey Sausage, Escarole and Sun-Dried Tomato Pasta 407
Salmon Penne with Peas and Lemon 408
Rotini with Fennel, Orange and Almonds 409
Roasted Cauliflower Rotini with Green Olives and Currants 410
Spaghetti Limone with Asparagus and Mushrooms 411
Spaghetti with Brussels Sprouts and Toasted Walnuts 412
Quick Pasta al Norma 413
Fast Pumpkin Pasta with Parmesan and Chives 414
Spaghetti with Tuna, Olives and Golden Raisins 415
Quinoa Spaghetti with Kale 416
Quinoa Spaghetti al Pomodoro 417
Wagon Wheels with Broccoli, Turkey and Parmesan 418
Fast Vegetable Lasagna 419
Pumpkin Mushroom Lasagna 420
Lasagna Rolls 421
Speedy Weeknight Lo Mein 422
Sesame Ginger Noodles 423
Thai Cashew Noodles 424
Chicken and Edamame Shiratake Noodles 425
Teriyaki Soba, Spinach and Tofu Noodles 426
Soba with Chicken in Green Tea Broth 427
Buckwheat Noodle Bowls with Beef and Snap Peas 428
Soba with Shrimp, Lime and Cilantro 429
Soba with Shrimp and Baby Bok Choy 430
Red Curry Shrimp Noodle Bowls 431

Red Pepper Pesto Capellini

Makes 4 servings

✪ Great for Steps 4 and 5

This tailored, pantry-ready pasta has just the right proportion of sauce to noodles.

Tips

An equal amount of almonds or walnuts may be used in place of the pine nuts.

Make sure to use fine sea salt in the water you use to cook the pasta. Conventional table salt contains chemicals and additives, whereas sea salt contains an abundance of naturally occurring trace minerals.

- **Blender or food processor**

8 oz	multigrain or whole wheat capellini (angel hair) pasta	250 g
1	jar (8 oz/227 mL) roasted red bell peppers, drained	1
1	clove garlic, minced	1
½ cup	packed fresh basil leaves, chopped, divided	125 mL
1 tbsp	pine nuts	15 mL
¼ tsp	fine sea salt	1 mL
2 tbsp	extra virgin olive oil	30 mL
¼ cup	freshly grated Romano or Parmesan cheese	60 mL

1. In a large pot of boiling salted water (see tip, at left), cook pasta according to package directions until al dente. Drain, reserving ¼ cup (60 mL) pasta water. Return pasta to pot.
2. Meanwhile, in blender, combine roasted peppers, garlic, half the basil, pine nuts, salt and oil; purée until smooth.
3. Add pesto to pasta, gently tossing to coat. If necessary, stir in enough of the reserved pasta water to moisten. Serve topped with cheese and the remaining basil.

▸ Health Note

Ounce for ounce, gram for gram, pine nuts contain more protein than any other nut or seed, as well as a variety of vitamins and nutrients, including beta-carotene (vitamin A) and vitamins E, B_1, B_2 and B_3, as well as essential amino acids, copper, iodine, iron, magnesium and zinc. In addition, recent research indicates that certain fatty acids in pine nuts may help curb appetite.

Nutrients per serving	
Calories	315
Total fat	10 g
Saturated fat	2 g
Cholesterol	10 mg
Sodium	292 mg
Carbohydrate	50 g
Fiber	6 g
Protein	11 g
Calcium	135 mg
Iron	2.1 mg

Capellini with Watercress, Carrots and Almonds

Makes 4 servings

✪ Great for Steps 1, 2, 3, 4 and 5

"Refreshing" may not be a word that comes up much when discussing pasta, but that's exactly how these noodles will strike you. A handful of almonds — rich in protein, minerals and vitamins E and B — in combination with toothsome multigrain pasta makes this dish main course–worthy, while watercress adds piquant emerald verve, vitamins and antioxidants.

Tip

An equal amount of arugula, roughly torn or chopped, may be used in place of the watercress.

8 oz	multigrain or whole wheat capellini (angel hair) pasta	250 g
1½ tbsp	extra virgin olive oil	22 mL
2	cloves garlic, thinly sliced	2
2 cups	shredded carrots	500 mL
6 cups	packed tender watercress sprigs	1.5 L
¼ tsp	fine sea salt	1 mL
¼ tsp	freshly cracked black pepper	1 mL
¼ cup	freshly squeezed lemon juice	60 mL
¼ cup	sliced almonds, toasted (see tip, page 409)	60 mL

1. In a large pot of boiling salted water (see tip, page 382), cook pasta according to package directions until al dente. Drain, reserving 2 tbsp (30 mL) pasta water. Return pasta to pot.
2. Meanwhile, in a large skillet, heat oil over medium-high heat. Add garlic and carrots; cook, stirring, for 1 to 2 minutes or until carrots are slightly softened. Remove from heat and stir in watercress.
3. To the pasta, add watercress mixture, salt, pepper, lemon juice and the reserved pasta water, tossing to combine. Serve sprinkled with almonds.

Superfood Spotlight

Watercress • Watercress is a powerhouse of nutrients — even if eaten in small quantities — and provides good amounts of vitamins C and K, potassium and calcium. It is a great source of carotenes and lutein, for eye health. Watercress is rich in a variety of plant chemicals that can help prevent or minimize cancers, including phenylethyl isothiocyanate, which can help block the action of cells linked with lung cancer. Watercress is also said to detoxify the liver and cleanse the blood, and its benzyl oils are powerful antibiotics. It can help improve night blindness and the light sensitivity associated with porphyria.

Nutrients per serving	
Calories	334
Total fat	11 g
Saturated fat	1 g
Cholesterol	130 mg
Sodium	246 mg
Carbohydrate	57 g
Fiber	8 g
Protein	11 g
Calcium	130 mg
Iron	2.3 mg

Greek Capellini with Shrimp, Tomatoes and Mint

Makes 4 servings

✪ Great for Steps 1, 3, 4 and 5

This fresh but filling pasta is full of flavor, with or without the shrimp. The aromatic mint leaves are ideal, but an equal amount of cilantro or flat-leaf (Italian) parsley will work.

Tip

Make sure to use fine sea salt in the water you use to cook the pasta. Conventional table salt contains chemicals and additives, whereas sea salt contains an abundance of naturally occurring trace minerals.

8 oz	multigrain or whole wheat capellini (angel hair) pasta	250 g
2 tsp	extra virgin olive oil	10 mL
2	cloves garlic, minced	2
8 oz	medium shrimp, peeled and deveined	250 g
2 cups	chopped tomatoes	500 mL
1/4 cup	pitted brine-cured black olives (such as kalamata), chopped	60 mL
2 tbsp	drained capers	30 mL
1/4 tsp	fine sea salt	1 mL
1/4 tsp	freshly cracked black pepper	1 mL
1/2 cup	packed fresh mint leaves, thinly sliced	125 mL
1/4 cup	crumbled feta cheese	60 mL

1. In a large pot of boiling salted water (see tip, at left), cook pasta according to package directions until al dente. Drain, reserving 1/3 cup (75 mL) pasta water.
2. In a large skillet, heat oil over medium-high heat. Add garlic and shrimp; cook, stirring, for 30 seconds. Add tomatoes, reduce heat and simmer, stirring occasionally, for 3 minutes or until thickened. Stir in pasta, olives, capers, salt, pepper and the reserved pasta water; simmer, stirring, for 1 minute. Serve sprinkled with mint and cheese.

▸ Health Note

Mint contains good amounts of vitamins A, B_{12} and C, folic acid, thiamine and riboflavin, as well as minerals such as calcium, copper, fluoride, iron, manganese, phosphorus, potassium, selenium and zinc.

Nutrients per serving	
Calories	344
Total fat	7 g
Saturated fat	2 g
Cholesterol	104 mg
Sodium	517 mg
Carbohydrate	52 g
Fiber	7 g
Protein	23 g
Calcium	128 mg
Iron	3.9 mg

Kamut Ditalini with Broccoli Rabe, Pesto and White Beans

Makes 4 servings

✪ Great for Steps 1, 2, 3, 4 and 5

The satisfaction value of this impressive pasta belies its short list of ingredients.

Tips

For the white beans, you could use Great Northern beans, cannellini (white kidney) beans or white pea (navy) beans.

If you cannot find Kamut ditalini, you can substitute any other small multigrain or whole wheat pasta shape.

If the pasta you're using takes less or more than 8 minutes to cook, adjust the total cooking time according to the package directions and add the broccoli rabe for the last 3 to 4 minutes.

Nutrients per serving	
Calories	373
Total fat	5 g
Saturated fat	1 g
Cholesterol	2 mg
Sodium	507 mg
Carbohydrate	68 g
Fiber	9 g
Protein	20 g
Calcium	161 mg
Iron	5.2 mg

8 oz	Kamut ditalini pasta	250 g
1 lb	broccoli rabe, trimmed and roughly chopped	500 g
1⅔ cups	reduced-sodium ready-to-use vegetable or chicken broth	400 mL
¼ tsp	hot pepper flakes	1 mL
1	can (14 to 19 oz/398 to 540 mL) white beans, drained and rinsed	1
¼ cup	basil pesto	60 mL
1 tbsp	white wine vinegar	15 mL

1. In a large pot of boiling salted water (see tip, page 384), cook pasta for 4 minutes. Add broccoli rabe and cook, stirring occasionally, for 3 to 4 minutes or until broccoli rabe is tender-crisp and pasta is al dente. Drain, reserving ½ cup (125 mL) pasta water. Return pasta mixture to pot.
2. Meanwhile, in a medium saucepan, combine broth and hot pepper flakes. Bring to a simmer over medium-high heat. Add beans, reduce heat and simmer, stirring occasionally, for about 3 minutes or until heated through.
3. To the pasta mixture, add bean mixture, pesto and vinegar, gently tossing to combine. If necessary, stir in enough of the reserved pasta water to moisten.

Farfalle with Swiss Chard, White Beans and Walnuts

Makes 4 servings

✪ Great for Steps 1, 2, 3, 4 and 5

I took a lead from a busy friend (and mother of four) who said she loves good recipes that have few ingredients but plenty of style; if they use ingredients from her CSA (community-supported agriculture) box, all the better. Check, check and check. Add one more check for the sensational nutrition.

8 oz	multigrain or whole wheat farfalle (bow-tie) pasta	250 g
1	large bunch red Swiss chard	1
1 tbsp	extra virgin olive oil	15 mL
6	cloves garlic, thinly sliced	6
1 tbsp	dried Italian seasoning	15 mL
1	can (14 to 19 oz/398 to 540 mL) cannellini (white kidney) beans, drained and rinsed	1
1/4 tsp	fine sea salt	1 mL
2 tsp	finely grated lemon zest	10 mL
2 tbsp	freshly squeezed lemon juice	30 mL
1/4 cup	chopped toasted walnuts	60 mL

1. In a large pot of boiling salted water (see tip, page 387), cook pasta according to package directions until al dente. Drain, reserving 1/4 cup (60 mL) pasta water.
2. Trim off tough stems from Swiss chard and discard. Trim tender stems and ribs from leaves and finely chop stems and ribs. Thinly slice leaves crosswise (to measure about 5 cups/1.25 L).
3. In the same pot, heat oil over medium heat. Add garlic and cook, stirring, for 30 seconds. Add Swiss chard and Italian seasoning; cook, stirring, for 2 to 3 minutes or until Swiss chard is just wilted. Stir in pasta, beans, salt, lemon zest, lemon juice and the reserved pasta water; cook, tossing, for 1 to 2 minutes or until pasta and beans are warmed through. Serve sprinkled with walnuts.

Superfood Spotlight

Walnuts • Unlike most nuts, walnuts are much richer in polyunsaturated fats than in monounsaturates. The type of polyunsaturates walnuts contain is mostly essential omega-3 fats, in the form of alpha-linolenic acid. An adequate and balanced intake of the omega fats has been linked with protection from aging, cardiovascular disease, cancers, arthritis, skin problems and diseases of the nervous system. For people who don't eat fish and fish oils, an intake of omega-3 fats from other sources, such as walnuts, flaxseeds and soy, is important.

Nutrients per serving	
Calories	263
Total fat	8 g
Saturated fat	1 g
Cholesterol	0 mg
Sodium	491 mg
Carbohydrate	38 g
Fiber	8 g
Protein	13 g
Calcium	88 mg
Iron	3.0 mg

Farfalle with Tuna and Tomatoes

Makes 4 servings

✪ Great for Steps 3, 4 and 5

The slightly sweet, almost flowery flavor of oregano adds delicate notes to this otherwise boldly flavored, Mediterranean-inspired pasta dish.

Tip

Make sure to use fine sea salt in the water you use to cook the pasta. Conventional table salt contains chemicals and additives, whereas sea salt contains an abundance of naturally occurring trace minerals.

8 oz	multigrain or whole wheat farfalle (bow-tie) pasta	250 g
1 tbsp	extra virgin olive oil	15 mL
1	can (14 to 15 oz/398 to 425 mL) diced tomatoes with Italian seasonings, with juice	1
1/2 cup	pitted brine-cured black olives (such as kalamata), quartered	125 mL
1	can (6 oz/170 g) water-packed tuna, with liquid	1
1/8 tsp	fine sea salt	0.5 mL
1 cup	packed fresh flat-leaf (Italian) parsley leaves, thinly sliced	250 mL
1 1/2 tsp	minced fresh oregano	7 mL
1 tbsp	finely grated lemon zest	15 mL
2 tbsp	freshly squeezed lemon juice	30 mL

1. In a large pot of boiling salted water (see tip, at left), cook pasta according to package directions until al dente. Drain, reserving 1/4 cup (60 mL) pasta water.
2. In a large, heavy skillet, heat oil over medium-high heat. Add tomatoes with juice, olives and the reserved pasta water. Bring to a simmer. Stir in pasta, tuna with liquid and salt; reduce heat and simmer for 1 minute, gently tossing to combine and break tuna up into bite-size pieces. Stir in parsley, oregano, lemon zest and lemon juice.

▶ Health Note

A mere 1/2 tsp (2 mL) of dried oregano contains the same amount of antioxidants as 3 cups (750 mL) of raw spinach.

Nutrients per serving	
Calories	210
Total fat	6 g
Saturated fat	1 g
Cholesterol	13 mg
Sodium	460 mg
Carbohydrate	25 g
Fiber	4 g
Protein	16 g
Calcium	72 mg
Iron	3.4 mg

Butternut Squash Fettuccine

Makes 4 servings

✪ Great for Steps 1, 2, 3, 4 and 5

This deeply flavored, autumnal pasta makes dinner duty a simple pleasure.

Tips

If you don't have honey on hand, you can use 1 tbsp (15 mL) packed light brown sugar instead.

Make sure to use fine sea salt in the water you use to cook the pasta. Conventional table salt contains chemicals and additives, whereas sea salt contains an abundance of naturally occurring trace minerals.

Nutrients per serving	
Calories	358
Total fat	7 g
Saturated fat	2 g
Cholesterol	10 mg
Sodium	436 mg
Carbohydrate	67 g
Fiber	10 g
Protein	11 g
Calcium	190 mg
Iron	2.9 mg

- **Preheat oven to 475°F (240°C)**
- **Large rimmed baking sheet, lined with foil and sprayed with nonstick cooking spray (preferably olive oil)**

1	large red onion, cut into 1-inch (2.5 cm) chunks	1
4 cups	cubed peeled butternut squash (1-inch/2.5 cm cubes)	1 L
2 tsp	dried rubbed sage	10 mL
1/2 tsp	fine sea salt	2 mL
1/2 tsp	freshly cracked black pepper	2 mL
4 tsp	extra virgin olive oil	20 mL
1 tbsp	liquid honey	15 mL
8 oz	multigrain or whole wheat fettuccine pasta	250 g
1/2 cup	packed fresh flat-leaf (Italian) parsley leaves, chopped	125 mL
1/4 cup	freshly grated Parmesan cheese	60 mL

1. On prepared baking sheet, toss red onion and squash with sage, salt, pepper, oil and honey; spread in a single layer. Roast in preheated oven for 20 to 25 minutes, stirring once or twice, until vegetables are golden brown and tender.
2. Meanwhile, in a large pot of boiling salted water (see tip, at left), cook pasta according to package directions until al dente. Drain, reserving 1/4 cup (60 mL) pasta water. Return pasta to pot.
3. To the pasta, add squash mixture and parsley, tossing to combine. If necessary, stir in enough of the reserved pasta water to moisten. Serve sprinkled with cheese.

Fusilli with Chickpeas, Tomatoes, Feta and Herbs

Makes 4 servings

✪ Great for Steps 1, 2, 3, 4 and 5

Nutty chickpeas — rich in protein, manganese, folate and fiber — add heft to this quick and easy pasta, while fresh herbs, feta and tomatoes add zing.

Tip

One 14- to 15-oz (398 to 425 mL) can of diced tomatoes, with juice, can be used in place of the cherry tomatoes. Bring to a boil in the skillet before adding the garlic, chickpeas and salt.

8 oz	multigrain or whole wheat fusilli, gemelli or rotini pasta	250 g
4 tsp	extra virgin olive oil	20 mL
2 cups	cherry or grape tomatoes	500 mL
2	cloves garlic, minced	2
1	can (14 to 19 oz/398 to 540 mL) chickpeas, drained and rinsed	1
1/4 tsp	fine sea salt	1 mL
3/4 cup	packed fresh mint leaves, chopped	175 mL
1/3 cup	packed fresh cilantro leaves, chopped	75 mL
1/4 cup	thinly sliced green onions	60 mL
1/2 cup	crumbled feta cheese	125 mL

1. In a large pot of boiling salted water (see tip, page 388), cook pasta according to package directions until al dente. Drain, reserving 2 tbsp (30 mL) pasta water. Return pasta to pot.
2. Meanwhile, in a large skillet, heat oil over medium-high heat. Add tomatoes and cook, stirring, for 5 minutes or until slightly browned and beginning to burst. Add garlic, chickpeas and salt; cook, stirring, for 4 to 5 minutes or until chickpeas are warmed through.
3. To the pasta, add tomato mixture, mint, cilantro, green onions and the reserved pasta water, tossing to combine. Serve sprinkled with cheese.

Nutrients per serving	
Calories	378
Total fat	9 g
Saturated fat	2 g
Cholesterol	17 mg
Sodium	537 mg
Carbohydrate	66 g
Fiber	10 g
Protein	16 g
Calcium	154 mg
Iron	3.3 mg

Falafel Fusilli with Spinach and Feta

Makes 4 servings

✪ Great for Steps 1, 2, 3, 4 and 5

This Mediterranean pantry pasta will become a weeknight standby. Gone is the grease from fast-food falafel; instead, the mixture here is sautéed and crumbled in a scant amount of heart-healthy olive oil, lending it a "meaty" texture and allowing its protein potential (ground chickpeas and spices) to shine. Freshness, as well as vitamins and antioxidants galore, comes from a heap of spinach, while a crumble of low-fat, high-flavor feta delivers piquancy.

Tip

Falafel mix is sold in boxes, typically shelved in the health food or international food sections of the supermarket, or in bulk at health food stores.

Nutrients per serving	
Calories	385
Total fat	9 g
Saturated fat	2 g
Cholesterol	11 mg
Sodium	540 mg
Carbohydrate	81 g
Fiber	11 g
Protein	19 g
Calcium	253 mg
Iron	7.1 mg

1 cup	dry falafel mix	250 mL
1 cup	water	250 mL
2 tsp	extra virgin olive oil	10 mL
8 oz	multigrain or whole wheat fusilli, gemelli or rotini pasta	250 g
1	package (10 oz/300 g) frozen chopped spinach, thawed and squeezed dry	1
2½ cups	reduced-sodium marinara sauce	625 mL
½ cup	packed fresh cilantro or flat-leaf (Italian) parsley leaves, chopped	125 mL
⅓ cup	crumbled feta cheese	75 mL

1. In a small bowl, combine falafel mix and water. Let stand for 15 minutes.
2. In a large skillet, heat oil over medium-high heat. Add falafel mixture and, using a spatula, spread out in pan. Cook for 3 to 4 minutes or until mixture begins to set and turn golden brown at edges. Using spatula, break mixture into smaller pieces; cook, stirring, for 3 to 5 minutes or until browned all over. Transfer to a plate.
3. Meanwhile, in a large pot of boiling salted water (see tip, page 388), cook pasta according to package directions until al dente. Drain, reserving ¼ cup (60 mL) pasta water. Return pasta to pot.
4. In the same skillet, combine spinach and marinara sauce. Heat over medium heat, stirring occasionally, until hot but not boiling.
5. Add spinach mixture to pasta, tossing to coat. Simmer over low heat, stirring occasionally, for 2 to 3 minutes or until warmed through. If necessary, stir in enough of the reserved pasta water to moisten. Stir in falafel mixture and cilantro. Serve sprinkled with cheese.

Fusilli with Red Lentils, Spinach and Feta

Makes 4 servings

✪ Great for Steps 1, 2, 3, 4 and 5

Lentils and pasta may sound like an unlikely partnership, but the combination is common — and beloved — in Northern África and the Middle East. Spinach, cumin, garlic and feta make the final dish sing.

Tips

Green or brown lentils may be used in place of the red lentils (see Cooking Legumes, page 438, for cooking instructions).

A 10-oz (300 g) package of frozen chopped spinach, thawed and squeezed dry, may be used in place of the fresh spinach.

2 tsp	extra virgin olive oil	10 mL
3	cloves garlic, minced	3
3 cups	chopped onions	750 mL
1 tsp	ground cumin	5 mL
1/4 tsp	fine sea salt	1 mL
1/8 tsp	freshly ground black pepper	0.5 mL
1 tbsp	red wine vinegar	15 mL
2/3 cup	dried red lentils, rinsed	150 mL
2 cups	water	500 mL
8 oz	multigrain or whole wheat fusilli or rotini pasta	250 g
6 cups	packed baby spinach (about 6 oz/175 g)	1.5 L
1/2 cup	crumbled feta cheese	125 mL

1. In a large skillet, heat oil over medium-high heat. Add garlic, onions, cumin, salt and pepper; reduce heat to medium-low, cover and cook, stirring occasionally, for 20 to 25 minutes or until onions are very tender and golden. Remove from heat and stir in vinegar.
2. Meanwhile, in a medium saucepan, combine lentils and water. Bring to a boil over medium-high heat. Reduce heat and simmer for about 22 minutes or until lentils are very tender but not mushy. Drain and add to onion mixture.
3. In a large pot of boiling salted water (see tip, page 388), cook pasta according to package directions until al dente. Drain, reserving 1/2 cup (125 mL) pasta water. Return pasta to pot.
4. To the pasta, add lentil mixture, spinach and enough of the reserved pasta water to wilt spinach and moisten pasta. Add cheese, tossing to combine.

Nutrients per serving	
Calories	246
Total fat	7 g
Saturated fat	3 g
Cholesterol	17 mg
Sodium	422 mg
Carbohydrate	35 g
Fiber	8 g
Protein	13 g
Calcium	167 mg
Iron	3.7 mg

Broccoli Rabe and Chicken Sausage Fusilli

Makes 4 servings

✪ Great for Steps 1, 3, 4 and 5

Broccoli rabe is tender-crisp, subtly bitter and utterly irresistible in combination with curly multigrain noodles and chicken.

Tip

This technique produces a tender-crisp broccoli rabe. If you prefer a more tender texture, blanch the chopped broccoli rabe in a pot of boiling water for 2 minutes or until bright green, then drain and add to skillet.

1 lb	broccoli rabe	500 g
8 oz	multigrain or whole wheat fusilli, rotini or gemelli pasta	250 g
1 tbsp	extra virgin olive oil	15 mL
4 oz	cooked chicken sausage, cut into 1/4-inch (0.5 cm) dice	125 g
3	cloves garlic, thinly sliced	3
1/4 cup	golden raisins, chopped	60 mL
1/2 tsp	fine sea salt	2 mL
1/4 tsp	hot pepper flakes	1 mL
2 tbsp	freshly squeezed lemon juice	30 mL

1. Cut broccoli rabe crosswise into 1-inch (2.5 cm) thick slices. Rinse well and drain, leaving water clinging to it.
2. In a large pot of boiling salted water (see tip, page 394), cook pasta according to package directions until al dente. Drain, reserving 1/4 cup (60 mL) pasta water. Return pasta to pot.
3. In a large skillet, heat oil over medium-high heat. Add sausage and cook, stirring, for 2 to 3 minutes or until browned. Using a slotted spoon, transfer to a plate.
4. In the same skillet, combine broccoli rabe, garlic, raisins, salt and hot pepper flakes; cook, stirring, for 6 to 10 minutes or until broccoli rabe is tender.
5. To pasta, add broccoli rabe mixture, lemon juice and the reserved pasta water. Cook, stirring, over medium heat for 1 minute.

▸ Health Note

Broccoli rabe, a ruffled-leaf member of the Brassica family, is a rich source of glucosinolates, which the body converts to cancer-fighting sulforaphanes and indoles.

Nutrients per serving	
Calories	354
Total fat	8 g
Saturated fat	2 g
Cholesterol	33 mg
Sodium	494 mg
Carbohydrate	62 g
Fiber	6 g
Protein	17 g
Calcium	117 mg
Iron	3.2 mg

Healthy Know-How

What Is the Glycemic Index?

Using a scale of 1 to 100, the glycemic index — or GI — is a numerical index of how your blood sugar is affected within 2 to 3 hours of eating foods that are high in carbohydrates and how those carbohydrates turn into blood glucose.

The glycemic index is about the quality of the carbohydrates, not the quantity. Foods that are digested and absorbed faster will have a higher glycemic index of 70 and above. Fifty-five and under is low GI, 56 to 69 is medium GI. High-GI foods include white bread, pasta and rice, low-fiber cereals and baked goods made with these items. Low-GI foods include fruit, vegetables, whole grains and legumes.

Many people have found the glycemic index to be a useful tool for losing weight: low-GI foods generally have less of an impact on blood sugar levels, providing sustained energy and a long-lasting feeling of fullness. If you want to try using the glycemic index, speak to your doctor.

Gemelli with Wilted Mustard Greens

Makes 4 servings

✪ Great for Steps 1, 2, 3, 4 and 5

For dinner in a hurry, look no further. Mustard greens are a great source of vitamins C and E, and the shaved Parmesan provides tryptophan.

Nutrients per serving	
Calories	341
Total fat	8 g
Saturated fat	2 g
Cholesterol	20 mg
Sodium	510 mg
Carbohydrate	54 g
Fiber	9 g
Protein	15 g
Calcium	343 mg
Iron	3.3 mg

8 oz	whole wheat gemelli, rotini or other spiral pasta	250 g
1 tbsp	extra virgin olive oil	15 mL
4	cloves garlic, minced	4
8 cups	packed chopped mustard greens, trimmed kale or trimmed Swiss chard leaves	2 L
1/2 tsp	fine sea salt	2 mL
1 tbsp	freshly squeezed lemon juice	15 mL
2 tsp	Dijon mustard	10 mL
1/2 cup	freshly grated Parmesan cheese	125 mL

1. In a large pot of boiling salted water (see tip, page 394), cook pasta according to package directions until al dente. Drain, reserving 1/4 cup (60 mL) pasta water. Return pasta to pot.
2. In a large skillet, heat oil over medium-high heat. Add garlic and cook, stirring, for 30 seconds. Add mustard greens and salt; cook, stirring, for 2 to 3 minutes or until greens are wilted.
3. To the pasta, add greens mixture, lemon juice, mustard and the reserved pasta water. Cook, stirring, over medium-high heat for 1 minute to heat through. Stir in cheese.

Multigrain Gemelli with Beets, Beet Greens and Goat Cheese

Makes 4 servings

✪ Great for Steps 1, 2, 3, 4 and 5

Think of this glorious pasta as a farmers' market homage. The straight-from-the-farm flavor of goat cheese, complemented by sweet beets and their gorgeous greens, is a salute to health, too.

Tips

An equal amount of chopped raisins or dried cranberries may be used in place of the currants.

Make sure to use fine sea salt in the water you use to cook the beets and pasta. Conventional table salt contains chemicals and additives, whereas sea salt contains an abundance of naturally occurring trace minerals.

Nutrients per serving	
Calories	382
Total fat	7 g
Saturated fat	2 g
Cholesterol	7 mg
Sodium	345 mg
Carbohydrate	82 g
Fiber	12 g
Protein	15 g
Calcium	115 mg
Iron	3.5 mg

1 tbsp	extra virgin olive oil	15 mL
4 cups	thinly sliced onions	1 L
6	beets (about 2 inches/5 cm in diameter), with green tops attached	6
3	cloves garlic, minced	3
1/4 tsp	fine sea salt	1 mL
8 oz	multigrain or whole wheat gemelli or rotini pasta	250 g
1/4 cup	dried currants	60 mL
2 tsp	balsamic vinegar	10 mL
2 oz	goat cheese, crumbled	60 g

1. In a large skillet, heat oil over medium heat. Add onions and cook, stirring occasionally, for about 25 minutes or until dark golden brown.
2. Meanwhile, trim leaves and stems from beets, reserving leaves and tender stems. Scrub beets. Rinse and spin-dry beet greens and tender stems, then coarsely chop. Peel beets and cut each into 8 wedges.
3. In a large pot of boiling salted water (see tip, at left), cook beets for about 10 minutes or until tender. Drain beets and transfer to a medium bowl.
4. Add garlic and salt to the onions; cook, stirring, for 2 minutes. Stir in beet greens; cover and cook for about 5 minutes or until tender.
5. In another large pot of boiling salted water, cook pasta according to package directions until al dente. Drain, reserving 1/4 cup (60 mL) pasta water. Return pasta to pot.
6. To the pasta, add onion mixture, beets, currants, vinegar and the reserved pasta water. Cook, tossing to combine, over medium-low heat for 1 minute. Serve sprinkled with cheese.

Gemelli with Ricotta, Peas and Lemon

Makes 4 servings

✪ Great for Steps 1, 2, 3, 4 and 5

Half the fun of making pasta is customizing your noodles with favorite toppings and sauces. But you likely won't change a thing about this dish: two kinds of peas, fresh lemon and tarragon sing spring.

Tip

If the pasta you're using takes less or more than 10 or 11 minutes to cook, adjust the total cooking time according to the package directions and add the sugar snap peas for the last 3 to 4 minutes.

8 oz	whole wheat gemelli, rotini or fusilli pasta	250 g
8 oz	sugar snap peas, strings removed	250 g
1 cup	frozen petite peas, thawed	250 mL
1 tbsp	chopped fresh tarragon	15 mL
$\frac{1}{2}$ tsp	fine sea salt	2 mL
1 cup	nonfat ricotta cheese	250 mL
2 tsp	finely grated lemon zest	10 mL
2 tbsp	freshly squeezed lemon juice	30 mL
1 tbsp	extra virgin olive oil	15 mL

1. In a large pot of boiling salted water (see tip, page 394), cook pasta for 7 minutes. Add sugar snap peas and cook for 3 to 4 minutes or until peas are tender-crisp and pasta is al dente. Drain, reserving $\frac{1}{2}$ cup (125 mL) pasta water. Return pasta mixture to pot.
2. To the pasta mixture, add petite peas, tarragon, salt, cheese, lemon zest, lemon juice and oil, gently tossing to coat. Stir in enough of the reserved pasta water to create a creamy sauce.

▶ Health Note

Sugar snap peas — an accidental hybrid that occurred in the 1960s — are high in vitamin C. Further, a 1-cup (250 mL) serving has 3 g of fiber.

Nutrients per serving	
Calories	340
Total fat	5 g
Saturated fat	1 g
Cholesterol	5 mg
Sodium	443 mg
Carbohydrate	61 g
Fiber	10 g
Protein	20 g
Calcium	263 mg
Iron	3.5 mg

Roasted Vegetable Linguine

Makes 6 servings

✪ Great for Steps 1, 2, 3, 4 and 5

Whole wheat linguine is a perfect complement to a quartet of garden vegetables: mushrooms, asparagus, red onion and tomatoes.

Tip

Make sure to use fine sea salt in the water you use to cook the pasta. Conventional table salt contains chemicals and additives, whereas sea salt contains an abundance of naturally occurring trace minerals.

Nutrients per serving	
Calories	234
Total fat	4 g
Saturated fat	0 g
Cholesterol	0 mg
Sodium	397 mg
Carbohydrate	40 g
Fiber	6 g
Protein	9 g
Calcium	58 mg
Iron	3.0 mg

- **Preheat oven to 450°F (230°C)**
- **Large roasting pan, lined with foil and sprayed with nonstick cooking spray (preferably olive oil)**

3	cloves garlic, minced	3
1	small red onion, cut into 1-inch (2.5 cm) chunks	1
12 oz	cremini mushrooms, trimmed and thickly sliced	375 g
12 oz	asparagus, trimmed and cut into 1-inch (2.5 cm) pieces	375 g
3/4 tsp	fine sea salt	3 mL
1/2 tsp	hot pepper flakes	2 mL
1 tbsp	extra virgin olive oil	15 mL
2 cups	cherry or grape tomatoes	500 mL
1/2 cup	dry white wine	125 mL
12 oz	whole wheat linguine or spaghetti pasta	375 g
1/2 cup	packed fresh basil leaves, thinly sliced	125 mL

1. In a large bowl, combine garlic, red onion, mushrooms, asparagus, salt, hot pepper flakes and oil. Spread in a single layer in prepared roasting pan. Roast in preheated oven for 18 to 21 minutes, stirring occasionally, until mushrooms and onions begin to brown. Add tomatoes and roast for 7 to 10 minutes or until tomatoes begin to burst and shrivel. Return vegetables to large bowl.
2. Add wine to the roasting pan, scraping up any browned bits from bottom of pan. Place pan over medium heat and simmer for 2 to 3 minutes (or return pan to oven for 5 minutes if pan is not stovetop-safe), until wine has evaporated by half.
3. Meanwhile, in a large pot of boiling salted water (see tip, at left), cook pasta according to package directions until al dente. Drain, reserving 1/3 cup (75 mL) pasta water. Return pasta to pot. Stir pasta water into wine in roasting pan.
4. To the pasta, add roasted vegetables and wine mixture. Cook, tossing, over medium-low heat for 1 minute or until heated through. Stir in basil.

Multigrain Linguine with Clam Sauce

Makes 6 servings

✪ Great for Steps 1, 3, 4 and 5

Chopping the parsley and garlic are the only steps for this pasta that take a bit of time. Yet the end results are wonderful: the pungent flavor of the garlic and fresh, grassy flavor of parsley brighten the flavor of the clams, melding all into a perfectly satisfying supper.

12 oz	multigrain or whole wheat linguine or spaghetti pasta	375 g
1 tbsp	extra virgin olive oil	15 mL
5	cloves garlic, minced	5
1	bottle (8 oz/227 mL) clam juice	1
1/2 cup	dry white wine	125 mL
3	cans (each 6 oz/170 g) minced clams, with liquid	3
1 cup	packed fresh flat-leaf (Italian) parsley leaves, chopped	250 mL
1/4 tsp	fine sea salt	1 mL
1/4 tsp	freshly cracked black pepper	1 mL
2 tbsp	freshly squeezed lemon juice	30 mL

1. In a large pot of boiling salted water (see tip, page 396), cook pasta according to package directions until al dente. Drain.
2. In a large skillet, heat oil over medium heat. Add garlic and cook, stirring, for 2 minutes or until golden. Stir in clam juice and wine. Drain the liquid from the clams into the skillet, reserving the clams. Simmer for 5 minutes. Stir in pasta and simmer for 1 minute. Stir in the reserved clams, parsley, salt, pepper and lemon juice.

Superfood Spotlight

Parsley • Flat-leaf (Italian) parsley and curly parsley have a similar nutritional profile. Parsley sprigs are often simply used as a garnish and then discarded, which is a pity because the leaves are a good source of several nutrients, including vitamin C and iron. Myristicin, an organic compound found in parsley, inhibits tumors in animals and has a strong antioxidant action, neutralizing carcinogens in the body, such as the dangerous compounds in tobacco smoke and barbecue smoke. Parsley is also an anticoagulant and contains compounds of oils that are linked with relief from menstrual problems such as pain, fluid retention and cramps.

Nutrients per serving	
Calories	403
Total fat	6 g
Saturated fat	1 g
Cholesterol	44 mg
Sodium	427 mg
Carbohydrate	91 g
Fiber	8 g
Protein	36 g
Calcium	302 mg
Iron	6.6 mg

Carrot Macaroni and Cheese

Makes 4 servings

✪ Great for Steps 1, 2, 3, 4 and 5

The carrots in this macaroni and cheese aren't sneaky so much as they are sidekicks, adding a velvety texture and understated sweetness to the sharp Cheddar cheese and hearty noodles.

Tips

The darker orange the carrot, the more carotenes it contains. Remove any green on the stalk end of the carrot before cooking, as this can be mildly toxic.

Make sure to use fine sea salt in the water you use to cook the pasta. Conventional table salt contains chemicals and additives, whereas sea salt contains an abundance of naturally occurring trace minerals.

Nutrients per serving	
Calories	262
Total fat	9 g
Saturated fat	5 g
Cholesterol	37 mg
Sodium	473 mg
Carbohydrate	27 g
Fiber	5 g
Protein	13 g
Calcium	297 mg
Iron	1.2 mg

- **Preheat oven to 350°F (180°C)**
- **Blender**
- **8-inch (20 cm) glass baking dish, sprayed with nonstick cooking spray**

12 oz	carrots, thinly sliced	375 g
1/2 cup	reduced-sodium ready-to-use vegetable or chicken broth	125 mL
8 oz	whole wheat macaroni pasta	250 g
1/4 tsp	fine sea salt	1 mL
1/8 tsp	freshly ground white or black pepper	0.5 mL
1 1/2 tsp	Dijon mustard	7 mL
1 1/4 cups	shredded extra-sharp (extra-old) Cheddar cheese, divided	300 mL

1. In a medium saucepan, combine carrots and broth. Bring to a boil over medium-high heat. Reduce heat to medium, cover and boil gently for about 30 minutes or until carrots are very soft.
2. Meanwhile, in a large pot of boiling salted water (see tip, at left), cook pasta according to package directions until al dente. Drain, reserving 1 cup (250 mL) pasta water. Return pasta to pot.
3. In blender, combine carrots and their cooking liquid, salt, pepper and mustard; purée until very smooth.
4. To the pasta, add carrot purée and the reserved pasta water. Cook, stirring, over medium heat for 3 to 5 minutes or until sauce is thickened and pasta is well coated. Stir in 1 cup (250 mL) of the cheese and cook, stirring, for about 1 minute or until cheese is melted. Transfer to prepared baking dish and sprinkle with the remaining cheese.
5. Bake in preheated oven for 18 to 23 minutes or until cheese is melted and lightly browned. Let cool for 5 to 10 minutes before serving.

▸ Health Note

You may be surprised to learn that whole wheat pasta has a lower glycemic index than whole wheat bread and has triple the fiber of regular pasta.

Multigrain Macaroni with Zucchini, Greek Yogurt and Romano

Makes 4 servings

✪ Great for Steps 1, 2, 3, 4 and 5

When zucchini is abundant in the garden, reach for this recipe. The zucchini — loaded with vitamin C, magnesium, beta-carotene, potassium and riboflavin — gets a quick steam when it's mixed into the hot pasta, allowing it to keep its emerald hue and delicate flavor.

Tip

Nonfat Greek yogurt may be used in this recipe, but for a creamier sauce that is still low in fat, opt for 2% Greek yogurt.

8 oz	multigrain or whole wheat macaroni	250 g
1 lb	small or medium zucchini, coarsely shredded	500 g
1 tbsp	extra virgin olive oil	15 mL
1⁄4 tsp	fine sea salt	1 mL
1⁄4 tsp	freshly cracked black pepper	1 mL
1⁄8 tsp	ground nutmeg	0.5 mL
2⁄3 cup	2% plain Greek yogurt	150 mL
1⁄2 cup	freshly grated Romano cheese, divided	125 mL

1. In a large pot of boiling salted water (see tip, page 398), cook pasta according to package directions until al dente. Drain, reserving 2 tbsp (30 mL) pasta water. Return pasta to pot. Stir in zucchini, cover and set aside.
2. In a large skillet, heat oil over medium-low heat. Add salt, pepper, nutmeg, yogurt, half the cheese and the reserved pasta water; cook, stirring, for 1 to 2 minutes or until just warmed through.
3. Add yogurt mixture to pasta mixture, gently tossing to combine. Serve sprinkled with the remaining cheese.

Nutrients per serving	
Calories	158
Total fat	9 g
Saturated fat	4 g
Cholesterol	13 mg
Sodium	392 mg
Carbohydrate	53 g
Fiber	2 g
Protein	12 g
Calcium	188 mg
Iron	1.2 mg

Moussaka Macaroni

Makes 4 servings

✪ Great for Steps 1, 3, 4 and 5

Moussaka is Greece's answer for an abundance of eggplant. Here, the favorite casserole is reinvented in a quick-to-the-table pasta loaded with all of the traditional flavors of the original.

Tip

Make sure to use fine sea salt in the water you use to cook the pasta. Conventional table salt contains chemicals and additives, whereas sea salt contains an abundance of naturally occurring trace minerals.

2 tsp	extra virgin olive oil	10 mL
1	large eggplant (about 1 lb/500 g), peeled and cut into 1/2-inch (1 cm) cubes	1
1 1/4 cups	chopped onions	300 mL
2	cloves garlic, minced	2
12 oz	extra-lean ground beef	375 g
1/2 tsp	fine sea salt	2 mL
1	can (28 oz/796 mL) crushed tomatoes	1
2 tsp	dried oregano	10 mL
1/2 tsp	ground cinnamon	2 mL
8 oz	whole wheat macaroni pasta	250 g
1/2 cup	packed fresh flat-leaf (Italian) parsley leaves, chopped	125 mL
1/2 cup	crumbled feta cheese	125 mL

1. In a Dutch oven or a large saucepan, heat oil over medium-high heat. Add eggplant and onions; cook, stirring, for 6 to 8 minutes or until softened. Transfer to a bowl.
2. Add garlic, beef and salt to the pan and cook, breaking up beef with a spoon, for 6 to 9 minutes or until beef is no longer pink. Drain off any fat. Stir in eggplant mixture, tomatoes, oregano and cinnamon. Bring to a boil. Reduce heat and simmer, stirring occasionally, for 20 to 25 minutes or until sauce is thickened and eggplant is very tender.
3. Meanwhile, in a large pot of boiling salted water (see tip, at left), cook pasta according to package directions until al dente. Drain, reserving 1/2 cup (125 mL) pasta water.
4. Add pasta to beef mixture. Simmer, stirring occasionally, for 2 minutes. If necessary, stir in enough of the reserved pasta water to moisten. Stir in parsley. Serve sprinkled with cheese.

Nutrients per serving	
Calories	404
Total fat	11 g
Saturated fat	3 g
Cholesterol	76 mg
Sodium	622 mg
Carbohydrate	82 g
Fiber	17 g
Protein	38 g
Calcium	221 mg
Iron	6.6 mg

Whole Wheat Orzo with Swiss Chard and Pecans

Makes 4 servings

✪ Great for Steps 1, 2, 3, 4 and 5

The perfect trio for a dinner dish: delicious, easy and healthy.

Tip

Other small whole wheat or multigrain pasta may be used in place of the orzo.

Nutrients per serving	
Calories	323
Total fat	13 g
Saturated fat	2 g
Cholesterol	7 mg
Sodium	300 mg
Carbohydrate	50 g
Fiber	7 g
Protein	12 g
Calcium	64 mg
Iron	2.6 mg

1	large bunch red Swiss chard	1
8 oz	whole wheat orzo pasta	250 g
1 tbsp	extra virgin olive oil	15 mL
1	large shallot, thinly sliced	1
1/4 tsp	fine sea salt	1 mL
2 tsp	sherry vinegar	10 mL
2 oz	goat cheese, crumbled	60 g
1/3 cup	chopped toasted pecans	75 mL

1. Trim off tough stems from Swiss chard and discard. Trim tender stems and ribs from leaves and finely chop stems and ribs. Thinly slice leaves crosswise (to measure about 5 cups/1.25 L). Set chopped stems and sliced leaves aside separately.
2. In a large pot of boiling salted water (see tip, page 400), cook pasta according to package directions until al dente. Drain, reserving 1/4 cup (60 mL) pasta water. Return pasta to pot.
3. Meanwhile, in a large skillet, heat oil over medium-high heat. Add shallot, Swiss chard stems and salt; cook, stirring, for 6 to 7 minutes or until stems are tender and slightly browned. Add Swiss chard leaves and cook, stirring, for about 2 minutes or until wilted. Stir in vinegar.
4. To the pasta, add cheese and enough of the reserved pasta water to create a creamy consistency. Stir in chard mixture. Serve sprinkled with pecans.

Healthy Know-How

Nutrition Tips for Kids

Good nutrition is essential for lifelong health, and it begins in childhood. But between peer pressure and a constant stream of advertisements for junk foods, getting children to eat well can be challenging — but not impossible. Children develop a natural preference for the foods they enjoy the most, so the challenge is to make healthy choices appealing. Here are some simple ways to make that happen:

- The childhood impulse to imitate is strong, so it's important to act as a role model for your kids. It's no good asking your child to eat fruit and vegetables while you gorge on potato chips and soda.
- Have regular family meals. Knowing dinner is served at approximately the same time every night and that the entire family will be sitting down together is comforting and enhances appetite. Breakfast is another great time for a family meal, especially since kids who eat breakfast tend to do better in school.
- Cook more meals at home. Home-cooked meals are healthier for the whole family and set a great example for kids about the importance of food. Restaurant meals tend to have more fat, sugar and salt. Save dining out for special occasions.
- Get kids involved. Children enjoy helping adults grocery shop, selecting what goes in their lunch box and preparing dinner. It's also a chance for you to teach them about the nutritional values of different foods and (for older children) how to read food labels.
- Make a variety of healthy snacks available. Keep plenty of fruits, vegetables, whole-grain snacks and healthy beverages (water, milk, pure fruit juice) around and easily accessible so kids become used to reaching for healthy snacks instead of empty-calorie snacks like soda, chips or cookies.
- Limit portion sizes. Don't insist that your child clean the plate, and never use food as a reward or bribe.
- Don't ban sweets entirely. A no-sweets rule is an invitation for cravings and overindulgence when your child is given the chance.

Asparagus Penne with Goat Cheese

Makes 4 servings

✪ Great for Steps 1, 2, 3, 4 and 5

Yes, a double-cheese pasta can still claim superfood status. The key? Use boldly flavored cheeses, such as goat cheese and Parmesan cheese, because even small amounts add a punch of flavor. Swap regular pasta for multigrain pasta, add a slew of delectable, nutrient-dense vegetables, and boast-worthy, superfood supper is in the bag.

Tip

Make sure to use fine sea salt in the water you use to cook the pasta. Conventional table salt contains chemicals and additives, whereas sea salt contains an abundance of naturally occurring trace minerals.

Nutrients per serving	
Calories	333
Total fat	10 g
Saturated fat	3 g
Cholesterol	19 mg
Sodium	407 mg
Carbohydrate	57 g
Fiber	9 g
Protein	16 g
Calcium	184 mg
Iron	2.5 mg

8 oz	multigrain or whole wheat penne pasta	250 g
1 tbsp	extra virgin olive oil	15 mL
1 cup	chopped red onion	250 mL
1 lb	asparagus, trimmed and cut into 1⁄2-inch (1 cm) pieces	500 g
1⁄2 tsp	fine sea salt	2 mL
1⁄2 tsp	hot pepper flakes	2 mL
1 tsp	finely grated lemon zest	5 mL
2 tbsp	freshly squeezed lemon juice	30 mL
2 1⁄2 oz	soft goat cheese, crumbled	75 g
1⁄4 cup	freshly grated Parmesan or Romano cheese	60 mL

1. In a large pot of boiling salted water (see tip, at left), cook pasta according to package directions until al dente. Drain, reserving 1⁄3 cup (75 mL) pasta water.
2. Meanwhile, in a large skillet, heat oil over medium-high heat. Add red onion and cook, stirring, for 5 to 6 minutes or until softened. Add asparagus, salt and hot pepper flakes; cook, stirring, for about 5 minutes or until asparagus is tender-crisp.
3. Stir in pasta, lemon zest, lemon juice and the reserved pasta water. Reduce heat to medium-low and cook, tossing to coat, for 1 minute. Add goat cheese, tossing until just melted. Serve sprinkled with Parmesan.

▸ Health Note

Lemon zest offers more than intense citrus flavor: it is also a potent source of vitamin C and the powerful antioxidant d-limonene, the latter of which may decrease the risk of cancer.

Penne with Hummus, Smoked Paprika and Chickpeas

Makes 4 servings

✪ Great for Steps 2, 3, 4 and 5

Hummus as a pasta sauce: why haven't we been doing this for years? Garlicky, creamy and incredibly convenient, it combines here with chickpeas, fire-roasted tomatoes and smoked paprika for one of the most delectable fast-food meals ever.

8 oz	whole wheat penne pasta	250 g
2 tsp	extra virgin olive oil	10 mL
1	can (14 to 19 oz/398 to 540 mL) chickpeas, drained and rinsed	1
1 tsp	hot or sweet smoked paprika	5 mL
1	can (14 to 15 oz/398 to 425 mL) diced fire-roasted tomatoes, with juice	1
$\frac{3}{4}$ cup	packed fresh cilantro leaves, chopped	175 mL
$\frac{1}{2}$ cup	hummus (store-bought or see page 105)	125 mL

1. In a large pot of boiling salted water (see tip, page 403), cook pasta according to package directions until al dente. Drain, reserving $\frac{1}{4}$ cup (60 mL) pasta water.
2. In a large skillet, heat oil over medium-high heat. Add chickpeas and paprika; cook, stirring, for 5 minutes or until chickpeas are crispy. Stir in pasta, tomatoes with juice and the reserved pasta water. Cook, tossing to coat, for 1 minute. Gently stir in cilantro and hummus.

Tip

If you can't find fire-roasted tomatoes, use regular diced tomatoes instead.

Nutrients per serving	
Calories	365
Total fat	6 g
Saturated fat	1 g
Cholesterol	0 mg
Sodium	505 mg
Carbohydrate	71 g
Fiber	12 g
Protein	15 g
Calcium	69 mg
Iron	4.0 mg

Penne with Chicken Sausage, Mustard and Basil

Makes 4 servings

✪ Great for Steps 3, 4 and 5

Rich and healthy — yes, the two do go together — this comforting sausage and pasta dish can be made with flat-leaf (Italian) parsley when basil is no longer in season.

Tip

A 5-oz (142 mL) can of evaporated skim milk yields 2⁄3 cup (150 mL).

8 oz	multigrain or whole wheat penne pasta	250 g
1 tsp	extra virgin olive oil	5 mL
8 oz	cooked chicken sausages (about 3 links), thinly sliced	250 g
1⁄8 tsp	fine sea salt	0.5 mL
Pinch	hot pepper flakes	Pinch
2⁄3 cup	evaporated skim milk	150 mL
3 tbsp	dry white wine	45 mL
1 1⁄2 tbsp	whole-grain Dijon mustard	22 mL
1⁄2 cup	packed fresh basil leaves, thinly sliced	125 mL

1. In a large pot of boiling salted water (see tip, page 403), cook pasta according to package directions until al dente. Drain, reserving 2 tbsp (30 mL) pasta water. Return pasta to pot.
2. Meanwhile, in a large skillet, heat oil over medium-high heat. Add sausages and cook, stirring, for 3 to 4 minutes or until browned. Add salt, hot pepper flakes, milk, wine and mustard; cook, scraping up browned bits from bottom of pan, for 3 to 4 minutes or until slightly thickened.
3. To the pasta, add sausage mixture, basil and the reserved pasta water, tossing to combine.

Nutrients per serving	
Calories	381
Total fat	8 g
Saturated fat	2 g
Cholesterol	45 mg
Sodium	593 mg
Carbohydrate	53 g
Fiber	6 g
Protein	18 g
Calcium	184 mg
Iron	2.3 mg

Chicken Sausage, Arugula and Tomato Penne

Makes 4 servings

✪ Great for Steps 1, 3, 4 and 5

Multiple textures and flavors — meaty sausages, peppery arugula, sweet-tart tomatoes and briny feta — combine in minutes for a pasta with "cooked all day" character.

Tip

Make sure to use fine sea salt in the water you use to cook the pasta. Conventional table salt contains chemicals and additives, whereas sea salt contains an abundance of naturally occurring trace minerals.

8 oz	multigrain or whole wheat penne pasta	250 g
2 tsp	extra virgin olive oil	10 mL
8 oz	cooked chicken sausages (about 3 links), thinly sliced	250 g
6	cloves garlic, minced	6
1/4 tsp	hot pepper flakes	1 mL
1	can (28 oz/796 mL) diced tomatoes, with juice	1
6 cups	packed arugula	1.5 L
1/2 cup	crumbled feta cheese	125 mL

1. In a large pot of boiling salted water (see tip, at left), cook pasta according to package directions until al dente. Drain, reserving 1/4 cup (60 mL) pasta water.
2. Meanwhile, in a large skillet, heat oil over medium-high heat. Add sausages and cook, stirring, for 3 to 4 minutes or until browned. Add garlic and hot pepper flakes; cook, stirring, for 30 seconds. Add tomatoes with juice and the reserved pasta water; simmer, stirring once or twice, for 2 minutes or until sauce is thickened.
3. Stir in pasta and arugula; simmer for 30 to 60 seconds or until arugula begins to wilt. Serve sprinkled with cheese.

Superfood Spotlight

Arugula • Arugula, a member of the Brassica family that grows wild across much of Europe, is closely related to the mustard plant. It is a small plant with elongated, serrated leaves. Today, much of the arugula we buy is cultivated, but wild arugula leaves contain more protective plant chemicals than cultivated hybrids. The leaves are rich in carotenes and are an excellent source of lutein and zeaxanthin for eye health, including prevention of cataracts. The indoles contained in arugula and other Brassicas are linked with protection from colon cancer. The leaves also supply good amounts of folate — especially important in pregnancy because it helps protect the fetus — and calcium for healthy bones and heart.

Nutrients per serving	
Calories	359
Total fat	10 g
Saturated fat	3 g
Cholesterol	42 mg
Sodium	603 mg
Carbohydrate	60 g
Fiber	8 g
Protein	21 g
Calcium	257 mg
Iron	3.9 mg

Turkey Sausage, Escarole and Sun-Dried Tomato Pasta

Makes 4 servings

✪ Great for Steps 1, 3, 4 and 5

Turkey sausage and sun-dried tomatoes make this pasta deliciously robust. The bittersweet edge of escarole ties the dish together — and eliminates the need to make a salad on the side.

Tip

An equal amount of packed tender watercress sprigs or arugula may be used in place of the escarole.

8 oz	multigrain or whole wheat penne pasta	250 g
2 tsp	extra virgin olive oil	10 mL
8 oz	Italian turkey sausage (bulk or casings removed)	250 g
2 cups	thinly sliced red onions	500 mL
8 cups	roughly chopped escarole (about 1 large head)	2 L
1/4 tsp	fine sea salt	1 mL
3 tbsp	thinly sliced drained oil-packed sun-dried tomatoes	45 mL
3 tbsp	freshly grated Romano or Parmesan cheese	45 mL

1. In a large pot of boiling salted water (see tip, page 406), cook pasta according to package directions until al dente. Drain, reserving 1/3 cup (75 mL) pasta water.
2. Meanwhile, in a large skillet, heat oil over medium-high heat. Add sausage and cook, breaking it up with a spoon, for 7 to 8 minutes or until no longer pink. Add red onions and cook, stirring, for 6 to 8 minutes or until softened. Add escarole and salt; cook, stirring, for 2 minutes or until mostly wilted.
3. Stir in pasta, sun-dried tomatoes and the reserved pasta water, tossing to combine. Cook, stirring, for 1 minute. Serve sprinkled with cheese.

Nutrients per serving	
Calories	348
Total fat	7 g
Saturated fat	2 g
Cholesterol	39 mg
Sodium	575 mg
Carbohydrate	59 g
Fiber	10 g
Protein	24 g
Calcium	182 mg
Iron	3.5 mg

Salmon Penne with Peas and Lemon

Makes 4 servings

✪ Great for Steps 1, 3, 4 and 5

Lemon, spinach and peas make mighty fine teammates for canned salmon and multigrain penne.

Tips

If fresh dill is not available, use 1½ tbsp (22 mL) dried dillweed.

Make sure to use fine sea salt in the water you use to cook the pasta. Conventional table salt contains chemicals and additives, whereas sea salt contains an abundance of naturally occurring trace minerals.

8 oz	multigrain or whole wheat penne pasta	250 g
1	can (15 oz/425 g) wild Alaskan salmon, drained and flaked (skin removed, if necessary)	1
6 cups	packed baby spinach (about 6 oz/175 g)	1.5 L
1½ cups	frozen petite peas	375 mL
¼ cup	chopped fresh dill	60 mL
¼ tsp	fine sea salt	1 mL
¼ tsp	freshly cracked black pepper	1 mL
1 tsp	finely grated lemon zest	5 mL
2 tbsp	freshly squeezed lemon juice	30 mL

1. In a large pot of boiling salted water (see tip, at left), cook pasta according to package directions until al dente. Drain, reserving ¼ cup (60 mL) pasta water. Return pasta to pot.
2. To the pasta, add salmon, spinach, peas, dill, salt, pepper, lemon zest, lemon juice and the reserved pasta water. Cook over medium-low heat, stirring occasionally, for 2 to 3 minutes or until warmed through and spinach is wilted.

▶ Health Note

Dill leaves are a good source of calcium, iron and magnesium, as well as vitamins A, C and E.

Nutrients per serving	
Calories	419
Total fat	11 g
Saturated fat	2 g
Cholesterol	53 mg
Sodium	338 mg
Carbohydrate	60 g
Fiber	11 g
Protein	33 g
Calcium	92 mg
Iron	4.0 mg

Rotini with Fennel, Orange and Almonds

Makes 4 servings

✪ Great for Steps 1, 2, 3, 4 and 5

Here, the nuanced flavor of licorice — from both fennel bulb and fennel fronds — takes the limelight in this streamlined pasta that is as comfortable on busy weeknights as it is for weekend get-togethers. Orange and almond are classic companions, highlighting fennel's flavorful charms.

Tip

To toast sliced almonds, place up to ½ cup (125 mL) almonds in a medium skillet set over medium heat. Cook, shaking the skillet, for 2 to 3 minutes or until almonds are golden brown and fragrant. Let cool completely before use.

8 oz	multigrain or whole wheat rotini pasta	250 g
1 tbsp	extra virgin olive oil	15 mL
4	cloves garlic, minced	4
2 cups	chopped fennel (about 1 large bulb), fronds reserved	500 mL
½ tsp	fine sea salt	2 mL
¼ cup	golden raisins, chopped	60 mL
1½ tsp	ground cumin	7 mL
1 tsp	finely grated orange zest	5 mL
¼ cup	freshly squeezed orange juice	60 mL
¼ cup	sliced almonds, toasted (see tip, at left)	60 mL

1. In a large pot of boiling salted water (see tip, page 408), cook pasta according to package directions until al dente. Drain, reserving ¼ cup (60 mL) pasta water.
2. Meanwhile, in a large skillet, heat oil over medium-high heat. Add garlic, fennel and salt; cook, stirring, for 5 to 6 minutes or until fennel is tender-crisp.
3. Stir in pasta, raisins, cumin, orange zest and orange juice; cook, stirring, for 2 minutes. If necessary, stir in enough of the reserved pasta water to moisten.
4. Chop enough of the reserved fennel fronds to measure ¼ cup (60 mL). Stir fennel fronds into pasta. Serve sprinkled with almonds.

Nutrients per serving	
Calories	357
Total fat	9 g
Saturated fat	1 g
Cholesterol	0 mg
Sodium	389 mg
Carbohydrate	63 g
Fiber	8 g
Protein	11 g
Calcium	87 mg
Iron	3.0 mg

Roasted Cauliflower Rotini with Green Olives and Currants

Makes 4 servings

✪ Great for Steps 1, 2, 3, 4 and 5

The caramelized nuttiness of roasted cauliflower, the briny bite of green olives and a hint of sweetness from dried currants are all anchored by the rustic flavor of whole wheat rotini.

Tip

An equal amount of chopped pitted brine-cured black olives (such as kalamata) may be used in place of the green olives.

- **Preheat oven to 450°F (230°C)**
- **Large rimmed baking sheet, lined with foil and sprayed with nonstick cooking spray (preferably olive oil)**

4 cups	roughly chopped cauliflower florets (about 1 medium head)	1 L
1⁄4 tsp	fine sea salt	1 mL
2 tsp	extra virgin olive oil	10 mL
8 oz	whole wheat rotini pasta	250 g
1⁄2 cup	packed fresh flat-leaf (Italian) parsley leaves, chopped	125 mL
1⁄4 cup	chopped pitted green olives	60 mL
3 tbsp	currants or chopped raisins	45 mL

1. On prepared baking sheet, toss cauliflower with salt and oil; spread in a single layer. Roast in preheated oven for 20 to 25 minutes, stirring once or twice, until golden brown and tender.
2. Meanwhile, in a large pot of boiling salted water (see tip, page 411), cook pasta according to package directions until al dente. Drain, reserving 1⁄4 cup (60 mL) pasta water. Return pasta to pot.
3. To the pasta, add roasted cauliflower, parsley, olives and currants, tossing to combine. If necessary, stir in enough of the reserved pasta water to moisten.

▶ Health Note

Olives have significant levels of monounsaturated fat, which helps fight against unhealthy cholesterol in the body and can protect the heart and blood vessels. Further, olives are high in vitamin E and flavonoids, both of which are known for their ability to attack free radicals, chemicals in the body that destroy the structure of cells and cause disease.

Nutrients per serving	
Calories	320
Total fat	6 g
Saturated fat	1 g
Cholesterol	0 mg
Sodium	353 mg
Carbohydrate	59 g
Fiber	9 g
Protein	10 g
Calcium	64 mg
Iron	2.8 mg

Spaghetti Limone with Asparagus and Mushrooms

Makes 6 servings

✪ Great for Steps 1, 2, 3, 4 and 5

Happiness is a bowlful of this sumptuous pasta, beautiful with hues of green and yellow and full of spring flavor from mushrooms, asparagus and lemon.

Tips

An equal amount of broccoli rabe, trimmed and cut into 1-inch (2.5 cm) pieces, may be used in place of the asparagus.

Make sure to use fine sea salt in the water you use to cook the pasta. Conventional table salt contains chemicals and additives, whereas sea salt contains an abundance of naturally occurring trace minerals.

Nutrients per serving	
Calories	251
Total fat	5 g
Saturated fat	1 g
Cholesterol	7 mg
Sodium	119 mg
Carbohydrate	42 g
Fiber	7 g
Protein	10 g
Calcium	126 mg
Iron	1.8 mg

12 oz	multigrain or whole wheat spaghetti pasta	375 g
1 tbsp	extra virgin olive oil	15 mL
1 cup	finely chopped onion	250 mL
1 lb	cremini or button mushrooms, trimmed and sliced	500 g
1½ cups	reduced-sodium ready-to-use vegetable broth	375 mL
1 tbsp	finely grated lemon zest	15 mL
⅓ cup	freshly squeezed lemon juice	75 mL
1 lb	asparagus, trimmed and cut into 1-inch (2.5 cm) pieces	500 g
¼ cup	freshly grated Parmesan cheese	60 mL

1. In a large pot of boiling salted water (see tip, at left), cook pasta according to package directions until al dente. Drain and return to pot.
2. Meanwhile, in a large skillet, heat oil over medium heat. Add onion and cook, stirring, for 1 minute. Add mushrooms and cook, stirring, for 5 to 6 minutes or until softened.
3. Stir in broth, lemon zest and lemon juice. Bring to a boil. Reduce heat and simmer, stirring occasionally, for about 6 minutes or until liquid is reduced by half. Add asparagus and simmer, stirring occasionally, for about 2 minutes or until bright green.
4. Add vegetable mixture to the pasta, tossing to combine. Cook over medium-low heat, stirring, for 1 minute. Serve sprinkled with cheese.

Spaghetti with Brussels Sprouts and Toasted Walnuts

Makes 4 servings

✪ Great for Steps 1, 2, 3, 4 and 5

Rich enough to qualify as comfort food, this quick pasta treatment of Brussels sprouts also appeals to those with a more refined palate.

Tip

The Brussels sprouts can be sliced with a kitchen knife, a mandoline or a food processor fitted with a slicing disk.

8 oz	multigrain or whole wheat spaghetti pasta	250 g
1 tbsp	extra virgin olive oil	15 mL
3	cloves garlic, minced	3
12 oz	Brussels sprouts, trimmed and very thinly sliced crosswise	375 g
½ tsp	fine sea salt	2 mL
¼ tsp	freshly cracked black pepper	1 mL
2 tsp	finely grated lemon zest	10 mL
2 tbsp	freshly squeezed lemon juice	30 mL
¼ cup	finely chopped toasted walnuts	60 mL

1. In a large pot of boiling salted water (see tip, page 411), cook pasta according to package directions until al dente. Drain, reserving ⅓ cup (75 mL) pasta water.
2. In a large skillet, heat oil over medium-high heat. Add garlic and cook, stirring, for 30 seconds. Add Brussels sprouts, salt and pepper; cook, stirring, for 3 to 4 minutes or until sprouts are tender and lightly browned. Stir in pasta, lemon zest, lemon juice and the reserved pasta water; cook, tossing to coat, for 1 minute. Serve sprinkled with walnuts.

Superfood Spotlight

Brussels Sprouts • Brussels sprouts are an important winter vegetable, providing high levels of vitamin C and many other immune-boosting nutrients. They are rich in sulforaphane, which is a detoxifier and has been shown to help the body clear potential carcinogens. Brussels sprouts help prevent DNA damage when eaten regularly and may help minimize the spread of breast cancer. They even contain small amounts of beneficial omega-3 fats and zinc, as well as selenium, a mineral many adults do not eat in the recommended daily amount. People who eat large quantities of Brussels sprouts and other Brassicas have a much lower risk of prostate, colorectal and lung cancer. Finally, Brussels sprouts are rich in indoles and other compounds that protect against cancer and help lower LDL "bad" cholesterol.

Nutrients per serving

Calories	377
Total fat	15 g
Saturated fat	1 g
Cholesterol	0 mg
Sodium	385 mg
Carbohydrate	58 g
Fiber	10 g
Protein	15 g
Calcium	77 mg
Iron	3.5 mg

Quick Pasta al Norma

Makes 4 servings

✪ Great for Steps 1, 2, 3, 4 and 5

When it comes to easy, satisfying dinners, this simplified take on pasta al Norma is hard to beat.

Tip

When selecting an eggplant, choose one with firm, shiny, blemish-free skin and a mostly green (not brown) stem top. The eggplant should feel heavier than it looks; the greater the moisture, the fresher the eggplant.

Nutrients per serving

Calories	321
Total fat	7 g
Saturated fat	2 g
Cholesterol	6 mg
Sodium	378 mg
Carbohydrate	60 g
Fiber	11 g
Protein	12 g
Calcium	120 mg
Iron	2.9 mg

- **Preheat oven to 500°F (260°C)**
- **Large rimmed baking sheet, lined with foil and sprayed with nonstick cooking spray (preferably olive oil)**

1	large eggplant, trimmed and cut into 1-inch (2.5 cm) cubes	1
1⁄4 tsp	fine sea salt	1 mL
2 tsp	extra virgin olive oil	10 mL
8 oz	multigrain or whole wheat spaghetti pasta	250 g
1⁄4 tsp	hot pepper flakes	1 mL
1 1⁄4 cups	reduced-sodium marinara sauce	300 mL
1⁄4 cup	freshly grated Romano cheese	60 mL
1⁄4 cup	packed fresh basil leaves, torn	60 mL

1. On prepared baking sheet, toss eggplant with salt and oil; spread in a single layer. Roast in preheated oven for 15 to 20 minutes or until tender and golden brown.
2. Meanwhile, in a large pot of boiling salted water (see tip, page 411), cook pasta according to package directions until al dente. Drain, reserving 1⁄4 cup (60 mL) pasta water. Return pasta to pot.
3. To the pasta, add roasted eggplant, hot pepper flakes, marinara sauce and the reserved pasta water, tossing to combine. Cook, stirring constantly, over medium-low heat for 5 to 6 minutes or until sauce is thickened. Serve sprinkled with cheese and basil.

Fast Pumpkin Pasta with Parmesan and Chives

Makes 4 servings

✪ Great for Steps 2, 3, 4 and 5

Pantry pasta, perfected: canned pumpkin and evaporated milk are the secrets to the lush sauce; the musky-mint flavor of sage adds instant depth.

8 oz	multigrain or whole wheat spaghetti pasta	250 g
3/4 cup	pumpkin purée (not pie filling)	175 mL
3/4 cup	reduced-sodium ready-to-use vegetable or chicken broth	175 mL
1/2 cup	evaporated skim milk	125 mL
2 tsp	dried rubbed sage	10 mL
1/4 tsp	fine sea salt	1 mL
4 tbsp	freshly grated Parmesan cheese, divided	60 mL
1/4 cup	minced fresh chives	60 mL

1. In a large pot of boiling salted water (see tip, page 415), cook pasta according to package directions until al dente. Drain, reserving 1/4 cup (60 mL) pasta water. Return pasta to pot.
2. Meanwhile, in a large saucepan, combine pumpkin, broth, milk, sage and salt. Heat over medium-low heat, stirring often, for 10 minutes or until slightly thickened.
3. To the pasta, add pumpkin mixture, half the cheese and the reserved pasta water, tossing to combine; cook, stirring, for 1 minute or until thickened. Serve sprinkled with chives and the remaining cheese.

Tip

An equal amount of thawed frozen winter squash purée may be used in place of the pumpkin purée.

Nutrients per serving	
Calories	313
Total fat	5 g
Saturated fat	2 g
Cholesterol	11 mg
Sodium	356 mg
Carbohydrate	55 g
Fiber	8 g
Protein	13 g
Calcium	229 mg
Iron	2.1 mg

Spaghetti with Tuna, Olives and Golden Raisins

Makes 4 servings

✪ Great for Steps 1, 3, 4 and 5

Caution: may require second helpings. The combination of salty, sweet, briny and fresh in this pasta is somewhat unexpected, but very pleasing.

8 oz	whole wheat linguine pasta	250 g
1 tbsp	extra virgin olive oil	15 mL
3	cloves garlic, minced	3
1 cup	chopped onion	250 mL
1/4 tsp	fine sea salt	1 mL
1/4 tsp	freshly cracked black pepper	1 mL
2	cans (each 6 oz/170 g) water-packed tuna, drained	2
1/3 cup	pitted brine-cured black olives (such as kalamata), roughly chopped	75 mL
1/3 cup	golden raisins, chopped	75 mL
1/2 cup	packed fresh flat-leaf (Italian) parsley leaves, chopped	125 mL

1. In a large pot of boiling salted water (see tip, at left), cook pasta according to package directions until al dente. Drain, reserving 1/4 cup (60 mL) pasta water.
2. Meanwhile, in a large, heavy skillet, heat oil over medium-high heat. Add garlic, onion, salt and pepper; cook, stirring, for 6 to 8 minutes or until onion is golden.
3. Stir in pasta, tuna, olives, raisins and the reserved pasta water; cook, stirring, for 1 minute or until some of the liquid is evaporated. Stir in parsley.

Tip

Make sure to use fine sea salt in the water you use to cook the pasta. Conventional table salt contains chemicals and additives, whereas sea salt contains an abundance of naturally occurring trace minerals.

Variation

Substitute 1 1/2 cups (375 mL) diced cooked chicken or turkey for the tuna.

Nutrients per serving	
Calories	409
Total fat	7 g
Saturated fat	1 g
Cholesterol	25 mg
Sodium	316 mg
Carbohydrate	63 g
Fiber	8 g
Protein	31 g
Calcium	71 mg
Iron	4.2 mg

Quinoa Spaghetti with Kale

Makes 4 servings

✪ Great for Steps 1, 2, 3, 4 and 5

This dish could easily pass muster as the definitively healthy pasta recipe. But it's the synchronicity of flavors that makes it worth making (often). A good-quality extra virgin olive oil makes all the difference, adding a mellow, grassy flavor that ties the other ingredients together.

Tip

Quinoa pastas are available in health food stores and in the health food section of well-stocked supermarkets. If you can't find quinoa spaghetti, use multigrain or whole wheat spaghetti.

1 lb	kale, stems and ribs removed, leaves very thinly sliced crosswise (about 8 cups/2 L)	500 g
8 oz	quinoa spaghetti pasta	250 g
1½ tbsp	extra virgin olive oil	22 mL
2 cups	thinly sliced red onions	500 mL
2	cloves garlic, minced	2
⅛ tsp	hot pepper flakes	0.5 mL
½ tsp	fine sea salt	2 mL
2 tsp	sherry vinegar or white wine vinegar	10 mL
¼ cup	freshly grated Parmesan cheese	60 mL

1. In a large pot of boiling salted water (see tip, page 415), cook kale for about 10 minutes or until just tender. Using a slotted spoon, transfer kale to a medium bowl.
2. In the same pot, return water to a boil. Cook pasta according to package directions until al dente. Drain, reserving ¼ cup (60 mL) pasta water. Return pasta to pot.
3. Meanwhile, in a large skillet, heat oil over medium-high heat. Add red onions and cook, stirring, for 6 to 8 minutes or until softened. Add garlic and hot pepper flakes; cook, stirring, for 1 minute. Add kale, reduce heat to medium and cook, stirring, for 2 minutes or until heated through. Remove from heat and stir in salt and vinegar.
4. To the pasta, add kale mixture and the reserved pasta water, tossing to combine. Cook, tossing, over medium-low heat for 1 minute. Serve sprinkled with cheese.

Superfood Spotlight

Kale • Kale is one of the most nutritious members of the Brassica family. It contains more calcium and iron than any other vegetable. A single portion provides twice the recommended daily amount of vitamin C, which helps the body absorb the vegetable's high iron content. One portion also contains about a fifth of the daily calcium requirement for an adult. Kale is rich in selenium, which helps fight cancer, and provides magnesium and vitamin E for a healthy heart and healthy, young-looking skin.

Nutrients per serving	
Calories	385
Total fat	9 g
Saturated fat	2 g
Cholesterol	10 mg
Sodium	213 mg
Carbohydrate	66 g
Fiber	9 g
Protein	15 g
Calcium	418 mg
Iron	5.8 mg

Quinoa Spaghetti al Pomodoro

Makes 4 servings

✪ Great for Steps 1, 2, 3, 4 and 5

If there is anything better than summer tomatoes, I don't know about it. Here, they are treated with simplicity: splashed with olive oil, balsamic vinegar and garlic, then left uncooked to draw out their flavor and sweetness. Quinoa pasta shifts the recipe from side dish to main dish.

Tip

Quinoa pastas are available in health food stores and in the health food section of well-stocked supermarkets. If you can't find quinoa spaghetti, use multigrain or whole wheat spaghetti.

Nutrients per serving	
Calories	644
Total fat	14 g
Saturated fat	2 g
Cholesterol	0 mg
Sodium	547 mg
Carbohydrate	124 g
Fiber	13 g
Protein	12 g
Calcium	43 mg
Iron	1.0 mg

2	cloves garlic, minced	2
4 cups	chopped tomatoes	1 L
1/2 tsp	fine sea salt	2 mL
1/4 tsp	freshly cracked black pepper	1 mL
2 tbsp	extra virgin olive oil	30 mL
1 tsp	balsamic vinegar	5 mL
12 oz	quinoa spaghetti pasta	375 g
2/3 cup	packed fresh basil leaves, thinly sliced	150 mL
2 tbsp	toasted pine nuts (optional)	30 mL

1. In a medium bowl, combine garlic, tomatoes, salt, pepper, oil and vinegar. Let stand for at least 10 minutes to blend the flavors.
2. Meanwhile, in a large pot of boiling salted water (see tip, page 415), cook pasta according to package directions until al dente. Drain, reserving 1/4 cup (60 mL) pasta water. Return pasta to pot.
3. To the pasta, add tomato mixture and the reserved pasta water. Cook over medium-low heat for 1 minute, tossing to combine. Serve sprinkled with basil and pine nuts (if using).

Wagon Wheels with Broccoli, Turkey and Parmesan

Makes 4 servings

✪ Great for Steps 1, 3, 4 and 5

And now for the kids' favorite portion of the menu. You won't get any arguments about cleaning plates with these yummy wagon wheels. Extra credit is in order, considering all of the good things going on in one pot.

Variation

Substitute lean ground chicken or extra-lean ground pork for the turkey.

Nutrients per serving	
Calories	400
Total fat	11 g
Saturated fat	4 g
Cholesterol	54 mg
Sodium	389 mg
Carbohydrate	50 g
Fiber	7 g
Protein	30 g
Calcium	150 mg
Iron	3.6 mg

8 oz	whole wheat wagon-wheel pasta or other medium-shape pasta	250 g
3 cups	small broccoli florets	750 mL
2 tsp	extra virgin olive oil	10 mL
12 oz	lean ground turkey	375 g
1 tbsp	dried Italian seasoning	15 mL
1/4 tsp	fine sea salt	1 mL
1/2 cup	reduced-sodium ready-to-use chicken or vegetable broth	125 mL
1/4 cup	freshly grated Parmesan cheese	60 mL

1. In a large pot of boiling salted water (see tip, page 415), cook pasta according to package directions until al dente. Add broccoli for the last minute of cooking. Drain, reserving 1/4 cup (60 mL) pasta water. Return pasta mixture to pot.
2. Meanwhile, in a large skillet, heat oil over medium-high heat. Add turkey, Italian seasoning and salt; cook, breaking turkey up with a spoon, for 7 to 8 minutes or until no longer pink. Add broth and cook, stirring occasionally, for 3 minutes.
3. To the pasta mixture, add turkey mixture and the reserved pasta water, tossing to combine. Cook, stirring, over medium-low heat for 3 minutes. Serve sprinkled with cheese.

Fast Vegetable Lasagna

Makes 6 servings

✪ Great for Steps 2, 3, 4 and 5

This creamy, gooey lasagna is sure to please a crowd, not to mention your wallet. The vegetables can be varied based on what you prefer or have on hand, as can the shredded cheese.

Variation

Vegan Lasagna: Replace the ricotta cheese with 16 oz (500 g) firm tofu, well drained and mashed with a fork, then seasoned with salt and pepper. Replace the mozzarella with an equal amount of non-dairy cheese alternative.

Nutrients per serving	
Calories	419
Total fat	10 g
Saturated fat	5 g
Cholesterol	27 mg
Sodium	396 mg
Carbohydrate	53 g
Fiber	9 g
Protein	31 g
Calcium	573 mg
Iron	3.0 mg

- **Preheat oven to 350°F (180°C)**
- **13- by 9-inch (33 by 23 cm) glass baking dish, sprayed with nonstick cooking spray (preferably olive oil)**

1	jar (26 oz/700 mL) reduced-sodium marinara sauce, divided	1
12	whole wheat oven-ready lasagna noodles	12
2 cups	nonfat ricotta cheese	500 mL
4 cups	thawed frozen mixed vegetables, chopped and patted dry with paper towels	1 L
2 cups	shredded mozzarella cheese	500 mL

1. Spread $\frac{1}{2}$ cup (125 mL) of the marinara sauce in prepared baking dish. Top with 4 lasagna noodles, breaking to fit as necessary. Gently spread one-third of the ricotta over noodles, then spread with one-third of the remaining sauce. Sprinkle one-third of the vegetables over sauce, then top with one-third of the mozzarella. Repeat layers two more times, starting with noodles and ending with mozzarella. Cover dish with foil.
2. Bake in preheated oven for 35 to 40 minutes or until noodles are tender. Remove foil and bake for 5 minutes or until cheese is golden brown. Let cool for 10 minutes before cutting.

Pumpkin Mushroom Lasagna

Makes 6 servings

✪ Great for Steps 1, 2, 3, 4 and 5

Ever adaptable lasagna is excellent with pumpkin and mushrooms. If you want to make the result more complex, substitute smoked Gouda cheese for the mozzarella.

Tip

If a 15-oz (425 mL) can of pumpkin isn't available, purchase a 28-oz (796 mL) can and measure out 1¾ cups (425 mL). Refrigerate extra pumpkin in an airtight container for up to 1 week.

Nutrients per serving	
Calories	373
Total fat	10 g
Saturated fat	4 g
Cholesterol	27 mg
Sodium	514 mg
Carbohydrate	47 g
Fiber	9 g
Protein	28 g
Calcium	593 mg
Iron	2.1 mg

- **Preheat oven to 375°F (190°C)**
- **11- by 7-inch (28 by 18 cm) glass baking dish, sprayed with nonstick cooking spray (preferably olive oil)**

2 tsp	extra virgin olive oil	10 mL
1 lb	cremini or button mushrooms, trimmed and sliced	500 g
1½ cups	chopped onions	375 mL
½ tsp	fine sea salt, divided	2 mL
1	can (15 oz/425 mL) pumpkin purée (not pie filling)	1
1 cup	evaporated skim milk	250 mL
2 tsp	dried rubbed sage	10 mL
9	whole wheat oven-ready lasagna noodles	9
1½ cups	nonfat ricotta cheese	375 mL
1 cup	shredded mozzarella cheese	250 mL
6 tbsp	freshly grated Parmesan cheese	90 mL

1. In a large skillet, heat oil over medium-high heat. Add mushrooms, onions and half the salt; cook, stirring, for 7 to 10 minutes or until vegetables are tender. Remove from heat.
2. In a small bowl, combine pumpkin, milk, sage and the remaining salt.
3. Spread ½ cup (125 mL) of the pumpkin sauce in prepared baking dish. Top with 3 noodles, overlapping slightly. Add ½ cup (125 mL) pumpkin sauce, spreading to edges of baking dish. Top with half the mushroom mixture, half the ricotta, half the mozzarella and 2 tbsp (30 mL) of the Parmesan. Repeat layers once more, starting with noodles and ending with Parmesan. Top with the remaining noodles and spread the remaining sauce over top.
4. Cover and bake in preheated oven for 45 minutes. Uncover and sprinkle with the remaining Parmesan. Bake for 10 to 15 minutes or until cheese is melted. Let cool for at least 15 minutes before cutting.

Lasagna Rolls

Makes 4 servings

✪ Great for Steps 1, 2, 3, 4 and 5

I predict you'll have this so-easy recipe committed to memory in no time. Add as few or as many additional fillings as you like, such as cooked sausage, pepperoni or black olives.

Variation

Vegan Lasagna Rolls: Replace the ricotta cheese with 8 oz (250 g) firm tofu, well drained and mashed with a fork, then seasoned with salt and pepper. Replace the mozzarella with an equal amount of non-dairy cheese alternative.

Nutrients per serving	
Calories	300
Total fat	5 g
Saturated fat	2 g
Cholesterol	13 mg
Sodium	264 mg
Carbohydrate	44 g
Fiber	8 g
Protein	21 g
Calcium	324 mg
Iron	2.9 mg

- **Preheat oven to 400°F (200°C)**
- **8-inch (20 cm) square glass baking dish, sprayed with nonstick cooking spray (preferably olive oil)**

8	whole wheat lasagna noodles	8
1 cup	nonfat ricotta cheese	250 mL
1½ cups	reduced-sodium marinara sauce	375 mL
2 cups	packed baby spinach	500 mL
½ cup	shredded mozzarella cheese	125 mL

1. In a large pot of boiling salted water (see tip, page 422), cook noodles according to package directions until al dente. Drain and gently pat noodles dry with paper towels.
2. Lay noodles flat on a work surface. Spread about 2 tbsp (30 mL) ricotta, 2 tbsp (30 mL) marinara sauce and a layer of spinach over each noodle. Starting at a short end, tightly roll up noodles. Place seam side down in prepared baking dish. Pour the remaining marinara sauce over rolls and sprinkle with cheese.
3. Bake in preheated oven for 20 to 24 minutes or until cheese is browned and bubbly.

Speedy Weeknight Lo Mein

Makes 4 side-dish servings

✪ Great for Steps 2, 3, 4 and 5

Turn the kitchen into your new favorite fast-food joint with these outstanding and easy noodles.

8 oz	quinoa spaghetti pasta or multigrain spaghetti pasta	250 g
1 tsp	ground ginger	5 mL
2 tbsp	reduced-sodium tamari or soy sauce	30 mL
2 tbsp	mirin or sherry	30 mL
1 tsp	toasted sesame oil	5 mL
2 tsp	vegetable oil	10 mL
10 oz	frozen stir-fry vegetables, thawed and patted dry	300 g
½ cup	thinly sliced green onions	125 mL

1. In a large pot of boiling salted water (see tip, at left), cook pasta according to package directions until al dente. Drain, reserving ¼ cup (60 mL) pasta water.
2. In a small cup, combine ginger, tamari, mirin and sesame oil.
3. In a large skillet, heat vegetable oil over medium-high heat. Add stir-fry vegetables and cook, stirring, for 3 minutes. Stir in pasta, ginger mixture and green onions; cook, tossing gently, for about 2 minutes or until heated through. If necessary, stir in enough of the reserved pasta water to moisten.

Tip

Make sure to use fine sea salt in the water you use to cook the noodles. Conventional table salt contains chemicals and additives, whereas sea salt contains an abundance of naturally occurring trace minerals.

Variation

To make the lo mein heartier, add 1 to 1½ cups (250 to 375 mL) cooked shrimp or diced cooked chicken when adding the pasta to the vegetables.

Nutrients per serving	
Calories	333
Total fat	6 g
Saturated fat	0 g
Cholesterol	0 mg
Sodium	390 mg
Carbohydrate	62 g
Fiber	6 g
Protein	8 g
Calcium	38 mg
Iron	1.2 mg

Sesame Ginger Noodles

Makes 6 side-dish servings

✪ Great for Steps 1, 2, 3, 4 and 5

Time to tear up the takeout menu: sesame oil stars in these easy-to-make, ready-in-a-flash noodles, lending its unmistakable, mildly nutty flavor and a wallop of nutrition — think copper, magnesium and calcium — to boot.

Tip

If the pasta you're using takes less or more than 8 minutes to cook, adjust the total cooking time according to the package directions and add the vegetables for the last 2 to 3 minutes.

12 oz	multigrain or whole wheat spaghetti pasta	375 mL
2	red bell peppers, thinly sliced	2
1	bunch broccoli, cut into florets, stalks peeled and thinly sliced (about 5 cups/1.25 L florets and stalks)	1
2	cloves garlic, minced	2
2 tbsp	minced gingerroot	30 mL
1⁄4 tsp	hot pepper flakes	1 mL
1⁄4 cup	unsweetened natural peanut butter or other nut butter	60 mL
3 tbsp	brown rice syrup or liquid honey	45 mL
2 tbsp	unseasoned rice vinegar	30 mL
2 tbsp	reduced-sodium tamari or soy sauce	30 mL
1 tbsp	toasted sesame oil	15 mL
2⁄3 cup	thinly sliced green onions	150 mL

1. In a large pot of boiling salted water (see tip, page 422), cook pasta for 5 minutes. Add red peppers and broccoli; cook for 2 to 3 minutes or until pasta is al dente and vegetables are tender-crisp. Drain, reserving 1⁄4 cup (60 mL) pasta water.
2. In a large bowl, whisk together garlic, ginger, hot pepper flakes, peanut butter, brown rice syrup, vinegar, tamari and sesame oil. Add pasta mixture, tossing to coat and adding enough of the reserved pasta water to thin, as necessary. Serve at room temperature or chilled, sprinkled with green onions.

Nutrients per serving	
Calories	208
Total fat	8 g
Saturated fat	1 g
Cholesterol	0 mg
Sodium	238 mg
Carbohydrate	29 g
Fiber	5 g
Protein	7 g
Calcium	41 mg
Iron	1.7 mg

Thai Cashew Noodles

Makes 4 servings

✪ Great for Steps 1, 2, 3, 4 and 5

Treat whole-grain spaghetti to Thai curry paste, whether mild or hot, and you will be rewarded with deeply satisfying noodles, balanced by crisp vegetables and buttery cashews.

Tips

Look for roasted cashews lightly seasoned with sea salt.

Make sure to use fine sea salt in the water you use to cook the pasta. Conventional table salt contains chemicals and additives, whereas sea salt contains an abundance of naturally occurring trace minerals.

- **Food processor or blender**

8 oz	multigrain or whole wheat spaghetti pasta	250 g
1/2 cup	packed fresh cilantro leaves, divided	125 mL
1/3 cup	unsweetened natural cashew or peanut butter	75 mL
2 tbsp	freshly squeezed lime juice	30 mL
2 tbsp	Thai red curry paste	30 mL
2 tsp	brown rice syrup or liquid honey	10 mL
1/4 tsp	fine sea salt	1 mL
1 1/2 cups	mung bean sprouts	375 mL
3/4 cup	shredded carrots	175 mL
1/3 cup	thinly sliced green onions	75 mL
1/3 cup	lightly salted roasted cashews, coarsely chopped	75 mL
1	lime, quartered	1

1. In a large pot of boiling salted water (see tip, at left), cook pasta according to package directions until al dente. Drain, reserving 1/2 cup (125 mL) pasta water. Rinse pasta under cold water until cool. Drain well.
2. In food processor, combine half the cilantro, cashew butter, lime juice, curry paste, brown rice syrup and the reserved pasta water; purée until smooth.
3. In a large bowl, toss pasta, cashew sauce, bean sprouts, carrots and green onions until well coated. Serve sprinkled with cashews and the remaining cilantro, with lime quarters on the side.

Superfood Spotlight

Cashews • Cashews are considerably lower in total fat than any other nut and can be useful as a dieter's snack. Much of the fat they do contain is monounsaturated oleic acid (the type found in olive oil), which has health benefits, including protection from heart and arterial disease. Cashews are also rich in important minerals, including magnesium for strong bones and heart health, immune-boosting zinc, and iron for healthy blood and energy. Like other nuts, cashews are linked with protection from cardiovascular diseases. People who regularly eat nuts are less likely to die from these diseases than people who never eat nuts.

Nutrients per serving	
Calories	477
Total fat	18 g
Saturated fat	3 g
Cholesterol	1 mg
Sodium	308 mg
Carbohydrate	66 g
Fiber	9 g
Protein	15 g
Calcium	42 mg
Iron	3.5 mg

Chicken and Edamame Shiratake Noodles

Makes 4 servings

✪ Great for Steps 1, 3, 4 and 5

Shiratake noodles — a no-carb, super-low-calorie pasta — are increasingly available in the refrigerator section of supermarkets. They are a snap to prepare and, like any noodle, can be prepared with countless flavor combinations. Here, they stay close to their Japanese origins with chicken, edamame and tamari.

Tip

If shiratake noodles are not available, use an equal amount of multigrain or whole wheat fettuccine pasta. Cook the pasta in a large pot of boiling salted water according to package directions before adding it to the skillet in step 4.

Nutrients per serving	
Calories	396
Total fat	6 g
Saturated fat	0 g
Cholesterol	50 mg
Sodium	599 mg
Carbohydrate	53 g
Fiber	6 g
Protein	34 g
Calcium	79 mg
Iron	5.0 mg

8 oz	shiratake fettuccine noodles	250 g
4 tsp	vegetable oil, divided	20 mL
12 oz	boneless skinless chicken breasts, cut into 1-inch (2.5 cm) pieces	375 g
2	cloves garlic, thinly sliced	2
1½ cups	thinly sliced red onions	375 mL
2 cups	shredded coleslaw mix (shredded cabbage and carrots)	500 mL
1 cup	frozen shelled edamame, thawed	250 mL
3 tbsp	reduced-sodium tamari or soy sauce	45 mL
2 tsp	brown rice syrup or liquid honey	10 mL
2 tsp	unseasoned rice vinegar	10 mL

1. Drain noodles and rinse under cold water for 1 minute. Drain and set aside.
2. In a large skillet, heat half the oil over medium-high heat. Add chicken and cook, stirring, for 3 to 5 minutes or until lightly browned. Transfer to a plate.
3. In the same skillet, heat the remaining oil over medium-high heat. Add garlic and red onions; cook, stirring, for 2 minutes. Add coleslaw and edamame; cook, stirring, for 3 to 4 minutes or until softened.
4. In a small cup, combine tamari, brown rice syrup and vinegar. Add to skillet, along with noodles, chicken and any accumulated juices, gently tossing to combine. Cook, stirring, for 3 to 4 minutes or until chicken is no longer pink inside.

Teriyaki Soba, Spinach and Tofu Noodles

Makes 4 servings

✪ Great for Steps 1, 2, 3, 4 and 5

Tamari adds "meaty" flavor (umami, or the fifth flavor) to this otherwise meatless tofu-noodle dish.

Tip

To toast sesame seeds, place up to 3 tbsp (45 mL) seeds in a medium skillet set over medium heat. Cook, shaking the skillet, for 3 to 5 minutes or until seeds are golden brown and fragrant. Let cool completely before use.

Nutrients per serving	
Calories	400
Total fat	11 g
Saturated fat	2 g
Cholesterol	0 mg
Sodium	567 mg
Carbohydrate	64 g
Fiber	7 g
Protein	22 g
Calcium	82 mg
Iron	5.8 mg

8 oz	soba (buckwheat) noodles	250 g
1/3 cup	reduced-sodium tamari or soy sauce	75 mL
2 tbsp	mirin or sherry	30 mL
2 tbsp	brown rice syrup or liquid honey	30 mL
1/2 tsp	toasted sesame oil	2 mL
2 tsp	vegetable oil	10 mL
1 lb	extra-firm or firm tofu, drained and cut into 1/2-inch (1 cm) cubes	500 g
3	cloves garlic, minced	3
6 cups	packed baby spinach (about 6 oz/175 g)	1.5 L
2 tbsp	minced gingerroot	30 mL
1/2 cup	thinly sliced green onions	125 mL
2 tbsp	toasted sesame seeds (see tip, at left)	30 mL

1. In a large pot of boiling salted water (see tip, page 427), cook noodles according to package directions until al dente. Drain.
2. Meanwhile, in a small bowl, whisk together tamari, mirin, brown rice syrup and sesame oil. Set aside.
3. In a large skillet, heat vegetable oil over medium-high heat. Add tofu and cook, stirring, for 3 to 5 minutes or until golden. Add garlic, spinach and ginger; cook, stirring, for 2 to 3 minutes or until spinach is wilted.
4. Divide noodles among four deep bowls. Top each portion with tofu mixture. Drizzle with tamari mixture and sprinkle with green onions and sesame seeds.

Soba with Chicken in Green Tea Broth

Makes 4 servings

✪ Great for Steps 1, 3, 4 and 5

It's been decades since pasta was considered exotic; now it's considered comfort food first and foremost. These soba noodles, infused with green tea and ginger and made dinner-worthy by the addition of chicken, maintain their homey pasta provenance, but with a Japanese twist.

Tip

Make sure to use fine sea salt in the water you use to cook the noodles. Conventional table salt contains chemicals and additives, whereas sea salt contains an abundance of naturally occurring trace minerals.

2 tbsp	minced gingerroot	30 mL
3 tbsp	reduced-sodium tamari or soy sauce	45 mL
2 tbsp	mirin or sherry	30 mL
1 tsp	toasted sesame oil	5 mL
8 oz	boneless skinless chicken breasts, cut into thin strips	250 g
8 oz	soba (buckwheat) noodles	250 g
3 cups	brewed green tea	750 mL
8 oz	snow peas, strings removed, cut lengthwise into julienne strips	250 g
2 tsp	unseasoned rice vinegar	10 mL
1/4 cup	thinly sliced green onions	60 mL

1. In a medium bowl, whisk together ginger, tamari, mirin and sesame oil. Add chicken and toss to coat. Let stand for 10 minutes.
2. Meanwhile, in a large pot of boiling salted water (see tip, at left), cook noodles according to package directions until al dente. Drain and divide among four deep bowls.
3. In the same pot, bring tea to a simmer over medium heat. Add chicken mixture and snow peas; simmer, stirring occasionally, for 3 to 4 minutes or until chicken is no longer pink inside. Stir in vinegar.
4. Spoon chicken mixture over noodles and sprinkle with green onions.

▸ Health Note

Green tea is chock full of catechin polyphenols, powerful antioxidants that are beneficial in lowering cholesterol and the risk of several cancers.

Nutrients per serving	
Calories	431
Total fat	4 g
Saturated fat	0 g
Cholesterol	33 mg
Sodium	532 mg
Carbohydrate	71 g
Fiber	5 g
Protein	25 g
Calcium	30 mg
Iron	4.5 mg

Buckwheat Noodle Bowls with Beef and Snap Peas

Makes 4 servings

✪ Great for Steps 1, 3, 4 and 5

Roast beef from the deli counter, coupled with hearty buckwheat noodles, makes these Japanese-inspired noodle bowls hearty and satisfying, in spite of their turbo assembly.

Tip

Make sure to use fine sea salt in the water you use to cook the noodles. Conventional table salt contains chemicals and additives, whereas sea salt contains an abundance of naturally occurring trace minerals.

8 oz	soba (buckwheat) noodles	250 g
2 tsp	vegetable oil	10 mL
12 oz	sugar snap peas, strings removed	375 g
1 cup	thinly sliced green onions, white and green parts separated	250 mL
1 tbsp	minced gingerroot	15 mL
1⁄4 tsp	hot pepper flakes	1 mL
2 tsp	cornstarch	10 mL
3 tbsp	reduced-sodium tamari or soy sauce	45 mL
1 tbsp	brown rice syrup or liquid honey	15 mL
2 tsp	unseasoned rice vinegar	10 mL
8 oz	thinly sliced lean deli roast beef, cut crosswise into 1⁄2-inch (1 cm) strips	250 g

1. In a large pot of boiling salted water (see tip, at left), cook noodles according to package directions until al dente. Drain, reserving 1⁄3 cup (75 mL) noodle water.
2. In a large skillet, heat oil over medium-high heat. Add peas, white parts of green onions, ginger and hot pepper flakes; cook, stirring, for 1 minute. Add the reserved noodle water and cook, stirring, for 1 to 2 minutes or until peas turn bright green.
3. In a small bowl, whisk together cornstarch, tamari, brown rice syrup and vinegar.
4. Reduce heat to medium and add cornstarch mixture to skillet. Bring to a simmer, stirring constantly. Add noodles and beef, gently tossing to combine. Simmer for 1 minute or until heated through. Serve sprinkled with green parts of green onions.

Nutrients per serving	
Calories	376
Total fat	7 g
Saturated fat	1 g
Cholesterol	31 mg
Sodium	554 mg
Carbohydrate	59 g
Fiber	6 g
Protein	26 g
Calcium	43 mg
Iron	6.5 mg

Soba with Shrimp, Lime and Cilantro

Makes 4 servings

✪ Great for Steps 1, 3, 4 and 5

A bowl of these noodles — fresh and vibrant with bright notes of citrus and herbs — is surprisingly hearty thanks to the protein-rich shrimp and the whole-grain goodness of the buckwheat noodles.

8 oz	soba (buckwheat) noodles	250 g
1 tbsp	vegetable oil	15 mL
12 oz	medium shrimp, peeled and deveined	375 g
2 tsp	Asian chile-garlic sauce	10 mL
1 tsp	finely grated lime zest	5 mL
2 tbsp	freshly squeezed lime juice	30 mL
1/4 cup	reduced-sodium tamari or soy sauce	60 mL
2 tsp	liquid honey or brown rice syrup	10 mL
1/2 cup	thinly sliced green onions	125 mL
1/3 cup	packed fresh cilantro leaves, chopped	75 mL

1. In a large pot of boiling salted water (see tip, page 428), cook noodles according to package directions until al dente. Drain.
2. Meanwhile, in a large skillet, heat oil over medium-high heat. Add shrimp and chile-garlic sauce; cook, stirring, for 2 to 3 minutes or until shrimp are pink, firm and opaque. Add lime zest and lime juice; cook, stirring, for 30 seconds.
3. In a medium bowl, combine tamari and honey. Add noodles and toss to coat.
4. Divide noodles among four deep bowls. Top with shrimp mixture, green onions and cilantro.

Nutrients per serving	
Calories	375
Total fat	6 g
Saturated fat	1 g
Cholesterol	143 mg
Sodium	519 mg
Carbohydrate	49 g
Fiber	4 g
Protein	29 g
Calcium	53 mg
Iron	4.9 mg

Soba with Shrimp and Baby Bok Choy

Makes 4 servings

✪ Great for Steps 1, 3, 4 and 5

Asian chile-garlic sauce brings pungent notes to this dish, tempered by cool, crisp baby bok choy and salty-sweet shrimp.

Tip

To make the shrimp seem more abundant, halve them lengthwise before cooking.

8 oz	soba (buckwheat) noodles	250 g
2 tsp	vegetable oil	10 mL
8 oz	medium shrimp, peeled and deveined	250 g
1/2 cup	thinly sliced green onions	125 mL
1 tbsp	minced gingerroot	15 mL
1 tsp	Asian chile-garlic sauce	5 mL
12 oz	baby bok choy, trimmed and cut crosswise into 1/2-inch (1 cm) slices	375 g
1 tbsp	water	15 mL
1/4 cup	hoisin sauce	60 mL

1. In a large pot of boiling salted water (see tip, page 431), cook noodles according to package directions until al dente. Drain, reserving 1/4 cup (60 mL) noodle water.
2. In a large skillet, heat oil over medium-high heat. Add shrimp, green onions, ginger and chile-garlic sauce; cook, stirring, for 2 to 3 minutes or until shrimp are pink, firm and opaque. Add bok choy and water; cover and cook for 1 to 2 minutes or until bok choy is wilted. Transfer to a plate.
3. Add noodles, hoisin sauce and the reserved noodle water to the skillet; cook, stirring to coat, for 30 seconds.
4. Divide noodles among four deep bowls. Top with shrimp mixture.

Nutrients per serving	
Calories	356
Total fat	5 g
Saturated fat	1 g
Cholesterol	96 mg
Sodium	546 mg
Carbohydrate	53 g
Fiber	5 g
Protein	24 g
Calcium	123 mg
Iron	5.0 mg

Red Curry Shrimp Noodle Bowls

Makes 4 servings

✪ Great for Steps 1, 3, 4 and 5

Shrimp, lime, coconut milk and curry paste coalesce in a complex-tasting pasta dish that's easily achieved with supermarket-ready ingredients.

Tip

Make sure to use fine sea salt in the water you use to cook the noodles. Conventional table salt contains chemicals and additives, whereas sea salt contains an abundance of naturally occurring trace minerals.

3/4 cup	light coconut milk	175 mL
3/4 cup	reduced-sodium ready-to-use chicken or vegetable broth	175 mL
3 tbsp	Thai red curry paste	45 mL
2 tsp	brown rice syrup or liquid honey	10 mL
8 oz	soba (buckwheat) noodles	250 g
12 oz	medium shrimp, peeled and deveined	375 g
1 tbsp	freshly squeezed lime juice	15 mL
2 tsp	fish sauce (nam pla)	10 mL
1 cup	mung bean sprouts (optional)	250 mL
1 cup	packed fresh cilantro leaves, chopped	250 mL

1. In a large pot, whisk together coconut milk, broth, curry paste and brown rice syrup. Bring to a simmer over medium heat. Reduce heat and simmer, stirring occasionally, for 7 to 8 minutes or until slightly thickened.
2. Meanwhile, in a large pot of boiling salted water (see tip, at left), cook noodles according to package directions until al dente. Drain.
3. Add shrimp to curry sauce and simmer, stirring occasionally, for 2 to 3 minutes or until pink, firm and opaque. Remove from heat and stir in lime juice and fish sauce.
4. Divide noodles among four deep bowls. Top with shrimp mixture, bean sprouts (if using) and cilantro.

Nutrients per serving	
Calories	385
Total fat	7 g
Saturated fat	4 g
Cholesterol	144 mg
Sodium	477 mg
Carbohydrate	50 g
Fiber	4 g
Protein	28 g
Calcium	57 mg
Iron	4.9 mg

Side Dishes

Roasting Vegetables 434
Cooking Legumes 436
Cooking Whole Grains 438
Asparagus with Tangerine Gremolata 440
Braised Baby Bok Choy 440
Healthy Know-How: Clean Eating 441
Steamed Broccoli with Tahini Miso Dressing 441
Skillet Brussels Sprouts with Toasted Pecans 442
Glazed Carrots with Mint 443
Garlicky Cauliflower Purée 443
Broiled Eggplant with Garlic Yogurt and Mint 444
Steamed Ginger Garlic Green Beans 445
Stir-Fried Mushrooms with Lemon and Parsley 445
Balsamic Roasted Red Onions 446
Sautéed Cherry Tomatoes 446
Collard Green Ribbons 447
Quick Sautéed Kale 448

Wilted Spinach with Garlic 448
Sautéed Swiss Chard 449
Roasted Oven Fries 450
Baked Parsnip Fries 451
Sweet Potato Fries. 451
Mashed Sweet Potatoes with Rosemary 452
Lima Bean Purée 452
Edamame Succotash 453
White Beans and Spinach 454
Cumin-Scented Black Beans and Quinoa 455
Jamaican Rice and Peas 456
Basic Brown Rice Pilaf 456
Spelt and Wild Mushroom Pilaf. 457
Bulgur Pilaf with Apricots and Coriander 458
Creamy Millet Polenta with Cheese and Chives 458
Kasha with Summer Vegetables 459

Roasting Vegetables

Five Tips for Perfectly Roasted Vegetables

1. **Roast in a very hot oven (450°F/230°C).** Vegetables cook quickly — many take only 15 to 20 minutes — but still have a chance to brown nicely on the outside by the time they become tender inside.
2. **Cut evenly.** It's very important to cut the vegetables into pieces of about the same size. Unevenly sized pieces won't roast and brown in the same amount of time, and you'll end up with both over-roasted and under-roasted vegetables.
3. **Line the pan.** To prevent sticking, line a large rimmed baking sheet or roasting pan with foil; otherwise, when you have to pry stuck vegetables off the baking sheet, all of the delicious caramelization gets left behind on the pan.
4. **Spread in a single layer, with lots of room.** Spread the vegetables in a single layer so that they are not touching. If they're crowded in the pan, they will steam (think pale and limp) rather than roast.
5. **Gently toss halfway through roasting.** For even browning, use a pancake turner or spatula to gently toss or turn the vegetables over halfway through the roasting time.

Vegetable	Amount	Preparation	Roasting Time at 450°F (230°C)
Asparagus	2 lbs (1 kg)	Trimmed	10 to 15 minutes
Beets, tops trimmed off	2 lbs (1 kg), about 6 medium	Whole, unpeeled, pricked with a fork, then peeled after roasting	1 hour
Bell peppers	2 lbs (1 kg)	1-inch (2.5 cm) wide strips	25 to 30 minutes
Broccoli	2 lbs (1 kg)	Stems trimmed, peeled and sliced into 1⁄4-inch (0.5 cm) rounds; florets split into 1 1⁄2-inch (4 cm) pieces	12 to 15 minutes
Brussels sprouts	2 lbs (1 kg)	Trimmed and quartered lengthwise	20 to 25 minutes
Butternut squash	2 lbs (1 kg)	Peeled and cut into 1-inch (2.5 cm) pieces	20 to 25 minutes
Carrots	2 lbs (1 kg)	Cut into 1-inch (2.5 cm) pieces	30 to 40 minutes
Cauliflower	1 1⁄2 lbs (750 g), about 1 medium	Cut into 1 1⁄2-inch (4 cm) florets	20 to 30 minutes

Vegetable	Amount	Preparation	Roasting Time at 450°F (230°C)
Eggplant	2 lbs (1 kg), about 2 medium	Cut into ½-inch (1 cm) thick slices	20 to 25 minutes
Fennel	2 lbs (1 kg), about 2 large bulbs	Trimmed and each bulb cut into 12 wedges	35 to 40 minutes
Green beans	2 lbs (1 kg)	Trimmed	20 to 30 minutes
Onions	2 lbs (1 kg), about 3 medium-large	Each onion cut into 12 wedges	20 to 30 minutes
Potatoes	2 lbs (1 kg)	Peeled and cut into 1½-inch (4 cm) pieces	35 to 40 minutes
Sweet potatoes	2 lbs (1 kg)	Peeled and cut into 1½-inch (4 cm) pieces	30 to 35 minutes
Turnips	2 lbs (1 kg), about 6 or 7 medium	Peeled and each cut into 6 wedges	45 to 50 minutes
Zucchini	2 lbs (1 kg)	Trimmed and cut in half crosswise, then each half quartered	15 to 20 minutes

Cooking Legumes

Legumes — beans, peas and lentils — are fundamental to myriad cuisines around the world, and for good reason. In addition to being delicious, versatile and inexpensive, they are nutrient powerhouses, packed with protein, vitamins and minerals, while simultaneously being low in fat and high in fiber. What more could you ask for in a healthy food?

Legume (1 cup/250 mL dry)	Water	Cooking Time	Yield
Adzuki (aduki) beans	4 cups (1 L)	45 to 55 minutes	3 cups (750 mL)
Anasazi beans	3 cups (750 mL)	45 to 55 minutes	2¼ cups (550 mL)
Black beans	4 cups (1 L)	65 to 75 minutes	2¼ cups (550 mL)
Black-eyed peas	3 cups (750 mL)	1 hour	2 cups (500 mL)
Cannellini (white kidney) beans	3 cups (750 mL)	45 minutes	2½ cups (625 mL)
Chickpeas (garbanzo beans)	4 cups (1 L)	1 to 2 hours	2 cups (500 mL)
Cranberry beans	3 cups (750 mL)	45 minutes	3 cups (750 mL)
Fava beans, skins removed	3 cups (750 mL)	40 to 50 minutes	1⅔ cups (400 mL)
Great Northern beans	3½ cups (875 mL)	1½ hours	2⅔ cups (650 mL)
Green peas, whole	6 cups (1.5 L)	1 to 2 hours	2 cups (500 mL)
Kidney beans	3 cups (750 mL)	1 hour	2¼ cups (550 mL)
Lentils, brown	2¼ cups (550 mL)	45 to 55 minutes	2¼ cups (550 mL)
Lentils, green	2 cups (500 mL)	30 to 45 minutes	2 cups (500 mL)
Lentils, red	3 cups (750 mL)	20 to 30 minutes	2½ cups (625 mL)
Lima beans, large	4 cups (1 L)	45 to 55 minutes	2 cups (500 mL)
Lima beans, small	4 cups (1 L)	50 to 60 minutes	3 cups (750 mL)
Lima beans, Christmas	4 cups (1 L)	1 hour	2 cups (500 mL)
Mung beans	2½ cups (625 mL)	1 hour	2 cups (500 mL)
Navy (white pea) beans	3 cups (750 mL)	45 to 60 minutes	2⅔ cups (650 mL)
Pink beans	3 cups (750 mL)	50 to 60 minutes	2¾ cups (675 mL)
Pinto beans	3 cups (750 mL)	1½ hours	2⅔ cups (650 mL)

Legume (1 cup/250 mL dry)	Water	Cooking Time	Yield
Soybeans	4 cups (1 L)	3 to 4 hours	3 cups (750 mL)
Split peas, green	4 cups (1 L)	45 minutes	2 cups (500 mL)
Split peas, yellow	4 cups (1 L)	1 to 1½ hours	2 cups (500 mL)

Cooking Directions

1. Rinse legumes under cold water. Discard any legumes that are discolored or badly formed, as well as any debris such as small rocks.
2. Place legumes in a large pot or bowl and fill with enough water to cover by about 3 inches (7.5 cm). Cover and let soak at room temperature for at least 8 hours or overnight. (Note: lentils and split peas do not require soaking; proceed from step 1 to step 4.)
3. Drain beans. Discard the soaking water and cook the beans in fresh water.
4. Return drained beans to pot and add the specified amount of water. Bring to a boil over high heat; reduce heat and boil gently, uncovered, for the specified cooking time, starting the timer once the water reaches a boil.

Quick-Soak Method

When presoaking legumes is not an option, wash and pick over legumes, then place them in a large pot and fill with enough water to cover by about 3 inches (7.5 cm). Bring to a boil and boil for 10 minutes (this will help remove toxins). Turn off heat, cover and let soak for 1 hour. Drain, discarding soaking water, then cook beans as directed above.

Tips

- Adding salt or acidic ingredients to the pot early in the cooking process can make legumes cook more slowly. For the best results, add any salt or acidic ingredients during the last 3 to 5 minutes of cooking time.
- Beans have a reputation for being somewhat difficult on the system, but some herbs and spices can make them easier to digest. Try adding bay leaf, cumin, winter or summer savory, or fresh epazote (available in Hispanic markets) during the cooking process. Alternatively, consider an East Indian tradition: chew on dried fennel seeds or drink a cup of fennel tea at the end of a legume meal to aid digestion.

Cooking Whole Grains

Whole grains make a perfect side dish, any time, any season. Convenient, inexpensive and incredibly delicious, they are rich in carbohydrates, the body's main fuel supply, as well as vitamins, minerals, fiber, antioxidants and phytonutrients. Add dried or fresh herbs, spices, nuts, seeds, cheeses or vegetables — the possibilities are almost endless.

But don't think of whole grains as merely side-dish fare. They are terrific for main dishes, too, as a satisfying foundation for meatless main dishes or to stretch a small amount of meat, fish or poultry. And when it comes to breakfast, options abound. Prepare any of the grains the night before, let cool, cover and refrigerate, then warm the next morning for an oh-so-satisfying breakfast in minutes. Top with the milk of your choice, yogurt, fresh fruit or a drizzle of maple syrup.

Grain (1 cup/250 mL dry)	Water	Cooking Time	Yield
Amaranth	2½ cups (625 mL)	20 to 25 minutes	2½ cups (625 mL)
Barley, pearl	3 cups (750 mL)	50 to 60 minutes	3½ cups (875 mL)
Buckwheat groats	2 cups (500 mL)	15 minutes	2½ cups (625 mL)
Bulgur	2 cups (250 mL)	15 minutes	2½ cups (625 mL)
Cornmeal, fine-grind	4¼ cups (1.05 L)	8 to 10 minutes	2½ cups (625 mL)
Cornmeal, polenta, coarse	4½ cups (1.125 L)	20 to 25 minutes	2½ cups (625 mL)
Farro	5 cups (1.25 L)	25 to 30 minutes	3 cups (750 mL)
Millet	3½ cups (875 mL)	20 to 25 minutes	3½ cups (875 mL)
Oat groats	3 cups (750 mL)	30 to 40 minutes	3½ cups (875 mL)
Quinoa	2 cups (500 mL)	15 to 20 minutes	2¾ cups (675 mL)
Rice, brown basmati	2½ cups (625 mL)	35 to 40 minutes	3 cups (750 mL)
Rice, long-grain brown	2½ cups (625 mL)	45 to 55 minutes	3 cups (750 mL)
Rice, short-grain brown	2⅓ cups (575 mL)	45 to 55 minutes	3 cups (750 mL)
Rye berries	4 cups (1 L)	1 hour	3 cups (750 mL)
Spelt	3½ cups (875 mL)	40 to 50 minutes	2½ cups (625 mL)
Teff	3 cups (750 mL)	15 to 20 minutes	3½ cups (875 mL)

Grain (1 cup/250 mL dry)	Water	Cooking Time	Yield
Triticale	3 cups (750 mL)	40 to 45 minutes	2½ cups (625 mL)
Wheat, cracked	2 cups (500 mL)	20 to 25 minutes	2¼ cups (550 mL)
Wheat berries	3 cups (750 mL)	60 to 75 minutes	2½ cups (625 mL)
Wild rice	3 cups (750 mL)	50 to 60 minutes	4 cups (1 L)

Cooking Directions

1. Combine grains and water in a medium saucepan. If desired, add ½ tsp (2 mL) fine sea salt. Cover and bring to a boil over high heat. Reduce heat and simmer for the specified cooking time.
2. Remove the lid and test the grains for tenderness. If more cooking is needed, cover and cook for 5 to 10 minutes, adding up to ¼ cup (60 mL) water if all the liquid has been absorbed.
3. Remove from heat and let stand, covered, for 5 minutes, then fluff with a fork.

Exceptions

- **Buckwheat groats:** Prepare as directed, but bring water to a boil before adding the groats. Return to a boil. Reduce heat and simmer for the specified cooking time.
- **Bulgur:** Bulgur can also be soaked, rather than cooked, for use in salads and other preparations. Place bulgur in a large bowl and cover with an equal amount of boiling water. Let stand for about 30 minutes or until water is absorbed. Fluff bulgur with a fork.
- **Farro:** Prepare as directed, but drain the excess water when farro is tender. Use immediately (no need to let stand).

Asparagus with Tangerine Gremolata

Makes 4 servings

✪ Great for Steps 1, 2 and 4

Nutrients per serving	
Calories	50
Total fat	2 g
Saturated fat	0 g
Cholesterol	0 mg
Sodium	251 mg
Carbohydrate	6 g
Fiber	3 g
Protein	3 g
Calcium	30 mg
Iron	0.5 mg

- **Steamer basket**

1 lb	asparagus, trimmed	500 g
2 tsp	extra virgin olive oil	10 mL
1	clove garlic, minced	1
2 tsp	finely grated tangerine zest	10 mL
½ tsp	fine sea salt	2 mL
2 tbsp	freshly squeezed tangerine juice	30 mL
1 tbsp	minced fresh flat-leaf (Italian) parsley	15 mL

1. Place asparagus in a steamer basket set over a large pot of boiling water. Cover and steam for 3 to 5 minutes or until tender. Remove with tongs and pat dry with paper towels.
2. In a large skillet, heat oil over medium-high heat. Add garlic and tangerine zest; cook, stirring, for 30 seconds. Add asparagus and toss to coat. Sprinkle with salt and drizzle with tangerine juice; cook, stirring, for 2 to 3 minutes or until asparagus is heated through. Serve sprinkled with parsley.

Braised Baby Bok Choy

Makes 4 servings

✪ Great for Steps 1, 2 and 4

Nutrients per serving	
Calories	40
Total fat	2 g
Saturated fat	0 g
Cholesterol	0 mg
Sodium	160 mg
Carbohydrate	5 g
Fiber	2 g
Protein	3 g
Calcium	184 mg
Iron	1.5 mg

2	cloves garlic, minced	2
⅛ tsp	hot pepper flakes	0.5 mL
1½ cups	reduced-sodium ready-to-use vegetable or chicken broth	375 mL
1½ lbs	baby bok choy, trimmed	750 g
¼ tsp	freshly ground black pepper	1 mL
1 tsp	toasted sesame oil	5 mL

1. In a large skillet, combine garlic, hot pepper flakes and broth. Bring to a simmer over medium-high heat. Arrange bok choy evenly in skillet. Reduce heat to medium-low, cover and simmer for about 5 minutes or until tender. Using tongs, transfer bok choy to a serving dish, cover and keep warm.
2. Increase heat to medium-high and boil broth mixture until reduced to about ¼ cup (60 mL), then stir in black pepper and sesame oil. Pour over bok choy.

Healthy Know-How

Clean Eating

In essence, clean eating means giving the body proper nutrition with healthy foods, and minimizing or eliminating processed foods. It involves consuming food in its most natural form (think whole foods). Those who eat clean usually follow a few simple principles:

- Avoid processed foods, especially those containing white flour and sugar.
- Avoid trans fat.
- Avoid soft drinks and juices that are high in sugar.
- Eat mini-meals every 3 to 4 hours and practice portion control.
- Consume plenty of fresh fruits and vegetables.
- Eat lean cuts of meat.

Steamed Broccoli with Tahini Miso Dressing

Makes 6 servings

✪ Great for Steps 1, 2 and 4

This easy side dish is as packed with nutrition as it is flavor.

Tip

This simple miso dressing can be used as a multi-purpose salad and vegetable dressing.

Nutrients per serving	
Calories	85
Total fat	5 g
Saturated fat	1 g
Cholesterol	0 mg
Sodium	160 mg
Carbohydrate	9 g
Fiber	4 g
Protein	5 g
Calcium	72 mg
Iron	1.5 mg

- Steamer basket

1½ lbs	broccoli (about 1 large bunch), tough stems trimmed off	750 g
1	clove garlic, minced	1
3 tbsp	tahini	45 mL
2 tbsp	water	30 mL
1 tbsp	yellow or white miso	15 mL
1 tsp	freshly squeezed lemon juice or unseasoned rice vinegar	5 mL

1. Cut broccoli into small florets. Use a vegetable peeler to peel the stem, then cut the stem crosswise into ¼-inch (0.5 cm) wide slices. Place in a steamer basket set over a large pot of boiling water. Cover and steam for 5 to 7 minutes or until tender. Transfer to a serving dish.
2. In a small bowl, whisk together garlic, tahini, water, miso and lemon juice. Drizzle over broccoli.

▸ Health Note

Broccoli is chock full of beta carotene — a powerful antioxidant that the body converts to vitamin A — and miso is a very good source of vitamin B_{12}.

Skillet Brussels Sprouts with Toasted Pecans

Makes 6 servings

✪ Great for Steps 1, 2 and 4

Miniature royalty of the cruciferous clan, Brussels sprouts strut their stuff in this modern, pecan-flecked side dish. Crunchy and slightly sweet when cooked quickly, the sprouts are an important part of the vegetable defense against cancer. They are also rich in calcium, folate and fiber.

Tip

When selecting Brussels sprouts, pick bright green, evenly shaped, firm bulbs that feel heavy for their size. Avoid sprouts that feel puffy or somewhat spongy, and any with black spotting or yellow leaves. Choosing sprouts that are similar in size will help them to cook evenly.

Nutrients per serving	
Calories	87
Total fat	5 g
Saturated fat	1 g
Cholesterol	0 mg
Sodium	148 mg
Carbohydrate	15 g
Fiber	5 g
Protein	4 g
Calcium	56 mg
Iron	1.9 mg

1½ lbs	Brussels sprouts	750 g
¼ tsp	fine sea salt	1 mL
⅛ tsp	freshly ground black pepper	0.5 mL
2 tbsp	freshly squeezed lemon juice	30 mL
2 tsp	liquid honey or agave nectar	10 mL
1 tbsp	extra virgin olive oil	15 mL
1	large shallot, thinly sliced	1
¼ cup	chopped toasted pecans	60 mL

1. Trim ends off Brussels sprouts, then separate the leaves from the cores and discard the cores.
2. In a small bowl, whisk together salt, pepper, lemon juice and honey. Set aside.
3. In a large skillet, heat oil over medium-high heat. Add shallot and cook, stirring, for 30 seconds. Add Brussels sprout leaves and cook, stirring, for 3 to 4 minutes or until softened but still bright green. Serve drizzled with dressing and sprinkled with pecans.

Glazed Carrots with Mint

Makes 6 servings

✪ Great for Steps 1, 2 and 4

Variation

Substitute parsnips for the carrots.

Nutrients per serving

Calories	78
Total fat	2 g
Saturated fat	1 g
Cholesterol	5 mg
Sodium	217 mg
Carbohydrate	15 g
Fiber	3 g
Protein	1 g
Calcium	37 mg
Iron	0.4 mg

1/2 cup	reduced-sodium ready-to-use vegetable or chicken broth	125 mL
1/2 cup	water	125 mL
1 1/2 tbsp	liquid honey	22 mL
1 tbsp	unsalted butter	15 mL
1/2 tsp	fine sea salt	2 mL
1 1/4 lbs	carrots, cut into 1/4-inch (0.5 cm) thick slices (about 8 medium)	625 g
1 tbsp	chopped fresh mint	15 mL
1 tsp	freshly squeezed lemon juice	5 mL

1. In a large skillet, combine broth, water, honey, butter and salt. Bring to a boil over medium-high heat, stirring occasionally. Add carrots, reduce heat to medium, cover and boil gently for 4 to 5 minutes or until just tender. Using a slotted spoon, transfer carrots to a dish.
2. Increase heat to medium-high and return cooking liquid to a boil. Boil until reduced to a glaze (about 2 tbsp/30 mL). Return carrots to the pan, reduce heat and simmer, stirring, until heated through and coated with glaze. Stir in mint and lemon juice.

Garlicky Cauliflower Purée

Makes 6 servings

✪ Great for Steps 1, 2 and 4

Nutrients per serving

Calories	44
Total fat	3 g
Saturated fat	0 g
Cholesterol	0 mg
Sodium	157 mg
Carbohydrate	5 g
Fiber	2 g
Protein	2 g
Calcium	23 mg
Iron	0.4 mg

- **Steamer basket**
- **Food processor**

4	cloves garlic	4
1	head cauliflower (2 to 2 1/2 lbs/1 to 1.25 kg), broken into florets	1
1/4 tsp	fine sea salt	1 mL
1/8 tsp	freshly ground black pepper	0.5 mL
3/4 cup	reduced-sodium ready-to-use vegetable or chicken broth	175 mL
1 tbsp	extra virgin olive oil	15 mL

1. Place garlic and cauliflower in a steamer basket set over a large pot of boiling water. Cover and steam for 7 to 9 minutes or until cauliflower is tender. Reserve steaming water.
2. In food processor, combine half the cauliflower mixture, salt, pepper, broth and oil; purée until smooth. Add the remaining cauliflower mixture and purée until smooth, adding a bit of the steaming water as needed to moisten.

Broiled Eggplant with Garlic Yogurt and Mint

Makes 6 servings

✪ Great for Steps 1, 2, 3 and 4

Eggplant broiled until it's luxuriously tender and slightly sweet from caramelization finds great flavor contrast with a simple sauce made with tangy yogurt, pungent garlic and fresh mint.

- **Preheat broiler, with rack set 4 to 6 inches (10 to 15 cm) from heat source**
- **Broiler pan, sprayed with nonstick cooking spray (preferably olive oil)**

2	eggplants (each about 1 lb/500 g), cut crosswise into 3⁄4-inch (2 cm) slices	2
	Nonstick cooking spray (preferably olive oil)	
1⁄2 tsp	fine sea salt, divided	2 mL
1	clove garlic, mashed (see tip, page 121)	1
1⁄2 cup	nonfat plain Greek yogurt	125 mL
2 tsp	freshly squeezed lemon juice	10 mL
1⁄4 cup	packed fresh mint leaves, chopped	60 mL

1. Place eggplant on prepared pan and spray generously with cooking spray. Sprinkle with half the salt. Broil for 15 to 20 minutes, turning occasionally, until very soft.
2. Meanwhile, in a small bowl, combine garlic, the remaining salt, yogurt and lemon juice.
3. Serve eggplant topped with garlic yogurt and sprinkled with mint.

Superfood Spotlight

Eggplant • Eggplant is a very good source of potassium and vitamins B_1 and B_6, and a good source of folic acid, magnesium, copper, manganese and niacin. Low in calories and an excellent source of dietary fiber, eggplant may also help lower cholesterol levels. Recently, researchers have discovered that eggplant skin contains an anthocyanin flavonoid called nasunin, which is a potent antioxidant and free-radical scavenger that protects cell membranes from damage. Nasunin also helps move excess iron out of the body.

Nutrients per serving

Calories	56
Total fat	0 g
Saturated fat	0 g
Cholesterol	0 mg
Sodium	245 mg
Carbohydrate	12 g
Fiber	6 g
Protein	4 g
Calcium	33 mg
Iron	0.5 mg

Steamed Ginger Garlic Green Beans

Makes 4 servings

✪ Great for Steps 1, 2 and 4

Nutrients per serving	
Calories	54
Total fat	2 g
Saturated fat	0 g
Cholesterol	0 mg
Sodium	203 mg
Carbohydrate	7 g
Fiber	3 g
Protein	3 g
Calcium	13 mg
Iron	0.4 mg

- **Steamer basket**

1 lb	green beans, trimmed	500 g
	Ice water	
3	cloves garlic, mashed (see tip, page 121)	3
1 tbsp	grated gingerroot	15 mL
2 tbsp	reduced-sodium tamari or soy sauce	30 mL
2 tsp	unseasoned rice vinegar	10 mL
1 tsp	toasted sesame oil	5 mL
1 tbsp	toasted sesame seeds (see tip, page 426)	15 mL

1. Place green beans in a steamer basket set over a large pot of boiling water. Cover and steam for 6 to 7 minutes or until tender. Transfer to a large bowl of ice water to stop the cooking. Drain and pat dry with paper towels.
2. In a medium bowl, whisk together garlic, ginger, tamari, vinegar and oil. Add beans and toss to coat. Serve sprinkled with sesame seeds.

Stir-Fried Mushrooms with Lemon and Parsley

Makes 4 servings

✪ Great for Steps 1, 2 and 4

Nutrients per serving	
Calories	68
Total fat	4 g
Saturated fat	1 g
Cholesterol	0 mg
Sodium	77 mg
Carbohydrate	8 g
Fiber	1 g
Protein	3 g
Calcium	31 mg
Iron	0.9 mg

1 tbsp	freshly squeezed lemon juice	15 mL
$1\frac{1}{2}$ tsp	reduced-sodium tamari or soy sauce	7 mL
1 tsp	liquid honey	5 mL
1 tbsp	extra virgin olive oil	15 mL
1 lb	cremini or button mushrooms, quartered	500 g
1	clove garlic, minced	1
$\frac{1}{3}$ cup	packed fresh flat-leaf (Italian) parsley leaves, chopped	75 mL

1. In a small bowl or cup, combine lemon juice, tamari and honey.
2. In a large skillet, heat oil over medium-high heat. Add mushrooms and cook, stirring, for 5 to 6 minutes or until golden brown. Add lemon juice mixture and garlic; cook, stirring, until sauce is absorbed. Serve sprinkled with parsley.

Balsamic Roasted Red Onions

Makes 6 servings

✪ Great for Steps 1, 2 and 4

Here, red onions move from the bench to the starting lineup in great style.

- **Preheat oven to 500°F (260°C)**
- **Large rimmed baking sheet, lined with foil and sprayed with nonstick cooking spray**

2 lbs	red onions, cut into narrow wedges	1 kg
1/4 tsp	fine sea salt	1 mL
1/4 tsp	freshly cracked black pepper	1 mL
2 tsp	extra virgin olive oil	10 mL
1 tbsp	unsalted butter	15 mL
1 1/2 tbsp	liquid honey or pure maple syrup	22 mL
3 tbsp	balsamic vinegar	45 mL
1 tbsp	chopped fresh flat-leaf (Italian) parsley	15 mL

1. In a large bowl, combine onions, salt, pepper and oil, tossing to coat. Spread in a single layer on prepared baking sheet. Roast in preheated oven for 40 to 45 minutes, turning two or three times, until onions are browned and tender.
2. Meanwhile, in a small skillet, melt butter over medium-high heat. Stir in honey. Remove pan from heat and stir in vinegar. Return to medium heat and bring to a simmer. Simmer for 1 to 2 minutes or until slightly thickened.
3. Arrange onions on a plate or platter. Drizzle glaze over top and sprinkle with parsley.

Nutrients per serving	
Calories	90
Total fat	3 g
Saturated fat	1 g
Cholesterol	5 mg
Sodium	103 mg
Carbohydrate	20 g
Fiber	3 g
Protein	2 g
Calcium	38 mg
Iron	0.4 mg

Sautéed Cherry Tomatoes

Makes 4 servings

✪ Great for Steps 1, 2 and 4

2 tsp	extra virgin olive oil	10 mL
2 cups	cherry or grape tomatoes	500 mL
1/8 tsp	fine sea salt	0.5 mL
1/8 tsp	freshly ground black pepper	0.5 mL
1 tbsp	finely chopped fresh flat-leaf (Italian) parsley, mint or cilantro	15 mL

1. In a large skillet, heat oil over medium-high heat. Add tomatoes, salt and pepper; cook, stirring, for 4 to 5 minutes or until skins begin to split. Serve sprinkled with parsley.

Nutrients per serving	
Calories	34
Total fat	3 g
Saturated fat	0 g
Cholesterol	0 mg
Sodium	76 mg
Carbohydrate	3 g
Fiber	1 g
Protein	1 g
Calcium	9 mg
Iron	0.3 mg

Collard Green Ribbons

Makes 4 servings

✪ Great for Steps 1, 2 and 4

Slicing collard greens into super-thin strips allows them to cook quickly while maintaining a bit of crunch and a glorious emerald hue.

1½ lbs	collard greens	750 g
1 tbsp	cider vinegar	15 mL
2 tsp	liquid honey or pure maple syrup	10 mL
1 tbsp	vegetable oil	15 mL
3	cloves garlic, minced	3
⅛ tsp	fine sea salt	0.5 mL
⅛ tsp	hot pepper flakes	0.5 mL

1. Stack half the collard greens. Using a very sharp knife, cut away the stems and tough portion of center ribs. Repeat with the remaining collard greens. Discard stems and ribs. Rinse and spin-dry leaves.
2. Stack half the collard leaves and roll them up crosswise into a tight cylinder. Cut the cylinder crosswise into ¼-inch (0.5 cm) thick slices. Repeat with the remaining leaves. Toss the collard ribbons to uncoil them. Set aside.
3. In a small bowl, whisk together vinegar and honey.
4. In a large skillet, heat oil over medium-high heat. Add garlic, salt and hot pepper flakes; cook, stirring, for 30 seconds. Add collard ribbons. Cook, tossing, for about 1 minute or until coated with oil and just wilted. Serve drizzled with vinegar mixture.

Superfood Spotlight

Collard Greens • As with other vegetables in the cabbage family, collard greens have many anticancer properties. Specifically, they are an excellent source of vitamins B_6 and C, carotenes, chlorophyll and manganese. One cup (250 mL) of collard greens provides more than 70% of the RDA for vitamin C. Collard greens are also a very good source of fiber and several minerals, including iron, copper and calcium, and a good source of vitamins B_1, B_2 and E.

Nutrients per serving

Calories	79
Total fat	3 g
Saturated fat	0 g
Cholesterol	0 mg
Sodium	299 mg
Carbohydrate	14 g
Fiber	6 g
Protein	4 g
Calcium	281 mg
Iron	2.4 mg

Quick Sautéed Kale

Makes 4 servings

✪ Great for Steps 1, 2 and 4

- Steamer basket

1 lb	kale, tough stems and ribs removed, leaves cut into 1⁄4-inch (0.5 cm) wide strips (about 8 cups/2 L)	500 g
1 tbsp	extra virgin olive oil	15 mL
1 cup	thinly sliced red onion	250 mL
2	cloves garlic, minced	2
Pinch	hot pepper flakes	Pinch
1⁄4 tsp	fine sea salt	1 mL
1 tbsp	red wine vinegar	15 mL

1. Place kale in a steamer basket set over a large pot of boiling water. Cover and steam for 8 to 10 minutes or until tender.
2. In a large skillet, heat oil over medium-high heat. Add red onion and cook, stirring, for 6 to 8 minutes or until golden. Add garlic and hot pepper flakes; cook, stirring, for 1 minute. Add kale, reduce heat to medium and cook, stirring occasionally, for 1 to 2 minutes or until heated through. Remove from heat and stir in salt and vinegar.

Nutrients per serving	
Calories	86
Total fat	3 g
Saturated fat	1 g
Cholesterol	0 mg
Sodium	256 mg
Carbohydrate	14 g
Fiber	3 g
Protein	4 g
Calcium	245 mg
Iron	3.5 mg

Wilted Spinach with Garlic

Makes 6 servings

✪ Great for Steps 2 and 4

2 tsp	extra virgin olive oil	10 mL
3	cloves garlic, thinly sliced lengthwise	3
2	packages (each 10 oz/300 g) baby spinach	2
1 tbsp	water	15 mL
1⁄8 tsp	fine sea salt	0.5 mL
1⁄8 tsp	freshly ground black pepper	0.5 mL
1⁄2 tsp	sherry vinegar or red wine vinegar	2 mL

1. In a large pot, heat oil over medium-high heat. Add garlic, spinach and water; cook, tossing with tongs, for about 2 minutes or until spinach is wilted but still bright green. Add salt, pepper and vinegar, gently tossing to combine.

▸ Health Note

Spinach is iron-rich, and garlic lowers cholesterol and blood pressure.

Nutrients per serving	
Calories	57
Total fat	2 g
Saturated fat	0 g
Cholesterol	0 mg
Sodium	186 mg
Carbohydrate	11 g
Fiber	5 g
Protein	3 g
Calcium	73 mg
Iron	3.2 mg

Sautéed Swiss Chard

Makes 8 servings

✪ Great for Steps 1, 2 and 4

Earthy, grassy Swiss chard makes a gorgeous, incredibly tasty side dish. It needs little adornment beyond a bit of olive oil and garlic.

3 lbs	Swiss chard (about 2 large bunches)	1.5 kg
1 tbsp	extra virgin olive oil	15 mL
2	onions, halved, then thinly sliced	2
3	cloves garlic, minced	3
1⁄4 tsp	fine sea salt	1 mL
1⁄4 tsp	freshly ground black pepper	1 mL

1. Trim stems and center ribs from Swiss chard, then cut stems and ribs crosswise into 1-inch (2.5 cm) pieces. Stack chard leaves, roll them up crosswise into a tight cylinder and cut the cylinder crosswise into 1-inch (2.5 cm) thick slices.
2. In a large, heavy pot, heat oil over medium heat. Add onions and cook, stirring, for 8 to 9 minutes or until golden. Stir in chard stems and ribs, garlic, salt and pepper. Cover and cook, stirring occasionally, for 8 to 10 minutes or until stems are tender.
3. Add half the chard leaves and cook, stirring, for 1 minute or until slightly wilted. Add the remaining leaves, cover and cook, stirring occasionally, for 4 to 6 minutes or until leaves are tender. Using a slotted spoon, transfer Swiss chard mixture to plates or a serving bowl.

Superfood Spotlight

Swiss Chard • Swiss chard is packed with nutrition and is one of the most powerful anticancer foods thanks to its combination of nutrients and soluble fiber. For starters, it is an excellent source of vitamins C, E and K, carotenes, chlorophyll, fiber and several minerals, including potassium, magnesium, iron and manganese. It is a good source of many other nutrients, including protein, vitamin B_6, calcium, thiamine, selenium, zinc, niacin and folate. Researchers note that the high level of vitamin K in Swiss chard is especially beneficial in the maintenance of bone health.

Nutrients per serving	
Calories	52
Total fat	1 g
Saturated fat	0 g
Cholesterol	0 mg
Sodium	232 mg
Carbohydrate	10 g
Fiber	4 g
Protein	4 g
Calcium	107 mg
Iron	3.9 mg

Roasted Oven Fries

Makes 6 servings

✪ Great for Steps 1, 2 and 4

Giving the vitamin-C-packed potato wedges a bath in hot water removes some of their starch, allowing them to become brown and crispy, like oil-cooked fries, while maintaining their superfood status.

- **Preheat oven to 475°F (240°C)**
- **Large rimmed baking sheet, lined with foil and sprayed with nonstick cooking spray**

1½ lbs	russet potatoes, peeled and cut lengthwise into ¼-inch (0.5 cm) thick wedges	750 g
	Hot water	
4 tsp	extra virgin olive oil	20 mL
4	cloves garlic, coarsely chopped	4
¾ tsp	fine sea salt	3 mL
½ tsp	freshly cracked black pepper	2 mL
1 tbsp	chopped fresh flat-leaf (Italian) parsley	15 mL

1. Place potatoes in a large bowl and add enough hot (not boiling) water to cover. Let stand for 10 minutes. Drain, pat dry and return to dry bowl.
2. Meanwhile, in a small skillet, heat oil over medium heat. Add garlic and cook, stirring, for 2 minutes or until golden. Using a slotted spoon, transfer garlic to a small bowl and set aside.
3. Pour garlic oil over potatoes, tossing to coat. Add salt and pepper, tossing to coat. Spread in a single layer on prepared baking sheet.
4. Bake in preheated oven for 18 to 20 minutes or until golden on the bottom. Turn potatoes over and bake for 10 minutes or until golden and crisp.
5. Stir parsley into the reserved garlic. Sprinkle over potatoes. Serve immediately.

Nutrients per serving	
Calories	100
Total fat	3 g
Saturated fat	1 g
Cholesterol	0 mg
Sodium	290 mg
Carbohydrate	21 g
Fiber	2 g
Protein	2 g
Calcium	19 mg
Iron	1.1 mg

Baked Parsnip Fries

Makes 4 servings

✪ Great for Steps 1, 2 and 4

Nutrients per serving	
Calories	95
Total fat	3 g
Saturated fat	1 g
Cholesterol	0 mg
Sodium	188 mg
Carbohydrate	20 g
Fiber	5 g
Protein	1 g
Calcium	45 mg
Iron	0.7 mg

- **Preheat oven to 400°F (200°C)**
- **Large rimmed baking sheet, lined with foil and sprayed with nonstick cooking spray**

1 lb	parsnips, cut into 3-inch (7.5 cm) long by 1⁄4-inch (0.5 cm) thick sticks	500 g
1⁄4 tsp	fine sea salt	1 mL
1⁄8 tsp	freshly ground black pepper	0.5 mL
1 tbsp	extra virgin olive oil	15 mL
1 tbsp	chopped fresh flat-leaf (Italian) parsley	15 mL

1. In a large bowl, combine parsnips, salt, pepper and oil, tossing to coat. Spread in a single layer on prepared baking sheet.
2. Bake in preheated oven for 15 minutes. Gently turn parsnips over and bake for 12 to 17 minutes or until crisp. Serve immediately, sprinkled with parsley.

Sweet Potato Fries

Makes 6 servings

✪ Great for Steps 1, 2 and 4

Sweet potatoes become incredibly tasty when roasted at a high temperature.

Nutrients per serving	
Calories	86
Total fat	3 g
Saturated fat	0 g
Cholesterol	0 mg
Sodium	213 mg
Carbohydrate	14 g
Fiber	2 g
Protein	1 g
Calcium	25 mg
Iron	0.5 mg

- **Preheat oven to 450°F (230°C)**
- **Large rimmed baking sheet, lined with foil and sprayed with nonstick cooking spray**

4	sweet potatoes (each about 8 oz/250 g), peeled and cut into 3-inch (7.5 cm) long by 1⁄4-inch (0.5 cm) thick sticks	4
1⁄2 tsp	fine sea salt	2 mL
1⁄4 tsp	freshly ground black pepper	1 mL
4 tsp	vegetable oil	20 mL

1. In a large bowl, combine sweet potatoes, salt, pepper and oil, tossing to coat. Spread in a single layer on prepared baking sheet.
2. Bake in preheated oven for 20 minutes. Gently turn sweet potatoes over and bake for 12 to 17 minutes or until crisp. Serve immediately.

Mashed Sweet Potatoes with Rosemary

Makes 6 servings

✪ Great for Steps 1, 2 and 4

Nutrients per serving	
Calories	102
Total fat	2 g
Saturated fat	0 g
Cholesterol	0 mg
Sodium	159 mg
Carbohydrate	25 g
Fiber	4 g
Protein	2 g
Calcium	46 mg
Iron	0.8 mg

2 lbs	sweet potatoes, peeled and diced	1 kg
2½ tsp	minced fresh rosemary	12 mL
¼ tsp	fine sea salt	1 mL
¼ tsp	freshly ground black pepper	1 mL
2 tsp	extra virgin olive oil	10 mL

1. Place sweet potatoes in a medium saucepan and cover with water. Bring to a boil over high heat. Boil for 8 minutes or until tender. Drain, reserving ⅓ cup (75 mL) of the cooking water.
2. In a large bowl, using an electric mixer on medium speed, beat sweet potatoes and reserved cooking liquid until smooth. Beat in rosemary, salt and pepper. Spoon into a bowl and drizzle with oil.

Lima Bean Purée

Makes 6 servings

✪ Great for Steps 2 and 4

Once puréed, lima beans taste rich and luxurious without being heavy.

Nutrients per serving	
Calories	131
Total fat	2 g
Saturated fat	1 g
Cholesterol	5 mg
Sodium	63 mg
Carbohydrate	26 g
Fiber	7 g
Protein	7 g
Calcium	65 mg
Iron	2.2 mg

- **Steamer basket**
- **Food processor**

4	cloves garlic	4
2	packages (each 10 oz/300 g) frozen baby lima beans	2
½ cup	packed fresh flat-leaf (Italian) parsley leaves	125 mL
¼ tsp	coarsely chopped fresh rosemary	1 mL
⅓ cup	reduced-sodium ready-to-use vegetable or chicken broth	75 mL
1 tbsp	unsalted butter	15 mL
	Freshly ground black pepper	

1. Place garlic and lima beans in a steamer basket set over a large pot of boiling water. Cover and steam for about 20 minutes or until beans are tender. Reserve steaming water.
2. In food processor, combine lima bean mixture, parsley, rosemary, broth and butter; purée until smooth, adding a bit of the steaming water as needed to moisten. Transfer to a serving bowl and season to taste with pepper.

Edamame Succotash

Makes 6 servings

✪ Great for Steps 1, 2, 3 and 4

Edamame (temporarily) abandons its Asian roots in this fresh, pretty side dish, to delicious effect.

Variation

Traditional Succotash: Substitute thawed frozen baby lima beans for the edamame, replace 1⁄3 cup (75 mL) of the broth with the same amount of 2% milk, and omit the lemon juice.

2 tsp	vegetable oil	10 mL
1 1⁄4 cups	fresh or thawed frozen corn kernels	300 mL
1 cup	frozen shelled edamame	250 mL
1⁄2 cup	chopped red bell pepper	125 mL
1⁄2 cup	chopped green onions, white and green parts separated	125 mL
1 tsp	dried thyme	5 mL
2⁄3 cup	reduced-sodium ready-to-use vegetable or chicken broth	150 mL
	Freshly ground black pepper	
1 tbsp	freshly squeezed lemon juice	15 mL

1. In a large skillet, heat oil over medium heat. Add corn, edamame, red pepper, white part of green onions and thyme; cook, stirring, for 3 minutes. Add broth, cover, leaving lid ajar, and boil gently for 7 to 10 minutes or until edamame is tender. Stir in green part of green onions, black pepper to taste and lemon juice.

Superfood Spotlight

Edamame • Rich in minerals and disease-preventing plant chemicals, edamame (fresh soybeans) are among the few plant sources of complete protein, making them an ideal food for vegetarians. Soybeans have been cultivated in China for over 10,000 years and are an excellent source of calcium, B vitamins, potassium, zinc and magnesium. They are a very good source of iron, although this iron can only be absorbed by the body if consumed with foods rich in vitamin C. Soy is rich in plant chemicals that offer protection from diseases, including breast and prostate cancers and heart disease. A regular intake of soybeans can also reduce menopausal symptoms.

Nutrients per serving	
Calories	79
Total fat	3 g
Saturated fat	0 g
Cholesterol	0 mg
Sodium	19 mg
Carbohydrate	10 g
Fiber	2 g
Protein	4 g
Calcium	23 mg
Iron	1.1 mg

White Beans and Spinach

Makes 4 servings

✪ Great for Steps 1, 2, 3 and 4

The round, rich taste of white beans perfectly complements earthy spinach in this Tuscan-inspired side dish.

Tip

For the white beans, you could use Great Northern beans, cannellini (white kidney) beans or white pea (navy) beans.

Variation

Spanish White Beans and Spinach: Add 2 tbsp (30 mL) chopped drained oil-packed sun-dried tomatoes and ½ tsp (2 mL) smoked hot or sweet paprika with the onion.

Nutrients per serving	
Calories	132
Total fat	2 g
Saturated fat	0 g
Cholesterol	0 mg
Sodium	244 mg
Carbohydrate	27 g
Fiber	8 g
Protein	8 g
Calcium	99 mg
Iron	3.3 mg

2 tsp	extra virgin olive oil	10 mL
2	cloves garlic, minced	2
1 cup	chopped onion	250 mL
1	can (14 to 19 oz/398 to 540 mL) white beans, drained and rinsed	1
8 cups	packed baby spinach (about 8 oz/250 g)	2 L
¼ tsp	fine sea salt	1 mL
⅛ tsp	freshly cracked black pepper	0.5 mL
¼ cup	water	60 mL

1. In a large skillet, heat oil over medium-high heat. Add garlic and onion; cook, stirring, for 6 to 8 minutes or until onion is golden. Add beans, spinach, salt, pepper and water; reduce heat to medium, cover and cook, stirring occasionally, for 4 to 5 minutes or until spinach is wilted.

Superfood Spotlight

White Beans • White beans are very high in fiber. Their soluble fiber helps lower cholesterol and prevent blood sugar levels from rising too rapidly after a meal, making them a good choice for dieters, as well as people with diabetes, insulin resistance and hypoglycemia. Their insoluble fiber helps prevent constipation and reduce the severity and symptoms of digestive disorders such as irritable bowel syndrome and diverticulitis. They are a good source of protein and are one of the best bean sources of calcium: one portion provides about 14% of a day's recommended intake. White beans are also very rich in magnesium, potassium, iron and zinc, and are a very good source of B vitamins and folate.

Cumin-Scented Black Beans and Quinoa

Makes 6 servings

✪ Great for Steps 1, 2, 3, 4 and 5

This protein-rich dish is wonderful plain, but is elevated further with some tomato salsa and crumbled queso fresco (or feta cheese) on top.

Tip

This dish also works well as a main dish, in which case it serves four.

Nutrients per serving	
Calories	154
Total fat	3 g
Saturated fat	0 g
Cholesterol	0 mg
Sodium	246 mg
Carbohydrate	29 g
Fiber	6 g
Protein	7 g
Calcium	48 mg
Iron	2.2 mg

2 tsp	vegetable oil	10 mL
1	red bell pepper, chopped	1
1½ cups	chopped white onions	375 mL
¾ cup	quinoa, rinsed	175 mL
1½ tsp	ground cumin	7 mL
¼ tsp	chipotle chile powder	1 mL
¼ tsp	fine sea salt	1 mL
1¼ cups	water	300 mL
1	can (14 to 19 oz/398 to 540 mL) black beans, drained and rinsed	1
½ cup	packed fresh cilantro leaves, chopped, divided	125 mL

1. In a medium saucepan, heat oil over medium-high heat. Add red pepper and onions; cook, stirring, for 5 to 6 minutes or until slightly softened.
2. Stir in quinoa, cumin, chipotle chile powder, salt and water. Bring to a boil. Reduce heat to medium-low, cover and simmer for 13 to 16 minutes or until quinoa is barely tender. Stir in beans and half the cilantro; simmer, uncovered, for 2 to 3 minutes or until liquid is absorbed. Serve sprinkled with the remaining cilantro.

Jamaican Rice and Peas

Makes 6 servings

✪ Great for Steps 2, 3, 4 and 5

Nutrients per serving	
Calories	201
Total fat	6 g
Saturated fat	4 g
Cholesterol	0 mg
Sodium	245 mg
Carbohydrate	37 g
Fiber	6 g
Protein	6 g
Calcium	30 mg
Iron	1.6 mg

1	clove garlic, minced	1
1 cup	long-grain brown rice	250 mL
1 tsp	dried thyme	5 mL
1/2 tsp	ground allspice	2 mL
1/2 tsp	fine sea salt	2 mL
1/4 tsp	freshly ground black pepper	1 mL
1	can (14 oz/400 mL) light coconut milk	1
3/4 cup	water	175 mL
1	can (14 to 19 oz/398 to 540 mL) dark red kidney beans, drained and rinsed	1

1. In a medium saucepan, combine garlic, rice, thyme, allspice, salt, pepper, coconut milk and water. Bring to a boil over medium-high heat. Reduce heat to low, cover and simmer for 45 to 50 minutes or until liquid is absorbed. Fluff with a fork.
2. Remove from heat and gently stir in beans. Cover and let stand for 5 minutes to warm the beans.

Basic Brown Rice Pilaf

Makes 6 servings

✪ Great for Steps 1, 2, 4 and 5

Even whole-grain skeptics will love this simple yet flavorful brown rice dish.

Nutrients per serving	
Calories	140
Total fat	3 g
Saturated fat	0 g
Cholesterol	0 mg
Sodium	63 mg
Carbohydrate	27 g
Fiber	2 g
Protein	3 g
Calcium	24 mg
Iron	0.6 mg

2 tsp	extra virgin olive oil	10 mL
1 cup	finely chopped celery	250 mL
1/2 cup	finely chopped onion	125 mL
1 cup	long-grain brown rice	250 mL
1/8 tsp	freshly ground black pepper	0.5 mL
2 cups	reduced-sodium ready-to-use chicken or vegetable broth	500 mL

1. In a large saucepan, heat oil over medium-high heat. Add celery and onion; cook, stirring, for 3 minutes. Add rice and cook, stirring, for 2 minutes.
2. Stir in pepper and broth. Bring to a boil. Reduce heat to low, cover and simmer for 40 to 45 minutes or until broth is absorbed. Let stand, covered, for 5 minutes, then fluff with a fork.

Spelt and Wild Mushroom Pilaf

Makes 6 servings

✪ Great for Steps 1, 2, 4 and 5

Spelt's rich, distinctive flavor is reminiscent of toasted nuts to some, roasted vegetables to others. Its toasty-nutty flavor goes well with both sweet and savory dishes, which is wonderful news, since it is full of heart-healthy fiber, rich in B vitamins and high in magnesium.

1 cup	spelt	250 mL
	Hot water	
3 tsp	extra virgin olive oil, divided	15 mL
3/4 cup	chopped onion	175 mL
1 1/2 tsp	minced fresh thyme	7 mL
1/2 tsp	fine sea salt	2 mL
1/4 tsp	freshly ground black pepper	1 mL
1 1/2 cups	reduced-sodium ready-to-use vegetable or chicken broth	375 mL
8 oz	mixed wild mushrooms (such as shiitake, cremini and oyster), coarsely chopped	250 g

1. Place spelt in a medium bowl and add enough hot water to cover. Cover and let stand for 1 hour. Drain and rinse with cold water, then drain again.
2. In a medium saucepan, heat 1 tsp (5 mL) of the oil over medium-high heat. Add onion and cook, stirring, for 5 to 6 minutes or until softened. Add spelt, thyme, salt and pepper; cook, stirring, for 1 minute.
3. Stir in broth and bring to a boil. Reduce heat to low, cover and simmer, stirring occasionally, for about 50 minutes or until spelt is tender.
4. In a large skillet, heat the remaining oil over medium-high heat. Add mushrooms and cook, stirring, for 5 to 7 minutes or until tender and beginning to brown. Stir into spelt mixture.

Superfood Spotlight

Thyme • The evergreen leaves of thyme have a powerful, aromatic flavor and strong antioxidant action because of the volatile oils and plant compounds they contain. The most important of these is thymol oil, which research has found can boost the effects of healthy omega-3 fats on the body (for example, the omega-3 DHA, found in fish oils, which has been shown to be important for healthy brain function). The oils in thyme are strongly antibacterial and can protect against food poisoning bugs such as *E. coli*, bacillus and staphylococcus. Finally, they are rich in flavonoids, which protect us against the diseases of aging and are a good source of vitamin C and iron.

Nutrients per serving	
Calories	139
Total fat	3 g
Saturated fat	1 g
Cholesterol	0 mg
Sodium	224 mg
Carbohydrate	25 g
Fiber	4 g
Protein	6 g
Calcium	26 mg
Iron	1.6 mg

Bulgur Pilaf with Apricots and Coriander

Makes 6 servings

✪ Great for Steps 1, 2, 4 and 5

Nutrients per serving	
Calories	137
Total fat	2 g
Saturated fat	0 g
Cholesterol	0 mg
Sodium	217 mg
Carbohydrate	29 g
Fiber	4 g
Protein	4 g
Calcium	28 mg
Iron	0.9 mg

2 tsp	extra virgin olive oil	10 mL
1½ cups	finely chopped onions	375 mL
1 cup	coarse bulgur	250 mL
½ cup	dried apricots, finely chopped	125 mL
1 tsp	ground coriander	5 mL
½ tsp	fine sea salt	2 mL
¼ tsp	freshly ground black pepper	1 mL
1¾ cups	water	425 mL
½ cup	packed fresh cilantro leaves, chopped	125 mL

1. In a large skillet, heat oil over medium-high heat. Add onions and cook, stirring, for 6 to 8 minutes or until softened. Add bulgur and cook, stirring, for 1 minute.
2. Stir in apricots, coriander, salt, pepper and water. Bring to a boil. Remove from heat, cover and let stand for about 30 minutes or until water is absorbed. Stir in cilantro.

Creamy Millet Polenta with Cheese and Chives

Makes 6 servings

✪ Great for Steps 4 and 5

1 cup	millet	250 mL
6 cups	reduced-sodium ready-to-use vegetable or chicken broth	1.5 L
½ cup	freshly grated Asiago or Parmesan cheese	125 mL
3 tbsp	minced fresh chives	45 mL
⅛ tsp	freshly ground black pepper	0.5 mL

1. In a medium saucepan, toast millet over medium heat, stirring constantly, for 2 to 3 minutes or until it smells toasty and begins to make a popping sound.
2. Stir in broth and bring to a boil. Reduce heat to low, cover and simmer, stirring every 5 to 6 minutes to prevent sticking, for 33 to 38 minutes or until millet appears very creamy. Remove from heat and stir in cheese, chives and pepper.

Nutrients per serving	
Calories	168
Total fat	5 g
Saturated fat	2 g
Cholesterol	13 mg
Sodium	232 mg
Carbohydrate	27 g
Fiber	4 g
Protein	6 g
Calcium	157 mg
Iron	1.4 mg

Kasha with Summer Vegetables

Makes 6 servings

✪ Great for Steps 1, 2, 4 and 5

With its assortment of tender spring vegetables, this quick-to-the-table side dish also makes a great meat-free lunch.

2 cups	reduced-sodium ready-to-use vegetable or chicken broth	500 mL
1	large egg, beaten lightly	1
1 cup	whole kasha (toasted buckwheat groats)	250 mL
3 tsp	extra virgin olive oil, divided	15 mL
2	cloves garlic, minced	2
1	red bell pepper, chopped	1
1 cup	chopped onion	250 mL
1	zucchini, cut into 1⁄4-inch (0.5 cm) dice	1
1 cup	fresh or thawed frozen corn kernels	250 mL
1⁄4 tsp	fine sea salt	1 mL
	Nonfat plain yogurt (optional)	

1. In a medium saucepan, bring broth to a boil over medium-high heat.
2. Meanwhile, in a small bowl, combine egg and kasha.
3. In a large, deep skillet, heat 1 tsp (5 mL) of the oil over medium heat. Add kasha mixture and cook, stirring to separate the grains, for 2 to 4 minutes or until golden. Remove from heat and gradually stir in broth. Reduce heat, cover tightly and simmer for 12 to 15 minutes or until liquid is absorbed.
4. Meanwhile, in a large skillet, heat the remaining oil over medium-high heat. Add garlic, red pepper and onion; cook, stirring, for 6 to 8 minutes or until softened. Add zucchini, corn and salt; cook, stirring, for 3 minutes or until zucchini is slightly softened.
5. Stir vegetable mixture into kasha mixture. Serve warm, with yogurt on the side, if desired.

▶ Health Note

Kasha (toasted buckwheat groats) contains a variety of flavonoids, most notably quercetin and rutin, which research indicates are especially promising in thwarting cancer.

Nutrients per serving

Calories	153
Total fat	3 g
Saturated fat	1 g
Cholesterol	30 mg
Sodium	160 mg
Carbohydrate	31 g
Fiber	5 g
Protein	5 g
Calcium	26 mg
Iron	1.2 mg

Breads

No-Knead Whole Wheat Bread. 462
Healthy Know-How: Carbohydrates 101 463
Quick Whole Wheat Walnut Bread 463
Whole Wheat Irish Soda Bread 464
Quick Pumpernickel Bread 465
Sunflower Spelt Bread. 466
Sesame and Green Onion Bread. 467
Skillet Cornbread. 468
Cardamom Carrot Bread 469
Pumpkin Bread 470
Spinach and Basil Bread 471
Whole Wheat Zucchini Bread 472
Amaranth Spice Bread. 473
Easy Raisin Rye Bread 474
Spiced Date Bread 475
Cranberry, Orange and Agave Bread 476

Fresh Apple Bread. 477
Applesauce Flax Bread 478
Banana Bran Bread 479
Whole Wheat Focaccia 480
Whole Wheat Pizza Dough 481
No-Knead Whole Wheat Dinner Rolls. 482
Whole Wheat Buttermilk Biscuits 483
Multi-Seed Spelt Biscuits. 484
Pumpkin Biscuits 485
Lemon Drop Scones 486
Maple Oat Drop Scones 487
Scottish Oat Cakes 488
Multi-Seed Supper Muffins 489
Maple Whole Wheat Muffins. 490
Gluten-Free Flax Muffins 491

No-Knead Whole Wheat Bread

Makes 16 slices

✪ Great for Step 5

Incredibly delicious, nearly foolproof and easy to make, this is definitely not your average homemade bread.

Tip

Vital wheat gluten can be found where flours are shelved in well-stocked supermarkets or at bulk food or health food stores. It helps develop the texture of the bread, and is a particular boon for whole-grain breads.

Storage Tip

Store the cooled bread, wrapped in foil or plastic wrap, in the refrigerator for up to 1 week. Alternatively, wrap it in plastic wrap, then foil, completely enclosing bread, and freeze for up to 3 months. Let thaw at room temperature for 4 to 6 hours before serving.

Nutrients per slice	
Calories	115
Total fat	3 g
Saturated fat	0 g
Cholesterol	0 mg
Sodium	178 mg
Carbohydrate	20 g
Fiber	3 g
Protein	4 g
Calcium	33 mg
Iron	1.6 mg

- **9- by 5-inch (23 by 12.5 cm) metal loaf pan, generously sprayed with nonstick cooking spray**

3 cups	whole wheat flour	750 mL
2 tbsp	vital wheat gluten	30 mL
2 tsp	quick-rising (instant) yeast	10 mL
1 tsp	fine sea salt	5 mL
1⅓ cups	lukewarm water	325 mL
¼ cup	vegetable oil	60 mL
¼ cup	dark (cooking) molasses	60 mL
	Nonstick cooking spray	

1. In a large bowl, whisk together flour, gluten, yeast and salt. Add water, oil and molasses. Using an electric mixer on high speed, beat for 3 minutes, scraping down sides of bowl as needed.
2. Spread dough evenly in prepared pan. Cover with plastic wrap sprayed with cooking spray and let rise in a warm, draft-free spot for 75 to 90 minutes or until dough just reaches rim of pan.
3. Meanwhile, preheat oven to 350°F (180°C).
4. Remove plastic wrap from pan. Bake for 40 to 45 minutes or until deep golden brown, tenting with foil after 25 minutes to prevent over-browning. Let cool in pan on a wire rack for 10 minutes, then transfer to the rack to cool.

Healthy Know-How

Carbohydrates 101

Of the three primary macronutrients (protein, fat and carbohydrates), we need carbohydrates in the greatest amounts because they are the body's main source of fuel in the form of glucose — all of our tissues and cells use glucose for energy. According to the USDA, 45% to 65% of calories should come from carbohydrates. Carbohydrates are essential for the proper function of the central nervous system, the kidneys, the brain and the muscles (including the heart), and are important in intestinal health and waste elimination.

Quick Whole Wheat Walnut Bread

Makes 16 slices

✪ Great for Steps 3, 4 and 5

Storage Tip

Store the cooled bread, wrapped in foil or plastic wrap, in the refrigerator for up to 1 week. Alternatively, wrap it in plastic wrap, then foil, completely enclosing bread, and freeze for up to 3 months. Let thaw at room temperature for 4 to 6 hours before serving.

Nutrients per slice	
Calories	142
Total fat	4 g
Saturated fat	1 g
Cholesterol	2 mg
Sodium	293 mg
Carbohydrate	25 g
Fiber	3 g
Protein	6 g
Calcium	93 mg
Iron	2.3 mg

- **Preheat oven to 350°F (180°C)**
- **9- by 5-inch (23 by 12.5 cm) metal loaf pan, sprayed with nonstick cooking spray**

3 cups	whole wheat flour	750 mL
2 tsp	baking soda	10 mL
1 tsp	fine sea salt	5 mL
2 cups	1% buttermilk	500 mL
1/2 cup	dark (cooking) molasses	125 mL
3/4 cup	chopped toasted walnuts	175 mL

1. In a large bowl, whisk together flour, baking soda and salt.
2. In a medium bowl, whisk together buttermilk and molasses until blended.
3. Add the buttermilk mixture to the flour mixture and stir until just blended. Gently fold in walnuts.
4. Spread batter evenly in prepared pan.
5. Bake in preheated oven for about 1 hour or until top is golden brown and a toothpick inserted in the center comes out clean. Let cool in pan on a wire rack for 10 minutes, then transfer to the rack to cool.

Variation

Substitute liquid honey for the molasses and chopped toasted pecans for the walnuts.

Whole Wheat Irish Soda Bread

Makes 16 slices

✪ Great for Steps 3 and 5

Irish soda bread is one of the easiest, healthiest breads you can bake, and it seems everyone has a favorite recipe. But the essential ingredients remain the same: flour, baking soda, salt and buttermilk. This one is gussied up with a bit of honey and whole wheat flour, but you can add more frills (see the variations, at right) if you like.

Storage Tip

Store the cooled bread, wrapped in foil or plastic wrap, in the refrigerator for up to 1 week. Alternatively, wrap it in plastic wrap, then foil, completely enclosing bread, and freeze for up to 3 months. Let thaw at room temperature for 4 to 6 hours before serving.

Nutrients per slice	
Calories	119
Total fat	1 g
Saturated fat	0 g
Cholesterol	2 mg
Sodium	289 mg
Carbohydrate	28 g
Fiber	3 g
Protein	6 g
Calcium	42 mg
Iron	1.2 mg

- **Preheat oven to 450°F (230°C)**
- **Large rimmed baking sheet, sprayed with nonstick cooking spray**

4 cups	whole wheat flour	1 L
3 tbsp	vital wheat gluten	45 mL
1 tsp	baking soda	5 mL
1 tsp	fine sea salt	5 mL
2 cups	1% buttermilk	500 mL
1/4 cup	liquid honey	60 mL

1. In a large bowl, whisk together flour, gluten, baking soda and salt.
2. In a medium bowl, whisk together buttermilk and honey until well blended.
3. Add the buttermilk mixture to the flour mixture and stir until just blended.
4. Transfer dough to prepared baking sheet and, with floured hands, form into a 2-inch (5 cm) high round. Using a serrated knife, cut a deep X in the top of the round.
5. Bake in preheated oven for 20 minutes. Reduce oven temperature to 400°F (200°C) and bake for 30 to 35 minutes or until loaf is brown on top and sounds hollow when tapped. Transfer loaf to a wire rack and let cool completely.

Variations

Caraway Currant Soda Bread: Gently fold in 3/4 cup (175 mL) currants and 1 1/2 tbsp (22 mL) caraway seeds at the end of step 3.

Sesame Soda Bread: Gently fold in 1/4 cup (60 mL) toasted sesame seeds (see tip, page 426) at the end of step 3.

Golden Raisin Soda Bread: Gently fold in 3/4 cup (175 mL) golden raisins and 1 tbsp (15 mL) finely grated orange zest at the end of step 3.

Quick Pumpernickel Bread

Makes 14 slices

✪ Great for Steps 3 and 5

My quick bread version of pumpernickel has all of the traditional flavor of the yeast kind, minus the fuss.

Tip

Use any variety of milk in this recipe, but to keep it relatively low in overall fat, opt for lower-fat or skim (nonfat) milk.

Storage Tip

Store the cooled bread, wrapped in foil or plastic wrap, in the refrigerator for up to 1 week. Alternatively, wrap it in plastic wrap, then foil, completely enclosing bread, and freeze for up to 3 months. Let thaw at room temperature for 4 to 6 hours before serving.

Nutrients per slice	
Calories	123
Total fat	4 g
Saturated fat	1 g
Cholesterol	1 mg
Sodium	297 mg
Carbohydrate	21 g
Fiber	4 g
Protein	4 g
Calcium	79 mg
Iron	1.8 mg

- **Preheat oven to 350°F (180°C)**
- **9- by 5-inch (23 by 12.5 cm) metal loaf pan, sprayed with nonstick cooking spray**

1¼ cups	dark or light rye flour	300 mL
1¼ cups	whole wheat flour	300 mL
2 tsp	baking powder	10 mL
1 tsp	baking soda	5 mL
1 tsp	fine sea salt	5 mL
1½ tsp	instant espresso powder	7 mL
¾ cup	nonfat plain yogurt	175 mL
⅓ cup	milk	75 mL
¼ cup	vegetable oil	60 mL
¼ cup	dark (cooking) molasses	60 mL
2 tbsp	caraway seeds (optional)	30 mL

1. In a large bowl, whisk together rye flour, whole wheat flour, baking powder, baking soda and salt.
2. In a medium bowl, whisk together espresso powder, yogurt, milk, oil and molasses until well blended.
3. Add the yogurt mixture to the flour mixture and stir until just blended.
4. Spread batter evenly in prepared pan. Sprinkle with caraway seeds (if using).
5. Bake in preheated oven for 50 to 55 minutes or until a toothpick inserted in the center comes out clean. Let cool in pan on a wire rack for 10 minutes, then transfer to the rack. Serve warm or let cool completely.

Variation

Vegan Quick Rye Bread: Replace the yogurt with plain soy yogurt and substitute plain non-dairy milk (such as soy, almond, rice or hemp) for the skim milk.

Sunflower Spelt Bread

Makes 16 slices

✪ Great for Steps 3, 4 and 5

Once you try spelt flour in baked goods, you'll wonder why you waited so long. Spelt is a very nutritious ancient grain with a nutty flavor. It is an excellent source of vitamin B_2, a very good source of manganese and a good source of niacin, thiamin and copper. When ground into flour, it yields incredibly delicious baked goods.

Storage Tip

Store the cooled bread, wrapped in foil or plastic wrap, in the refrigerator for up to 3 days. Alternatively, wrap it in plastic wrap, then foil, completely enclosing bread, and freeze for up to 3 months. Let thaw at room temperature for 4 to 6 hours before serving.

Nutrients per slice	
Calories	150
Total fat	6 g
Saturated fat	1 g
Cholesterol	2 mg
Sodium	291 mg
Carbohydrate	23 g
Fiber	3 g
Protein	7 g
Calcium	66 mg
Iron	1.3 mg

- **Preheat oven to 400°F (200°C)**
- **Large rimmed baking sheet, sprayed with nonstick cooking spray**

2 cups	whole-grain spelt flour	500 mL
1¾ cups	whole wheat flour	425 mL
⅔ cup	lightly salted roasted sunflower seeds	150 mL
2 tsp	fennel seeds (optional)	10 mL
2 tsp	baking soda	10 mL
1 tsp	fine sea salt	5 mL
1¾ cups	1% buttermilk	425 mL
¼ cup	extra virgin olive oil	60 mL

1. In a large bowl, whisk together spelt flour, whole wheat flour, sunflower seeds, fennel seeds (if using), baking soda and salt.
2. In a medium bowl, whisk together buttermilk and oil until well blended.
3. Add the buttermilk mixture to the flour mixture and stir until just blended.
4. Transfer dough to prepared baking sheet and, with floured hands, form into a 2-inch (5 cm) high round. Using a serrated knife, cut a deep X in the top of the round.
5. Bake in preheated oven for 35 to 40 minutes or until loaf is brown on top and sounds hollow when tapped. Transfer loaf to a wire rack and let cool completely.

Superfood Spotlight

Sunflower Seeds • Sunflower seeds, usually sold shelled, are one of the world's main sources of vegetable oil. They are rich in polyunsaturated fats, plant sterols (which have a cholesterol-lowering effect) and various minerals, including iron, magnesium and selenium. They are very rich in vitamin E, an antioxidant that neutralizes the free radicals that, in excess, can damage the body's cells and speed up the aging process. Vitamin E also helps protect against inflammatory conditions such as asthma and rheumatoid arthritis and is linked with a lower risk of cardiovascular disease and with protection from colon cancer.

Sesame and Green Onion Bread

Makes 12 slices

✪ Great for Steps 3, 4 and 5

This bread was inspired by the sesame and green onion pancakes at one of my favorite Chinese restaurants. The green onions lend moisture and a delicate onion flavor to the bread, along with high levels of vitamins A and C.

Storage Tip

Store the cooled bread, wrapped in foil or plastic wrap, in the refrigerator for up to 3 days. Alternatively, wrap it in plastic wrap, then foil, completely enclosing bread, and freeze for up to 3 months. Let thaw at room temperature for 4 to 6 hours before serving.

Nutrients per slice	
Calories	129
Total fat	5 g
Saturated fat	0 g
Cholesterol	14 mg
Sodium	165 mg
Carbohydrate	16 g
Fiber	2 g
Protein	4 g
Calcium	60 mg
Iron	0.6 mg

- **Preheat oven to 350°F (180°C)**
- **9- by 5-inch (23 by 12.5 cm) metal loaf pan, sprayed with nonstick cooking spray**

2 cups	whole wheat pastry flour	500 mL
2¼ tsp	baking powder	11 mL
1 tsp	baking soda	5 mL
½ tsp	fine sea salt	2 mL
1	large egg	1
1¼ cups	nonfat plain yogurt	300 mL
¼ cup	vegetable oil	60 mL
2 tbsp	toasted sesame oil	30 mL
1 tbsp	brown rice syrup or liquid honey	15 mL
1 cup	chopped green onions	250 mL
2 tbsp	sesame seeds	30 mL

1. In a large bowl, whisk together flour, baking powder, baking soda and salt.
2. In a medium bowl, whisk together egg, yogurt, vegetable oil, sesame oil and brown rice syrup until well blended.
3. Add the egg mixture to the flour mixture and stir until just blended. Gently fold in green onions.
4. Spread batter evenly in prepared pan. Sprinkle with sesame seeds.
5. Bake in preheated oven for 45 to 50 minutes or until top is golden brown and a toothpick inserted in the center comes out clean. Let cool in pan on a wire rack for 10 minutes, then transfer to the rack. Serve warm or let cool completely.

Skillet Cornbread

Makes 12 slices

✪ Great for Steps 3 and 5

It's worth seeking out stone-ground cornmeal — it has a fuller corn flavor and more health benefits.

Tip

If you don't have a cast-iron skillet, use a 9-inch (23 cm) metal baking pan instead. Do not preheat the pan; simply spray it with nonstick cooking spray or rub it with oil. The bread will not be as crusty as when baked in the skillet.

Storage Tip

Store the cooled bread, wrapped in foil or plastic wrap, in the refrigerator for up to 3 days. Alternatively, wrap it in plastic wrap, then foil, completely enclosing bread, and freeze for up to 3 months. Let thaw at room temperature for 4 to 6 hours before serving.

Nutrients per slice	
Calories	149
Total fat	6 g
Saturated fat	1 g
Cholesterol	14 mg
Sodium	264 mg
Carbohydrate	23 g
Fiber	2 g
Protein	4 g
Calcium	73 mg
Iron	0.6 mg

- **Preheat oven to 400°F (200°C)**
- **9-inch (23 cm) cast-iron skillet, oiled**

1¾ cups	whole wheat pastry flour	425 mL
1 cup	cornmeal (preferably stone-ground)	250 mL
2 tsp	baking powder	10 mL
½ tsp	fine sea salt	2 mL
½ tsp	baking soda	1 mL
1	large egg	1
1½ cups	1% buttermilk	375 mL
¼ cup	vegetable oil	60 mL
3 tbsp	pure maple syrup or brown rice syrup	45 mL

1. Place prepared skillet in preheated oven for 10 minutes while you prepare the batter.
2. In a large bowl, whisk together flour, cornmeal, baking powder, salt and baking soda.
3. In a medium bowl, whisk together egg, buttermilk, oil and maple syrup until well blended.
4. Add the egg mixture to the flour mixture and stir until just blended.
5. Carefully spread batter evenly in hot skillet.
6. Bake for 22 to 25 minutes or until golden and a toothpick inserted in the center comes out clean. Let cool in skillet on a wire rack for 10 minutes, then transfer to the rack. Serve warm or let cool completely.

Cardamom Carrot Bread

Makes 12 slices

✪ Great for Steps 1, 2, 3, 4 and 5

Carrots not only make this quick, easy bread moist, they also contain fiber and a broad range of vitamins and minerals.

Tip

An equal amount of white whole wheat flour may be used in place of the whole wheat pastry flour. Alternatively, use half whole wheat flour and half unbleached all-purpose flour.

Storage Tip

Store the cooled bread, wrapped in foil or plastic wrap, in the refrigerator for up to 3 days. Alternatively, wrap it in plastic wrap, then foil, completely enclosing bread, and freeze for up to 3 months. Let thaw at room temperature for 4 to 6 hours before serving.

Nutrients per slice	
Calories	166
Total fat	7 g
Saturated fat	1 g
Cholesterol	0 mg
Sodium	216 mg
Carbohydrate	30 g
Fiber	2 g
Protein	3 g
Calcium	69 mg
Iron	0.6 mg

- **Preheat oven to 350°F (180°C)**
- **9- by 5-inch (23 by 12.5 cm) metal loaf pan, sprayed with nonstick cooking spray**

1½ cups	whole wheat pastry flour	375 mL
2 tsp	baking powder	10 mL
1 tsp	ground cardamom	5 mL
½ tsp	baking soda	2 mL
½ tsp	fine sea salt	2 mL
1 cup	nonfat plain yogurt	250 mL
½ cup	liquid honey	125 mL
⅓ cup	vegetable oil	75 mL
1 tsp	finely grated orange zest	5 mL
2 cups	shredded carrots	500 mL
½ cup	golden raisins	125 mL
⅓ cup	chopped pistachios	75 mL

1. In a large bowl, whisk together flour, baking powder, cardamom, baking soda and salt.
2. In a medium bowl, whisk together yogurt, honey, oil and orange zest until well blended.
3. Add the yogurt mixture to the flour mixture and stir until just blended. Gently fold in carrots, raisins and pistachios.
4. Spread batter evenly in prepared pan.
5. Bake in preheated oven for 50 to 55 minutes or until top is golden brown and a toothpick inserted in the center comes out clean. Let cool in pan on a wire rack for 10 minutes, then transfer to the rack to cool.

Pumpkin Bread

Makes 14 slices

✪ Great for Steps 2, 3, 4 and 5

What can pumpkin do for quick bread? How about add richness, deep flavor and moisture, with a minimum of calories and no fat. Meet your new go-to pumpkin bread.

Storage Tip

Store the cooled bread, wrapped in foil or plastic wrap, in the refrigerator for up to 3 days. Alternatively, wrap it in plastic wrap, then foil, completely enclosing bread, and freeze for up to 3 months. Let thaw at room temperature for 4 to 6 hours before serving.

Nutrients per slice	
Calories	167
Total fat	8 g
Saturated fat	1 g
Cholesterol	13 mg
Sodium	107 mg
Carbohydrate	24 g
Fiber	3 g
Protein	5 g
Calcium	36 mg
Iron	0.7 mg

- **Preheat oven to 350°F (180°C)**
- **9- by 5-inch (23 by 12.5 cm) metal loaf pan, sprayed with nonstick cooking spray**

1¾ cups	whole wheat pastry flour	425 mL
1 tbsp	pumpkin pie spice	15 mL
1 tsp	baking powder	5 mL
¼ tsp	baking soda	1 mL
¼ tsp	fine sea salt	1 mL
1	large egg	1
1¼ cups	pumpkin purée (not pie filling)	300 mL
⅔ cup	pure maple syrup, brown rice syrup or liquid honey	150 mL
⅓ cup	vegetable oil	75 mL
⅓ cup	1% buttermilk	75 mL
1 tsp	vanilla extract	5 mL
1 cup	chopped toasted walnuts	250 mL

1. In a large bowl, whisk together flour, pumpkin pie spice, baking powder, baking soda and salt.
2. In a medium bowl, whisk together egg, pumpkin, maple syrup, oil, buttermilk and vanilla until well blended.
3. Add the egg mixture to the flour mixture and stir until just blended. Gently fold in walnuts.
4. Spread batter evenly in prepared pan.
5. Bake in preheated oven for about 1 hour or until golden and a toothpick inserted in the center comes out clean. Let cool in pan on a wire rack for 10 minutes, then transfer to the rack to cool.

Spinach and Basil Bread

Makes 12 slices

✪ Great for Steps 2, 3, 4 and 5

A fantastic supper bread, this pretty loaf is also soup's best friend. Spinach delivers generous doses of vitamin C, folate and carotene, but basil shares the limelight. In addition to being a good source of vitamin A, the essential oils in the leaves contain eugenol, which has an anti-inflammatory effect.

Storage Tip

Store the cooled bread, wrapped in foil or plastic wrap, in the refrigerator for up to 3 days. Alternatively, wrap it in plastic wrap, then foil, completely enclosing bread, and freeze for up to 3 months. Let thaw at room temperature for 4 to 6 hours before serving.

Nutrients per slice	
Calories	116
Total fat	5 g
Saturated fat	1 g
Cholesterol	0 mg
Sodium	223 mg
Carbohydrate	18 g
Fiber	3 g
Protein	4 g
Calcium	107 mg
Iron	0.9 mg

- **Preheat oven to 350°F (180°C)**
- **9- by 5-inch (23 by 12.5 cm) metal loaf pan, sprayed with nonstick cooking spray**

2¼ cups	whole wheat pastry flour	550 mL
2½ tsp	baking powder	12 mL
2½ tsp	dried basil	12 mL
¾ tsp	garlic powder	3 mL
½ tsp	baking soda	2 mL
½ tsp	fine sea salt	2 mL
1 cup	nonfat plain yogurt	250 mL
¼ cup	extra virgin olive oil	60 mL
1 tbsp	liquid honey or brown rice syrup	15 mL
1	package (10 oz/300 g) frozen chopped spinach, thawed and squeezed dry	1

1. In a large bowl, whisk together flour, baking powder, basil, garlic powder, baking soda and salt.
2. In a medium bowl, whisk together yogurt, oil and honey until well blended. Stir in spinach.
3. Add the yogurt mixture to the flour mixture and stir until just blended.
4. Spread batter evenly in prepared pan.
5. Bake in preheated oven for 45 to 50 minutes or until a toothpick inserted in the center comes out clean. Let cool in pan on a wire rack for 15 minutes, then transfer to the rack. Serve warm or let cool completely.

Variation

Substitute a 12-oz (340 mL) jar of roasted red bell peppers, drained, patted dry and chopped, for the frozen spinach. Replace the basil with 1½ tsp (7 mL) dried oregano.

Whole Wheat Zucchini Bread

Makes 12 slices

✪ Great for Steps 1, 2, 3, 4 and 5

Zucchini keeps this bread incredibly moist. It's amazing how something so humble and so nutritious can also be so scrumptious.

Storage Tip

Store the cooled bread, wrapped in foil or plastic wrap, in the refrigerator for up to 5 days. Alternatively, wrap it in plastic wrap, then foil, completely enclosing bread, and freeze for up to 3 months. Let thaw at room temperature for 4 to 6 hours before serving.

- **Preheat oven to 350°F (180°C)**
- **9- by 5-inch (23 by 12.5 cm) metal loaf pan, sprayed with nonstick cooking spray**

1½ cups	whole wheat flour	375 mL
1 tsp	ground cinnamon	5 mL
½ tsp	baking powder	2 mL
½ tsp	baking soda	2 mL
½ tsp	fine sea salt	2 mL
1	large egg	1
¾ cup	liquid honey	175 mL
⅓ cup	vegetable oil	75 mL
⅓ cup	unsweetened applesauce	75 mL
¼ cup	nonfat plain yogurt	60 mL
2 tsp	vanilla extract	10 mL
1¼ cups	shredded zucchini	300 mL
½ cup	finely chopped walnuts (optional)	125 mL

1. In a large bowl, whisk together flour, cinnamon, baking powder, baking soda and salt.
2. In a medium bowl, whisk together egg, honey, oil, applesauce, yogurt and vanilla until well blended.
3. Add the egg mixture to the flour mixture and stir until just blended. Gently fold in zucchini and walnuts (if using).
4. Spread batter evenly in prepared pan.
5. Bake in preheated oven for 40 to 45 minutes or until golden and a toothpick inserted in the center comes out clean. Let cool in pan on a wire rack for 10 minutes, then transfer to the rack to cool.

▸ Health Note

Zucchini is packed with vitamins A and C. In addition, it is a good source of the B-complex vitamins, including thiamin, pyridoxine and riboflavin, and minerals such as iron, manganese, phosphorus, zinc and potassium. Potassium is an important component of cell and body fluids, helping to control heart rate and blood pressure.

Nutrients per slice	
Calories	175
Total fat	6 g
Saturated fat	1 g
Cholesterol	15 mg
Sodium	192 mg
Carbohydrate	30 g
Fiber	2 g
Protein	3 g
Calcium	23 mg
Iron	0.8 mg

Amaranth Spice Bread

Makes 14 slices

✪ Great for Steps 4 and 5

Amaranth is a tiny grain that dates back hundreds of years to the Aztecs in Mexico. It offers a particularly high-quality protein and is high in fiber. What I love best about it, though, is that its toasty, nutty flavor makes it a delicious (and inexpensive) alternative to nuts in a wide range of baking recipes.

Storage Tip

Store the cooled bread, wrapped in foil or plastic wrap, in the refrigerator for up to 5 days. Alternatively, wrap it in plastic wrap, then foil, completely enclosing bread, and freeze for up to 3 months. Let thaw at room temperature for 4 to 6 hours before serving.

Nutrients per slice	
Calories	154
Total fat	5 g
Saturated fat	1 g
Cholesterol	0 mg
Sodium	152 mg
Carbohydrate	29 g
Fiber	4 g
Protein	4 g
Calcium	112 mg
Iron	2.5 mg

- **9- by 5-inch (23 by 12.5 cm) metal loaf pan, sprayed with nonstick cooking spray**

3/4 cup	chopped dried figs or raisins	175 mL
1/2 cup	whole-grain amaranth	125 mL
1/3 cup	ground flax seeds (flaxseed meal)	75 mL
1 1/2 cups	boiling water	375 mL
2 cups	whole wheat pastry flour	500 mL
2 1/2 tsp	pumpkin pie spice	12 mL
2 tsp	baking powder	10 mL
1 tsp	ground ginger	5 mL
1/2 tsp	fine sea salt	2 mL
1/2 cup	dark (cooking) molasses	125 mL
1/4 cup	vegetable oil	60 mL
1 tsp	vanilla extract	5 mL

1. In a medium bowl, combine figs, amaranth, flax seeds and boiling water. Let stand for 20 minutes.
2. Preheat oven to 350°F (180°C).
3. In a large bowl, whisk together flour, pumpkin pie spice, baking powder, ginger and salt.
4. Stir molasses, oil and vanilla into fig mixture until well blended.
5. Add the fig mixture to the flour mixture and stir until just blended.
6. Spread batter evenly in prepared pan.
7. Bake for 50 to 55 minutes or until a toothpick inserted in the center comes out clean. Let cool in pan on a wire rack for 10 minutes, then transfer to the rack to cool.

Superfood Spotlight

Figs • Figs are usually sold dried, as fresh figs are easily damaged and have a very short shelf life. Figs contain a good amount of fiber (most of it soluble, which helps protect against heart disease) and sterols, which help lower blood cholesterol. They are also a good source of vitamin B_6, with small amounts of other B vitamins, folate and several other vitamins and minerals. Dried figs are a concentrated source of potassium and are rich in calcium, magnesium and iron.

Easy Raisin Rye Bread

Makes 14 slices

✪ Great for Steps 3, 4 and 5

A slice of this mildly sweet bread is a perfect way to start your morning. Rye flour lends it a rich nuttiness, as well as high levels of fiber and manganese.

Tip

This recipe is vegan if you use the non-dairy milk and brown rice syrup.

Storage Tip

Store the cooled bread, wrapped in foil or plastic wrap, in the refrigerator for up to 5 days. Alternatively, wrap it in plastic wrap, then foil, completely enclosing bread, and freeze for up to 3 months. Let thaw at room temperature for 4 to 6 hours before serving.

Nutrients per slice	
Calories	138
Total fat	5 g
Saturated fat	1 g
Cholesterol	1 mg
Sodium	174 mg
Carbohydrate	25 g
Fiber	5 g
Protein	4 g
Calcium	65 mg
Iron	1.3 mg

- **Preheat oven to 350°F (180°C)**
- **9- by 5-inch (23 by 12.5 cm) metal loaf pan, sprayed with nonstick cooking spray**

2 cups	light or dark rye flour	500 mL
4 tsp	baking powder	20 mL
1 tsp	ground cinnamon	5 mL
1⁄2 tsp	fine sea salt	2 mL
2⁄3 cup	milk or plain non-dairy milk	150 mL
1⁄3 cup	vegetable oil	75 mL
1⁄4 cup	liquid honey or brown rice syrup	60 mL
3⁄4 cup	raisins	175 mL

1. In a large bowl, whisk together flour, baking powder, cinnamon and salt.
2. In a medium bowl, whisk together milk, oil and honey until well blended.
3. Add the milk mixture to the flour mixture and stir until just blended. Gently fold in raisins.
4. Spread batter evenly in prepared pan.
5. Bake in preheated oven for 45 to 50 minutes or until tops are golden and a toothpick inserted in the center comes out clean. Let cool in pan on a wire rack for 10 minutes, then transfer to the rack to cool.

▸ Health Note

Rye flour provides the body with lignans, naturally occurring plant compounds that may help reduce the risk of breast and prostate cancer.

Spiced Date Bread

Makes 12 slices

✪ Great for Steps 3, 4 and 5

Move over, candy — dates, with their honey-like sweetness, are in town. Beyond sheer deliciousness, dates are a great source of dietary fiber and are one of the best natural sources of potassium. They also provide a variety of B vitamins: thiamin, riboflavin, niacin, vitamin B_6 and pantothenic acid.

Storage Tip

Store the cooled bread, wrapped in foil or plastic wrap, in the refrigerator for up to 5 days. Alternatively, wrap it in plastic wrap, then foil, completely enclosing bread, and freeze for up to 3 months. Let thaw at room temperature for 4 to 6 hours before serving.

- **9- by 5-inch (23 by 12.5 cm) metal loaf pan, sprayed with nonstick cooking spray**

3/4 cup	1% buttermilk	175 mL
1 tsp	ground cinnamon	5 mL
1 tsp	ground ginger	5 mL
1/4 tsp	ground nutmeg	1 mL
1 cup	chopped pitted dates	250 mL
1 1/2 cups	whole wheat pastry flour	375 mL
1 1/2 tsp	baking soda	7 mL
1/4 tsp	fine sea salt	1 mL
2	large eggs	2
1/2 cup	brown rice syrup or liquid honey	125 mL
2 tbsp	vegetable oil	30 mL

1. In a small saucepan, combine buttermilk, cinnamon, ginger and nutmeg. Bring to a simmer over medium-high heat. Stir in dates, remove from heat, cover and let stand for 20 minutes.
2. Preheat oven to 350°F (180°C).
3. In a large bowl, whisk together flour, baking soda and salt.
4. Stir eggs, brown rice syrup and oil into date mixture until well blended.
5. Add the egg mixture to the flour mixture and stir until just blended.
6. Spread batter evenly in prepared pan.
7. Bake for 50 to 55 minutes or until a toothpick inserted in the center comes out clean. Let cool in pan on a wire rack for 10 minutes, then transfer to the rack to cool.

Nutrients per slice	
Calories	148
Total fat	3 g
Saturated fat	1 g
Cholesterol	24 mg
Sodium	205 mg
Carbohydrate	32 g
Fiber	2 g
Protein	4 g
Calcium	37 mg
Iron	0.5 mg

Cranberry, Orange and Agave Bread

Makes 14 slices

✪ Great for Steps 1, 2, 4 and 5

The cranberry is praised for its sauce capabilities at the Thanksgiving table, but the ruby fruit is underappreciated as a health food. Cranberries are teamed with whole-grain flour and antioxidant-rich orange zest and juice to create this bread, destined to be a favorite.

Storage Tip

Store the cooled bread, wrapped in foil or plastic wrap, in the refrigerator for up to 3 days. Alternatively, wrap it in plastic wrap, then foil, completely enclosing bread, and freeze for up to 3 months. Let thaw at room temperature for 4 to 6 hours before serving.

Nutrients per slice	
Calories	114
Total fat	2 g
Saturated fat	0 g
Cholesterol	13 mg
Sodium	213 mg
Carbohydrate	26 g
Fiber	2 g
Protein	2 g
Calcium	27 mg
Iron	0.3 mg

- **Preheat oven to 350°F (180°C)**
- **9- by 5-inch (23 by 12.5 cm) metal loaf pan, sprayed with nonstick cooking spray**

2 cups	whole wheat pastry flour	500 mL
1½ tsp	baking powder	7 mL
¾ tsp	fine sea salt	3 mL
½ tsp	baking soda	2 mL
1	large egg	1
1 tbsp	finely grated orange zest	15 mL
¾ cup	freshly squeezed orange juice	175 mL
⅔ cup	agave nectar or liquid honey	150 mL
2 tbsp	vegetable oil	30 mL
1⅔ cups	fresh or thawed frozen cranberries, coarsely chopped	400 mL

1. In a large bowl, whisk together flour, baking powder, salt and baking soda.
2. In a medium bowl, whisk together egg, orange zest, orange juice, agave nectar and oil until well blended.
3. Add the egg mixture to the flour mixture and stir until just blended. Gently fold in cranberries.
4. Spread batter evenly in prepared pan.
5. Bake in preheated oven for about 1 hour or until golden and a toothpick inserted in the center comes out clean. Let cool in pan on a wire rack for 10 minutes, then transfer to the rack to cool.

Superfood Spotlight

Cranberries • Bright red cranberries have a variety of health benefits. They boost the work of the kidneys and can help prevent or alleviate urinary tract infections. This is partly because they contain quinic acid, which increases the acidity of the urine, and partly because of the tannins they contain, which are antibacterial. The same compounds may also help protect against stomach ulcers and heart disease. In addition, cranberries have a high soluble fiber content, which may help reduce "bad" cholesterol and protect against heart disease. They are loaded with disease-fighting antioxidants and are a good source of vitamin C, manganese and potassium.

Fresh Apple Bread

Makes 12 slices

✪ Great for Steps 1, 2, 4 and 5

Humble apples are rich in a flavonoid called quercetin, which has been shown to reduce allergic reactions and inflammation. Don't bother peeling the apples: keeping the peel on boosts the bread's already high fiber content, and the bits of peel become very tender upon baking.

Storage Tip

Store the cooled bread, wrapped in foil or plastic wrap, in the refrigerator for up to 3 days. Alternatively, wrap it in plastic wrap, then foil, completely enclosing bread, and freeze for up to 3 months. Let thaw at room temperature for 4 to 6 hours before serving.

Nutrients per slice	
Calories	157
Total fat	6 g
Saturated fat	1 g
Cholesterol	0 mg
Sodium	195 mg
Carbohydrate	28 g
Fiber	3 g
Protein	2 g
Calcium	20 mg
Iron	0.7 mg

- **Preheat oven to 350°F (180°C)**
- **Blender or immersion blender**
- **9- by 5-inch (23 by 12.5 cm) metal loaf pan, sprayed with nonstick cooking spray**

1½ cups	whole wheat flour	375 mL
1 tsp	ground cinnamon	5 mL
1 tsp	baking powder	5 mL
½ tsp	baking soda	2 mL
½ tsp	fine sea salt	2 mL
½ tsp	ground nutmeg	2 mL
3 tbsp	ground flax seeds (flaxseed meal)	45 mL
½ cup	water	125 mL
⅔ cup	brown rice syrup or liquid honey	150 mL
⅓ cup	vegetable oil	75 mL
1½ tsp	vanilla extract	7 mL
1½ cups	chopped apples (unpeeled)	375 mL

1. In a large bowl, whisk together flour, cinnamon, baking powder, baking soda, salt and nutmeg.
2. In blender (or in a tall cup, using an immersion blender), combine flax seeds and water; process for 1 minute or until thickened and frothy. Add brown rice syrup, oil and vanilla. Process for 2 minutes or until well blended and frothy.
3. Add the flax seed mixture to the flour mixture and stir until just blended. Gently fold in apples.
4. Spread batter evenly in prepared pan.
5. Bake in preheated oven for 55 to 60 minutes or until top is golden brown and a toothpick inserted in the center comes out clean. Let cool in pan on a wire rack for 10 minutes, then transfer to the rack to cool.

Variation

Substitute chopped pears (unpeeled) for the apples.

Applesauce Flax Bread

Makes 12 slices

✪ Great for Steps 4 and 5

Whether you use store-bought applesauce or make your own, you'll find it a challenge to stop eating this pure comfort bread after just one slice.

Storage Tip

Store the cooled bread, wrapped in foil or plastic wrap, in the refrigerator for up to 5 days. Alternatively, wrap it in plastic wrap, then foil, completely enclosing bread, and freeze for up to 3 months. Let thaw at room temperature for 4 to 6 hours before serving.

- **Preheat oven to 350°F (180°C)**
- **9- by 5-inch (23 by 12.5 cm) metal loaf pan, sprayed with nonstick cooking spray**

2 cups	whole wheat flour	500 mL
1⁄3 cup	ground flax seeds (flaxseed meal)	75 mL
2 tsp	baking powder	10 mL
2 tsp	ground cinnamon	10 mL
1⁄2 tsp	baking soda	2 mL
1⁄2 tsp	fine sea salt	2 mL
1 1⁄3 cups	unsweetened applesauce	325 mL
2⁄3 cup	brown rice syrup or liquid honey	150 mL
3 tbsp	vegetable oil	45 mL
1 tsp	vanilla extract	5 mL
1⁄2 cup	raisins	125 mL

1. In a large bowl, whisk together flour, flax seeds, baking powder, cinnamon, baking soda and salt.
2. In a medium bowl, whisk together applesauce, brown rice syrup, oil and vanilla until well blended.
3. Add the applesauce mixture to the flour mixture and stir until just blended. Gently fold in raisins.
4. Spread batter evenly in prepared pan.
5. Bake in preheated oven for 50 to 55 minutes or until top is golden brown and a toothpick inserted in the center comes out clean. Let cool in pan on a wire rack for 10 minutes, then transfer to the rack to cool.

▸ Health Note

Applesauce contains quercetin, an antioxidant bioflavonoid that research indicates may reduce the risk of several cancers.

Nutrients per slice

Calories	179
Total fat	4 g
Saturated fat	0 g
Cholesterol	0 mg
Sodium	223 mg
Carbohydrate	39 g
Fiber	4 g
Protein	4 g
Calcium	39 mg
Iron	1.1 mg

Banana Bran Bread

Makes 16 slices

✪ Great for Steps 1, 2, 3, 4 and 5

Everybody needs a great banana bread recipe in their repertoire, and this one fits the bill, with fantastic flavor and a tender, moist texture. As a bonus, you'll reap the rewards of high fiber from the bran and whole wheat flour, potassium and vitamin A from the bananas, and protein and calcium from the yogurt.

Storage Tip

Store the cooled bread, wrapped in foil or plastic wrap, in the refrigerator for up to 5 days. Alternatively, wrap it in plastic wrap, then foil, completely enclosing bread, and freeze for up to 3 months. Let thaw at room temperature for 4 to 6 hours before serving.

Nutrients per slice	
Calories	122
Total fat	4 g
Saturated fat	0 g
Cholesterol	0 mg
Sodium	174 mg
Carbohydrate	24 g
Fiber	3 g
Protein	3 g
Calcium	22 mg
Iron	0.8 mg

- **Preheat oven to 350°F (180°C)**
- **9- by 5-inch (23 by 12.5 cm) metal loaf pan, sprayed with nonstick cooking spray**

1¼ cups	whole wheat flour	300 mL
1¼ cups	natural bran	300 mL
1½ tsp	baking soda	7 mL
1 tsp	baking powder	5 mL
½ tsp	fine sea salt	2 mL
½ tsp	ground nutmeg	2 mL
1 cup	mashed bananas	250 mL
¾ cup	nonfat plain yogurt	175 mL
½ cup	pure maple syrup, brown rice syrup or liquid honey	125 mL
¼ cup	vegetable oil	60 mL

1. In a large bowl, whisk together flour, bran, baking soda, baking powder, salt and nutmeg.
2. In a medium bowl, combine bananas, yogurt, maple syrup and oil until well blended.
3. Add the banana mixture to the flour mixture and stir until just blended.
4. Spread batter evenly in prepared pan.
5. Bake in preheated oven for 55 to 60 minutes or until top is golden brown and a toothpick inserted in the center comes out clean. Let cool in pan on a wire rack for 10 minutes, then transfer to the rack to cool.

Superfood Spotlight

Nutmeg • Nutmeg is the fruit of an evergreen that is native to Indonesia and now grown in several countries. The spice is made from the seed of this fruit. Like many other spices, nutmeg has antibacterial action and can help protect us from food poisoning bacteria, such as *E. coli*. The spice has been used to treat Crohn's disease, an inflammatory condition of the bowel, and it is said that the essential oil of the fruit can help painful gums.

Whole Wheat Focaccia

Makes 24 slices

✪ Great for Steps 4 and 5

The taste and texture of this rosemary-scented focaccia make it a winner, but the whole wheat flour — high in fiber, magnesium and tryptophan — elevates it to star status.

Storage Tip

Store the cooled focaccia, wrapped in foil or plastic wrap, at room temperature for up to 2 days. Alternatively, wrap it in plastic wrap, then foil, completely enclosing bread, and freeze for up to 3 months. Let thaw at room temperature for 4 to 6 hours before serving.

Nutrients per slice

Calories	66
Total fat	3 g
Saturated fat	0 g
Cholesterol	0 mg
Sodium	117 mg
Carbohydrate	11 g
Fiber	2 g
Protein	3 g
Calcium	5 mg
Iron	0.6 mg

- **Large baking sheet, sprayed with nonstick cooking spray (preferably olive oil)**

2 cups	lukewarm water	500 mL
4 tbsp	extra virgin olive oil, divided	60 mL
1 tbsp	liquid honey or brown rice syrup	15 mL
2¼ tsp	active dry yeast	11 mL
3 cups	whole wheat flour	750 mL
3 tbsp	vital wheat gluten	45 mL
1 tsp	fine sea salt	5 mL
	Nonstick cooking spray (preferably olive oil)	
1 tbsp	chopped fresh rosemary	15 mL

1. In a large bowl, combine water, 3 tbsp (45 mL) of the oil, and honey. Sprinkle with yeast. Let stand for about 5 minutes or until foamy.
2. Using a wooden spoon, stir in flour, gluten and salt until blended and sticky. Transfer to a large bowl sprayed with cooking spray. Cover with plastic wrap sprayed with cooking spray. Let rise in a warm, draft-free spot for about 50 minutes or until doubled in bulk.
3. Turn dough out onto a well-floured surface. With floured hands, knead for 30 to 60 seconds or until smooth. Transfer dough to prepared baking sheet and pat into a 13- by 11-inch (33 by 28 cm) rectangle. Cover with a kitchen towel and let rise in a warm, draft-free spot for 1 hour.
4. Meanwhile, preheat oven to 425°F (220°C).
5. Poke indentations all over top of bread with your fingertips. Brush dough with the remaining oil and sprinkle with rosemary.
6. Bake for 25 to 30 minutes or until golden brown. Let cool on pan on a wire rack for at least 20 minutes before slicing.

Whole Wheat Pizza Dough

Makes two 1-lb (500 g) balls

✪ Great for Step 5

Enjoy nutritious and delicious pizza any time by making a batch (or two) of this fantastic dough and freezing it in 1-lb (500 g) balls. One batch of dough makes enough for two large pizza shells or eight individual ones.

Tip

For recipes using this dough, see pages 241–247.

2 cups	lukewarm water	500 mL
1/4 cup	vegetable oil	60 mL
2 tbsp	liquid honey or brown rice syrup	30 mL
1 1/2 tbsp	active dry yeast	22 mL
4 cups	whole wheat flour	1 L
3 tbsp	vital wheat gluten	45 mL
1 1/2 tsp	fine sea salt	7 mL
	Nonstick cooking spray	

1. In a large bowl, combine water, oil and honey. Sprinkle with yeast. Let stand for about 5 minutes or until foamy.
2. Using a wooden spoon, stir in flour, gluten and salt until blended and sticky. Transfer to a large bowl sprayed with cooking spray. Cover with plastic wrap sprayed with cooking spray. Let rise in a warm, draft-free spot for about 1 hour or until dough is doubled in bulk.
3. Turn dough out onto a well-floured surface. With floured hands, knead for 30 to 60 seconds or until smooth. Divide into two equal balls.
4. Use immediately or, to freeze, set balls of dough on a plate, far enough apart that they do not touch. Freeze for about 1 hour or until firm. Transfer each ball to a freezer bag and freeze for up to 3 months. To thaw, place the frozen ball of dough in a medium bowl coated with nonstick cooking spray (to prevent sticking). Loosely cover with plastic wrap and thaw overnight in the refrigerator. Let dough come to room temperature (about 30 minutes) before rolling.

Nutrients per 1/8 dough ball	
Calories	138
Total fat	4 g
Saturated fat	0 g
Cholesterol	0 mg
Sodium	214 mg
Carbohydrate	25 g
Fiber	4 g
Protein	5 g
Calcium	11 mg
Iron	1.2 mg

No-Knead Whole Wheat Dinner Rolls

Makes 12 rolls

✪ Great for Steps 3 and 5

These whole wheat rolls will impress one and all with their tender texture and nutty flavor. Don't tell anyone how incredibly easy they were to prepare!

Tip

Use any variety of milk in this recipe, but to keep it relatively low in overall fat, opt for lower-fat or skim (nonfat) milk.

Storage Tip

Store the cooled rolls, wrapped in foil or plastic wrap, at room temperature for up to 3 days. Alternatively, wrap them in plastic wrap, then foil, completely enclosing rolls, and freeze for up to 3 months. Let thaw at room temperature for 4 to 6 hours before serving.

Nutrients per roll	
Calories	116
Total fat	4 g
Saturated fat	0 g
Cholesterol	15 mg
Sodium	103 mg
Carbohydrate	19 g
Fiber	2 g
Protein	4 g
Calcium	10 mg
Iron	0.9 mg

- **12-cup muffin pan, sprayed with nonstick cooking spray**

1 cup	lukewarm milk	250 mL
3 tbsp	vegetable oil	45 mL
2 tbsp	liquid honey or pure maple syrup	30 mL
2¼ tsp	active dry yeast	11 mL
2¼ cups	whole wheat flour	550 mL
2 tsp	vital wheat gluten	10 mL
½ tsp	fine sea salt	2 mL
1	large egg, at room temperature, beaten	1
	Nonstick cooking spray	

1. In a large bowl, combine milk, oil and honey. Sprinkle with yeast. Let stand for about 5 minutes or until foamy.
2. Using a wooden spoon, stir in flour, gluten, salt and egg until blended and sticky. Transfer to a large bowl sprayed with cooking spray. Cover with plastic wrap sprayed with cooking spray. Let rise in a warm, draft-free spot for about 1 hour or until doubled in bulk.
3. Gently fold dough with a wooden spoon to deflate it. Divide equally among prepared muffin cups. Let rise in a warm, draft-free spot for about 1 hour or until doubled in bulk.
4. Meanwhile, preheat oven to 400°F (200°C).
5. Bake for 15 to 20 minutes or until golden brown. Let cool in pan on a wire rack for 3 minutes, then transfer to the rack to cool.

▸ Health Note

In a 2003 study in the *American Journal of Clinical Nutrition*, Harvard Medical School researchers who had followed 74,000 women over a 12-year period found that those who consumed the most dietary fiber from whole grains were 49% less likely to gain weight than those who ate foods made from refined grains.

Whole Wheat Buttermilk Biscuits

Makes 12 biscuits

✪ Great for Steps 3 and 5

Who knew whole wheat biscuits could be so, well, fabulous? They've got great substance, too, with a satisfyingly golden exterior and a pillowy interior that begs for a drizzle of honey. Buttermilk is the key ingredient to the flavor and texture.

Storage Tip

Store the cooled biscuits in an airtight container at room temperature for up to 2 days or in the freezer for up to 3 months. Let thaw at room temperature for 1 to 2 hours before serving.

Nutrients per biscuit	
Calories	91
Total fat	3 g
Saturated fat	1 g
Cholesterol	6 mg
Sodium	239 mg
Carbohydrate	14 g
Fiber	2 g
Protein	3 g
Calcium	50 mg
Iron	0.2 mg

- **Preheat oven to 425°F (220°C)**
- **Large rimmed baking sheet, lined with parchment paper**

2 cups	whole wheat pastry flour	500 mL
2 tsp	baking powder	10 mL
1/2 tsp	baking soda	2 mL
1/2 tsp	fine sea salt	2 mL
2 tbsp	cold unsalted butter, cut into small pieces	30 mL
3/4 cup	1% buttermilk	175 mL
1 tbsp	vegetable oil	15 mL
1 tbsp	liquid honey or pure maple syrup	15 mL
1 tbsp	1% buttermilk	15 mL

1. In a large bowl, whisk together flour, baking powder, baking soda and salt. Using a pastry blender or two knives, cut in butter until crumbly.
2. In a small bowl, whisk together 3/4 cup (175 mL) buttermilk, oil and honey until well blended.
3. Add the buttermilk mixture to the flour mixture and stir until just blended.
4. Turn dough out onto a lightly floured surface and knead briefly until dough comes together. Gently pat into an 8- by 6-inch (20 by 15 cm) rectangle about 3/4 inch (2 cm) thick. Cut into twelve 2-inch (5 cm) squares and place 2 inches (5 cm) apart on prepared baking sheet. Brush with 1 tbsp (15 mL) buttermilk.
5. Bake in preheated oven for 12 to 16 minutes or until golden brown. Transfer biscuits to a wire rack and let cool slightly. Serve warm.

▸ Health Note

Buttermilk is a good source of calcium and protein. It is also rich in vitamins A, B_{12}, E and K, potassium, phosphorous, selenium and essential probiotics.

Multi-Seed Spelt Biscuits

Makes 16 biscuits

✪ Great for Steps 3, 4 and 5

Spelt is a very nutritious ancient grain with a nutty flavor. When ground into flour, it yields incredibly delicious baked goods.

Storage Tip

Store the cooled biscuits in an airtight container at room temperature for up to 2 days or in the freezer for up to 3 months. Let thaw at room temperature for 1 to 2 hours before serving.

- **Preheat oven to 450°F (230°C)**
- **Large rimmed baking sheet, lined with parchment paper**

2 cups	whole-grain spelt flour	500 mL
½ cup	stone-ground cornmeal	125 mL
1 tbsp	sesame seeds	15 mL
1 tbsp	poppy seeds	15 mL
1 tbsp	fennel seeds	15 mL
1½ tsp	baking soda	7 mL
½ tsp	baking powder	2 mL
½ tsp	fine sea salt	2 mL
¼ cup	cold non-hydrogenated vegetable shortening, cut into small pieces	60 mL
1 cup	1% buttermilk	250 mL
2 tbsp	liquid honey or brown rice syrup	30 mL

1. In a large bowl, whisk together flour, cornmeal, sesame seeds, poppy seeds, fennel seeds, baking soda, baking powder and salt. Using a pastry blender or two knives, cut in shortening until crumbly.
2. In a small bowl, whisk together buttermilk and honey until well blended.
3. Add the buttermilk mixture to the flour mixture and stir until just blended.
4. Turn dough out onto a lightly floured surface and knead briefly until dough comes together. Gently pat into an 8-inch (20 cm) square about ½ inch (1 cm) thick. Cut into sixteen 2-inch (5 cm) squares and place 2 inches (5 cm) apart on prepared baking sheet.
5. Bake in preheated oven for 13 to 17 minutes or until golden brown. Transfer biscuits to a wire rack and let cool slightly. Serve warm.

▶ Health Note

Spelt is an excellent source of vitamin B_2, a very good source of manganese and a good source of niacin, thiamin and copper.

Nutrients per biscuit

Calories	118
Total fat	5 g
Saturated fat	1 g
Cholesterol	1 mg
Sodium	205 mg
Carbohydrate	18 g
Fiber	2 g
Protein	4 g
Calcium	66 mg
Iron	0.8 mg

Pumpkin Biscuits

Makes 12 biscuits

✪ Great for Steps 2, 3, 4 and 5

Pumpkin adds lovely color, subtle sweetness and moisture to these biscuits, with few calories and zero fat.

Tip

Use any variety of milk in this recipe, but to keep it relatively low in overall fat, opt for lower-fat or skim (nonfat) milk.

Storage Tip

Store the cooled biscuits in an airtight container at room temperature for up to 2 days or in the freezer for up to 3 months. Let thaw at room temperature for 1 to 2 hours before serving.

- **Preheat oven to 400°F (200°C)**
- **Large rimmed baking sheet, lined with parchment paper**

2 cups	whole wheat pastry flour	500 mL
2 tsp	baking powder	10 mL
1 tsp	ground cinnamon	5 mL
1/2 tsp	fine sea salt	2 mL
1/3 cup	cold non-hydrogenated vegetable shortening, cut into small pieces	75 mL
1 cup	pumpkin purée (not pie filling)	250 mL
1/3 cup	milk	75 mL
1 tbsp	pure maple syrup or liquid honey	15 mL

1. In a large bowl, whisk together flour, baking powder, cinnamon and salt. Using a pastry blender or two knives, cut in shortening until crumbly.
2. In a small bowl, whisk together pumpkin, milk and maple syrup until well blended.
3. Add the pumpkin mixture to the flour mixture and stir until just blended.
4. Turn dough out onto a lightly floured surface and knead briefly until dough comes together. Gently pat into an 8- by 6-inch (20 by 15 cm) rectangle about 3/4 inch (2 cm) thick. Cut into twelve 2-inch (5 cm) squares and place 2 inches (5 cm) apart on prepared baking sheet.
5. Bake in preheated oven for 13 to 17 minutes or until golden brown. Transfer biscuits to a wire rack and let cool slightly. Serve warm.

▸ Health Note

Pumpkin is chock full of powerful antioxidants known as carotenoids, organic pigments that may help ward off heart disease and various types of cancer, as well as cataracts and macular degeneration.

Nutrients per biscuit	
Calories	111
Total fat	5 g
Saturated fat	1 g
Cholesterol	1 mg
Sodium	228 mg
Carbohydrate	15 g
Fiber	3 g
Protein	3 g
Calcium	46 mg
Iron	0.4 mg

Lemon Drop Scones

Makes 12 scones

✪ Great for Steps 3, 4 and 5

Honey gives these scones a gentle boost of sweetness, yogurt provides the tender texture and fresh lemon adds a bright zing.

Tip

An equal amount of white whole wheat flour may be used in place of the whole wheat pastry flour. Alternatively, use half whole wheat flour and half unbleached all-purpose flour.

Storage Tip

Store the cooled scones in an airtight container at room temperature for up to 2 days or in the freezer for up to 3 months. Let thaw at room temperature for 1 to 2 hours before serving.

Nutrients per scone	
Calories	119
Total fat	4 g
Saturated fat	2 g
Cholesterol	23 mg
Sodium	179 mg
Carbohydrate	19 g
Fiber	2 g
Protein	3 g
Calcium	61 mg
Iron	0.3 mg

- **Preheat oven to 400°F (200°C)**
- **Large rimmed baking sheet, lined with parchment paper**

2 cups	whole wheat pastry flour	500 mL
2 tsp	baking powder	10 mL
1/2 tsp	baking soda	2 mL
1/4 tsp	fine sea salt	1 mL
1	large egg	1
1 cup	nonfat plain yogurt	250 mL
1/4 cup	liquid honey	60 mL
3 tbsp	unsalted butter, melted	45 mL
2 tsp	finely grated lemon zest	10 mL
2 tbsp	freshly squeezed lemon juice	30 mL
1 tbsp	vegetable oil	15 mL

1. In a large bowl, whisk together flour, baking powder, baking soda and salt.
2. In a medium bowl, whisk together egg, yogurt, honey, butter, lemon zest, lemon juice and oil until well blended.
3. Add the egg mixture to the flour mixture and stir until just blended.
4. Drop dough by 1/4 cup (60 mL) measures 2 inches (5 cm) apart on prepared baking sheet.
5. Bake in preheated oven for 14 to 19 minutes or until tops are golden brown and a toothpick inserted in the center comes out clean. Let cool on pan on a wire rack for 5 minutes, then transfer to the rack to cool for 5 minutes. Serve warm or let cool completely.

Variations

Replace the butter and oil with 1/4 cup (60 mL) coconut oil, warmed.

Use the zest and juice of any citrus fruit, such as orange, tangerine or lime.

Gently fold in 1/2 cup (125 mL) raisins, dried cranberries, chopped dates or dried cherries at the end of step 3.

For an extra burst of lemon flavor, combine 1/2 cup (125 mL) confectioners' (icing) sugar, 1/2 tsp (2 mL) finely grated lemon zest and 1 tbsp (15 mL) freshly squeezed lemon juice. Drizzle glaze over warm scones.

Maple Oat Drop Scones

Makes 12 scones

✪ Great for Steps 3, 4 and 5

Tangy buttermilk is the catalyst that makes a trio of flavors — maple, cinnamon and vanilla — jump out of the tender interiors of these lovely oat scones.

Tip

An equal amount of white whole wheat flour may be used in place of the whole wheat pastry flour. Alternatively, use half whole wheat flour and half unbleached all-purpose flour.

Storage Tip

Store the cooled scones in an airtight container at room temperature for up to 2 days or in the freezer for up to 3 months. Let thaw at room temperature for 1 to 2 hours before serving.

Nutrients per scone	
Calories	159
Total fat	7 g
Saturated fat	3 g
Cholesterol	22 mg
Sodium	249 mg
Carbohydrate	24 g
Fiber	3 g
Protein	4 g
Calcium	73 mg
Iron	0.7 mg

- **Preheat oven to 400°F (200°C)**
- **Large rimmed baking sheet, lined with parchment paper**

2¼ cups	whole wheat pastry flour	550 mL
1 cup	large-flake (old-fashioned) rolled oats	250 mL
2½ tsp	baking powder	12 mL
1 tsp	ground cinnamon	5 mL
¾ tsp	baking soda	3 mL
½ tsp	fine sea salt	2 mL
1	large egg	1
1 cup	1% buttermilk	250 mL
¼ cup	unsalted butter, melted and cooled slightly	60 mL
¼ cup	pure maple syrup	60 mL
2 tbsp	vegetable oil	30 mL
1 tbsp	vanilla extract	15 mL

1. In a large bowl, whisk together flour, oats, baking powder, cinnamon, baking soda and salt.
2. In a medium bowl, whisk together egg, buttermilk, butter, maple syrup, oil and vanilla until well blended.
3. Add the egg mixture to the flour mixture and stir until just blended.
4. Drop dough by ⅓ cup (75 mL) measures 2 inches (5 cm) apart on prepared baking sheet.
5. Bake in preheated oven for 16 to 21 minutes or until tops are golden brown and a toothpick inserted in the center comes out clean. Let cool on pan on a wire rack for 5 minutes, then transfer to the rack to cool for 5 minutes. Serve warm or let cool completely.

Variations

Replace the butter and oil with 6 tbsp (90 mL) of coconut oil, warmed.

Gently fold in ½ cup (125 mL) raisins, dried cranberries, chopped dates or dried cherries at the end of step 3.

Scottish Oat Cakes

Makes 24 oat cakes

✪ Great for Steps 4 and 5

Combining the crunch of a cracker with the tenderness of an oat scone, these little numbers are especially delectable. Spread them with jam or marmalade in the morning, top them with cheese at lunch, or serve them alongside soup at supper. And for heaven's sake, make sure they are present at teatime.

Storage Tip

Store the cooled oat cakes in an airtight container at room temperature for up to 5 days or in the freezer for up to 3 months. Let thaw at room temperature for 1 to 2 hours before serving.

- **Preheat oven to 325°F (160°C)**
- **Food processor**
- **2½-inch (6 cm) round cookie cutter**
- **Large rimmed baking sheet, lined with parchment paper**

2 cups	large-flake (old-fashioned) rolled oats	500 mL
½ cup	whole wheat flour	125 mL
½ tsp	baking powder	2 mL
½ tsp	fine sea salt	2 mL
1	large egg, lightly beaten	1
2 tbsp	unsalted butter, melted	30 mL
2 tbsp	liquid honey	30 mL

1. In food processor, process oats until coarsely ground.
2. In a large bowl, whisk together ground oats, flour, baking powder and salt. Using a wooden spoon, stir in egg, butter and honey until just blended.
3. Turn dough out onto a floured surface and roll out to a ¼-inch (0.5 cm) thick rectangle. Using the cookie cutter, cut dough into circles, rerolling scraps. Place 1 inch (2.5 cm) apart on prepared baking sheet.
4. Bake in preheated oven for 20 to 25 minutes or until golden and set at the edges. Let cool on pan on a wire rack for 5 minutes, then transfer to the rack. Serve warm or let cool completely.

Variations

For an extra touch of sweetness, sprinkle the rounds with turbinado (raw) sugar before baking.

For a more savory finish, sprinkle the unbaked rounds with sea salt flakes.

Nutrients per oat cake	
Calories	51
Total fat	2 g
Saturated fat	1 g
Cholesterol	10 mg
Sodium	68 mg
Carbohydrate	8 g
Fiber	1 g
Protein	1 g
Calcium	5 mg
Iron	0.4 mg

Multi-Seed Supper Muffins

Makes 12 muffins

✪ Great for Steps 3, 4 and 5

An assortment of seeds — flax, sesame and poppy — adds intriguing flavor and crunch, not to mention antioxidants and protein, to these quick and simple supper muffins.

Tip

Use any variety of milk in this recipe, but to keep it relatively low in overall fat, opt for lower-fat or skim (nonfat) milk.

Storage Tip

Store the cooled muffins in an airtight container at room temperature for up to 2 days or in the freezer for up to 3 months. Let thaw at room temperature for 1 to 2 hours before serving.

- **Preheat oven to 400°F (200°C)**
- **12-cup muffin pan, sprayed with nonstick cooking spray**

2 cups	whole wheat pastry flour	500 mL
3 tbsp	sesame seeds, divided	45 mL
2 tbsp	flax seeds	30 mL
1 tbsp	poppy seeds	15 mL
1 tbsp	baking powder	15 mL
1/2 tsp	fine sea salt	2 mL
1	large egg	1
1/4 cup	extra virgin olive oil	60 mL
2 tsp	Dijon mustard	10 mL
1 1/4 cups	milk	300 mL

1. In a large bowl, whisk together flour, 2 tbsp (30 mL) of the sesame seeds, flax seeds, poppy seeds, baking powder and salt.
2. In a medium bowl, whisk together egg, oil and mustard until well blended. Whisk in milk until blended.
3. Add the egg mixture to the flour mixture and stir until just blended.
4. Divide batter equally among prepared muffin cups. Sprinkle with the remaining sesame seeds.
5. Bake in preheated oven for 16 to 20 minutes or until tops are golden and a toothpick inserted in the center comes out clean. Let cool in pan on a wire rack for 5 minutes, then transfer to the rack. Serve warm or let cool completely.

Superfood Spotlight

Sesame Seeds • Sesame seeds contain two special types of fiber, sesamin and sesamolin, which are members of the lignans group and can lower "bad" cholesterol and help prevent high blood pressure. Sesamin is a powerful antioxidant in its own right and has been shown to protect the liver from damage. Plant sterols contained in sesame seeds also have a cholesterol-lowering action. The seeds are particularly rich in copper, which may be of use to arthritis sufferers because it is thought to have an anti-inflammatory action, reducing pain and swelling. Finally, sesame seeds provide iron, zinc, calcium and potassium in varying quantities.

Nutrients per muffin	
Calories	131
Total fat	7 g
Saturated fat	1 g
Cholesterol	17 mg
Sodium	203 mg
Carbohydrate	14 g
Fiber	2 g
Protein	4 g
Calcium	94 mg
Iron	0.5 mg

Maple Whole Wheat Muffins

Makes 12 muffins

✪ Great for Steps 3 and 5

Maple syrup gives these versatile whole wheat muffins a gentle boost of sweetness and flavor. Buttermilk makes them a good source of calcium, while whole wheat flour provides vitamins B and E.

Storage Tip

Store the cooled muffins in an airtight container at room temperature for up to 2 days or in the freezer for up to 3 months. Let thaw at room temperature for 1 to 2 hours before serving.

Nutrients per muffin	
Calories	158
Total fat	6 g
Saturated fat	1 g
Cholesterol	17 mg
Sodium	231 mg
Carbohydrate	25 g
Fiber	2 g
Protein	4 g
Calcium	51 mg
Iron	0.8 mg

- **Preheat oven to 400°F (200°C)**
- **12-cup muffin pan, sprayed with nonstick cooking spray**

2 cups	whole wheat flour	500 mL
1 tsp	baking soda	5 mL
1/2 tsp	fine sea salt	2 mL
1	large egg	1
1/2 cup	pure maple syrup, brown rice syrup or liquid honey	125 mL
1/3 cup	vegetable oil	75 mL
1 tsp	vanilla extract	5 mL
1 1/3 cups	1% buttermilk	325 mL

1. In a large bowl, whisk together flour, baking soda and salt.
2. In a medium bowl, whisk together egg, maple syrup, oil and vanilla until well blended. Whisk in buttermilk until blended.
3. Add the egg mixture to the flour mixture and stir until just blended.
4. Divide batter equally among prepared muffin cups.
5. Bake in preheated oven for 15 to 20 minutes or until tops are golden and a toothpick inserted in the center comes out clean. Let cool in pan on a wire rack for 3 minutes, then transfer to the rack to cool.

Variation

Gently fold in 3/4 cup (175 mL) chopped dried fruit (such as figs, dates, cranberries, apples or raisins) or chopped toasted nuts (such as pecans, walnuts or almonds) at the end of step 3.

Gluten-Free Flax Muffins

Makes 12 muffins

✪ Great for Steps 3, 4 and 5

Gluten-free baking can look a bit fussy, and the reality is that some recipes are, requiring three or more varieties of flour and some complicated steps. But this one is limited to two flours and scraps the fuss entirely. The result is an irresistible muffin that can be varied any which way with flavors you love (see variations, below).

Storage Tip

Store the cooled muffins in an airtight container at room temperature for up to 2 days or in the freezer for up to 3 months. Let thaw at room temperature for 1 to 2 hours before serving.

Nutrients per muffin	
Calories	163
Total fat	6 g
Saturated fat	1 g
Cholesterol	31 mg
Sodium	179 mg
Carbohydrate	22 g
Fiber	3 g
Protein	5 g
Calcium	27 mg
Iron	0.6 mg

- **Preheat oven to 375°F (190°C)**
- **12-cup muffin pan, sprayed with nonstick cooking spray**

3/4 cup	brown rice flour	175 mL
3/4 cup	buckwheat flour	175 mL
1/2 cup	ground flax seeds (flaxseed meal)	125 mL
1 tsp	baking soda	5 mL
1/4 tsp	fine sea salt	1 mL
2	large eggs	2
1 cup	1% buttermilk	250 mL
1/2 cup	unsweetened applesauce	125 mL
1/3 cup	liquid honey or brown rice syrup	75 mL
1/4 cup	vegetable oil	60 mL

1. In a large bowl, whisk together brown rice flour, buckwheat flour, flax seeds, baking soda and salt.
2. In a medium bowl, whisk together eggs, buttermilk, applesauce, honey and oil until well blended.
3. Add the egg mixture to the flour mixture and stir until just blended.
4. Divide batter equally among prepared muffin cups.
5. Bake in preheated oven for 25 to 30 minutes or until tops are golden and a toothpick inserted in the center comes out clean. Let cool in pan on a wire rack for 5 minutes, then transfer to the rack to cool.

Variations

Cinnamon Raisin Muffins: Add 1 tsp (5 mL) ground cinnamon to the flour mixture. Gently fold in 1/2 cup (125 mL) raisins at the end of step 3.

Dried Berry Muffins: Add 1/2 tsp (2 mL) almond extract to the egg mixture. Gently fold in 1/2 cup (125 mL) dried blueberries or cranberries at the end of step 3.

Spice Muffins: Add 1 tsp (5 mL) ground cinnamon, 1 tsp (5 mL) ground ginger, 1/4 tsp (1 mL) ground nutmeg and 1/8 tsp (0.5 mL) ground cloves to the flour mixture.

Natural Sugar Sweets

Decadent Chocolate Cake . . . 494
Whole Wheat Maple Bundt Cake . . . 495
Yogurt Cake with Fresh Berries . . . 496
Honey Apple Cake . . . 497
Whole Wheat Maple Applesauce Cake . . . 498
Spiced Carrot Cake with Currants . . . 499
Fresh Ginger Gingerbread . . . 500
Healthy Know-How: Go Nuts for Good Health . . . 501
Five-Minute Cheesecake Cups with Raspberries . . . 501
Maple Pumpkin Micro-Pies . . . 502
Berry Peach Crumbles . . . 503
Cherry Clafouti . . . 504
Baked Apples with Walnuts and Dried Cherries . . . 505
Honey-Roasted Plums with Ricotta . . . 506
Minted Fruit Salad . . . 507
Goat Cheese and Pistachio–Stuffed Dates . . . 507
Cocoa Truffles . . . 508
No-Bake Raspberry Thumbprints . . . 509
Oatmeal Cookies . . . 510
Maple Spice Cookies . . . 511
Soft Apple Cookies . . . 512
Pumpkin Cranberry Cookies . . . 513

Whole Wheat and Olive Oil Biscotti 514
Double Almond Chocolate Biscotti 515
Crispy Brown Rice Treats 516
Date Bars 517
Black Bean Brownies 518
Ricotta Pudding with Strawberry Coulis 519
Maple Brown Rice Pudding with Dried Cherries 520
Strawberry Mousse 520
Chocolate Pudding 521
Lemon Blackberry Fool 522
All-Natural Fruit Gelatin (*Kanten*) 523
Kiwi Sorbet 523
Chocolate Gelato 524
Vanilla Cashew Ice Cream 525
Blueberry Lemon Nice Cream 526
Healthy Know-How: Dietary Fat 101 527
Instant Strawberry Frozen Yogurt 527
Lemon Raspberry Yogurt Cones 528
Blueberry Yogurt Pops 529
Very Berry Ice Pops 530
Chocolate-Dipped Frozen Bananas 531
Cashew Vanilla "Whipped Cream" 532

Decadent Chocolate Cake

Makes 8 servings

✪ Great for Steps 4 and 5

It is a stunning but true fact that many people are able to will themselves not to eat chocolate — all for the sake of their health and waistlines. For such folks, I offer this cake. Easy to make, grand to eat and, yes, good for you, too, it is a recipe I suspect you will make again and again.

Storage Tip

Store the cooled cake, loosely wrapped in foil or waxed paper, at room temperature for up to 1 week. Alternatively, wrap it in plastic wrap, then foil, completely enclosing cake, and freeze for up to 6 months. Let thaw at room temperature for 4 to 6 hours before serving.

Nutrients per serving	
Calories	224
Total fat	11 g
Saturated fat	1 g
Cholesterol	0 mg
Sodium	274 mg
Carbohydrate	30 g
Fiber	1 g
Protein	1 g
Calcium	6 mg
Iron	0.4 mg

- **Preheat oven to 350°F (180°C)**
- **8-inch (20 cm) square metal baking pan, sprayed with nonstick baking spray with flour**

1½ cups	whole wheat pastry flour	375 mL
¼ cup	unsweetened cocoa powder (not Dutch process)	60 mL
¾ tsp	baking soda	3 mL
½ tsp	fine sea salt	2 mL
½ cup	vegetable oil	125 mL
2 tsp	cider or white vinegar	10 mL
1½ tsp	vanilla extract	7 mL
1 cup	water	250 mL
¾ cup	brown rice syrup or liquid honey	175 mL

1. In a large bowl, whisk together flour, cocoa powder, baking soda and salt.
2. Using the end of a wooden spoon, make one large and two small holes in flour mixture. Add oil to large hole, vinegar to one of the small holes and vanilla to the other small hole. Pour water and brown rice syrup over top and stir until just blended.
3. Immediately pour batter into prepared pan.
4. Bake in preheated oven for 27 to 32 minutes or until a toothpick inserted in the center comes out clean. Let cool completely in pan on a wire rack.

Whole Wheat Maple Bundt Cake

Makes 12 servings

✪ Great for Steps 4 and 5

Though this modern version of a homespun cake pairs wonderfully with fresh fruit (think berries, peaches and apples), it is perhaps at its finest served straight-up.

Tip

This cake is also delicious made with liquid honey instead of maple syrup.

Storage Tip

Store the cooled cake at room temperature in a cake keeper, or loosely wrapped in foil or plastic wrap, for up to 3 days. Alternatively, wrap it in plastic wrap, then foil, completely enclosing cake, and freeze for up to 6 months. Let thaw at room temperature for 4 to 6 hours before serving.

Nutrients per serving	
Calories	261
Total fat	9 g
Saturated fat	1 g
Cholesterol	0 mg
Sodium	294 mg
Carbohydrate	48 g
Fiber	3 g
Protein	4 g
Calcium	86 mg
Iron	0.5 mg

- **Preheat oven to 325°F (160°C)**
- **10-inch (25 cm) Bundt pan, greased and floured with whole wheat pastry flour**

3½ cups	whole wheat pastry flour	875 mL
2 tsp	baking powder	10 mL
2 tsp	baking soda	10 mL
2 tsp	ground cinnamon	10 mL
½ tsp	fine sea salt	2 mL
1½ cups	pure maple syrup	375 mL
⅔ cup	vegetable oil	150 mL
2 tbsp	vanilla extract	30 mL
1 tbsp	cider or white vinegar	15 mL

1. In a large bowl, whisk together flour, baking powder, baking soda, cinnamon and salt.
2. Add maple syrup, oil, vanilla and vinegar to flour mixture. Using an electric mixer on medium speed, beat for 1 minute, until blended. Scrape sides and bottom of bowl with a spatula. Beat on high speed for 2 minutes.
3. Spread batter evenly in prepared pan.
4. Bake in preheated oven for about 55 minutes or until a piece of uncooked spaghetti inserted in the center comes out with a few moist crumbs attached. Let cool in pan on a wire rack for 10 minutes, then invert cake onto rack to cool completely.

Yogurt Cake with Fresh Berries

Makes 12 servings

✪ Great for Steps 1, 3, 4 and 5

This light-as-can-be cake has an easy sophistication. An ample amount of yogurt, chock full of calcium and protein, is part of the cake's secret, as well its healthfulness. Fresh berries, high in vitamin C and manganese, are the perfect complement.

Storage Tip

Store the cooled cake at room temperature in a cake keeper, or loosely wrapped in foil or plastic wrap, for up to 3 days. Alternatively, wrap it in plastic wrap, then foil, completely enclosing cake, and freeze for up to 6 months. Let thaw at room temperature for 4 to 6 hours before serving.

Nutrients per serving	
Calories	219
Total fat	7 g
Saturated fat	1 g
Cholesterol	45 mg
Sodium	125 mg
Carbohydrate	40 g
Fiber	2 g
Protein	5 g
Calcium	61 mg
Iron	0.5 mg

- **Preheat oven to 350°F (180°C)**
- **9-inch (23 cm) square metal baking pan, sprayed with nonstick cooking spray**

2 cups	whole wheat pastry flour	500 mL
1½ tsp	baking powder	7 mL
½ tsp	baking soda	2 mL
¼ tsp	fine sea salt	1 mL
3	large eggs, at room temperature	3
1 cup	nonfat plain yogurt	250 mL
1 cup	liquid honey	250 mL
⅓ cup	vegetable oil	75 mL
1 tbsp	finely grated orange or lemon zest	15 mL
2 cups	berries (such as raspberries, blackberries, blueberries, sliced strawberries or a combination)	500 mL

1. In a large bowl, whisk together flour, baking powder, baking soda and salt.
2. Add eggs, yogurt, honey, oil and orange zest to flour mixture. Using an electric mixer on medium-low speed, beat for 1 minute, until blended. Scrape sides and bottom of bowl with a spatula. Beat on medium speed for 1 minute.
3. Spread batter evenly in prepared pan.
4. Bake in preheated oven for 45 minutes or until a toothpick inserted in the center comes out with a few moist crumbs attached. Let cool in pan on a wire rack for 10 minutes, then invert cake onto rack to cool completely. Cut into squares and serve with berries.

Honey Apple Cake

Makes 12 servings

✪ Great for Steps 1, 3, 4 and 5

Though it's quite irresistible when still warm from the oven, this moist apple cake is perfect potluck or picnic food, since it's also terrific cold or at room temperature.

Tip

Pure maple syrup may be used in place of the honey.

Storage Tip

Store the cooled cake at room temperature in a cake keeper, or loosely wrapped in foil or plastic wrap, for up to 3 days. Alternatively, wrap it in plastic wrap, then foil, completely enclosing cake, and freeze for up to 6 months. Let thaw at room temperature for 4 to 6 hours before serving.

Nutrients per serving	
Calories	204
Total fat	6 g
Saturated fat	1 g
Cholesterol	31 mg
Sodium	225 mg
Carbohydrate	36 g
Fiber	3 g
Protein	4 g
Calcium	66 mg
Iron	0.6 mg

- **Preheat oven to 350°F (180°C)**
- **9-inch (23 cm) square metal baking pan, sprayed with nonstick baking spray with flour**

2½ cups	whole wheat pastry flour	625 mL
2 tsp	baking powder	10 mL
2 tsp	ground cinnamon	10 mL
½ tsp	fine sea salt	2 mL
½ tsp	baking soda	2 mL
2	large eggs, at room temperature	2
1 cup	1% buttermilk	250 mL
¾ cup	liquid honey	175 mL
¼ cup	vegetable oil	60 mL
2 tsp	vanilla extract	10 mL
2 cups	chopped peeled tart-sweet apples (such as Gala, Braeburn or Golden Delicious)	500 mL

1. In a large bowl, whisk together flour, baking powder, cinnamon, salt and baking soda.
2. In a medium bowl, whisk together eggs, buttermilk, honey, oil and vanilla until well blended.
3. Add the egg mixture to the flour mixture and stir until just blended. Gently fold in apples.
4. Spread batter evenly in prepared pan.
5. Bake in preheated oven for 45 to 50 minutes or until a toothpick inserted in the center comes out with a few moist crumbs attached. Let cool in pan on a wire rack for 10 minutes, then invert cake onto rack to cool slightly or completely.

Whole Wheat Maple Applesauce Cake

Makes 12 servings

✪ Great for Steps 4 and 5

A perfect ending to any meal, this homey cake is made even better with whole wheat flour. And it will remind you why you still love applesauce as much now as you did when you were three.

Storage Tip

Store the cooled cake at room temperature in a cake keeper, or loosely wrapped in foil or plastic wrap, for up to 3 days. Alternatively, wrap it in plastic wrap, then foil, completely enclosing cake, and freeze for up to 6 months. Let thaw at room temperature for 4 to 6 hours before serving.

Nutrients per serving	
Calories	189
Total fat	6 g
Saturated fat	1 g
Cholesterol	30 mg
Sodium	205 mg
Carbohydrate	34 g
Fiber	3 g
Protein	4 g
Calcium	16 mg
Iron	1.0 mg

- **Preheat oven to 350°F (180°C)**
- **9-inch (23 cm) square metal baking pan, sprayed with nonstick cooking spray**

2 cups	whole wheat flour	500 mL
1½ tsp	ground cinnamon	7 mL
1 tsp	baking soda	5 mL
½ tsp	fine sea salt	2 mL
2	large eggs, at room temperature	2
1 cup	unsweetened applesauce	250 mL
¾ cup	pure maple syrup or liquid honey	175 mL
¼ cup	vegetable oil	60 mL
1 tsp	vanilla extract	5 mL
½ cup	chopped pecans (optional)	125 mL

1. In a large bowl, whisk together flour, cinnamon, baking soda and salt.
2. Add eggs, applesauce, maple syrup, oil and vanilla to flour mixture. Using an electric mixer on medium-low speed, beat for 1 minute, until blended. Scrape sides and bottom of bowl with a spatula. Beat on medium speed for 1 minute.
3. Spread batter evenly in prepared pan. If desired, sprinkle with pecans.
4. Bake in preheated oven for 32 to 38 minutes or until a toothpick inserted in the center comes out with a few moist crumbs attached. Let cool completely in pan on a wire rack.

Spiced Carrot Cake with Currants

Makes 16 servings

✪ Great for Steps 1, 4 and 5

A classic cake takes a healthy turn with whole wheat pastry flour, oats and maple syrup.

Tip

An equal amount of white whole wheat flour may be used in place of the whole wheat pastry flour. Alternatively, use half whole wheat flour and half unbleached all-purpose flour.

Storage Tip

Store the cooled cake at room temperature in a cake keeper, or loosely wrapped in foil or plastic wrap, for up to 3 days. Alternatively, wrap it in plastic wrap, then foil, completely enclosing cake, and freeze for up to 6 months. Let thaw at room temperature for 4 to 6 hours before serving.

Nutrients per serving	
Calories	187
Total fat	7 g
Saturated fat	2 g
Cholesterol	0 mg
Sodium	195 mg
Carbohydrate	32 g
Fiber	3 g
Protein	4 g
Calcium	39 mg
Iron	0.9 mg

- **Preheat oven to 325°F (160°C)**
- **Food processor**
- **9-inch (23 cm) square metal baking pan, sprayed with nonstick baking spray with flour**

1 cup	quick-cooking rolled oats	250 mL
1 cup	chopped walnuts or pecans	250 mL
1 cup	whole wheat pastry flour	250 mL
2 tsp	baking powder	10 mL
1 tsp	baking soda	5 mL
1 tsp	ground cinnamon	5 mL
½ tsp	ground ginger	2 mL
½ tsp	fine sea salt	2 mL
2 cups	shredded carrots	500 mL
⅔ cup	dried currants	150 mL
½ cup	unsweetened flaked coconut	125 mL
1 cup	pure maple syrup, brown rice syrup or liquid honey	250 mL
2 tsp	vanilla extract	10 mL

1. In food processor, combine oats and walnuts; pulse until coarsely ground.
2. In a large bowl, whisk together oat mixture, flour, baking powder, baking soda, cinnamon, ginger and salt.
3. In a medium bowl, combine carrots, currants, coconut, maple syrup and vanilla.
4. Add the carrot mixture to the flour mixture and stir with a wooden spoon until blended.
5. Spread batter evenly in prepared pan.
6. Bake in preheated oven for 50 to 60 minutes or until a toothpick inserted in the center comes out with a few moist crumbs attached. Let cool completely in pan on a wire rack.

Fresh Ginger Gingerbread

Makes 10 servings

✪ Great for Steps 3, 4 and 5

Even if you're not a ginger lover, you're going to love this gingerbread. Freshly grated gingerroot and the rounded complexity of dark molasses lend it a rich flavor and an intoxicating scent.

Tips

An equal amount of white whole wheat flour may be used in place of the whole wheat pastry flour. Alternatively, use half whole wheat flour and half unbleached all-purpose flour.

For a milder-flavored cake, use pure maple syrup, brown rice syrup or additional liquid honey in place of the molasses.

Storage Tip

See page 499.

Nutrients per serving	
Calories	182
Total fat	8 g
Saturated fat	1 g
Cholesterol	19 mg
Sodium	120 mg
Carbohydrate	30 g
Fiber	1 g
Protein	3 g
Calcium	106 mg
Iron	2.5 mg

- **Preheat oven to 350°F (180°C)**
- **9-inch (23 cm) round metal baking pan, sprayed with nonstick cooking spray**

1¼ cups	whole wheat pastry flour	300 mL
1 tsp	ground cinnamon	5 mL
½ tsp	baking soda	2 mL
⅛ tsp	ground cloves	0.5 mL
⅛ tsp	fine sea salt	0.5 mL
2 tbsp	grated gingerroot	30 mL
1	large egg, at room temperature	1
½ cup	1% buttermilk	125 mL
½ cup	dark (cooking) molasses	125 mL
⅓ cup	vegetable oil	75 mL
⅓ cup	liquid honey	75 mL
1 tbsp	confectioners' (icing) sugar (optional)	15 mL

1. In a large bowl, whisk together flour, cinnamon, baking soda, cloves and salt.
2. Add ginger, egg, buttermilk, molasses, oil and honey to flour mixture. Using an electric mixer on medium-low speed, beat for 1 minute, until blended. Scrape sides and bottom of bowl with a spatula. Beat on medium speed for 1 minute.
3. Spread batter evenly in prepared pan.
4. Bake in preheated oven for 25 to 30 minutes or until a toothpick inserted in the center comes out with a few moist crumbs attached. Let cool in pan on a wire rack for 10 minutes, then invert cake onto rack to cool completely. If desired, sprinkle confectioners' sugar over top of cooled cake.

Healthy Know-How

Go Nuts for Good Health

Rich in polyunsaturated and monounsaturated fatty acids, walnuts, almonds and many other nuts can reduce blood cholesterol and help keep blood vessels healthy. According to the U.S. Food and Drug Administration, eating a handful (1½ oz/45 g) of nuts a day may reduce your risk of heart disease.

Although it varies by nut, most nuts contain at least some of these heart-healthy substances:

- **Unsaturated fats.** For reasons that are still not clear to researchers, monounsaturated and polyunsaturated fats help lower "bad" cholesterol levels.
- **Omega-3 fatty acids.** Many nuts are rich in omega-3 fatty acids, which, like the omega-3s found in oily fish, protect the heart.
- **Fiber.** Nuts are rich in fiber, which helps lower your cholesterol, makes you feel full longer and may play a role in preventing diabetes.
- **Vitamin E.** Many nuts have high levels of vitamin E, which can reduce the chances of heart disease by preventing the development of plaques in your arteries.
- **Plant sterols.** Some nuts contain plant sterols, a substance that may help lower cholesterol. Plant sterols are sometimes added to margarine and juice to increase their health benefits.
- **L-arginine.** Nuts provide l-arginine, a compound that may improve arterial health.

Five-Minute Cheesecake Cups with Raspberries

Makes 2 servings

✪ Great for Steps 1, 3 and 4

Nutrients per serving	
Calories	167
Total fat	4 g
Saturated fat	0 g
Cholesterol	5 mg
Sodium	321 mg
Carbohydrate	22 g
Fiber	1 g
Protein	17 g
Calcium	115 mg
Iron	0.8 mg

- **Food processor**
- **Two 6-oz (175 mL) ramekins or dessert glasses**

1 cup	nonfat cottage cheese	250 mL
1 tbsp	agave nectar or liquid honey	15 mL
½ tsp	vanilla extract	2 mL
⅔ cup	raspberries	150 mL
2 tbsp	finely chopped lightly salted roasted pistachios	30 mL

1. In food processor, combine cottage cheese, agave nectar and vanilla; purée until smooth.
2. Divide mixture between ramekins. Top with raspberries and pistachios.

Maple Pumpkin Micro-Pies

Makes 16 servings

✪ Great for Steps 2 and 4

These maple-pumpkin mini sweets — crispy, creamy and wonderfully spiced — are easy enough for a weeknight dessert and good enough for company.

Tips

These are best eaten soon after baking.

An equal amount of ground cinnamon may be used in place of the pumpkin pie spice.

Nutrients per serving	
Calories	43
Total fat	0 g
Saturated fat	0 g
Cholesterol	1 mg
Sodium	46 mg
Carbohydrate	11 g
Fiber	1 g
Protein	1 g
Calcium	7 mg
Iron	0.4 mg

- **Preheat oven to 400°F (200°C)**
- **Baking sheet, lined with parchment paper**

1 cup	pumpkin purée (not pie filling)	250 mL
1/4 cup	pure maple syrup, liquid honey or brown rice syrup	60 mL
1 tsp	pumpkin pie spice	5 mL
16	wonton wrappers	16
	Nonstick cooking spray	
1 tbsp	turbinado (raw) sugar	15 mL

1. In a medium bowl, whisk together pumpkin, maple syrup and pumpkin pie spice.
2. Place one wonton wrapper on a work surface. Spoon 1 tbsp (15 mL) filling into center of wrapper. Using a pastry brush or a fingertip, moisten the edges of the wrapper with water. Fold in half to form a triangle, pressing the edges to seal. Repeat with the remaining wontons and filling.
3. Arrange filled wontons on prepared baking sheet. Lightly spray both sides of wontons with cooking spray and sprinkle tops with turbinado sugar.
4. Bake in preheated oven for 14 minutes. Carefully turn wontons over and bake for 4 to 5 minutes or until golden. Let cool on pan on a wire rack.

Berry Peach Crumbles

Makes 4 servings

✪ Great for Steps 1, 2, 4 and 5

Summer's bounty gets even better when it's combined into a crumble-topped dessert.

Tip

Ripe peaches are soft, delicate and prone to bruising, which can make them difficult to peel. Fortunately, there's an easy way to do it. Fill a saucepan with enough water to fully submerge the peaches, and bring to a boil over high heat. Working with one peach at a time, use a slotted spoon to lower the peach into the boiling water for 30 to 45 seconds. Remove the peach and immediately submerge it in an ice water bath. You should then be able to easily pull off the skin of the peach with your fingers or a paring knife.

Nutrients per serving	
Calories	153
Total fat	6 g
Saturated fat	1 g
Cholesterol	0 mg
Sodium	2 mg
Carbohydrate	28 g
Fiber	2 g
Protein	2 g
Calcium	23 mg
Iron	1.0 mg

- **Preheat oven to 375°F (190°C)**
- **Four 6-oz (175 mL) ramekins, sprayed with nonstick cooking spray**
- **Rimmed baking sheet**

1 cup	blackberries or raspberries	250 mL
1 cup	diced peeled peaches (see tip, at left)	250 mL
1 tsp	cornstarch	5 mL
4 tsp	freshly squeezed orange juice	20 mL
1/2 tsp	vanilla extract	2 mL
1/4 cup	whole wheat flour	60 mL
1/4 cup	large-flake (old-fashioned) rolled oats	60 mL
2 tbsp	packed brown sugar	30 mL
1 tsp	ground cinnamon	5 mL
1/8 tsp	ground nutmeg	0.5 mL
1 1/2 tbsp	vegetable oil	22 mL
2 tsp	liquid honey	10 mL

1. In a medium bowl, gently toss blackberries, peaches, cornstarch, orange juice and vanilla.
2. In a small bowl, whisk together flour, oats, brown sugar, cinnamon and nutmeg. Add oil and honey, mixing with your fingertips until moist and crumbly.
3. Place prepared ramekins on baking sheet. Spoon fruit mixture into ramekins. Sprinkle with flour mixture.
4. Bake in preheated oven for 20 to 25 minutes or until fruit is bubbling and topping is golden brown. Let cool to room temperature before serving.

▸ Health Note

Blueberries get plenty of (well-deserved) bravado for their superfood attributes, but peaches are worth noting, too. In particular, peaches are a good source of lutein, the phytochemical that gives a red, orange or yellow color to fruits and vegetables. Lutein is especially beneficial in the prevention of heart disease, macular degeneration and cancer.

Cherry Clafouti

Makes 12 servings

✪ Great for Steps 2, 3, 4 and 5

Clafouti is something of a cross between a flan and a fruit-filled pancake. Traditional versions embrace cherries, but any fruit can be used, including apples, pears, peaches or plums. It will puff up dramatically during baking, then collapse. Let it cool slightly before serving, then chill the leftovers for a delicious breakfast treat the next morning.

Tips

A 9-inch (23 cm) glass pie plate may be used in place of the square baking dish. Cut the cooled clafouti into 12 wedges.

Use any variety of milk in this recipe, but to keep it relatively low in overall fat, opt for lower-fat or skin (nonfat) milk.

Nutrients per serving	
Calories	101
Total fat	3 g
Saturated fat	1 g
Cholesterol	47 mg
Sodium	146 mg
Carbohydrate	16 g
Fiber	1 g
Protein	4 g
Calcium	47 mg
Iron	0.5 mg

- **Preheat oven to 350°F (180°C)**
- **9-inch (23 cm) square glass baking dish, sprayed with nonstick cooking spray**
- **Blender, food processor or immersion blender**

3 cups	pitted fresh or frozen dark cherries, thawed and patted dry	750 mL
3	large eggs, at room temperature	3
1¼ cups	milk	300 mL
⅓ cup	liquid honey	75 mL
1 tsp	almond extract	5 mL
⅔ cup	whole wheat pastry flour	150 mL
⅛ tsp	fine sea salt	0.5 mL
2 tbsp	sliced almonds	30 mL
1 tbsp	confectioners' (icing) sugar (optional)	15 mL

1. Arrange cherries in prepared baking dish.
2. In blender (or in a tall cup, using an immersion blender), combine eggs, milk, honey and almond extract; process until just blended. Add flour and salt; pulse until just blended.
3. Pour batter evenly over cherries and sprinkle with almonds.
4. Bake in preheated oven for 45 to 50 minutes or until puffed and golden. Let cool in baking dish on a wire rack for about 20 minutes. If desired, sprinkle with confectioners' sugar. Cut into 12 squares and serve warm.

▸ Health Note

A growing body of science suggests that cherries, enjoyed fresh, dried, frozen or as juice, have among the highest levels of disease-fighting antioxidants of any fruits. They also contain other important nutrients, such as beta carotene (19 times more than blueberries or strawberries), vitamin C, potassium, magnesium, iron, fiber and folate. In addition, emerging evidence links cherries to many important health benefits, from helping to ease the pain of arthritis and gout to reducing risk factors for heart disease, diabetes and certain cancers.

Baked Apples with Walnuts and Dried Cherries

Makes 4 servings

✪ Great for Steps 1, 2, 3 and 4

After a rich main course in the colder months, you'll love the minimalist sensibility of these baked apples.

Tip

Other varieties of dried fruit, such as cranberries, blueberries or raisins, may be used in place of the cherries.

Storage Tip

Store the cooled apples, loosely covered in foil or plastic wrap, in the refrigerator for up to 1 day. Serve cold, or warm in the microwave on Medium (50%) for about 1 minute.

Nutrients per serving	
Calories	291
Total fat	6 g
Saturated fat	0 g
Cholesterol	0 mg
Sodium	92 mg
Carbohydrate	64 g
Fiber	7 g
Protein	5 g
Calcium	45 mg
Iron	1.2 mg

- **Preheat oven to 350°F (180°C)**
- **9-inch (23 cm) square glass baking dish or glass pie plate**

4	tart-sweet apples (such as Braeburn, Gala or Fuji), cored	4
1⁄3 cup	dried cherries	75 mL
1⁄3 cup	chopped toasted walnuts or pecans	75 mL
1⁄3 cup	crushed gingersnap cookies	75 mL
4 tbsp	pure maple syrup or liquid honey	60 mL
4 tbsp	nonfat plain Greek yogurt	60 mL

1. Using a vegetable peeler, peel top inch (2.5 cm) of apples. Place apples, top side up, in baking dish.
2. In a small bowl, combine cherries, walnuts and gingersnaps. Stuff cherry mixture into apple cavities. Drizzle 1 tbsp (15 mL) maple syrup over each apple.
3. Bake in preheated oven, brushing occasionally with accumulated juices, for 45 to 55 minutes or until apples are tender.
4. Transfer apples to a plate and pour pan juices over top. Serve each apple dolloped with 1 tbsp (15 mL) yogurt.

Honey–Roasted Plums with Ricotta

Makes 4 servings

✪ Great for Steps 1, 2, 3 and 4

A classic pairing like ricotta and honey invites fresh plums, roasted until their sweetness intensifies, to make this simple dish a symphony of flavor.

Tip

See page 29 for instructions on toasting nuts.

Nutrients per serving	
Calories	180
Total fat	2 g
Saturated fat	0 g
Cholesterol	7 mg
Sodium	110 mg
Carbohydrate	32 g
Fiber	2 g
Protein	13 g
Calcium	277 mg
Iron	0.5 mg

- **Preheat oven to 400°F (200°C)**
- **Large rimmed baking sheet, lined with parchment paper**

8	large red or purple plums, each cut into 8 wedges	8
2 tbsp	liquid honey, divided	30 mL
1⅓ cups	nonfat ricotta cheese	325 mL
2 tbsp	chopped toasted walnuts	30 mL

1. In a medium bowl, gently toss plums and half the honey. Arrange in a single layer on prepared baking sheet.
2. Roast in preheated oven for 15 to 20 minutes or until browned at the edges. Let cool completely on pan.
3. In a small bowl, combine cheese and the remaining honey.
4. Divide cheese mixture among four dessert dishes. Top with roasted plums and walnuts.

Superfood Spotlight

Plums • Plums come in many colors, from the more common red and purple varieties to yellow and white. They contain neochlorogenic and chlorogenic acids, phenolic compounds that are particularly effective at neutralizing free radicals, which contribute to disease and the aging process. These compounds seem to be especially beneficial in their antioxidant action on the fatty tissues in the brain, and help prevent damage to fats circulating in the blood. Raw red and purple plums are also rich in anthocyanins, the pigments that help prevent heart disease and cancers. Plums have a high water content and a low glycemic index, making them an excellent choice for dieters and diabetics, and are a good source of carotenes, for cancer protection and eye health.

Minted Fruit Salad

Makes 6 servings

✪ Great for Steps 1, 2 and 4

Nutrients per serving	
Calories	69
Total fat	0 g
Saturated fat	0 g
Cholesterol	0 mg
Sodium	3 mg
Carbohydrate	17 g
Fiber	4 g
Protein	1 g
Calcium	35 mg
Iron	0.6 mg

$1\frac{1}{2}$ cups	quartered hulled strawberries	375 mL
$1\frac{1}{2}$ cups	blackberries	375 mL
1 cup	fresh pineapple chunks, (see tip, page 367)	250 mL
1 cup	diced kiwifruit	250 mL
1 cup	loosely packed mint leaves, chopped	250 mL
1 tbsp	freshly squeezed lemon juice	15 mL
1 tbsp	agave nectar or liquid honey	15 mL

1. In a large bowl, gently toss strawberries, blackberries, pineapple, kiwi, mint, lemon juice and agave nectar. Serve within 1 to 2 hours.

▸ Health Note

The freshest blackberries have a shiny, plump appearance; if they look dull, they are likely to be past their prime, and their vitamin C content will be lower.

Goat Cheese and Pistachio–Stuffed Dates

Makes 8 servings

✪ Great for Steps 3 and 4

This three-ingredient dessert manages to be both everyday and upscale.

Nutrients per serving	
Calories	80
Total fat	1 g
Saturated fat	1 g
Cholesterol	1 mg
Sodium	12 mg
Carbohydrate	18 g
Fiber	2 g
Protein	1 g
Calcium	21 mg
Iron	0.3 mg

8 tsp	soft goat cheese	40 mL
1 tbsp	finely chopped lightly salted roasted pistachios	15 mL
8	large Medjool dates, pitted	8

1. In a small bowl, combine cheese and pistachios.
2. Stuff each date with a heaping teaspoon (5 mL) of the cheese mixture.

Superfood Spotlight

Pistachios • Pistachios are rich in beta-sitosterols, which can help lower "bad" cholesterol and may protect against cancer, and are a good source of both insoluble and soluble fiber, which offer benefits for the blood cholesterol profile and may help prevent certain cancers and symptoms of digestive problems, such as constipation and irritable bowel syndrome. Pistachios are also a good source of protein and are lower in fat than other types of nuts. They are rich in potassium, and contain a range of minerals and B vitamins.

Cocoa Truffles

Makes 2 dozen truffles

✪ Great for Step 4

Cocoa powder is nothing if not versatile: you can transform it into a quick chocolate sauce, make it into hot cocoa in minutes or use it as the base for cookies. But if you're feeling even mildly industrious, use it to make these cocoa truffles. I promise, you won't be sorry. The combination of nuts, dates and cocoa powder produces a deeply flavored, not-too-sweet confection.

Storage Tip

Store the truffles in an airtight container in the refrigerator for up to 1 week.

Nutrients per truffle	
Calories	108
Total fat	7 g
Saturated fat	1 g
Cholesterol	0 mg
Sodium	30 mg
Carbohydrate	13 g
Fiber	2 g
Protein	2 g
Calcium	10 mg
Iron	0.4 mg

- **Food processor**

2 cups	pecan halves	500 mL
	Cold water	
2 cups	packed chopped pitted dates	500 mL
2⁄3 cup	unsweetened cocoa powder (preferably natural cocoa)	150 mL
1⁄4 tsp	fine sea salt	1 mL
1 tbsp	vanilla extract	15 mL

1. Place pecans in a medium bowl and add enough cold water to cover. Let soak for 4 to 6 hours to soften. Drain well.
2. In food processor, pulse softened pecans until chopped. Add dates, cocoa powder, salt and vanilla; process until almost smooth, stopping once or twice to scrape sides of bowl.
3. Transfer pecan mixture to a medium bowl. Cover and refrigerate for at least 2 hours or until firm enough to roll.
4. Roll pecan mixture into 1-inch (2.5 cm) balls.

No-Bake Raspberry Thumbprints

Makes 3 dozen cookies

✪ Great for Steps 3, 4 and 5

A hearty dose of oats and natural nut butter balances the mild sweetness of these no-bake charmers. Consider the recipe a blueprint for countless variations: change the nut butter, juice and jam according to your whims or what's on hand.

- **Food processor**
- **Large baking sheet, lined with parchment paper**

3/4 cup	chopped pitted dates	175 mL
	Hot water	
3 cups	large-flake (old-fashioned) rolled oats	750 mL
1/2 cup	unsweetened flaked coconut	125 mL
1/2 tsp	ground cinnamon	2 mL
1/4 tsp	fine sea salt	1 mL
1 tsp	finely grated orange zest	5 mL
1/4 cup	freshly squeezed orange juice	60 mL
1 1/2 cups	unsweetened natural almond butter	375 mL
1/3 cup	raspberry or other fruit jam sweetened with fruit juice	75 mL

1. Place dates in a medium bowl and add enough hot water to cover. Let soak for 15 minutes. Drain, reserving 1/2 cup (125 mL) soaking liquid.
2. Meanwhile, in food processor, combine oats, coconut, cinnamon and salt; pulse until coarsely ground. Transfer to a large bowl.
3. In food processor, combine soaked dates, the reserved soaking liquid, orange zest and orange juice; purée until smooth.
4. Add the date mixture and almond butter to the oat mixture, mixing with a wooden spoon or your hands to make a cohesive dough.
5. Roll dough into thirty-six 1-inch (2.5 cm) balls. Place on prepared baking sheet. Using your thumb, make a small indentation in the center of each ball. Loosely cover with foil or plastic wrap and refrigerate for at least 1 hour, until chilled, or store in an airtight container in the refrigerator for up to 1 week. Just before serving, spoon 1/4 tsp (1 mL) jam into each indentation.

Tips

You can use any unsweetened natural nut or seed butter, such as peanut butter, cashew butter or sunflower butter, in place of the almond butter.

There's no need to clean the food processor bowl between steps 2 and 3.

Nutrients per cookie	
Calories	82
Total fat	7 g
Saturated fat	1 g
Cholesterol	0 mg
Sodium	43 mg
Carbohydrate	6 g
Fiber	2 g
Protein	3 g
Calcium	44 mg
Iron	0.6 mg

Oatmeal Cookies

Makes about 30 cookies

✪ Great for Steps 3, 4 and 5

It's likely you've nibbled one too many cookies whose sweetness overpowers the flavors of the other ingredients. These oatmeal cookies couldn't be more of a contrast. The restrained, mellow sweetness from dates and brown rice syrup still allows the toasty flavor of the oats and walnuts to come through.

Storage Tip

Store the cooled cookies in an airtight container at room temperature for up to 3 days.

Nutrients per cookie	
Calories	81
Total fat	5 g
Saturated fat	0 g
Cholesterol	6 mg
Sodium	60 mg
Carbohydrate	11 g
Fiber	1 g
Protein	2 g
Calcium	8 mg
Iron	0.4 mg

- **Preheat oven to 350°F (180°C)**
- **Food processor**
- **2 large baking sheets, lined with parchment paper**

1 cup	chopped pitted dates	250 mL
1 cup	chopped walnuts or pecans	250 mL
1 cup	large-flake (old-fashioned) rolled oats	250 mL
3/4 cup	whole wheat pastry flour	175 mL
1/2 tsp	ground cinnamon	2 mL
1/2 tsp	fine sea salt	2 mL
1/4 tsp	baking soda	1 mL
1	large egg, at room temperature	1
1/4 cup	brown rice syrup, pure maple syrup or liquid honey	60 mL
1/4 cup	unsweetened applesauce	60 mL
1/4 cup	vegetable oil	60 mL
1 tsp	vanilla extract	5 mL

1. In food processor, combine dates and walnuts; pulse until finely chopped.
2. In a large bowl, whisk together oats, flour, cinnamon, salt and baking soda. Stir in date mixture, egg, brown rice syrup, applesauce, oil and vanilla until just blended.
3. Drop by tablespoonfuls (15 mL) onto prepared baking sheet, spacing them 2 inches (5 cm) apart. Flatten slightly with your fingertips.
4. Bake in preheated oven for 20 to 25 minutes or until just set at the center. Let cool on a wire rack for 2 minutes, then transfer to the rack to cool.

Maple Spice Cookies

Makes about 30 cookies

✪ Great for Steps 4 and 5

Although these aromatic cookies may bring to mind winter holidays, they are worth baking — and eating — throughout the year.

Tip

An equal amount of white whole wheat flour may be used in place of the whole wheat pastry flour. Alternatively, use half whole wheat flour and half unbleached all-purpose flour.

Storage Tip

Store the cooled cookies in an airtight container at room temperature for up to 3 days.

Nutrients per cookie	
Calories	73
Total fat	4 g
Saturated fat	0 g
Cholesterol	0 mg
Sodium	35 mg
Carbohydrate	10 g
Fiber	1 g
Protein	1 g
Calcium	9 mg
Iron	0.3 mg

- **Preheat oven to 350°F (180°C)**
- **Large baking sheet, lined with parchment paper**

2 cups	large-flake (old-fashioned) rolled oats	500 mL
1 cup	whole wheat pastry flour	250 mL
1 tsp	ground cinnamon	5 mL
1⁄4 tsp	ground nutmeg	1 mL
1⁄4 tsp	fine sea salt	1 mL
1⁄4 tsp	baking soda	1 mL
1⁄2 cup	vegetable oil	125 mL
1⁄2 cup	pure maple syrup	125 mL
2 tsp	vanilla extract	10 mL

1. In a large bowl, whisk together oats, flour, cinnamon, nutmeg, salt and baking soda. Stir in oil, maple syrup and vanilla until just blended.
2. Drop by tablespoonfuls (15 mL) onto prepared baking sheet, spacing them 2 inches (5 cm) apart. Flatten slightly with your fingertips.
3. Bake in preheated oven for 12 to 15 minutes or until just set at the center. Let cool on a wire rack for 5 minutes, then transfer to the rack to cool.

Soft Apple Cookies

Makes about 42 cookies

✪ Great for Steps 1, 4 and 5

These tender spiced cookies are reminiscent of apple pie. A double dose of apple in the batter — applesauce and chopped fresh apples — keeps them exceptionally moist.

Tip

An equal amount of white whole wheat flour may be used in place of the whole wheat pastry flour. Alternatively, use half whole wheat flour and half unbleached all-purpose flour.

Storage Tip

Store the cooled cookies in an airtight container at room temperature for up to 3 days.

Nutrients per cookie	
Calories	56
Total fat	2 g
Saturated fat	0 g
Cholesterol	0 mg
Sodium	59 mg
Carbohydrate	10 g
Fiber	1 g
Protein	1 g
Calcium	20 mg
Iron	0.6 mg

- **Preheat oven to 325°F (160°C)**
- **2 large baking sheets, lined with parchment paper**

2½ cups	whole wheat pastry flour	625 mL
¾ cup	natural cane sugar	175 mL
1½ tsp	baking powder	7 mL
1 tsp	baking soda	5 mL
1 tsp	ground ginger	5 mL
1 tsp	ground cinnamon	5 mL
¼ tsp	ground nutmeg	1 mL
¼ tsp	fine sea salt	1 mL
⅓ cup	vegetable oil	75 mL
¼ cup	unsweetened applesauce	60 mL
¼ cup	dark (cooking) molasses	60 mL
1 cup	finely chopped peeled tart-sweet apples (such as Braeburn, Gala or Pippin)	250 mL

1. In a large bowl, whisk together flour, sugar, baking powder, baking soda, ginger, cinnamon, nutmeg and salt. Stir in oil, applesauce and molasses until just blended. Gently fold in apples.
2. Drop by tablespoonfuls (15 mL) onto prepared baking sheet, spacing them 2 inches (5 cm) apart.
3. Bake in preheated oven for 12 to 15 minutes or until just set at the center. Let cool on a wire rack for 5 minutes, then transfer to the rack to cool.

Superfood Spotlight

Apples • In recent years, scientific evidence has shown that the old proverb "An apple a day keeps the doctor away" may indeed be true. Although apples don't provide any particular vitamins or minerals (with the exception of potassium), they do contain high levels of various plant chemicals, including the flavonoid quercetin, which has anticancer and anti-inflammatory properties. Apples are also a valuable source of pectin, a soluble fiber that can help lower LDL ("bad") cholesterol and help prevent colon cancer.

Pumpkin Cranberry Cookies

Makes 3 dozen cookies

✪ Great for Steps 4 and 5

Be the hit of the party when you arrive with a platter of these crowd-pleasing pumpkin cookies. They'll satisfy guests far beyond taste alone.

Tip

For a milder-flavored cookie, use liquid honey, pure maple syrup or brown rice syrup in place of the molasses.

Storage Tip

Store the cooled cookies in an airtight container at room temperature for up to 3 days.

- **Preheat oven to 350°F (180°C)**
- **2 large baking sheets, lined with parchment paper**

1⅓ cups	whole wheat pastry flour	325 mL
1 tsp	baking powder	5 mL
1 tsp	ground cinnamon	5 mL
¾ tsp	ground ginger	3 mL
½ tsp	baking soda	2 mL
½ tsp	fine sea salt	2 mL
¼ tsp	ground nutmeg	1 mL
¾ cup	natural cane sugar	175 mL
2	large eggs, at room temperature	2
¾ cup	pumpkin purée (not pie filling)	175 mL
¼ cup	vegetable oil	60 mL
¼ cup	dark (cooking) molasses	60 mL
1 cup	dried cranberries or raisins	250 mL

1. In a large bowl, whisk together flour, baking powder, cinnamon, ginger, baking soda, salt and nutmeg.
2. In a medium bowl, whisk together sugar, eggs, pumpkin, oil and molasses until blended.
3. Add the pumpkin mixture to the flour mixture, stirring until just blended. Gently fold in cranberries.
4. Drop by tablespoonfuls (15 mL) onto prepared baking sheet, spacing them 2 inches (5 cm) apart.
5. Bake in preheated oven for 10 to 12 minutes or until just set at the center. Let cool on a wire rack for 5 minutes, then transfer to the rack to cool.

Nutrients per cookie	
Calories	68
Total fat	2 g
Saturated fat	0 g
Cholesterol	10 mg
Sodium	72 mg
Carbohydrate	12 g
Fiber	1 g
Protein	1 g
Calcium	24 mg
Iron	0.8 mg

Whole Wheat and Olive Oil Biscotti

Makes 3 dozen cookies

✪ Great for Steps 3, 4 and 5

Olive oil may sound like an unusual ingredient for biscotti, but it's actually quite traditional in many regions of Italy.

Tips

For the nuts, try walnuts, pecans, hazelnuts, pistachios or almonds. For the dried fruit, try raisins, cherries or chopped apricots.

The biscotti will continue to harden after the second bake, as they cool.

Storage Tip

Store the cooled biscotti in an airtight container at room temperature for up to 5 days.

Nutrients per cookie	
Calories	81
Total fat	5 g
Saturated fat	0 g
Cholesterol	10 mg
Sodium	32 mg
Carbohydrate	10 g
Fiber	1 g
Protein	2 g
Calcium	12 mg
Iron	0.5 mg

- **Preheat oven to 300°F (150°C)**
- **Large baking sheet, lined with parchment paper**

1¾ cups	whole wheat pastry flour	425 mL
1 tsp	baking powder	5 mL
¼ tsp	fine sea salt	1 mL
1¼ cups	coarsely chopped nuts	300 mL
¾ cup	chopped dried fruit	175 mL
¾ cup	natural cane sugar or granulated sugar	175 mL
2	large eggs, at room temperature	2
¼ cup	extra virgin olive oil	60 mL
2 tsp	vanilla extract	10 mL

1. In a medium bowl, whisk together flour, baking powder and salt. Stir in nuts and dried fruit.
2. In a large bowl, whisk together sugar, eggs, oil and vanilla until blended. Gradually add the flour mixture, stirring until just blended. Divide dough in half.
3. Place dough halves on prepared baking sheet and, using moistened hands, shape into two parallel 12- by 2-inch (30 by 5 cm) rectangles, spaced about 3 inches (7.5 cm) apart.
4. Bake in preheated oven for 30 to 35 minutes or until golden and center is set. Let cool on pan on a wire rack for 15 minutes.
5. Cut rectangles crosswise into ½-inch (1 cm) slices. Place slices, cut side down, on baking sheet. Bake for 8 to 10 minutes or until edges are dark golden. Let cool on pan for 1 minute, then transfer to wire racks to cool completely.

▸ Health Note

Studies conducted at Brigham and Women's Hospital in Boston and the Harvard School of Public Health revealed that three times as many people who were trying to lose weight were able to stick to a diet if it included moderate fat content in the form of nuts and seeds. Researchers suggested that the fat, protein and fiber in nuts helped dieters feel full longer, so many felt less deprived and ate less during the day.

Another study by the Harvard School of Public Health reported a 30% reduced risk of type 2 diabetes in women who ate five or more 1-oz (30 g) servings of nuts per week, as compared with women who rarely or never ate nuts.

Double Almond Chocolate Biscotti

Makes 3 dozen cookies

✪ Great for Steps 3, 4 and 5

Combining two classic dessert flavors — chocolate and almond — these biscotti are always in fashion.

Tips

An equal amount of white whole wheat flour may be used in place of the whole wheat pastry flour. Alternatively, use half whole wheat flour and half unbleached all-purpose flour.

The biscotti will continue to harden after the second bake, as they cool.

Storage Tip

Store the cooled biscotti in an airtight container at room temperature for up to 5 days.

Nutrients per cookie	
Calories	64
Total fat	3 g
Saturated fat	0 g
Cholesterol	10 mg
Sodium	55 mg
Carbohydrate	9 g
Fiber	1 g
Protein	2 g
Calcium	18 mg
Iron	0.4 mg

- **Preheat oven to 325°F (160°C)**
- **Large baking sheet, lined with parchment paper**

1½ cups	whole wheat pastry flour	375 mL
⅓ cup	unsweetened cocoa powder (not Dutch process)	75 mL
¾ tsp	baking soda	3 mL
¼ tsp	fine sea salt	1 mL
⅓ cup	unsweetened natural almond butter	75 mL
⅔ cup	brown rice syrup or liquid honey	150 mL
2	large eggs, at room temperature	2
¾ tsp	almond extract	3 mL
½ cup	slivered almonds	125 mL

1. In a medium bowl, whisk together flour, cocoa powder, baking soda and salt.
2. In a large bowl, using an electric mixer on medium speed, beat almond butter and brown rice syrup until blended. Add eggs and almond extract, beating on low speed until just blended.
3. Add the flour mixture to the egg mixture, stirring until just blended. Gently fold in almonds.
4. Place dough halves on prepared baking sheet and, using moistened hands, shape into two parallel 12- by 2-inch (30 by 5 cm) rectangles, spaced about 3 inches (7.5 cm) apart.
5. Bake in preheated oven for 30 to 35 minutes or until center is set. Let cool on pan on a wire rack for 15 minutes.
6. Cut rectangles crosswise into ½-inch (1 cm) slices. Place slices, cut side down, on baking sheet. Bake for 8 to 10 minutes or until centers are set. Let cool on pan for 1 minute, then transfer to wire racks to cool completely.

▸ Health Note

Cornell University food scientists discovered that cocoa powder has nearly twice the antioxidants of red wine and up to three times the antioxidants of green tea. Moreover, research studies from the past decade have shown a link between cocoa and cardiovascular health, with a reduced risk of blood clots, strokes and heart attacks.

Crispy Brown Rice Treats

Makes 16 bars

✪ Great for Steps 3, 4 and 5

It's always a good idea to have a few no-nonsense recipes in your repertoire. Crispy rice treats are just that, and with some simple ingredient swaps and additions, this variation on the classic offers good health and great taste in equal measure.

Tip

For the dried fruit, try raisins, cranberries, cherries or chopped apricots. For the nut or seed butter, try almond butter, peanut butter or sunflower butter.

Storage Tip

Store the rice treats in an airtight container at room temperature for up to 3 days.

Nutrients per bar	
Calories	92
Total fat	4 g
Saturated fat	0 g
Cholesterol	0 mg
Sodium	31 mg
Carbohydrate	14 g
Fiber	1 g
Protein	2 g
Calcium	0 mg
Iron	0.1 mg

- **9-inch (23 cm) square metal baking pan, sprayed with nonstick cooking spray**

4 cups	crisp brown rice cereal	1 L
1/2 cup	finely chopped dried fruit	125 mL
1/2 cup	unsweetened natural nut or seed butter	125 mL
1/3 cup	brown rice syrup or liquid honey	75 mL
2 tsp	vanilla extract	10 mL

1. In a large bowl, combine rice cereal and dried fruit.
2. In a small saucepan, over medium-low heat, heat nut butter and brown rice syrup for 2 to 3 minutes or until warm and blended. Remove from heat and stir in vanilla.
3. Add the nut butter mixture to the cereal mixture, stirring until combined. Spread in prepared baking pan. Cover and refrigerate for 1 hour or until set. Cut into 16 bars.

Date Bars

Makes 16 bars

✪ Great for Steps 4 and 5

Date bars have long been favorite curl-up-with-a-cup-of-tea options, and this version is no different.

Tip

For the best results, use whole pitted dates and chop them yourself. Pre-chopped dates are typically tossed with oat flour (to prevent sticking) and sugar. In addition, they tend to be fairly hard. If pre-chopped dates are the only option available, give them a quick rinse in hot (not boiling) water to remove any coatings and soften them slightly.

Storage Tip

Store the cooled bars in an airtight container in the refrigerator for up to 5 days.

Nutrients per bar	
Calories	90
Total fat	4 g
Saturated fat	0 g
Cholesterol	0 mg
Sodium	31 mg
Carbohydrate	14 g
Fiber	1 g
Protein	2 g
Calcium	0 mg
Iron	0.1 mg

- **Preheat oven to 375°F (190°C)**
- **Blender or food processor**
- **8-inch (20 cm) square metal baking pan, sprayed with nonstick cooking spray**

1¼ cups	quick-cooking rolled oats	300 mL
½ cup	whole wheat flour	125 mL
½ tsp	ground cardamom or cinnamon	2 mL
½ tsp	baking powder	2 mL
¼ tsp	fine sea salt	1 mL
⅔ cup	chopped pitted dates, divided	150 mL
1 tsp	finely grated orange zest	5 mL
¼ cup	freshly squeezed orange juice	60 mL
¼ cup	vegetable oil	60 mL
1	large egg, at room temperature	1

1. In a medium bowl, whisk together oats, flour, cardamom, baking powder and salt.
2. In a blender, combine half the dates, orange zest, orange juice and oil; purée until very smooth. Add egg and blend until just combined.
3. Add the date mixture to the flour mixture, stirring until just blended. Gently fold in the remaining dates.
4. Spread batter evenly in prepared pan.
5. Bake in preheated oven for 15 to 20 minutes or until golden brown and set at the center. Let cool completely in pan on a wire rack. Cut into 16 bars.

Black Bean Brownies

Makes 16 squares

✪ Great for Steps 2, 3 and 4

Black bean brownies are all the rage, but not all versions are worthy of the "brownie" moniker. This very fudgy option is.

Tip

Lining a pan with foil is easy. Begin by turning the pan upside down. Tear off a piece of foil longer than the pan, then mold the foil over the pan. Remove the foil and set it aside. Flip the pan over and gently fit the shaped foil into the pan, allowing the foil to hang over the sides (the overhang ends will work as "handles" when the contents of the pan are removed).

Storage Tip

Store the cooled brownies in an airtight container in the refrigerator for up to 3 days.

Nutrients per square	
Calories	147
Total fat	7 g
Saturated fat	4 g
Cholesterol	32 mg
Sodium	154 mg
Carbohydrate	18 g
Fiber	2 g
Protein	4 g
Calcium	22 mg
Iron	0.9 mg

- **Preheat oven to 350°F (180°C)**
- **Food processor**
- **8-inch (20 cm) square metal baking pan, lined with foil (see tip, at left) and sprayed with nonstick cooking spray**

3 cups	rinsed drained canned black beans	750 mL
1/3 cup	unsweetened cocoa powder (not Dutch process)	75 mL
1/8 tsp	fine sea salt	0.5 mL
2	large eggs, at room temperature	2
2	large egg whites, at room temperature	2
1/3 cup	warmed virgin coconut oil or melted unsalted butter	75 mL
1/3 cup	brown rice syrup or liquid honey	75 mL
2 tsp	vanilla extract	10 mL
1/2 cup	bittersweet (dark) or semisweet chocolate chips, roughly chopped	125 mL
1/3 cup	finely chopped toasted pecans or walnuts (optional)	75 mL

1. In food processor, combine beans, cocoa powder, salt, eggs, egg whites, coconut oil, brown rice syrup and vanilla; purée until smooth.
2. Spread bean mixture in prepared pan. Sprinkle with chocolate chips and pecans (if using).
3. Bake in preheated oven for 30 to 35 minutes or until just set at the center. Let cool completely in pan on a wire rack. Using foil liner, lift mixture from pan and invert onto a cutting board; peel off foil and cut into 16 squares.

Ricotta Pudding with Strawberry Coulis

Makes 6 servings

✪ Great for Steps 1, 3 and 4

Napped with a luscious — and ridiculously simple — strawberry coulis, this mix-and-bake ricotta pudding is so delicious it will have everyone asking for the recipe.

Tip

Choose strawberries that look plump and glossy; dull ones are usually past their prime. Store strawberries in the refrigerator in a container with air holes for up to 3 days. Bring them to room temperature for the best flavor.

Nutrients per serving	
Calories	163
Total fat	2 g
Saturated fat	1 g
Cholesterol	97 mg
Sodium	160 mg
Carbohydrate	20 g
Fiber	1 g
Protein	14 g
Calcium	288 mg
Iron	0.7 mg

- **Preheat oven to 375°F (190°C)**
- **Blender or food processor**
- **9-inch (23 cm) glass pie plate, sprayed with nonstick cooking spray (preferably olive oil)**

3	large eggs	3
2 cups	nonfat ricotta cheese	500 mL
4 tbsp	liquid honey, divided	60 mL
2 tsp	vanilla extract	10 mL
1/8 tsp	fine sea salt	0.5 mL
2 cups	quartered hulled strawberries	500 mL
1 tbsp	water	15 mL
2 tsp	balsamic vinegar	10 mL

1. In blender, combine eggs, ricotta, 3 tbsp (45 mL) of the honey, vanilla and salt; purée for 1 to 2 minutes or until very smooth. Pour into prepared pie plate.
2. Bake in preheated oven for 22 to 26 minutes or until golden and just set at the center. Let cool on a wire rack.
3. Meanwhile, in clean blender, combine strawberries, the remaining honey, water and vinegar; purée until smooth. Cover and refrigerate for at least 30 minutes, until chilled, or for up to 1 day.
4. Cut pudding into wedges and serve with strawberry coulis.

Superfood Spotlight

Strawberries • Strawberries rank very high in antioxidant activity. They are extremely rich in vitamin C (an average portion contains the entire recommended daily amount for an adult), which boosts the immune system and helps to heal wounds, prevent arterial damage, promote iron absorption and strengthen blood vessel walls. Strawberries also contain antioxidant phenolic plant chemicals, such as anthocyanins and ellagic acid, which can block cancer cells and help prevent some cancers. Finally, they contain good amounts of fiber, folate and potassium.

Maple Brown Rice Pudding with Dried Cherries

Makes 6 servings

✪ Great for Steps 3, 4 and 5

Nutrients per serving

Calories	193
Total fat	2 g
Saturated fat	1 g
Cholesterol	5 mg
Sodium	77 mg
Carbohydrate	40 g
Fiber	5 g
Protein	4 g
Calcium	102 mg
Iron	0.8 mg

2 cups	cooked medium- or short-grain brown rice (see page 438), cooled	500 mL
3⁄4 cup	dried cherries, cranberries or raisins	175 mL
1⁄2 tsp	ground cinnamon	2 mL
1⁄8 tsp	fine sea salt	0.5 mL
11⁄2 cups	milk	375 mL
1⁄4 cup	pure maple syrup	60 mL
1 tsp	vanilla extract	5 mL

1. In a medium saucepan, combine rice, cherries, cinnamon, salt, milk and maple syrup. Bring to a simmer over medium-high heat. Reduce heat and simmer, stirring constantly, for 20 to 25 minutes or until thickened. Remove from heat and stir in vanilla. Let cool to room temperature. Serve at room temperature, or cover and refrigerate until cold.

Strawberry Mousse

Makes 6 servings

✪ Great for Steps 1, 2, 3 and 4

If you like strawberries, you'll love this creamy mousse.

Nutrients per serving

Calories	156
Total fat	2 g
Saturated fat	0 g
Cholesterol	0 mg
Sodium	54 mg
Carbohydrate	31 g
Fiber	2 g
Protein	4 g
Calcium	35 mg
Iron	0.9 mg

- **Food processor**
- **Six 6-oz (175 mL) ramekins or dessert glasses**

1 cup	unsweetened apple juice	250 mL
1⁄3 cup	agave nectar or liquid honey	75 mL
1⁄4 cup	cornstarch	60 mL
1⁄8 tsp	fine sea salt	0.5 mL
21⁄2 cups	chopped strawberries	625 mL
12⁄3 cups	drained soft silken tofu	400 mL

1. In a medium saucepan, whisk together apple juice, agave nectar, cornstarch and salt. Bring to a simmer over medium heat, whisking often. Reduce heat and simmer, whisking constantly, for 30 seconds or until thickened (mixture will be very thick). Remove from heat and let cool for 10 minutes.
2. In food processor, combine apple juice mixture, strawberries and tofu; purée until creamy and smooth.
3. Divide mousse among ramekins. Cover and refrigerate for at least 4 hours, until chilled, or for up to 1 day.

Chocolate Pudding

Makes 6 servings

✪ Great for Steps 3 and 4

Cashews, cocoa and pumpkin may sound like unlikely bedfellows — especially to make a chocolate pudding — but this dish disproves the assumption.

Tip

If a 15-oz (425 mL) can of pumpkin isn't available, purchase a 28-oz (796 mL) can and measure out 1¾ cups (425 mL). Refrigerate extra pumpkin in an airtight container for up to 1 week.

- **Blender or food processor**
- **Six 6-oz (175 mL) ramekins or dessert glasses**

1 cup	chopped pitted dates	250 mL
¾ cup	raw cashews	175 mL
	Very hot water	
1	can (15 oz/425 mL) pumpkin purée (not pie filling)	1
¾ cup	light coconut milk	175 mL
½ cup	unsweetened cocoa powder (not Dutch process)	125 mL
1 tsp	vanilla extract	5 mL
	Raspberries (optional)	

1. Place dates and cashews in a medium bowl and add enough very hot water to cover. Let soak for 1 hour to soften. Drain well.
2. In blender, combine date mixture, pumpkin and coconut milk; purée for 1 to 2 minutes or until very smooth. Add cocoa powder and vanilla; process for 1 minute or until well blended.
3. Divide mixture among ramekins. Cover and refrigerate for at least 1 hour, until chilled, or for up to 1 day. Garnish with raspberries, if desired.

Nutrients per serving	
Calories	212
Total fat	9 g
Saturated fat	4 g
Cholesterol	0 mg
Sodium	12 mg
Carbohydrate	36 g
Fiber	8 g
Protein	6 g
Calcium	41 mg
Iron	2.8 mg

Lemon Blackberry Fool

Makes 4 servings

✪ Great for Steps 1, 2, 3 and 4

A fool can be many things, but when it comes to food, it's traditionally a British dessert made of lightly sweetened, puréed fruit that is haphazardly mixed into whipped cream. Swap out the whipped cream for luscious Greek yogurt, and the dessert becomes a superfood sensation.

Tips

This recipe is very versatile. For example, you can swap in other berries or any other juicy fruit for the blackberries, and/or use lime or orange zest and juice in place of the lemon.

Blackberries freeze well, so pack them into lidded containers or open-freeze them on a tray and then pack them into plastic bags.

Nutrients per serving	
Calories	154
Total fat	0 g
Saturated fat	0 g
Cholesterol	0 mg
Sodium	43 mg
Carbohydrate	28 g
Fiber	3 g
Protein	11 g
Calcium	93 mg
Iron	0.4 mg

1½ cups	fresh or thawed frozen blackberries	375 mL
2 tsp	chopped fresh mint or basil (optional)	10 mL
4 tbsp	agave nectar or liquid honey, divided	60 mL
2 cups	nonfat plain Greek yogurt	500 mL
1 tbsp	finely grated lemon zest	15 mL
1 tbsp	freshly squeezed lemon juice	15 mL

1. In a medium bowl, mash berries with mint (if using) and 1 tbsp (15 mL) of the agave nectar.
2. In another medium bowl, whisk together yogurt, the remaining agave nectar, lemon zest and lemon juice until smooth.
3. Fold all but ½ cup (125 mL) mashed berries into yogurt mixture, creating a marbled effect.
4. Divide yogurt mixture among four small glasses or glass dessert cups. Top with the reserved mashed berries. Serve immediately.

Superfood Spotlight

Blackberries • Juicy blackberries are small powerhouses of health. Their deep purple color denotes that they are rich in several compounds, including antioxidants, anthocyanins and ellagic acid, that can help beat heart disease, cancer and the signs of aging. In addition, blackberries are rich in fiber and minerals, including magnesium, zinc, iron and calcium. Their high vitamin E content helps protect the heart and keeps skin healthy. Like other berries, blackberries are a good source of vitamin C, which boosts the immune system. They are also a good source of folate, which is beneficial for healthy blood.

All-Natural Fruit Gelatin *(Kanten)*

Makes 4 servings

✪ Great for Steps 2 and 4

Nutrients per serving	
Calories	54
Total fat	0 g
Saturated fat	0 g
Cholesterol	0 mg
Sodium	75 mg
Carbohydrate	13 g
Fiber	0 g
Protein	0 g
Calcium	14 mg
Iron	0.3 mg

1 cup	unsweetened apple juice	250 mL
1 cup	unsweetened grape juice	250 mL
2 tbsp	agar-agar flakes	30 mL
1⁄8 tsp	fine sea salt	0.5 mL

1. In a small saucepan, whisk together apple juice, grape juice, agar-agar and salt. Bring to a simmer over medium-high heat, whisking constantly. Reduce heat and simmer, whisking constantly, for 10 to 12 minutes or until agar-agar is completely dissolved.
2. Divide apple juice mixture among four small dessert cups or ramekins. Refrigerate for about 1 hour, until set.

Kiwi Sorbet

Makes 8 servings

✪ Great for Steps 1, 2 and 4

Frozen flawlessness is but four ingredients away.

Nutrients per serving	
Calories	128
Total fat	0 g
Saturated fat	0 g
Cholesterol	0 mg
Sodium	2 mg
Carbohydrate	32 g
Fiber	2 g
Protein	1 g
Calcium	23 mg
Iron	0.2 mg

- **Food processor or blender**
- **Ice cream maker**

3 cups	chopped kiwifruit	750 mL
2⁄3 cup	agave nectar or liquid honey	150 mL
1⁄3 cup	water	75 mL
1 tbsp	freshly squeezed lime juice	15 mL

1. In food processor, combine kiwi, agave nectar, water and lime juice; process until smooth.
2. Pour into ice cream maker and freeze according to manufacturer's instructions.
3. Spoon into an airtight container, cover and freeze for 8 hours, until firm, or for up to 1 day.

Variation

Replace the kiwifruit with chopped pineapple, diced mango, chopped strawberries, blueberries, diced peaches or diced apricots.

Chocolate Gelato

Makes 8 servings

✪ Great for Steps 3 and 4

This chocolate gelato, made decadently rich with coconut milk and cocoa powder in place of dairy and chocolate, is a triumph.

- **Ice cream maker**

2⁄3 cup	unsweetened cocoa powder (not Dutch process)	150 mL
2	cans (each 14 oz/398 mL) light coconut milk, divided	2
1 tsp	vanilla extract	5 mL
3⁄4 cup	agave nectar	175 mL
2 tbsp	cornstarch	30 mL
1⁄8 tsp	fine sea salt	0.5 mL

1. In a large bowl, whisk together cocoa, 2⁄3 cup (150 mL) of the coconut milk and vanilla to make a smooth paste.
2. In a medium saucepan, whisk together the remaining coconut milk, agave nectar, cornstarch and salt. Bring to a simmer over medium heat, whisking gently. Reduce heat and simmer, whisking constantly, for 2 to 3 minutes or until mixture begins to thicken. Pour over cocoa paste, whisking until blended and smooth. Cover and refrigerate for at least 4 hours or until cold.
3. Pour into ice cream maker and freeze according to manufacturer's instructions.
4. Spoon into an airtight container, cover and freeze for 4 hours, until firm, or for up to 3 days.

Superfood Spotlight

Cocoa Powder • Cocoa powder is made from cocoa beans, which are rich in antioxidant flavonoids, fiber and minerals. Cocoa powder is also low in sodium, high in potassium and full of mood-boosting compounds. The antioxidants in cocoa powder have garnered the most attention from researchers in recent years, because they can have an anticoagulant action, protecting against the oxidation of cholesterol in the body. It's important to note, however, that most of the research conducted on the health benefits of cocoa powder were performed on natural or non-alkalized cocoa (not Dutch-process cocoa powder). Alkalization is a process used to mellow the flavor of cocoa, but it also destroys the polyphenolic compounds.

Nutrients per serving	
Calories	182
Total fat	8 g
Saturated fat	6 g
Cholesterol	0 mg
Sodium	54 mg
Carbohydrate	32 g
Fiber	2 g
Protein	1 g
Calcium	9 mg
Iron	1.0 mg

Vanilla Cashew Ice Cream

Makes 4 servings

✪ Great for Steps 3 and 4

At last, a creamy, dreamy vanilla ice cream that (within moderation) is good for you — and may even help keep your weight in check. The secret is in the cashews, which are blended at high speed until thick and velvety, resulting in a taste akin to the heavy cream used in traditional ice cream.

- **Blender**
- **Ice cream maker**

1 cup	raw cashews	250 mL
1⁄8 tsp	fine sea salt	0.5 mL
2 cups	ice water	500 mL
1⁄4 cup	agave nectar or liquid honey	60 mL
1 tbsp	vanilla extract	15 mL

1. In blender, combine cashews, salt, ice water, agave nectar and vanilla; purée on high speed for 2 minutes.
2. Pour into ice cream maker and freeze according to manufacturer's instructions.
3. Spoon into an airtight container, cover and freeze for 4 hours, until firm, or for up to 3 days.

▶ Health Note

Cashews are high in protein, monounsaturated fats and fiber, so they're both filling and satisfying. Studies have shown that people who eat nuts on a daily basis are less likely to gain weight and have a tendency to be thinner, on average, than those who don't.

Nutrients per serving	
Calories	237
Total fat	14 g
Saturated fat	2 g
Cholesterol	0 mg
Sodium	75 mg
Carbohydrate	27 g
Fiber	1 g
Protein	6 g
Calcium	12 mg
Iron	2.2 mg

Blueberry Lemon Nice Cream

Makes 8 servings

✪ Great for Steps 1, 2, 3 and 4

Bursting with blueberry flavor, this beautifully colored frozen dessert — made as rich and creamy as ice cream thanks to cashew "cream" — is celebratory of summer. Double scoop, anyone?

Tip

Although this recipe can be made in either a blender or food processor, the former is preferable because it will produce a creamier dessert.

- **Blender or food processor**
- **Ice cream maker**

2¼ cups	blueberries	550 mL
¾ cup	raw cashews	175 mL
⅛ tsp	fine sea salt	0.5 mL
1¼ cups	ice water	300 mL
1 tbsp	finely grated lemon zest	15 mL
¼ cup	freshly squeezed lemon juice	60 mL
¼ cup	agave nectar or liquid honey	60 mL

1. In blender, combine blueberries, cashews, salt, ice water, lemon zest, lemon juice and agave nectar; purée until smooth.
2. Pour into ice cream maker and freeze according to manufacturer's instructions.
3. Spoon into an airtight container, cover and freeze for 4 hours, until firm, or for up to 3 days.

▶ Health Note

Blueberries and cashews are abundant in antioxidants, those free radical scavengers that help to protect cells from damage.

Nutrients per serving

Calories	127
Total fat	6 g
Saturated fat	1 g
Cholesterol	0 mg
Sodium	38 mg
Carbohydrate	19 g
Fiber	2 g
Protein	3 g
Calcium	9 mg
Iron	0.9 mg

Healthy Know-How

Dietary Fat 101

Fat, just like carbohydrates and protein, provides calories, or energy. Fat is required to transport vitamins A, D, E and K, produce hormones, store energy, maintain healthy skin and protect organs. Fat also gives flavor and texture to foods.

Although too little fat in the diet can cause serious problems, too much fat is a more common concern in North America. Too much dietary fat can increase the risk of obesity, heart disease, cancer and diabetes. An excess of any macronutrient, be it carbohydrate, protein or fat, can lead to weight gain; however, since fat provides more than double the calories per gram that carbohydrate or protein provide, a high-fat diet often leads to excess weight gain. Certain types of fat (trans fats and saturated fats) can also have a dangerous impact on heart health, and should be kept to a minimum in the diet.

Instant Strawberry Frozen Yogurt

Makes 4 servings

✪ Great for Steps 1, 2, 3 and 4

Tip

Although this recipe can be made in either a blender or food processor, the former is preferable because it will produce a creamier dessert.

Nutrients per serving	
Calories	276
Total fat	0 g
Saturated fat	0 g
Cholesterol	0 mg
Sodium	17 mg
Carbohydrate	81 g
Fiber	4 g
Protein	4 g
Calcium	44 mg
Iron	1.3 mg

- **Blender or food processor**

3½ cups	frozen strawberries, thawed for 10 minutes	875 mL
⅓ cup	agave nectar or liquid honey	75 mL
½ cup	nonfat plain Greek yogurt	125 mL
1 tbsp	freshly squeezed lemon juice	15 mL

1. In blender, combine strawberries and agave nectar; process until coarsely chopped. Add yogurt and lemon juice; pulse until smooth and creamy, scraping down the sides once or twice. Serve immediately in small dessert dishes.

Lemon Raspberry Yogurt Cones

Makes 2 servings

✪ Great for Steps 1, 2, 3 and 4

Fresh, creamy and crunchy all at once, this quick and clever dessert cone is worth making any time, with whatever fruit is on hand. A touch of lemon juice complements the yogurt and raspberries beautifully.

Tips

Look for organic sugar cones in the health food section of the supermarket or at health food stores.

Raspberries do not keep for long, so they should be eaten within a day or two of purchase. They do freeze very well, though, if packed in containers rather than plastic bags. Never wash raspberries before storing unless absolutely necessary, as they break down very quickly when wet.

Nutrients per serving	
Calories	177
Total fat	1 g
Saturated fat	0 g
Cholesterol	0 mg
Sodium	78 mg
Carbohydrate	35 g
Fiber	0 g
Protein	11 g
Calcium	81 mg
Iron	0.5 mg

1 cup	nonfat plain Greek yogurt	250 mL
2 tbsp	liquid honey or agave nectar	30 mL
1 tbsp	freshly squeezed lemon juice	15 mL
2	sugar ice cream cones	2
$\frac{1}{2}$ cup	raspberries	125 mL

1. In a small bowl, whisk together yogurt, honey and lemon juice until smooth.
2. Spoon $\frac{1}{2}$ cup (125 mL) yogurt mixture into each cone and top with raspberries. Serve immediately.

Superfood Spotlight

Raspberries • Packed with vitamin C, high in fiber and loaded with antioxidants to protect the heart, raspberries are one of the most nutritious fruits. They are best eaten raw, because cooking or processing destroys some of these antioxidants, especially anthocyanins. Anthocyanins are red and purple pigments that have been shown to help prevent heart disease and cancer and may help prevent varicose veins. Raspberries also contain high levels of ellagic acid, a compound with anticancer properties. In addition, they contain good amounts of iron, which the body absorbs well because of their high levels of vitamin C.

Blueberry Yogurt Pops

Makes 8 pops

✪ Great for Steps 1, 2, 3 and 4

Blue heaven. Why restrict delectable blueberries to muffins and pies? Here, they shine in cool, creamy ice pops guaranteed to thrill.

- **Blender**
- **8-serving ice-pop mold**

1 cup	fresh or thawed frozen blueberries	250 mL
2/3 cup	unsweetened apple juice	150 mL
2/3 cup	nonfat plain yogurt	150 mL
1/2 tsp	vanilla extract	2 mL

1. In blender, combine blueberries, apple juice, yogurt and vanilla; purée until smooth.
2. Pour blueberry mixture into ice-pop molds, insert sticks and freeze for 4 to 6 hours, until solid, or for up to 3 days. If necessary, briefly dip bases of mold in hot water to loosen and unmold.

▶ Health Note

The pigments that give blueberries their beautiful hue are also what make them so healthful. Berries contain phytochemicals and flavonoids that may help to prevent some forms of cancer, as well as lutein, which is important for healthy vision.

Tip

You can use 4-oz (125 mL) paper cups as ice-pop molds. Place them on a baking sheet, then fill until almost full. Cover with foil, then make a small slit to insert ice-pop sticks or small bamboo skewers and freeze as directed.

Variation

Peaches and Cream Pops: Substitute chopped peeled peaches for the blueberries and freshly squeezed orange juice for the apple juice.

Nutrients per pop	
Calories	28
Total fat	0 g
Saturated fat	0 g
Cholesterol	0 mg
Sodium	12 mg
Carbohydrate	6 g
Fiber	1 g
Protein	1 g
Calcium	27 mg
Iron	0.1 mg

Very Berry Ice Pops

Makes 8 pops

✪ Great for Steps 1, 2 and 4

These ice pops are a serious ode to summer fruit.

Tip

You can use 4-oz (125 mL) paper cups as ice-pop molds. Place them on a baking sheet, then fill until almost full. Cover with foil, then make a small slit to insert ice-pop sticks or small bamboo skewers and freeze as directed.

Nutrients per pop	
Calories	69
Total fat	0 g
Saturated fat	0 g
Cholesterol	0 mg
Sodium	1 mg
Carbohydrate	18 g
Fiber	1 g
Protein	1 g
Calcium	8 mg
Iron	0.2 mg

- **Blender**
- **8-serving ice-pop mold**

1½ cups	hulled fresh strawberries or thawed frozen strawberries	375 mL
1 cup	fresh or thawed frozen blueberries	250 mL
1 cup	fresh or thawed frozen raspberries	250 mL
⅓ cup	agave nectar or liquid honey	75 mL

1. In blender, combine strawberries, blueberries, raspberries and agave nectar; purée until smooth. Strain through a fine-mesh sieve to remove seeds.
2. Pour strawberry mixture into ice-pop molds, insert sticks and freeze for 4 to 6 hours, until solid, or for up to 3 days. If necessary, briefly dip bases of mold in hot water to loosen and unmold.

Chocolate-Dipped Frozen Bananas

Makes 6 servings

✪ Great for Steps 1, 2 and 4

Here, sweet bananas get the chocolate treatment. Topping the chocolate is a sprinkle of toasted coconut.

Tip

To toast coconut, preheat oven to 300°F (150°C). Spread coconut in a thin, even layer on an ungreased baking sheet. Bake for 15 to 20 minutes, stirring every 5 minutes, until golden brown and fragrant. Transfer to a plate and let cool completely.

Storage Tip

After the chocolate coating has set, wrap the bananas individually in foil and store in the freezer for up to 3 days.

Nutrients per serving	
Calories	214
Total fat	11 g
Saturated fat	9 g
Cholesterol	0 mg
Sodium	2 mg
Carbohydrate	41 g
Fiber	2 g
Protein	4 g
Calcium	4 mg
Iron	0.3 mg

- **6 wooden ice-pop sticks**
- **Baking sheet, lined with parchment paper**

3	large firm-ripe bananas, halved crosswise	3
1 cup	semisweet chocolate chips	250 mL
1⁄3 cup	unsweetened shredded coconut, toasted (see tip, at left)	75 mL

1. Carefully push an ice-pop stick into the cut end of each banana half, leaving about 2 inches (5 cm) of the stick poking out. Place bananas on prepared baking sheet. Freeze for 30 to 45 minutes or until just solid.
2. Place chocolate chips in a medium microwave-safe bowl and microwave on High, stopping to stir every 20 to 30 seconds, until completely melted and smooth.
3. Place coconut in a wide, shallow bowl.
4. Dip frozen bananas in chocolate, turning to coat evenly, then sprinkle with coconut, allowing excess coconut to fall back into the bowl. Return dipped bananas to baking sheet. Freeze for 15 to 20 minutes or until chocolate is set.

▶ Health Note

Coconut contains a very healthy type of fat called medium-chain triglycerides (MCTs). Although MCTs are a form of saturated fat, research indicates that they have special characteristics, including antiviral and antimicrobial properties, making coconut a good choice for supporting the immune system.

Cashew Vanilla "Whipped Cream"

Makes 6 servings

✪ Great for Steps 3 and 4

This whipped dessert topping manages the near-impossible feat of being velvety and creamy without any cream. A touch of vanilla extract adds a final soupçon of richness. Use it wherever you might use whipped cream — atop fruit or on any number of desserts.

Storage Tip

Store in an airtight container in the refrigerator for up to 3 days.

Nutrients per serving

Calories	72
Total fat	5 g
Saturated fat	1 g
Cholesterol	0 mg
Sodium	1 mg
Carbohydrate	6 g
Fiber	0 g
Protein	2 g
Calcium	4 mg
Iron	0.7 mg

- **Blender**

½ cup	raw cashews	125 mL
½ cup	ice water	125 mL
1 tbsp	agave nectar or liquid honey	15 mL
½ tsp	vanilla extract	2 mL

1. In blender, combine cashews, ice water, agave nectar and vanilla; purée on high speed until smooth and creamy, stopping to scrape down the sides once or twice.

▶ Health Note

A mere ¼ cup (60 mL) of cashews supplies almost 25% of the daily requirement for magnesium, which plays an important role in maintaining a healthy blood pressure and in building and maintaining bone health. Studies have shown that people with low magnesium levels are at higher risk of heart disease. Magnesium is also an important mineral for diabetics, because it reduces insulin resistance.

Index

A

agar flakes, 41
  All-Natural Fruit Gelatin (*Kanten*), 523
almonds, 84. *See also* nuts
  Almond Flax Seed Energy Cookies, 84
  Breakfast Polenta with Cherries and Almonds, 57
  Capellini with Watercress, Carrots and Almonds, 383
  Cheese, Almond and Mushroom Muffins, 68
  Chicken Salad Sandwiches with Apricots and Almonds, 219
  Double Almond Chocolate Biscotti, 515
  Quinoa Cranberry Granola, 60
  Rotini with Fennel, Orange and Almonds, 409
  Seared Striped Bass with Broccoli and Almond Quinoa, 343
amaranth, 20–21, 438
  Amaranth Spice Bread, 473
apples and applesauce, 478, 512
  Applesauce Flax Bread, 478
  Baked Apples with Walnuts and Dried Cherries, 505
  Carrot Oat Breakfast Cookies, 73
  Chicken with Sautéed Apples and Swiss Chard, 298
  Chunky Applesauce, 63
  Cinnamon Apple Chips, 92
  Creamy Cashew Maple Dip with Apples, 108
  Fresh Apple Bread, 477
  Gluten-Free Flax Muffins, 491
  Honey Apple Cake, 497
  Kale, Apple and Walnut Slaw, 128
  Red Lentil Mulligatawny, 184
  Soft Apple Cookies, 512
  Waldorf Salad, 114
  Whole Wheat Maple Applesauce Cake, 498
  Whole Wheat Zucchini Bread, 472
  Winter Red Cabbage Slaw, 127
apricots, 219. *See also* fruit
  Bulgur Pilaf with Apricots and Coriander, 458
  Chicken Salad Sandwiches with Apricots and Almonds, 219
  Moroccan-Spiced Ground Turkey with Apricot Couscous, 322
  Pistachio and Citrus Couscous Salad, 144
  Sunflower Apricot Go-Bars, 70
artichoke hearts
  Artichoke and Ricotta Pizza, 243
  Cannellini and Artichoke Sandwiches, 217
  Portobello Pizzas, 273
  Provençal Chicken and Orzo Salad, 157
arugula, 332, 406. *See also* greens; watercress
  Arugula, Watermelon and Feta Salad, 117
  Chicken Sausage, Arugula and Tomato Penne, 406
  Delicata Squash with Quinoa Stuffing, 262
  Farro Salad with Arugula and Tomatoes, 146
  Grilled Steak with Arugula and Parmesan, 332
  Lentil, Walnut and Arugula Spread, 100
  Mushroom, Pepper and Arugula Pizza, 246
  Portobello Pesto Burgers, 233
  Seared Salmon with Warm Lentil and Arugula Salad, 359
  Shaved Beet Salad with Pistachios and Goat Cheese, 132
  Sweet Potato, Lentil and Arugula Salad, 134
  Tuna with Farro and Fennel, 370
  Tunisian Tuna and Egg Salad Pitas, 225
  Turkish Tomato, Pepper and Herb Salad, 126
  Winter White Bean, Cauliflower and Arugula Salad, 135
asparagus, 245, 434
  Asparagus and Goat Cheese Pizza, 245
  Asparagus Penne with Goat Cheese, 403
  Asparagus with Tangerine Gremolata, 440
  Barley Risotto with Asparagus and Lemon, 266
  Broccoli, Asparagus and Chicken Stir-Fry, 304
  Foil-Roasted Halibut and Asparagus, 351
  Roasted Vegetable Linguine, 396
  Shrimp and Asparagus Stir-Fry, 374
  Spaghetti Limone with Asparagus and Mushrooms, 411
  Spring Vegetable Chicken Quinoa, 315
  Swedish Salmon, Asparagus and Potato Omelet, 361
  Tuna and Asparagus Frittata, 371
avocado, 138
  Avocado and Egg Breakfast Wraps, 56
  Balsamic Tuna Salad in Avocado Halves, 160
  Black Bean Avocado Salsa, 98
  California Sushi Roll Salad, 138
  Chicken with Cherry Tomato and Avocado Salsa, 300
  Green Club Sandwich, 216
  Grilled Steak Tacos with Avocado and Cumin Lime Slaw, 334
  Scandinavian Breakfast Toasts with Smoked Salmon and Avocado, 64
  Shrimp, Grapefruit and Watercress Salad, 163
  Smoked Turkey, Avocado and Mango Wraps, 231
  Spicy Salsa Joes, 221
  Spicy Skillet Chicken with Avocado Mango Salsa, 301
  Spinach, Avocado and Orange Salad, 115

B

bananas
  Banana and Toasted Millet Muffins, 67
  Banana Bran Bread, 479
  Banana Buttermilk Smoothie, 74
  Berry Protein Shake, 74
  Cashew Butter and Banana Wraps, 229
  Chocolate-Dipped Frozen Bananas, 531
  Green Machine Smoothie, 76
  Multigrain Cranberry Breakfast Cookies, 72
  Pumpkin Smoothie, 77
barley, 22, 140, 266, 438. *See also* farro
  Barley, Mushroom and Kale Stew, 204
  Barley, Parsley and Walnut Salad, 140
  Barley Risotto with Asparagus and Lemon, 266
  French Green Bean, Barley and Tomato Salad, 139
  Mushroom and Barley Soup, 188
  White Bean Bajane with Thyme Barley, 259
beans, dried, 28, 207, 260, 318, 436–37, 454
  Best Black Bean Burgers, 234
  Black Bean and Spinach Burritos, 226
  Black Bean Avocado Salsa, 98
  Black Bean Brownies, 518
  Black Bean Chili–Topped Sweet Potatoes, 251
  Black Bean Chipotle Chili, 207
  Black Bean Pumpkin Soup, 186
  Black Bean Tacos, 277
  Bulgur Burgers, 236
  Butternut Squash, White Bean and Kale Stew, 202
  Cannellini and Artichoke Sandwiches, 217
  Cannellini Beans with Shrimp and Roasted Peppers, 377
  Chicken and Black Bean Chilaquiles, 316
  Cuban Chicken with Black Beans and Brown Rice, 311
  Cumin-Scented Black Beans and Quinoa, 455
  Farfalle with Swiss Chard, White Beans and Walnuts, 386

beans, dried (*continued*)
Jamaican Rice and Peas, 456
Kamut Ditalini with Broccoli Rabe, Pesto and White Beans, 385
Lean Beef and Bean Cowboy Chili, 212
Lima Bean Purée, 452
Middle Eastern Eggplant Spread, 104
Pasta e Fagioli, 201
Quick Kale and Quinoa Minestrone, 177
Quinoa and Black Bean Salad, 147
Speedy Southwest Black Bean and Quinoa Skillet, 260
Spicy Three-Bean Salad, 136
Sweet Potato, Swiss Chard and Black Bean Chili, 208
Texas BBQ Turkey Burgers, 237
Tuna and White Bean Salad, 160
Turkey Sausage, Spinach and Chickpea Ragù (variation), 319
Turkey Sausage with Mustard Greens and Kidney Beans, 318
Tuscan Farro and White Bean Soup, 187
White Bean Bajane with Thyme Barley, 259
White Bean Garlic Spread, 98
White Beans and Spinach, 454
White Turkey Chili, 210
Winter Squash and Goat Cheese Enchiladas, 275
Winter White Bean, Cauliflower and Arugula Salad, 135
beans, green, 435
Basil Coconut Tofu Curry, 290
French Green Bean, Barley and Tomato Salad, 139
Green Bean Salad with Toasted Hazelnuts, 125
Steamed Ginger Garlic Green Beans, 445
Summer Salmon Panzanella, 159
Summer Vegetable Orzo Soup, 189
Vegetable Minestrone, 176
beef
Beef and Quinoa Power Burgers, 238
Beef and Snow Pea Soup, 198
Buckwheat Noodle Bowls with Beef and Snap Peas, 428
Cuban Braised Beef with Brown Rice and Mango, 331
Grilled Steak Tacos with Avocado and Cumin Lime Slaw, 334
Grilled Steak with Arugula and Parmesan, 332
Japanese Ginger Beef Bowls, 333
Lean Beef and Bean Cowboy Chili, 212
Middle Eastern Beef, Bulgur and Chickpea Soup, 199
Middle Eastern Meatballs with Feta Sauce, 339
Moussaka Macaroni, 400
Persian Ground Beef Kebabs, 338
Picadillo, 335
Quick Beef Ragù with Spaghetti Squash, 336
Quick Moroccan Beef and Chickpea Chili, 213
Southeast Asian Roast Beef Wraps, 232
Spiced Beef Keema with Chickpeas and Green Peas, 337
Spicy Salsa Joes (variation), 221
Texas BBQ Turkey Burgers (variation), 237
Vietnamese Pho, 197
beets, 434
Beet Soup with Fresh Ginger, 166
Halibut with Beets and Beet Greens, 352
Multigrain Gemelli with Beets, Beet Greens and Goat Cheese, 394
Roasted Beet and Beet Greens Salad, 118
Roasted Beet and Hummus Heroes, 216
Shaved Beet Salad with Pistachios and Goat Cheese, 132
Shredded Beet, Carrot and Mint Salad, 129
Swiss Chard Spring Rolls with Sesame Lime Dipping Sauce, 109
berries. *See also* fruit; *specific berries*
Berry Peach Crumbles, 503
Berry Protein Shake, 74
Five-Minute Cheesecake Cups with Raspberries, 501
Gluten-Free Flax Muffins (variation), 491
Greek Yogurt, Grain and Blackberry Parfaits, 63
Kiwi Sorbet (variation), 523
Lemon Blackberry Fool, 522
Lemon Raspberry Yogurt Cones, 528
PB&J Energy Balls, 86
Power Granola, 59
Super Antioxidant Smoothie, 75
Super C Smoothie, 75
Very Berry Ice Pops, 530
Yogurt Cake with Fresh Berries, 496
blueberries, 48, 526, 529. *See also* berries
Blueberry Lemon Nice Cream, 526
Blueberry Yogurt Pops, 529
Quinoa Blueberry Breakfast Cookies, 71
Quinoa Blueberry Pancakes, 48
Whole-Grain Blueberry Maple Muffins, 65
bok choy
Asian Chicken Noodle Soup, 194
Bok Choy and Mushroom Soup, 167
Bok Choy Salad with Miso Ginger Dressing, 119
Braised Baby Bok Choy, 440
Soba with Shrimp and Baby Bok Choy, 430
Stir-Fried Tofu with Bok Choy and Spinach, 292
broccoli, 168, 434, 441
Broccoli, Asparagus and Chicken Stir-Fry, 304
Broccoli and Spinach Enchiladas, 274
Broccoli Carrot Slaw with Cranberries and Sunflower Seeds, 129
Garden Pasta Salad, 154
Power Pitas with Eggs and Vegetables, 54
Seared Striped Bass with Broccoli and Almond Quinoa, 343
Sesame Ginger Noodles, 423
Soba and Tofu Salad with Carrot Miso Dressing, 152
Steamed Broccoli with Tahini Miso Dressing, 441
Thai Tempeh with Broccoli and Snow Peas, 295
Wagon Wheels with Broccoli, Turkey and Parmesan, 418
broccoli rabe, 392
Broccoli Rabe and Chicken Sausage Fusilli, 392
Kamut Ditalini with Broccoli Rabe, Pesto and White Beans, 385
Spaghetti Limone with Asparagus and Mushrooms (tip), 411
Brussels sprouts, 412, 434
Brussels Sprouts Salad with Maple Mustard Dressing, 120
Lemony Brussels Sprouts Slaw, 128
Skillet Brussels Sprouts with Toasted Pecans, 442
Spaghetti with Brussels Sprouts and Toasted Walnuts, 412
buckwheat, 20, 21, 438. *See also* noodles
Gluten-Free Flax Muffins, 491
Kasha with Summer Vegetables, 459
bulgur, 21, 141, 438
Bulgur Burgers, 236
Bulgur Pilaf with Apricots and Coriander, 458
Bulgur Salad with Oranges, Cashews and Fresh Mint, 142
Lentil and Bulgur Salad with Grapes and Mint, 143
Middle Eastern Beef, Bulgur and Chickpea Soup, 199
Middle Eastern Meatballs with Feta Sauce, 339
Moroccan-Spiced Shrimp (variation), 376
Mushroom- and Bulgur-Stuffed Peppers, 264
Tabbouleh, 141
Tabbouleh Soup with Lentils and Bulgur, 185

C

cabbage, 154. *See also* coleslaw mix
Garden Pasta Salad, 154
Grilled Tilapia Tacos with Mango Salsa, 366
Minted Sprout Salad, 132
Napa Cabbage and Ginger Slaw, 127
Roasted Pork Tenderloin with Pear Slaw, 323

Thai Chicken Salad, 158
Winter Red Cabbage Slaw, 127
capers, 40–41
carrots, 73, 169, 188, 434. *See also* coleslaw mix
Broccoli Carrot Slaw with Cranberries and Sunflower Seeds, 129
California Vegetable Wraps, 228
Capellini with Watercress, Carrots and Almonds, 383
Cardamom Carrot Bread, 469
Carrot and Feta Fritters with Minted Yogurt Sauce, 268
Carrot Macaroni and Cheese, 398
Carrot Oat Breakfast Cookies, 73
Glazed Carrots with Mint, 443
Goat Cheese, Carrot and Golden Raisin Sandwich, 217
Lentil Patties with Herbed Yogurt Sauce, 271
Minted Sprout Salad, 132
Miso Soup with Soba and Vegetables, 192
Moroccan Carrot Salad, 130
Napa Cabbage and Ginger Slaw, 127
Provençal Poached Sea Scallops, 373
Shredded Beet, Carrot and Mint Salad, 129
Soba and Tofu Salad with Carrot Miso Dressing, 152
Spiced Carrot Cake with Currants, 499
Velvety Carrot Soup, 169
cashews, 85, 424, 525, 526, 532. *See also* nut butters
Blueberry Lemon Nice Cream, 526
Bulgur Salad with Oranges, Cashews and Fresh Mint, 142
Carob Energy Nuggets, 87
Cashew Oat Cakes with Spicy Tomato Sauce, 270
Cashew Vanilla "Whipped Cream," 532
Chocolate Pudding, 521
Creamy Cashew Maple Dip with Apples, 108
Grilled Eggplant with Chickpeas and Cashew Yogurt Sauce, 257
Persian Brown Rice and Cashew Salad, 137
Quinoa Cashew Power Balls, 85
Thai Cashew Noodles, 424
Vanilla Cashew Ice Cream, 525
cauliflower, 170, 282, 434
Garlicky Cauliflower Purée, 443
Indian-Spiced Cauliflower, Spinach and Tofu Scramble, 291
Roasted Cauliflower and Radicchio Salad, 122
Roasted Cauliflower Rotini with Green Olives and Currants, 410
Roasted Cauliflower Soup, 170
Skillet-Roasted Cauliflower Omelet, 282
Warm Cauliflower and Parsley Salad, 121
Winter White Bean, Cauliflower and Arugula Salad, 135
celery, 209
Miso Chicken with Crunchy Herb Salad, 302
Spicy Three-Bean Salad, 136
Waldorf Salad, 114
cheese, 32. *See also specific cheeses (below)*
Broccoli and Spinach Enchiladas, 274
Carrot Macaroni and Cheese, 398
Cheese, Almond and Mushroom Muffins, 68
Cottage Cheese Pancakes with Yogurt and Jam, 47
Creamy Millet Polenta with Cheese and Chives, 458
Eggplant Parmesan Melts, 277
Fast Vegetable Lasagna, 419
Five-Minute Cheesecake Cups with Raspberries, 501
Gemelli with Ricotta, Peas and Lemon, 395
Herbed Cheese, Turkey and Sprouts Sandwiches, 221
Honey-Roasted Plums with Ricotta, 506
Lasagna Rolls, 421
Multigrain Macaroni with Zucchini, Greek Yogurt and Romano, 399
Portobello Pizzas, 273
Pumpkin Mushroom Lasagna, 420
Ricotta Pudding with Strawberry Coulis, 519
Seared Halloumi with Chickpea Salsa and Herbed Couscous, 278
Spinach and Ricotta Bruschetta, 64
Spinach Mushroom Quesadillas, 276
Swiss Chard, Cherry Tomato and Ricotta Bake, 280
cheese, feta, 53
Arugula, Watermelon and Feta Salad, 117
Carrot and Feta Fritters with Minted Yogurt Sauce, 268
Cherry Tomato, Avocado and Cucumber Pitas (variation), 224
Chopped Greek Salad, 119
Falafel Fusilli with Spinach and Feta, 390
Favorite Frittata, 53
Fusilli with Chickpeas, Tomatoes, Feta and Herbs, 389
Fusilli with Red Lentils, Spinach and Feta, 391
Greek Chicken with Cherry Tomatoes and Feta, 299
Greek Grilled Shrimp with Feta and Dill, 375
Greek Pizza, 244
Greek Salad Frittata, 283
Greek Salad Pitas, 224
Middle Eastern Meatballs with Feta Sauce, 339
Moussaka Macaroni, 400
Skillet-Roasted Cauliflower Omelet, 282
Spinach and Feta Crustless Quiche, 287
Spinach-Stuffed Mushrooms, 110
cheese, goat
Asparagus and Goat Cheese Pizza, 245
Asparagus Penne with Goat Cheese, 403
Fresh Herb Goat Cheese Spread, 105
Goat Cheese, Carrot and Golden Raisin Sandwich, 217
Goat Cheese, Edamame and Roasted Pepper Wraps, 228
Goat Cheese and Pistachio-Stuffed Dates, 507
Mesclun Salad with Dates and Goat Cheese, 117
Multigrain Gemelli with Beets, Beet Greens and Goat Cheese, 394
Orzo Salad with Fennel, Radishes and Goat Cheese, 155
Quinoa-Stuffed Poblano Chiles, 263
Shaved Beet Salad with Pistachios and Goat Cheese, 132
Whole Wheat Orzo with Swiss Chard and Pecans, 401
Winter Squash and Goat Cheese Enchiladas, 275
cheese, Parmesan
Farro Risotto with Swiss Chard and Parmesan, 267
Fast Pumpkin Pasta with Parmesan and Chives, 414
Gemelli with Wilted Mustard Greens, 393
Grilled Steak with Arugula and Parmesan, 332
Lemony Chickpea and Quinoa Soup with Parmesan, 181
Wagon Wheels with Broccoli, Turkey and Parmesan, 418
cherries, 81, 504. *See also* berries; fruit
Baked Apples with Walnuts and Dried Cherries, 505
Breakfast Polenta with Cherries and Almonds, 57
Cherry Clafouti, 504
Chewy Cherry Granola Bars, 81
Maple Brown Rice Pudding with Dried Cherries, 520
Sautéed Pork Chops with Balsamic Onions, Kale and Cherries, 327
Swiss Chard, Cherry and Pecan Salad, 115
Waldorf Salad, 114
Wheat Berry, Pecan and Cherry Salad, 151
chicken, 298. *See also* turkey
Asian Chicken Noodle Soup, 194
Broccoli, Asparagus and Chicken Stir-Fry, 304
Broccoli Rabe and Chicken Sausage Fusilli, 392

chicken (*continued*)
Chicken and Black Bean Chilaquiles, 316
Chicken and Edamame Shiratake Noodles, 425
Chicken and Zucchini Spiedini with Salsa Verde, 310
Chicken Biryani, 314
Chicken Salad Sandwiches with Apricots and Almonds, 219
Chicken Sausage, Arugula and Tomato Penne, 406
Chicken Sausage and Black-Eyed Peas, 317
Chicken Shwarma, 308
Chicken Souvlaki, 307
Chicken with Cherry Tomato and Avocado Salsa, 300
Chicken with Sautéed Apples and Swiss Chard, 298
Couscous Paella with Shrimp and Chicken Sausage, 378
Cuban Chicken with Black Beans and Brown Rice, 311
Greek Chicken with Cherry Tomatoes and Feta, 299
Jamaican Chicken Couscous, 312
Japanese Sesame Chicken Skewers, 309
Mediterranean Tuna Sandwich (variation), 222
Miso Chicken with Crunchy Herb Salad, 302
Penne with Chicken Sausage, Mustard and Basil, 405
Pineapple Mint Chicken, 313
Provençal Chicken and Orzo Salad, 157
Pumpkin, Sausage and Smoked Gouda Pizza, 247
Soba with Chicken in Green Tea Broth, 427
Spaghetti with Tuna, Olives and Golden Raisins (variation), 415
Speedy Weeknight Lo Mein (variation), 422
Spiced Chicken and Couscous Soup, 195
Spicy Chicken, Spinach and Peanut Stir-Fry, 305
Spicy Skillet Chicken with Avocado Mango Salsa, 301
Spring Vegetable Chicken Quinoa, 315
Stir-Fried Pork and Peppers with Buckwheat Noodles (variation), 329
Stir-Fried Tangerine Chicken, 306
Thai Chicken and Basil, 303
Thai Chicken Salad, 158
Vietnamese-Style Chicken Sandwiches, 220

chickpeas, 145
Brown Rice, Greens and Miso Soup, 191
Butternut Squash Farro with Chickpeas and Cranberries, 258
Chickpea Potato Masala, 252
Chopped Greek Salad, 119
Fusilli with Chickpeas, Tomatoes, Feta and Herbs, 389
Greek Salad Pitas, 224
Grilled Eggplant with Chickpeas and Cashew Yogurt Sauce, 257
Hummus, Traditional, 105
Indian-Spiced Chickpea Chili, 209
Indian-Spiced Quinoa, Watercress and Chickpea Salad, 150
Lemony Chickpea and Quinoa Soup with Parmesan, 181
Middle Eastern Beef, Bulgur and Chickpea Soup, 199
Middle Eastern Couscous, Date and Chickpea Salad, 145
Middle Eastern Meatballs with Feta Sauce, 339
Okra, Chickpea and Tomato Tagine, 255
Penne with Hummus, Smoked Paprika and Chickpeas, 404
Quick Moroccan Beef and Chickpea Chili, 213
Quinoa and Chickpea Wraps, 229
Red Lentil and Kale Stew, 203
Seared Halloumi with Chickpea Salsa and Herbed Couscous, 278
Spiced Beef Keema with Chickpeas and Green Peas, 337
Spicy, Crispy Roasted Chickpeas, 89
Spicy Chickpea Burgers, 235
Spicy Punjabi Chickpeas with Mint Radish Raita, 256
Spicy Three-Bean Salad, 136
Spring Vegetable Tagine, 254
Tuna and White Bean Salad (variation), 160
Tunisian Chickpea, Quinoa and Lentil Soup, 182
Turkey Sausage, Spinach and Chickpea Ragù, 319
Zucchini and Chickpea Salad, 136

chocolate and cocoa powder, 38, 515, 524
Black Bean Brownies, 518
Carob Energy Nuggets (variation), 87
Chocolate Cake, Decadent, 494
Chocolate-Dipped Frozen Bananas, 531
Chocolate Gelato, 524
Chocolate Pudding, 521
Cocoa Truffles, 508
Double Almond Chocolate Biscotti, 515

citrus fruits, 38, 403. *See also specific fruits*
Lemon Drop Scones, 486
Pistachio and Citrus Couscous Salad, 144
Shrimp, Grapefruit and Watercress Salad, 163

coconut, 531. *See also* coconut milk
Carob Energy Nuggets, 87
Chewy Cherry Granola Bars, 81
Chickpea Potato Masala, 252
Chocolate-Dipped Frozen Bananas, 531
No-Bake Raspberry Thumbprints, 509
Spiced Carrot Cake with Currants, 499

coconut milk, 33
Basil Coconut Tofu Curry, 290
Chocolate Gelato, 524
Chocolate Pudding, 521
Halibut with Coconut Lime Sauce, 353
Jamaican Rice and Peas, 456
One-Pot Eggplant, Mushroom and Potato Curry, 250
Red Curry Shrimp Noodle Bowls, 431
Red Lentil Dal Spread, 99
Red Lentil Mulligatawny, 184
Sweet Potato and Spinach Curry with Quinoa, 261
Sweet Potato Bisque with West Indian Spices, 173
Thai Curry Pumpkin Soup, 171
Thai Pumpkin and Brown Rice Risotto, 265
Thai Tempeh with Broccoli and Snow Peas, 295

coleslaw mix. *See also* cabbage; carrots
Black Bean Tacos, 277
Chicken and Edamame Shiratake Noodles, 425
Chipotle Tilapia Tacos with Pineapple, 367
Grilled Salmon Sandwiches with Creamy Lime Coleslaw, 223
Grilled Steak Tacos with Avocado and Cumin Lime Slaw, 334
Korean Sesame Soy Pork with Quick Kimchi Slaw, 328
Southeast Asian Roast Beef Wraps, 232
Vietnamese-Style Chicken Sandwiches, 220

corn, 275, 316. *See also* cornmeal and hominy
Black Bean Avocado Salsa, 98
Edamame and Corn Salad, 124
Edamame Succotash, 453
Kasha with Summer Vegetables, 459
Oven-BBQ Salmon with Fresh Corn Basil Relish, 356
Speedy Southwest Black Bean and Quinoa Skillet, 260
Summer Vegetable Orzo Soup, 189

cornmeal and hominy, 20, 438
Breakfast Polenta with Cherries and Almonds, 57
Green Chile and Pork Pozole, 211
Multigrain Pancake and Waffle Mix, 44
Multi-Seed Spelt Biscuits, 484
Skillet Cornbread, 468

couscous, 378. *See also* pasta
Couscous Paella with Shrimp and Chicken Sausage, 378
Jamaican Chicken Couscous, 312
Mediterranean Grilled Tilapia and Whole Wheat Couscous, 364
Middle Eastern Couscous, Date and Chickpea Salad, 145

Moroccan-Spiced Ground Turkey with Apricot Couscous, 322
Moroccan-Spiced Shrimp, 376
Pistachio and Citrus Couscous Salad, 144
Seared Halloumi with Chickpea Salsa and Herbed Couscous, 278
Spiced Chicken and Couscous Soup, 195
cranberries, 476. *See also* berries
Broccoli Carrot Slaw with Cranberries and Sunflower Seeds, 129
Butternut Squash Farro with Chickpeas and Cranberries, 258
Cranberry, Orange and Agave Bread, 476
Delicata Squash with Quinoa Stuffing, 262
Multigrain Cranberry Breakfast Cookies, 72
Oats and Dried Fruit Breakfast Bars, 69
Pumpkin Cranberry Cookies, 513
Quinoa Cranberry Granola, 60
Turkey, Kale and Cranberry Wraps, 230
Winter Red Cabbage Slaw, 127
cucumber
California Sushi Roll Salad, 138
California Vegetable Wraps, 228
Cherry Tomato, Avocado and Cucumber Pitas, 224
Chicken Souvlaki, 307
Chopped Greek Salad, 119
Farmers' Market Gazpacho, 175
Greek Salad Pitas, 224
Greek Yogurt Dip with Fresh Squash "Chips," 107
Grilled Striped Bass with Kiwi and Cucumber Salsa, 342
Pistachio and Citrus Couscous Salad, 144
Tabbouleh, 141
Thai Chicken Salad, 158
Thai Salmon Burgers, 240

D

dates, 36–37. *See also* fruit
Chocolate Pudding, 521
Cocoa Truffles, 508
Date Bars, 517
Goat Cheese and Pistachio-Stuffed Dates, 507
Mesclun Salad with Dates and Goat Cheese, 117
Middle Eastern Couscous, Date and Chickpea Salad, 145
Oatmeal Cookies, 510
Persian Brown Rice and Cashew Salad, 137
Spiced Date Bread, 475

E

edamame, 453
Chicken and Edamame Shiratake Noodles, 425
Cod with Roasted Tomatoes and Edamame Mash, 348
Edamame and Corn Salad, 124
Edamame Basil Spread, 102
Edamame Succotash, 453
Goat Cheese, Edamame and Roasted Pepper Wraps, 228
Roasted Salt and Pepper Edamame, 89
eggplant, 435, 444
Broiled Eggplant with Garlic Yogurt and Mint, 444
Easy Ratatouille with Poached Eggs, 279
Eggplant Parmesan Melts, 277
Grilled Eggplant with Chickpeas and Cashew Yogurt Sauce, 257
Middle Eastern Eggplant Spread, 104
Moussaka Macaroni, 400
One-Pot Eggplant, Mushroom and Potato Curry, 250
Quick Pasta al Norma, 413
Roasted Vegetable Salsa, 96
Tofu and Eggplant Stir-Fry, 289
eggs, 30–31, 56, 287
Avocado and Egg Breakfast Wraps, 56
Baked Eggs in Marinara, 52
Easy Ratatouille with Poached Eggs, 279
Egg Salad Sandwiches on Dark Rye, 218
Favorite Frittata, 53
Greek Salad Frittata, 283
Herbed Deviled Eggs, 111
Microwave Poached Eggs, 52
Niçoise Salad Wraps, 232
Persian Zucchini Frittata, 284
Picadillo, 335
Power Pitas with Eggs and Vegetables, 54
Quinoa, Mushroom and Green Onion Frittata, 286
Quinoa Kale Breakfast Casserole, 57
Red Lentil Frittata, 285
Sicilian Tuna and Rice Salad, 161
Skillet-Roasted Cauliflower Omelet, 282
Spanish Sweet Potato Tortilla with Roasted Pepper Sauce, 281
Spinach and Feta Crustless Quiche, 287
Spinach Egg Drop Soup, 193
Swedish Salmon, Asparagus and Potato Omelet, 361
Swiss Chard, Cherry Tomato and Ricotta Bake, 280
Tuna and Asparagus Frittata, 371
Tunisian Tuna and Egg Salad Pitas, 225

F

farro, 21, 438. *See also* barley
Butternut Squash Farro with Chickpeas and Cranberries, 258
Farro Risotto with Swiss Chard and Parmesan, 267
Farro Salad with Arugula and Tomatoes, 146
Farro Stew with Spring Peas and Mint, 205
Tabbouleh (variation), 141
Tuna with Farro and Fennel, 370
Tuscan Farro and White Bean Soup, 187
fennel, 435
Fennel, Orange and Olive Salad, 116
Orzo Salad with Fennel, Radishes and Goat Cheese, 155
Rotini with Fennel, Orange and Almonds, 409
Tuna with Farro and Fennel, 370
White Bean Bajane with Thyme Barley, 259
fish. *See also* salmon; seafood; tuna
Baked Trout with Shiitake Mushrooms and Ginger, 369
Black Cod with Fresh Herb Sauce, 344
Broiled Herbed Trout Fillets, 368
Broiled Mahi Mahi with Red Pepper Harissa, 354
Chipotle Tilapia Tacos with Pineapple, 367
Cod Poached in Tapenade Tomato Broth, 347
Cod with Roasted Tomatoes and Edamame Mash, 348
Foil-Roasted Halibut and Asparagus, 351
Garam Masala–Spiced Tilapia with Watermelon Salsa, 365
Ginger Soy Cod, 347
Grilled Black Cod with North African Salsa, 346
Grilled Striped Bass with Kiwi and Cucumber Salsa, 342
Grilled Tilapia Tacos with Mango Salsa, 366
Halibut with Beets and Beet Greens, 352
Halibut with Coconut Lime Sauce, 353
Herbed Cod Cakes, 349
Lemon Dill Tilapia in Foil, 363
Mediterranean Grilled Tilapia and Whole Wheat Couscous, 364
Red Fish Stew, 206
Seared Striped Bass with Broccoli and Almond Quinoa, 343
Whole Grain–Crusted Fish Sticks, 350
flax seeds (ground), 29, 31
Almond Flax Seed Energy Cookies, 84
Amaranth Spice Bread, 473
Applesauce Flax Bread, 478
Banana and Toasted Millet Muffins, 67
Carrot Oat Breakfast Cookies, 73
Fresh Apple Bread, 477
Gluten-Free Flax Muffins, 491
Multigrain Pancake and Waffle Mix, 44
Oats and Dried Fruit Breakfast Bars, 69
Overnight Oatmeal, 58

flax seeds (*continued*)
Power Granola, 59
Pumpkin Maple Waffles, 51
Toasted Oat Muesli with Dried Fruit and Pecans, 61
Walnut Flax Waffles, 50
Whole Grain–Crusted Fish Sticks, 350
Yogurt Bran Muffins, 66
fruit, 9, 23–27, 178, 272, 506. *See also* berries; fruit juices; *specific fruits*
Amaranth Spice Bread, 473
Cottage Cheese Pancakes with Yogurt and Jam, 47
Crispy Brown Rice Treats, 516
Fruit and Nut Raw Energy Bars, 82
Gluten-Free Flax Muffins (variation), 491
Honey-Roasted Plums with Ricotta, 506
Jamaican Chicken Couscous, 312
Lemon Drop Scones (variation), 486
Maple Oat Drop Scones (variation), 487
Maple Whole Wheat Muffins (variation), 490
Minted Fruit Salad, 507
Moroccan Carrot Salad, 130
Moroccan-Spiced Shrimp, 376
Multigrain Gemelli with Beets, Beet Greens and Goat Cheese, 394
No-Bake Raspberry Thumbprints, 509
Oats and Dried Fruit Breakfast Bars, 69
Pomegranate and Quinoa Salad with Sunflower Seeds (variation), 149
Provençal Chicken and Orzo Salad, 157
Roasted Cauliflower Rotini with Green Olives and Currants, 410
Spiced Carrot Cake with Currants, 499
Toasted Oat Muesli with Dried Fruit and Pecans, 61
Whole Wheat and Olive Oil Biscotti, 514
Whole Wheat Irish Soda Bread (variation), 464
fruit juices, 10
All-Natural Fruit Gelatin (*Kanten*), 523
Blueberry Yogurt Pops, 529
Papaya Pineapple Smoothie, 76
Pistachio and Citrus Couscous Salad, 144
Pumpkin Smoothie, 77
Strawberry Mousse, 520

G

grapes, 143
Green Machine Smoothie, 76
Lentil and Bulgur Salad with Grapes and Mint, 143
Waldorf Salad, 114
greens, 447. *See also* beets; *specific greens*
Beef and Quinoa Power Burgers, 238
Brown Rice, Greens and Miso Soup, 191
Collard Green Ribbons, 447
Egg Salad Sandwiches on Dark Rye, 218
Goat Cheese, Carrot and Golden Raisin Sandwich, 217
Green Club Sandwich, 216
Green Machine Smoothie, 76
Miso Chicken with Crunchy Herb Salad, 302
Tofu Salad Sandwiches, 218
Turkey Sausage, Escarole and Sun-Dried Tomato Pasta, 407

K

kale, 416. *See also* greens
Barley, Mushroom and Kale Stew, 204
Butternut Squash, White Bean and Kale Stew, 202
Crispy Kale Chips, 91
Kale, Apple and Walnut Slaw, 128
Lentil, Mushroom and Kale Burritos, 227
Quick Kale and Quinoa Minestrone, 177
Quick Sautéed Kale, 448
Quinoa Kale Breakfast Casserole, 57
Quinoa Spaghetti with Kale, 416
Red Lentil and Kale Stew, 203
Sautéed Pork Chops with Balsamic Onions, Kale and Cherries, 327
Turkey, Kale and Cranberry Wraps, 230
Vegetable Minestrone, 176
Kamut, 21
Kamut Ditalini with Broccoli Rabe, Pesto and White Beans, 385
kiwifruit
Green Machine Smoothie, 76
Grilled Striped Bass with Kiwi and Cucumber Salsa, 342
Kiwi Sorbet, 523
Minted Fruit Salad, 507

L

lemon, 363. *See also* citrus fruits
Barley Risotto with Asparagus and Lemon, 266
Blueberry Lemon Nice Cream, 526
Gemelli with Ricotta, Peas and Lemon, 395
Lemon Blackberry Fool, 522
Lemon Dill Tilapia in Foil, 363
Lemon Drop Scones, 486
Lemon Raspberry Yogurt Cones, 528
Lemony Brussels Sprouts Slaw, 128
Lemony Chickpea and Quinoa Soup with Parmesan, 181
Lemony Lentil and Quinoa Salad, 148
Salmon Penne with Peas and Lemon, 408
Spaghetti Limone with Asparagus and Mushrooms, 411
Spicy Tuna Cakes with Lemony Spinach, 372
lentils, 28, 99, 203, 227, 436–37
French Lentil Soup, 183
Fusilli with Red Lentils, Spinach and Feta, 391
Koshari, 253
Lemony Lentil and Quinoa Salad, 148
Lentil, Mushroom and Kale Burritos, 227
Lentil, Walnut and Arugula Spread, 100
Lentil and Bulgur Salad with Grapes and Mint, 143
Lentil Patties with Herbed Yogurt Sauce, 271
Red Lentil and Kale Stew, 203
Red Lentil Dal Spread, 99
Red Lentil Frittata, 285
Red Lentil Mulligatawny, 184
Seared Salmon with Warm Lentil and Arugula Salad, 359
Swedish Yellow Split Pea Soup with Fresh Dill (tip), 179
Sweet Potato, Lentil and Arugula Salad, 134
Tabbouleh Soup with Lentils and Bulgur, 185
Tunisian Chickpea, Quinoa and Lentil Soup, 182
lettuce, 335. *See also* greens
Asian Lettuce Wraps, 321
Carrot and Feta Fritters with Minted Yogurt Sauce, 268
Chicken Salad Sandwiches with Apricots and Almonds, 219
Chopped Greek Salad, 119
Lentil Patties with Herbed Yogurt Sauce, 271
Mesclun Salad with Dates and Goat Cheese, 117
Miso Chicken with Crunchy Herb Salad, 302
Niçoise Salad Wraps, 232
Picadillo, 335
Salmon Cakes with Buttermilk Dressing and Mixed Greens, 362
Smoked Turkey, Avocado and Mango Wraps, 231
lime. *See also* citrus fruits
Grilled Salmon Sandwiches with Creamy Lime Coleslaw, 223
Grilled Steak Tacos with Avocado and Cumin Lime Slaw, 334
Halibut with Coconut Lime Sauce, 353
Lemon Drop Scones (variation), 486
Soba with Shrimp, Lime and Cilantro, 429
Swiss Chard Spring Rolls with Sesame Lime Dipping Sauce, 109

M

mango, 231
  Chipotle Tilapia Tacos with Pineapple (variation), 367
  Cuban Braised Beef with Brown Rice and Mango, 331
  Grilled Tilapia Tacos with Mango Salsa, 366
  Kiwi Sorbet (variation), 523
  Smoked Turkey, Avocado and Mango Wraps, 231
  Spicy Skillet Chicken with Avocado Mango Salsa, 301
  Thai Salmon Burgers, 240
maple syrup, 36
millet, 21–22, 438
  Banana and Toasted Millet Muffins, 67
  Creamy Millet Polenta with Cheese and Chives, 458
mushrooms, 167, 233, 273
  Baked Trout with Shiitake Mushrooms and Ginger, 369
  Barley, Mushroom and Kale Stew, 204
  Bok Choy and Mushroom Soup, 167
  Brown Rice, Greens and Miso Soup, 191
  Cheese, Almond and Mushroom Muffins, 68
  Lentil, Mushroom and Kale Burritos, 227
  Mushroom, Pepper and Arugula Pizza, 246
  Mushroom and Barley Soup, 188
  Mushroom- and Bulgur-Stuffed Peppers, 264
  One-Pot Eggplant, Mushroom and Potato Curry, 250
  Portobello Pesto Burgers, 233
  Portobello Pizzas, 273
  Pumpkin Mushroom Lasagna, 420
  Quinoa, Mushroom and Green Onion Frittata, 286
  Roasted Vegetable Linguine, 396
  Skillet Pizza Marinara (variation), 241
  Soba and Tofu Salad with Carrot Miso Dressing, 152
  Spaghetti Limone with Asparagus and Mushrooms, 411
  Spelt and Wild Mushroom Pilaf, 457
  Spinach-Stuffed Mushrooms, 110
  Stir-Fried Mushrooms with Lemon and Parsley, 445
  Tofu Scramble, 54
mustard greens, 325. *See also* greens
  Chicken Sausage and Black-Eyed Peas, 317
  Gemelli with Wilted Mustard Greens, 393
  Honey Mustard Pork Tenderloin with Mustard Greens, 325
  Turkey Sausage with Mustard Greens and Kidney Beans, 318
  Turkey Soup with Sweet Potatoes and Mustard Greens, 196

N

noodles, 23. *See also* pasta
  Buckwheat Noodle Bowls with Beef and Snap Peas, 428
  Chicken and Edamame Shiratake Noodles, 425
  Miso Soup with Soba and Vegetables, 192
  Red Curry Shrimp Noodle Bowls, 431
  Soba and Tofu Salad with Carrot Miso Dressing, 152
  Soba with Chicken in Green Tea Broth, 427
  Soba with Shrimp, Lime and Cilantro, 429
  Soba with Shrimp and Baby Bok Choy, 430
  Stir-Fried Pork and Peppers with Buckwheat Noodles, 329
  Teriyaki Soba, Spinach and Tofu Noodles, 426
nut butters, 30. *See also* nuts; seed butters
  Almond Flax Seed Energy Cookies, 84
  Cashew Butter and Banana Wraps, 229
  Chewy Cherry Granola Bars, 81
  Crispy Brown Rice Treats, 516
  Double Almond Chocolate Biscotti, 515
  Multigrain Cranberry Breakfast Cookies, 72
  No-Bake Raspberry Thumbprints, 509
  PB&J Energy Balls, 86
  Sesame Ginger Noodles, 423
  Sesame Peanut Vegetable Noodle Salad, 153
  Southeast Asian Roast Beef Wraps, 232
  Thai Cashew Noodles, 424
  Thai Chicken Salad, 158
  Thai Tempeh with Broccoli and Snow Peas, 295
  Walnut Quinoa Power Bars, 83
nuts, 29, 125, 501, 514. *See also* nut butters; *specific types of nuts*
  Fruit and Nut Raw Energy Bars, 82
  Green Bean Salad with Toasted Hazelnuts, 125
  Maple Whole Wheat Muffins (variation), 490
  Oats and Dried Fruit Breakfast Bars, 69
  Sweet and Spicy Nuts and Seeds, 88
  Tamari Seed and Nut Mix, 88
  Whole Wheat and Olive Oil Biscotti, 514

O

oats, 22, 46, 438
  Banana Buttermilk Smoothie, 74
  Berry Peach Crumbles, 503
  Carrot Oat Breakfast Cookies, 73
  Cashew Oat Cakes with Spicy Tomato Sauce, 270
  Chewy Cherry Granola Bars, 81
  Creamy Broccoli Soup, 168
  Crunchy Vanilla Granola Bars, 80
  Date Bars, 517
  Maple Oat Drop Scones, 487
  Maple Spice Cookies, 511
  Multigrain Cranberry Breakfast Cookies, 72
  Multigrain Pancake and Waffle Mix, 44
  No-Bake Raspberry Thumbprints, 509
  Oatmeal Buttermilk Pancakes, 46
  Oatmeal Cookies, 510
  Oats and Dried Fruit Breakfast Bars, 69
  Overnight Oatmeal, 58
  PB&J Energy Balls, 86
  Power Granola, 59
  Quinoa Cranberry Granola, 60
  Scottish Oat Cakes, 488
  Spiced Carrot Cake with Currants, 499
  Sunflower Apricot Go-Bars, 70
  Toasted Oat Muesli with Dried Fruit and Pecans, 61
  Walnut Quinoa Power Bars (variation), 83
  Whole-Grain Blueberry Maple Muffins, 65
onions, 191, 435
  Balsamic Roasted Red Onions, 446
  Farro Risotto with Swiss Chard and Parmesan, 267
  Fusilli with Red Lentils, Spinach and Feta, 391
  Ginger Soy Cod, 347
  Japanese Ginger Beef Bowls, 333
  Multigrain Gemelli with Beets, Beet Greens and Goat Cheese, 394
  Quinoa, Mushroom and Green Onion Frittata, 286
  Quinoa-Stuffed Poblano Chiles, 263
  Red Lentil Dal Spread, 99
  Sautéed Pork Chops with Balsamic Onions, Kale and Cherries, 327
  Sesame and Green Onion Bread, 467
  Shrimp and Asparagus Stir-Fry, 374
  Spicy Chicken, Spinach and Peanut Stir-Fry, 305
  Spring Vegetable Chicken Quinoa, 315
  Spring Vegetable Tagine, 254
  Stir-Fried Pork and Peppers with Buckwheat Noodles, 329
  Turkey Sausage, Escarole and Sun-Dried Tomato Pasta, 407
oranges, 75, 116. *See also* fruit juices; tangerines
  Bulgur Salad with Oranges, Cashews and Fresh Mint, 142
  Cranberry, Orange and Agave Bread, 476
  Fennel, Orange and Olive Salad, 116
  Jamaican Chicken Couscous, 312

oranges (*continued*)
Moroccan Carrot Salad (variation), 130
Roasted Beet and Beet Greens Salad, 118
Rotini with Fennel, Orange and Almonds, 409
Spinach, Avocado and Orange Salad, 115
Super C Smoothie, 75

P

papaya, 76
Crab and Papaya Salad with Mint Dressing, 162
Papaya Pineapple Smoothie, 76
parsnips
Baked Parsnip Fries, 451
Glazed Carrots with Mint (variation), 443
pasta, 14, 22–23, 378, 398. *See also* couscous; noodles
Asian Chicken Noodle Soup, 194
Asparagus Penne with Goat Cheese, 403
Broccoli Rabe and Chicken Sausage Fusilli, 392
Butternut Squash Fettuccine, 388
Capellini with Watercress, Carrots and Almonds, 383
Carrot Macaroni and Cheese, 398
Chicken Sausage, Arugula and Tomato Penne, 406
Curried Orzo Soup, 190
Falafel Fusilli with Spinach and Feta, 390
Farfalle with Swiss Chard, White Beans and Walnuts, 386
Farfalle with Tuna and Tomatoes, 387
Fast Pumpkin Pasta with Parmesan and Chives, 414
Fast Vegetable Lasagna, 419
Fusilli with Chickpeas, Tomatoes, Feta and Herbs, 389
Fusilli with Red Lentils, Spinach and Feta, 391
Garden Pasta Salad, 154
Gemelli with Ricotta, Peas and Lemon, 395
Gemelli with Wilted Mustard Greens, 393
Greek Capellini with Shrimp, Tomatoes and Mint, 384
Kamut Ditalini with Broccoli Rabe, Pesto and White Beans, 385
Koshari, 253
Lasagna Rolls, 421
Moussaka Macaroni, 400
Multigrain Gemelli with Beets, Beet Greens and Goat Cheese, 394
Multigrain Linguine with Clam Sauce, 397
Multigrain Macaroni with Zucchini, Greek Yogurt and Romano, 399
Orzo Salad with Fennel, Radishes and Goat Cheese, 155
Pasta e Fagioli, 201
Penne with Chicken Sausage, Mustard and Basil, 405
Penne with Hummus, Smoked Paprika and Chickpeas, 404
Provençal Chicken and Orzo Salad, 157
Pumpkin Mushroom Lasagna, 420
Quick Pasta al Norma, 413
Quinoa Spaghetti al Pomodoro, 417
Quinoa Spaghetti with Kale, 416
Red Pepper Pesto Capellini, 382
Roasted Cauliflower Rotini with Green Olives and Currants, 410
Roasted Vegetable Linguine, 396
Rotini with Fennel, Orange and Almonds, 409
Salmon Penne with Peas and Lemon, 408
Sesame Ginger Noodles, 423
Sesame Peanut Vegetable Noodle Salad, 153
Spaghetti Limone with Asparagus and Mushrooms, 411
Spaghetti with Brussels Sprouts and Toasted Walnuts, 412
Spaghetti with Tuna, Olives and Golden Raisins, 415
Speedy Weeknight Lo Mein, 422
Summer Vegetable Orzo Soup, 189
Thai Cashew Noodles, 424
Turkey Sausage, Escarole and Sun-Dried Tomato Pasta, 407
Vegetable Minestrone, 176
Vietnamese Pho, 197
Wagon Wheels with Broccoli, Turkey and Parmesan, 418
Whole Wheat Orzo with Swiss Chard and Pecans, 401
peaches, 503
Berry Peach Crumbles, 503
Blueberry Yogurt Pops (variation), 529
Kiwi Sorbet (variation), 523
peanuts, 86. *See also* nut butters
PB&J Energy Balls, 86
Sesame Peanut Vegetable Noodle Salad, 153
Spicy Chicken, Spinach and Peanut Stir-Fry, 305
Tamari Seed and Nut Mix, 88
Thai Chicken Salad, 158
pears, 323
Cinnamon Apple Chips (variation), 92
Fresh Apple Bread (variation), 477
Roasted Pork Tenderloin with Pear Slaw, 323
peas, dried, 28, 179, 436–37. *See also* chickpeas
Black-Eyed Pea Soup with Indian Spices, 180
Chicken Sausage and Black-Eyed Peas, 317
Swedish Yellow Split Pea Soup with Fresh Dill, 179
peas, green, 205, 254, 395
Barley Risotto with Asparagus and Lemon, 266
Beef and Snow Pea Soup, 198
Buckwheat Noodle Bowls with Beef and Snap Peas, 428
Couscous Paella with Shrimp and Chicken Sausage, 378
Farro Stew with Spring Peas and Mint, 205
Gemelli with Ricotta, Peas and Lemon, 395
Green Pea and Radish Salad, 124
One-Pan Shrimp Pilau, 379
Salmon Penne with Peas and Lemon, 408
Soba and Tofu Salad with Carrot Miso Dressing, 152
Soba with Chicken in Green Tea Broth, 427
So-Easy Spring Pea Soup, 178
Spiced Beef Keema with Chickpeas and Green Peas, 337
Spring Vegetable Chicken Quinoa, 315
Spring Vegetable Tagine, 254
Thai Tempeh with Broccoli and Snow Peas, 295
pecans. *See also* nuts; walnuts
Cocoa Truffles, 508
Fruit and Nut Raw Energy Bars, 82
Power Granola, 59
Skillet Brussels Sprouts with Toasted Pecans, 442
Swiss Chard, Cherry and Pecan Salad, 115
Toasted Oat Muesli with Dried Fruit and Pecans, 61
Wheat Berry, Pecan and Cherry Salad, 151
Whole Wheat Orzo with Swiss Chard and Pecans, 401
peppers, bell, 246, 309, 434. *See also* peppers, roasted red; vegetables
Crab and Papaya Salad with Mint Dressing, 162
Egg Salad Sandwiches on Dark Rye, 218
Japanese Sesame Chicken Skewers, 309
Mushroom, Pepper and Arugula Pizza, 246
Mushroom- and Bulgur-Stuffed Peppers, 264
Sesame Ginger Noodles, 423
Spicy Chicken, Spinach and Peanut Stir-Fry, 305
Stir-Fried Pork and Peppers with Buckwheat Noodles, 329
Tofu Scramble, 54
Tuna and Asparagus Frittata (variation), 371
peppers, chile
Chicken with Cherry Tomato and Avocado Salsa, 300
Green Chile and Pork Pozole, 211
Grilled Striped Bass with Kiwi and Cucumber Salsa, 342
Napa Cabbage and Ginger Slaw, 127
Pineapple Salsa, 97
Quinoa-Stuffed Poblano Chiles, 263
Spicy Chickpea Burgers, 235

Spicy Punjabi Chickpeas with Mint Radish Raita, 256
Spicy Three-Bean Salad, 136
peppers, roasted red (bell)
Artichoke and Ricotta Pizza (variation), 243
Broiled Mahi Mahi with Red Pepper Harissa, 354
Cannellini Beans with Shrimp and Roasted Peppers, 377
Chard and Red Pepper Salad with Tahini Yogurt Dressing, 123
Farro Salad with Arugula and Tomatoes, 146
Goat Cheese, Edamame and Roasted Pepper Wraps, 228
Greek Chicken with Cherry Tomatoes and Feta (variation), 299
Grilled Black Cod with North African Salsa, 346
Middle Eastern Eggplant Spread, 104
Muhammara (Syrian Red Pepper Walnut Spread), 103
Red Fish Stew, 206
Red Pepper Pesto Capellini, 382
Spanish Sweet Potato Tortilla with Roasted Pepper Sauce, 281
Spinach and Basil Bread (variation), 471
Turkish Tomato, Pepper and Herb Salad, 126
pineapple, 97. *See also* fruit juices
Chipotle Tilapia Tacos with Pineapple, 367
Kiwi Sorbet (variation), 523
Minted Fruit Salad, 507
Pineapple Mint Chicken, 313
Pineapple Salsa, 97
Seared Salmon with Fresh Pineapple Salsa, 358
pistachios, 507
Cardamom Carrot Bread, 469
Five-Minute Cheesecake Cups with Raspberries, 501
Goat Cheese and Pistachio-Stuffed Dates, 507
Pistachio and Citrus Couscous Salad, 144
Shaved Beet Salad with Pistachios and Goat Cheese, 132
pitas
Cherry Tomato, Avocado and Cucumber Pitas, 224
Chicken Souvlaki, 307
Garlic Pita Chips, 90
Greek Salad Pitas, 224
Power Pitas with Eggs and Vegetables, 54
Tunisian Tuna and Egg Salad Pitas, 225
pork
Beef and Quinoa Power Burgers (variation), 238
Chipotle Maple Pork with Sweet Potato and Spinach Hash, 326
Green Chile and Pork Pozole, 211
Honey Mustard Pork Tenderloin with Mustard Greens, 325
Korean Sesame Soy Pork with Quick Kimchi Slaw, 328
Lean Beef and Bean Cowboy Chili (variation), 212
Roasted Pork Tenderloin with Pear Slaw, 323
Sautéed Pork Chops with Balsamic Onions, Kale and Cherries, 327
Spicy Salsa Joes (variation), 221
Stir-Fried Pork and Peppers with Buckwheat Noodles, 329
Texas BBQ Turkey Burgers (variation), 237
Thai-Style Pork with Brown Jasmine Rice, 330
Wagon Wheels with Broccoli, Turkey and Parmesan (variation), 418
White Turkey Chili (variation), 210
potatoes, 435. *See also* sweet potatoes
Chickpea Potato Masala, 252
Mustard Dill Red Potato Salad, 133
One-Pot Eggplant, Mushroom and Potato Curry, 250
Roasted Oven Fries, 450
Salmon Chowder, 200
Spanish Sweet Potato Tortilla with Roasted Pepper Sauce (tip), 281
Swedish Salmon, Asparagus and Potato Omelet, 361
Tuscan Farro and White Bean Soup, 187
pumpkin, 51, 171, 485. *See also* squash
Black Bean Pumpkin Soup, 186
Chocolate Pudding, 521
Fast Pumpkin Pasta with Parmesan and Chives, 414
Maple Pumpkin Micro-Pies, 502
Pumpkin, Sausage and Smoked Gouda Pizza, 247
Pumpkin Biscuits, 485
Pumpkin Bread, 470
Pumpkin Cranberry Cookies, 513
Pumpkin Maple Waffles, 51
Pumpkin Mushroom Lasagna, 420
Pumpkin Pepita Hummus, 106
Pumpkin Smoothie, 77
Pumpkin Yogurt with Quinoa Crunch, 62
Thai Curry Pumpkin Soup, 171
Thai Pumpkin and Brown Rice Risotto, 265
Winter Squash and Goat Cheese Enchiladas, 275

Q

quinoa, 22, 60, 293, 438. *See also* quinoa pasta
Beef and Snow Pea Soup (tip), 198
Cumin-Scented Black Beans and Quinoa, 455
Delicata Squash with Quinoa Stuffing, 262
Indian-Spiced Quinoa, Watercress and Chickpea Salad, 150
Koshari (variation), 253
Lemony Chickpea and Quinoa Soup with Parmesan, 181
Lemony Lentil and Quinoa Salad, 148
Moroccan-Spiced Shrimp (variation), 376
Pomegranate and Quinoa Salad with Sunflower Seeds, 149
Quick Kale and Quinoa Minestrone, 177
Quick Quinoa Stir-Fry with Vegetables and Tofu, 293
Quinoa, Mushroom and Green Onion Frittata, 286
Quinoa and Black Bean Salad, 147
Quinoa and Chickpea Wraps, 229
Quinoa Blueberry Breakfast Cookies, 71
Quinoa Blueberry Pancakes, 48
Quinoa Cashew Power Balls, 85
Quinoa Cranberry Granola, 60
Quinoa Crunch, 62
Quinoa Kale Breakfast Casserole, 57
Quinoa-Stuffed Poblano Chiles, 263
Quinoa Vegetable Cakes, 269
Seared Striped Bass with Broccoli and Almond Quinoa, 343
Speedy Southwest Black Bean and Quinoa Skillet, 260
Spring Vegetable Chicken Quinoa, 315
Sweet Potato and Spinach Curry with Quinoa, 261
Tabbouleh (variation), 141
Toasted Quinoa Porridge, 58
Tunisian Chickpea, Quinoa and Lentil Soup, 182
quinoa pasta, 23
Quinoa Spaghetti al Pomodoro, 417
Quinoa Spaghetti with Kale, 416
Speedy Weeknight Lo Mein, 422

R

radishes
California Vegetable Wraps, 228
Farro Stew with Spring Peas and Mint, 205
Greek Salad Pitas, 224
Green Pea and Radish Salad, 124
Orzo Salad with Fennel, Radishes and Goat Cheese, 155
Spicy Punjabi Chickpeas with Mint Radish Raita, 256
raisins, 314. *See also* fruit
Almond Flax Seed Energy Cookies, 84
Applesauce Flax Bread, 478
Cardamom Carrot Bread, 469
Carrot Oat Breakfast Cookies, 73
Easy Raisin Rye Bread, 474
Gluten-Free Flax Muffins (variation), 491
Goat Cheese, Carrot and Golden Raisin Sandwich, 217
Spaghetti with Tuna, Olives and Golden Raisins, 415

rice, 21, 379, 438. *See also* rice flour
Asian Lettuce Wraps, 321
Basic Brown Rice Pilaf, 456
Black Bean and Spinach Burritos, 226
Brown Rice, Greens and Miso Soup, 191
California Sushi Roll Salad, 138
Chicken Biryani, 314
Cuban Braised Beef with Brown Rice and Mango, 331
Cuban Chicken with Black Beans and Brown Rice, 311
Jamaican Rice and Peas, 456
Japanese Ginger Beef Bowls, 333
Koshari, 253
Maple Brown Rice Pudding with Dried Cherries, 520
One-Pan Shrimp Pilau, 379
Persian Brown Rice and Cashew Salad, 137
Red Lentil Mulligatawny, 184
Sicilian Tuna and Rice Salad, 161
Thai Pumpkin and Brown Rice Risotto, 265
Thai-Style Pork with Brown Jasmine Rice, 330
rice flour, 20
Gluten-Free Flax Muffins, 491
rye flour, 474
Easy Raisin Rye Bread, 474
Quick Pumpernickel Bread, 465

S

salmon, 359. *See also* fish
Grilled Salmon Sandwiches with Creamy Lime Coleslaw, 223
Grilled Salmon with Mustard Maple Vinaigrette, 355
Hoisin Salmon, 358
Mediterranean Tuna Sandwich (variation), 222
Oven-BBQ Salmon with Fresh Corn Basil Relish, 356
Salmon Cakes with Buttermilk Dressing and Mixed Greens, 362
Salmon Chowder, 200
Salmon Penne with Peas and Lemon, 408
Scandinavian Breakfast Toasts with Smoked Salmon and Avocado, 64
Seared Salmon with Fresh Pineapple Salsa, 358
Seared Salmon with Warm Lentil and Arugula Salad, 359
Spice-Crusted Salmon with Mint Raita, 357
Summer Salmon Panzanella, 159
Swedish Salmon, Asparagus and Potato Omelet, 361
Thai Red Curry–Glazed Salmon, 360
Thai Salmon Burgers, 240
sausage. *See* chicken; turkey
seafood. *See also* fish; shrimp
Crab and Papaya Salad with Mint Dressing, 162
Multigrain Linguine with Clam Sauce, 397
Provençal Poached Sea Scallops, 373
Salmon Chowder, 200
seed butters, 30. *See also* seeds
Crispy Brown Rice Treats, 516
Sunflower Apricot Go-Bars, 70
seeds, 514. *See also* seed butters; sunflower seeds
Japanese Sesame Chicken Skewers, 309
Multi-Seed Spelt Biscuits, 484
Multi-Seed Supper Muffins, 489
Pumpkin Pepita Hummus, 106
Sweet and Spicy Nuts and Seeds, 88
Tamari Seed and Nut Mix, 88
Whole Wheat Irish Soda Bread (variation), 464
sesame oil, 35, 302
shrimp, 374
Cannellini Beans with Shrimp and Roasted Peppers, 377
Couscous Paella with Shrimp and Chicken Sausage, 378
Greek Capellini with Shrimp, Tomatoes and Mint, 384
Greek Grilled Shrimp with Feta and Dill, 375
Moroccan-Spiced Shrimp, 376
One-Pan Shrimp Pilau, 379
Red Curry Shrimp Noodle Bowls, 431
Shrimp, Grapefruit and Watercress Salad, 163
Shrimp and Asparagus Stir-Fry, 374
Soba with Shrimp, Lime and Cilantro, 429
Soba with Shrimp and Baby Bok Choy, 430
Speedy Weeknight Lo Mein (variation), 422
spelt and spelt flour, 20, 22, 438, 484
Multi-Seed Spelt Biscuits, 484
Spelt and Wild Mushroom Pilaf, 457
Sunflower Spelt Bread, 466
spinach, 287, 305, 448. *See also* greens
Avocado and Egg Breakfast Wraps, 56
Black Bean and Spinach Burritos, 226
Broccoli and Spinach Enchiladas, 274
Bulgur Burgers, 236
Cannellini and Artichoke Sandwiches, 217
Chipotle Maple Pork with Sweet Potato and Spinach Hash, 326
Curried Orzo Soup, 190
Falafel Fusilli with Spinach and Feta, 390
Favorite Frittata, 53
Fusilli with Red Lentils, Spinach and Feta, 391
Indian-Spiced Cauliflower, Spinach and Tofu Scramble, 291
Lasagna Rolls, 421
Miso Soup with Soba and Vegetables, 192
Quinoa Vegetable Cakes, 269
Salmon Penne with Peas and Lemon, 408
Skillet Pizza Marinara, 241
Spicy Chicken, Spinach and Peanut Stir-Fry, 305
Spicy Tuna Cakes with Lemony Spinach, 372
Spinach, Avocado and Orange Salad, 115
Spinach and Basil Bread, 471
Spinach and Feta Crustless Quiche, 287
Spinach and Ricotta Bruschetta, 64
Spinach Egg Drop Soup, 193
Spinach Mushroom Quesadillas, 276
Spinach-Stuffed Mushrooms, 110
Stir-Fried Tofu with Bok Choy and Spinach, 292
Super Antioxidant Smoothie, 75
Sweet Potato and Spinach Curry with Quinoa, 261
Tempeh Fajita Wraps, 230
Teriyaki Soba, Spinach and Tofu Noodles, 426
Turkey Sausage, Spinach and Chickpea Ragù, 319
White Bean Bajane with Thyme Barley, 259
White Beans and Spinach, 454
Wilted Spinach with Garlic, 448
sprouts. *See also* Brussels sprouts
Asian Lettuce Wraps, 321
California Vegetable Wraps, 228
Herbed Cheese, Turkey and Sprouts Sandwiches, 221
Minted Sprout Salad, 132
Swiss Chard Spring Rolls with Sesame Lime Dipping Sauce, 109
Thai Cashew Noodles, 424
Vietnamese Pho, 197
squash, 172, 336, 434. *See also* pumpkin; zucchini
Butternut Squash, White Bean and Kale Stew, 202
Butternut Squash Farro with Chickpeas and Cranberries, 258
Butternut Squash Fettuccine, 388
Butternut Squash Soup with Sage and Thyme, 172
Delicata Squash with Quinoa Stuffing, 262
Greek Yogurt Dip with Fresh Squash "Chips," 107
Quick Beef Ragù with Spaghetti Squash, 336
Winter Squash and Goat Cheese Enchiladas, 275
strawberries, 519. *See also* berries
Instant Strawberry Frozen Yogurt, 527
Ricotta Pudding with Strawberry Coulis, 519
Strawberry Mousse, 520

sunflower seeds, 30, 236, 466. *See also* sprouts
Broccoli Carrot Slaw with Cranberries and Sunflower Seeds, 129
Bulgur Burgers, 236
Pomegranate and Quinoa Salad with Sunflower Seeds, 149
Sunflower Apricot Go-Bars, 70
Sunflower Spelt Bread, 466
Walnut Quinoa Power Bars (variation), 83
sweet potatoes, 91, 435
Black Bean Chili–Topped Sweet Potatoes, 251
Chipotle Maple Pork with Sweet Potato and Spinach Hash, 326
Mashed Sweet Potatoes with Rosemary, 452
Southwestern Sweet Potato Salad, 133
Spanish Sweet Potato Tortilla with Roasted Pepper Sauce, 281
Sweet Potato, Lentil and Arugula Salad, 134
Sweet Potato, Swiss Chard and Black Bean Chili, 208
Sweet Potato and Spinach Curry with Quinoa, 261
Sweet Potato Bisque with West Indian Spices, 173
Sweet Potato Chips, 91
Sweet Potato Fries, 451
Turkey Soup with Sweet Potatoes and Mustard Greens, 196
Swiss chard, 449. *See also* greens
Chard and Red Pepper Salad with Tahini Yogurt Dressing, 123
Chicken with Sautéed Apples and Swiss Chard, 298
Farfalle with Swiss Chard, White Beans and Walnuts, 386
Farro Risotto with Swiss Chard and Parmesan, 267
Sautéed Swiss Chard, 449
Stuffed Swiss Chard Leaves, 320
Sweet Potato, Swiss Chard and Black Bean Chili, 208
Swiss Chard, Cherry and Pecan Salad, 115
Swiss Chard, Cherry Tomato and Ricotta Bake, 280
Swiss Chard Spring Rolls with Sesame Lime Dipping Sauce, 109
Whole Wheat Orzo with Swiss Chard and Pecans, 401

T

tangerines, 306. *See also* oranges
Asparagus with Tangerine Gremolata, 440
Lemon Drop Scones (variation), 486
Stir-Fried Tangerine Chicken, 306
tempeh, 29
Tempeh Fajita Wraps, 230
Tempeh with Moroccan Tomato Sauce, 294
Thai Chicken Salad (variation), 158
Thai Tempeh with Broccoli and Snow Peas, 295
Vietnamese-Style Chicken Sandwiches (variation), 220
tofu, 28–29.
Berry Protein Shake, 74
Bok Choy and Mushroom Soup, 167
Crispy Baked Tofu, 288
Fast Vegetable Lasagna (variation), 419
Indian-Spiced Cauliflower, Spinach and Tofu Scramble, 291
Lasagna Rolls (variation), 421
Miso Soup with Soba and Vegetables, 192
Oven-Baked Tofu "Fries," 94
Power Pitas with Eggs and Vegetables, 54
Quick Quinoa Stir-Fry with Vegetables and Tofu, 293
Soba and Tofu Salad with Carrot Miso Dressing, 152
Stir-Fried Tofu with Bok Choy and Spinach, 292
Strawberry Mousse, 520
Teriyaki Soba, Spinach and Tofu Noodles, 426
Tofu and Eggplant Stir-Fry, 289
Tofu Salad Sandwiches, 218
Tofu Scramble, 54
Vietnamese Pho (variation), 197
White Bean Garlic Spread, 98
tomatoes, 26–27, 174. *See also* tomatoes, cherry or grape
Black Bean Avocado Salsa, 98
Chicken Sausage, Arugula and Tomato Penne, 406
Classic Tomato Soup, 174
Cod Poached in Tapenade Tomato Broth, 347
Cuban Braised Beef with Brown Rice and Mango, 331
Eggplant Parmesan Melts, 277
Farfalle with Tuna and Tomatoes, 387
Farmers' Market Gazpacho, 175
Greek Capellini with Shrimp, Tomatoes and Mint, 384
Green Club Sandwich, 216
Lean Beef and Bean Cowboy Chili, 212
Moroccan-Spiced Shrimp, 376
Moussaka Macaroni, 400
Okra, Chickpea and Tomato Tagine, 255
Pizza Margherita, 242
Quick Moroccan Beef and Chickpea Chili, 213
Quinoa and Black Bean Salad, 147
Quinoa Spaghetti al Pomodoro, 417
Red Fish Stew, 206
Roasted Vegetable Salsa, 96
Spiced Beef Keema with Chickpeas and Green Peas, 337
Spiced Chicken and Couscous Soup, 195
Summer Vegetable Orzo Soup, 189
Sweet Potato, Swiss Chard and Black Bean Chili, 208
Tabbouleh, 141
Tabbouleh Soup with Lentils and Bulgur, 185
Tempeh with Moroccan Tomato Sauce, 294
Turkey Sausage, Escarole and Sun-Dried Tomato Pasta, 407
tomatoes, cherry or grape
Cherry Tomato, Avocado and Cucumber Pitas, 224
Chicken with Cherry Tomato and Avocado Salsa, 300
Chopped Greek Salad, 119
Cod with Roasted Tomatoes and Edamame Mash, 348
Farro Salad with Arugula and Tomatoes, 146
French Green Bean, Barley and Tomato Salad, 139
Fusilli with Chickpeas, Tomatoes, Feta and Herbs, 389
Garden Pasta Salad, 154
Greek Chicken with Cherry Tomatoes and Feta, 299
Greek Pizza, 244
Greek Salad Frittata, 283
Greek Salad Pitas, 224
Orzo Salad with Fennel, Radishes and Goat Cheese, 155
Roasted Vegetable Linguine, 396
Sautéed Cherry Tomatoes, 446
Seared Halloumi with Chickpea Salsa and Herbed Couscous, 278
Summer Salmon Panzanella, 159
Swiss Chard, Cherry Tomato and Ricotta Bake, 280
Tuna and White Bean Salad (variation), 160
Tunisian Tuna and Egg Salad Pitas, 225
Turkish Tomato, Pepper and Herb Salad, 126
tortillas, 316
Avocado and Egg Breakfast Wraps, 56
Black Bean and Spinach Burritos, 226
Black Bean Tacos, 277
Broccoli and Spinach Enchiladas, 274
California Vegetable Wraps, 228
Cashew Butter and Banana Wraps, 229
Chicken and Black Bean Chilaquiles, 316
Chipotle Tilapia Tacos with Pineapple, 367
Goat Cheese, Edamame and Roasted Pepper Wraps, 228
Grilled Steak Tacos with Avocado and Cumin Lime Slaw, 334
Grilled Tilapia Tacos with Mango Salsa, 366
Lentil, Mushroom and Kale Burritos, 227
Niçoise Salad Wraps, 232

tortillas (*continued*)
Oven Tortilla Chips, 90
Quinoa and Chickpea Wraps, 229
Smoked Turkey, Avocado and Mango Wraps, 231
Southeast Asian Roast Beef Wraps, 232
Spinach Mushroom Quesadillas, 276
Tempeh Fajita Wraps, 230
Turkey, Kale and Cranberry Wraps, 230
Winter Squash and Goat Cheese Enchiladas, 275
tuna, 370
Anytime Tuna Burgers, 239
Balsamic Tuna Salad in Avocado Halves, 160
Farfalle with Tuna and Tomatoes, 387
Mediterranean Tuna Sandwich, 222
Niçoise Salad Wraps, 232
Sicilian Tuna and Rice Salad, 161
Spaghetti with Tuna, Olives and Golden Raisins, 415
Spicy Tuna Cakes with Lemony Spinach, 372
Tuna and Asparagus Frittata, 371
Tuna and White Bean Salad, 160
Tuna with Farro and Fennel, 370
Tunisian Tuna and Egg Salad Pitas, 225
turkey. *See also* chicken
Asian Lettuce Wraps, 321
Beef and Quinoa Power Burgers (variation), 238
Herbed Cheese, Turkey and Sprouts Sandwiches, 221
Lean Beef and Bean Cowboy Chili (variation), 212
Moroccan-Spiced Ground Turkey with Apricot Couscous, 322
Portobello Pizzas, 273
Smoked Turkey, Avocado and Mango Wraps, 231
Spicy Salsa Joes, 221
Stuffed Swiss Chard Leaves, 320
Texas BBQ Turkey Burgers, 237
Thai-Style Pork with Brown Jasmine Rice (variation), 330
Turkey, Kale and Cranberry Wraps, 230
Turkey Sausage, Escarole and Sun-Dried Tomato Pasta, 407
Turkey Sausage, Spinach and Chickpea Ragù, 319
Turkey Sausage with Mustard Greens and Kidney Beans, 318
Turkey Soup with Sweet Potatoes and Mustard Greens, 196
Wagon Wheels with Broccoli, Turkey and Parmesan, 418
White Turkey Chili, 210

V

vegetables, 9, 23–27, 122, 178, 272, 434–35. *See also specific vegetables*
Fast Vegetable Lasagna, 419
Kasha with Summer Vegetables, 459
Okra, Chickpea and Tomato Tagine, 255
Power Pitas with Eggs and Vegetables, 54
Quick Quinoa Stir-Fry with Vegetables and Tofu, 293
Quinoa Vegetable Cakes, 269
Sesame Peanut Vegetable Noodle Salad, 153
Speedy Weeknight Lo Mein, 422
Spring Vegetable Chicken Quinoa, 315
Spring Vegetable Tagine, 254
Vegetable Minestrone, 176

W

walnuts, 386. *See also* nuts; pecans
Baked Apples with Walnuts and Dried Cherries, 505
Barley, Parsley and Walnut Salad, 140
Carrot Oat Breakfast Cookies, 73
Farfalle with Swiss Chard, White Beans and Walnuts, 386
Kale, Apple and Walnut Slaw, 128
Lemony Brussels Sprouts Slaw, 128
Lentil, Walnut and Arugula Spread, 100
Muhammara (Syrian Red Pepper Walnut Spread), 103
Oatmeal Cookies, 510
Pumpkin Bread, 470
Quick Whole Wheat Walnut Bread, 463
Spaghetti with Brussels Sprouts and Toasted Walnuts, 412
Spiced Carrot Cake with Currants, 499
Walnut Flax Waffles, 50
Walnut Quinoa Power Bars, 83
watercress, 383. *See also* arugula; greens
Anytime Tuna Burgers, 239
Capellini with Watercress, Carrots and Almonds, 383
Grilled Salmon with Mustard Maple Vinaigrette, 355
Shrimp, Grapefruit and Watercress Salad, 163
Turkey Sausage, Escarole and Sun-Dried Tomato Pasta (tip), 407
watermelon, 365
Arugula, Watermelon and Feta Salad, 117
Garam Masala–Spiced Tilapia with Watermelon Salsa, 365
wheat and wheat berries, 22, 439. *See also* bulgur
Wheat Berry, Pecan and Cherry Salad, 151

Z

zucchini, 435, 472. *See also* squash
Chicken and Zucchini Spiedini with Salsa Verde, 310
Easy Ratatouille with Poached Eggs, 279
Kasha with Summer Vegetables, 459
Multigrain Macaroni with Zucchini, Greek Yogurt and Romano, 399
Persian Zucchini Frittata, 284
Roasted Vegetable Salsa, 96
Spring Vegetable Tagine, 254
Summer Vegetable Orzo Soup, 189
Whole Wheat Zucchini Bread, 472
Zucchini and Chickpea Salad, 136

Library and Archives Canada Cataloguing in Publication

Saulsbury, Camilla V.
5 easy steps to healthy cooking : 500 recipes for lifelong wellness / Camilla V. Saulsbury.

Includes index.
ISBN 978-0-7788-0296-9

1. Cooking. 2. Health. 3. Cookbooks. I. Title. II. Title: Five easy steps to healthy cooking.

TX714.S337 2012 641.5'63 C2011-907442-7